D1313616

# DETERMINANTS OF FERTILITY IN DEVELOPING COUNTRIES

Volume 2

*Fertility Regulation and
Institutional Influences*

Academic Press Rapid Manuscript Reproduction

This is a volume in
STUDIES IN POPULATION

A complete list of titles in this series appears at the end of this volume.

# DETERMINANTS OF FERTILITY IN DEVELOPING COUNTRIES

## Volume 2
### *Fertility Regulation and Institutional Influences*

PANEL ON FERTILITY DETERMINANTS
COMMITTEE ON POPULATION AND DEMOGRAPHY
COMMISSION ON BEHAVIORAL AND SOCIAL SCIENCES AND EDUCATION
NATIONAL RESEARCH COUNCIL

Edited by

## Rodolfo A. Bulatao
*National Research Council*
*Washington, D.C.*

## Ronald D. Lee
*University of California, Berkeley*
*Berkeley, California*

with

## Paula E. Hollerbach
## John Bongaarts
*Population Council*
*New York, New York*

**ACADEMIC PRESS   1983**

*A Subsidiary of Harcourt Brace Jovanovich, Publishers*

New York     London
Paris   San Diego   San Francisco   São Paulo   Sydney   Tokyo   Toronto

NOTICE:   The project that is the subject of this report was approved by the Governing Board of the National Research Council, whose members are drawn from the councils of the National Academy of Sciences, the National Academy of Engineering, and the Institute of Medicine. The members of the panel responsible for the report were chosen for their special competences and with regard for appropriate balance.

This report has been reviewed by a group other than the authors according to procedures approved by a Report Review Committee consisting of members of the National Academy of Sciences, the National Academy of Engineering, and the Institute of Medicine.

The National Research Council was established by the National Academy of Sciences in 1916 to associate the broad community of science and technology with the Academy's purposes of furthering knowledge and of advising the federal government. The Council operates in accordance with general policies determined by the Academy under the authority of its congressional charter of 1863, which establishes the Academy as a private, nonprofit, self-governing membership corporation. The Council has become the principal operating agency of both the National Academy of Sciences and the National Academy of Engineering in the conduct of their services to the government, the public, and the scientific and engineering communities. It is administered jointly by both Academies and the Institute of Medicine. The National Academy of Engineering and the Institute of Medicine were established in 1964 and 1970, respectively, under the charter of the National Academy of Sciences.

ACADEMIC PRESS, INC.
111 Fifth Avenue, New York, New York 10003

*United Kingdom Edition published by*
ACADEMIC PRESS, INC. (LONDON) LTD.
24/28 Oval Road, London NW1  7DX

Library of Congress Cataloging in Publication Data

Determinants of fertility in developing countries.

(Studies in population)
Contents: v. 1. Supply and demand for children--v. 2. Fertility regulation and institutional influences. 1. Fertility, Human--Developing countries. 2. Family size--Developing countries. 3. Birth control--Developing countries. I. Bulatao, Rodolfo A., Date  . II. Lee, Ronald Demos, Date     .   III. National Research Council (U.S.). Committee on Population and Demography.  Panel on Fertility Determinants. [DNLM: 1. Fertility. 2. Developing countries.  WP 656 D479] HB901.D48   1983      304.6'32'091724      83-17135 ISBN 0-12-140502-8 (v.2 alk. paper)

PRINTED IN THE UNITED STATES OF AMERICA

83 84 85 86     9 8 7 6 5 4 3 2 1

# Contents

CONTRIBUTORS     ix
PANEL ON FERTILITY DETERMINANTS     xi
COMMITTEE ON POPULATION AND DEMOGRAPHY     xiii
PREFACE     xv

## FERTILITY REGULATION AND ITS COSTS

**1  Fertility Regulation and Its Costs: A Critical Essay**     1
*Albert I. Hermalin*

**2  Birth Control Methods and Their Effects on Fertility**     54
*John A. Ross*

**3  Monetary and Health Costs of Contraception**     89
*S. Bruce Schearer*

**4  Normative and Psychic Costs of Contraception**     151
*Donald J. Bogue*

**5  Abortion: Its Prevalence, Correlates, and Costs**     193
*Henry P. David*

**6  Infanticide as Deliberate Fertility Regulation**     245
*Susan C. M. Scrimshaw*

**7  Population Programs and Fertility Regulation**     267
*W. Parker Mauldin*

**8** **Diffusion Processes Affecting Fertility Regulation** 295

　　*Robert D. Retherford and James A. Palmore*


## FERTILITY DECISION-MAKING PROCESSES

**9** **Fertility Decision-Making Processes: A Critical Essay** 340

　　*Paula E. Hollerbach*

**10** **Cultural Influences on Fertility Decision Styles** 381

　　*Terence H. Hull*

**11** **Communication, Power, and the Influence of Social Networks in Couple Decisions on Fertility** 415

　　*Linda J. Beckman*

**12** **Sequential Fertility Decision Making and the Life Course** 444

　　*N. Krishnan Namboodiri*


## NUPTIALITY AND FERTILITY

**13** **The Impact of Age at Marriage and Proportions Marrying on Fertility** 473

　　*Peter C. Smith*

**14** **The Impact of Forms of Families and Sexual Unions and Dissolution of Unions on Fertility** 532

　　*Thomas K. Burch*


## SOCIAL INSTITUTIONS AND FERTILITY CHANGE

**15** **Modernization and Fertility: A Critical Essay** 562

　　*Richard A. Easterlin*

16  **Effects of Education and Urbanization
    on Fertility**                                              587
    *Susan H. Cochrane*

17  **Effects of Societal and Community Institutions
    on Fertility**                                              627
    *Joseph E. Potter*

18  **Effects of Culture on Fertility:
    Anthropological Contributions**                             666
    *Robert A. LeVine and Susan C. M. Scrimshaw*

19  **Statistical Studies of Aggregate Fertility Change:
    Time Series of Cross Sections**                             696
    *Toni Richards*

20  **Cohort and Period Measures of Changing Fertility**        737
    *Norman B. Ryder*

## CONCLUSION

21  **An Overview of Fertility Determinants in Developing
    Countries**                                                 757
    *Rodolfo A. Bulatao and Ronald D. Lee*

22  **An Agenda for Research on the Determinants of
    Fertility in the Developing Countries**                     788

**ABSTRACTS**                                                   831

# Contributors

*Numbers in parentheses indicate the pages on which the authors' contributions begin.*

LINDA J. BECKMAN (415) *Department of Psychiatry and School of Public Health, University of California, Los Angeles, California 90024*

DONALD J. BOGUE (151) *Community and Family Study Center, University of Chicago, Chicago, Illinois 60637*

RODOLFO A. BULATAO\* (757) *National Research Council, Washington, D.C. 20418*

THOMAS K. BURCH (532) *Department of Sociology, University of Western Ontario, London N6A 5C2, Ontario, Canada*

SUSAN H. COCHRANE (587) *The World Bank, Washington, D.C. 20433*

HENRY P. DAVID (193) *Transnational Family Research Institute, 8307 Whitman Drive, Bethesda, Maryland 20817*

RICHARD A. EASTERLIN (562) *Department of Economics, University of Southern California, Los Angeles, California 90089-0152*

ALBERT I. HERMALIN (1) *Department of Sociology and Population Studies Center, University of Michigan, Ann Arbor, Michigan 48109*

PAULA E. HOLLERBACH (340) *Center for Policy Studies, Population Council, One Dag Hammarskjold Plaza, New York, New York 10007*

TERENCE H. HULL (381) *International Population Dynamics Program, Department of Demography, Australian National University, Canberra, A.C.T. 2600, Australia*

RONALD D. LEE (757) *Graduate Group in Demography, University of California, Berkeley, California 94720*

ROBERT A. LEVINE (666) *Graduate School of Education, Harvard University, Cambridge, Massachusetts 02138*

W. PARKER MAULDIN (267) *Population Sciences, Rockefeller Foundation, 1133 Avenue of the Americas, New York, New York 10036.*

\**Present address:* The World Bank, Washington, D.C. 20433; on leave from East-West Population Institute, East-West Center, Honolulu, Hawaii 96848

N. KRISHNAN NAMBOODIRI (444) *Department of Sociology, University of North Carolina, Chapel Hill, North Carolina 27514*

JAMES A. PALMORE (295) *Population Studies Program, University of Hawaii, and East-West Population Institute, East-West Center, Honolulu, Hawaii 96848*

JOSEPH E. POTTER (627) *El Colegio de Mexico, Camino al Ajusco No. 20, Mexico City, Mexico*

ROBERT D. RETHERFORD (295) *East-West Population Institute, East-West Center, Honolulu, Hawaii 96848*

TONI RICHARDS (696) *Office of Population Research, Princeton University, Princeton, New Jersey 08540*

JOHN A. ROSS (54) *Advisor to the National Family Planning Coordinating Board, Government of Indonesia, and Department of Clinical Public Health, Columbia University, New York, New York 10032*

NORMAN B. RYDER (737) *Office of Population Research, Princeton University, Princeton, New Jersey 08540*

S. BRUCE SCHEARER (89) *Population Resource Center, 622 Third Avenue, New York, New York 10017*

SUSAN C. M. SCRIMSHAW (245, 666) *Departments of Public Health and Anthropology, University of California, Los Angeles, Los Angeles, California 90024*

PETER C. SMITH (473) *East-West Population Institute, East-West Center, Honolulu, Hawaii 96848*

# Panel on Fertility Determinants

xi

# Committee on Population and Demography

Members of the panel and the committee participated in this project in their individual capacities; their organizational affiliations are provided for identification only, and the views and designations used in this report are not necessarily those of the organizations mentioned.

# Preface

These two volumes review the research evidence about determinants of fertility differentials and fertility change in the developing countries. Following a scheme set out in the introductory chapter, the first volume discusses supply and demand for children and the second discusses fertility regulation and its costs, fertility decisions, nuptiality, and the effects of social institutions. The second volume also contains a summary chapter and an agenda for further research.

Fertility and its determinants have been urgent topics for research in recent decades with the rapid expansion in world population. Attempts to control population growth have focused on reducing fertility, with some apparent effect. The peak rate of growth in the world's population has now been passed, but growth is still at a high level in almost all the developing countries. In absolute numbers, the increase in the world's population continues to rise; according to United Nations medium projections, more people will be added each year for the next 50 years than were added in 1980. Long-term trends in population therefore still pose considerable problems.

These volumes are an attempt to summarize and integrate scientific knowledge about the determinants of the fertility levels that contribute to continued population growth. It was prepared by the Panel on Fertility Determinants of the Committee on Population and Demography. This panel was created by the Commission on Behavioral and Social Sciences and Education of the National Research Council in response to a request from the Agency for International Development to assess research in this area and make recommendations for further work. In addition to this report, the panel has prepared studies of several developing countries and a few illustrative cross-national analyses.

Part of the background for the panel reports was provided by previous work of the Committee on Population and Demography and its other panels to pin down actual fertility levels and trends in selected developing countries; this work, also supported by the Agency for International

Development, is detailed in a series of country reports from the National Academy Press, and the demographic methodology developed for this purpose is laid out in a volume issued by the United Nations.

The causes of fertility reductions in some developing nations, as well as the causes of continued high fertility in others, are strongly debated. What contribution is made to lower fertility by such factors as lower infant mortality levels, improvements in the status of women, and spreading knowledge of and access to efficient methods of contraception and abortion, and what contribution is made to higher fertility by such factors as cultural and religious norms, the economic benefits children provide, and traditional reluctance to interfere with reproduction—all these matters continue to be investigated by researchers in several fields. To encompass such research, the panel was of necessity a heterogeneous group, including scholars from several disciplines: anthropology, demography, economics, epidemiology, psychology, sociology, and statistics. This report contains many perspectives, generally congenial but occasionally contrasting, held together, one would like to say, by a carefully crafted framework, though an act of will may be at least part of the truth.

To design and prepare the report, the panel formed a working group composed of Ronald D. Lee (Chair), Paula E. Hollerbach, John Bongaarts, and Rodolfo A. Bulatao. This group drew upon the analytical framework prepared by a separate working group (chaired by Ronald Freedman), devised the scheme for the volumes, and, with much advice and suggestions from the panel, solicited the help of 42 authors to prepare the individual papers of the report.

Each author received an early version of the analytical framework and a description of that part of it he or she was expected to develop. It is an indication of the good sense of this group that, working within this imposed structure, they were able to focus on substantive problems and summarize important areas of research.

The papers were reviewed, often unmercifully, at several levels. The working group reviewed all the papers and panel members reviewed papers in their areas, in many cases suggesting extensive improvements that authors took with surprisingly good grace. At the working group's request, additional reviews were carried out by other researchers, including Bryan Boulier, Mead Cain, Ruth Dixon, Peter Lindert, Geoffrey McNicoll, Eva Mueller, Dorothy Nortman, Toni Richards, Michele G. Shedlin, Christopher Tietze, and Hania Zlotnik. For the panel's parent Committee on Population and Demography, Conrad Taeuber and Samuel Preston undertook the daunting task of reviewing the entire collection. The concluding section was also reviewed by the Commission on Behavioral and Social Sciences and Education. The sum of these reviews was a considerable improvement, for many of the papers, in concept and precision.

Ensuring that the mountain of often dense scientific prose in fact contained readable English sentences was mainly the responsibility of Rona Briere, who performed this task with vigor and understanding. Carol Bradford Ward assisted in keeping all the pieces of the work together and moving on track. Elaine McGarraugh handled production editing details. Among several who worked at the alternately intriguing and boring task of typing and correcting drafts, Carole Turley and Solveig Padilla deserve special acknowledgment.

Finally, although the views expressed in the papers are those of the authors rather than of the organizations to which they are affiliated, those organizations nevertheless contributed considerably by making time and resources available. Their incalculable contribution is hereby acknowledged.

W. PARKER MAULDIN, *Chair*
*Panel on Fertility Determinants*

Part I
# FERTILITY REGULATION AND ITS COSTS

# Chapter 1
# Fertility Regulation and Its Costs: A Critical Essay

ALBERT I. HERMALIN*

## INTRODUCTION

This paper investigates the motivation for and the costs of fertility control as determinants of fertility regulation, which is one part of the conceptual framework guiding these volumes. On occasion it will be necessary to touch on other parts of the framework as well, such as supply and demand, social and economic structure, and individual socioeconomic characteristics; at other times the relationship of fertility control to actual fertility will be addressed. Though often not designed with the present framework in mind, a large number of empirical studies treat topics relevant to this discussion, such as the levels, patterns, and correlates of contraceptive use and abortion; the effectiveness, costs, and safety of specific contraceptive methods; and the efficacy of family planning programs and other policies in regulating fertility. The strategy adopted here is to hew closely to the framework as a base from which to review such research and to derive implications for future efforts. Though this strategy may prove less comprehensive than some alternatives, it should provide a more systematic overview. A number of topics receiving only brief attention here are treated in more detail in subsequent chapters, and these will be noted. In addition, a brief

*This paper has benefited from suggestions by Ronald Freedman, Mark Montgomery, and four anonymous reviewers. Portions of this paper reflect ideas that have emerged from ongoing collaborative research with Barbara Entwisle and William M. Mason. None of the aforementioned are responsible for remaining deficiencies. Mary Scott provided valuable assistance in preparing the manuscript.

summary of major trends and data sources will be provided
for readers who may not be familiar with these materials.


## BASIC CONCEPTS

The conceptual framework for these volumes attributes to
each couple a demand for some number of surviving
children; this demand serves as a reference point for
assessing the sufficiency of their supply (or likely
number of surviving children) at any given point. Once
supply reaches or exceeds the desired number, the couple
is motivated to some degree to control their fertility.
Whether they do so or not is influenced by the means of
fertility regulation available and their costs. The
latter include economic costs (monetary and time), social-
opinion costs (the possibility of violating existing
social norms and facing sanctions), and health and psychic
costs (the results of trying something new that may be to
some degree risky or unpleasant). These costs are a function of both individual and social-structural characteristics: a couple's economic position, social standing,
and other traits partly determine their regulation costs;
at the same time, a community[1] may raise or lower costs
by encouraging or discouraging use of control methods, by
affecting their accessibility, and by establishing pricing
mechanisms. Even in its narrowest sense, therefore, the
study of regulation costs must involve both individual-
and community-level characteristics.

The influence of social organization, however, extends
beyond costs. Social, economic, cultural, and environmental factors influence both the demand for and the
supply of children for a couple and therefore influence
motivation to control. Demographic transition theory is
a theory of societal change, not of individual accounting.
Changes in social and industrial structure, levels of
literacy, and urbanization are viewed as providing induce-
ments for reducing family size and thus sharply lowering
the desired number of children (see, e.g., Coale, 1973;
Lee and Bulatao, in these volumes). At the same time,
social control is viewed as important in regulating the
supply of children through customs and norms affecting
such behaviors as age at marriage, widow remarriage,
postpartum abstinence, and breastfeeding (see Freedman,
1975, and Lesthaeghe, 1980, for general discussion and
specific examples).

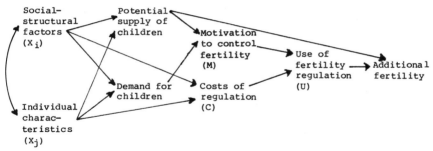

FIGURE 1  Basic Model of Factors Determining Additional
Fertility

Figure 1 shows a basic model of the fertility-
determining factors outlined above.  A number of
observations on this model will serve to frame the
remainder of this discussion.

First, the model posits two sets of exogenous or
predetermined variables:

- socioeconomic-structural factors--including such
  elements as level of development; family planning
  program policy and inputs; community social
  organization; and norms, laws, and customs governing
  abortion, breastfeeding, and marriage.
- individual characteristics--including socioeconomic
  status (e.g., education), biological elements (e.g.,
  fecundity), and demographic characteristics (age,
  marital status, and so on).

These two sets of variables have direct effects only on
demand, supply, and regulation costs; these in turn
determine directly or indirectly the remaining variables--
motivation to control, fertility regulation, and fertility.  The exogenous variables influencing demand and
supply, and therefore motivation to control, need not be
the same as those that influence costs.  The model is
block-recursive:  variables can be affected only by those
to their left.

Second, demand and supply define rather than cause
motivation to control.  As stated earlier, if supply
exceeds demand, motivation is presumed to exist; if
supply is less than demand, motivation is absent.  From
this standpoint, supply and demand are components of
motivation; once they have been measured, the degree of

motivation is known.  Thus motivation does not mean
"determination" or "resolve" in the usual sense of those
words.  An important implication is that the exogenous
factors are determinants of motivation only if they are
determinants of supply or demand.

Third, the difference between potential supply at a
given point and actual fertility is worth noting.  Potential supply is the number of surviving children a woman
would have without parity-specific regulating behavior.
This reflects levels of natural fertility (see Bongaarts
and Menken, in these volumes; Knodel, in these volumes)
and infant and child mortality.  If no fertility regulation has taken place, a woman's actual number of surviving
children is equal to her potential supply.  The two measures diverge with regulation to an extent determined by
its duration and effectiveness.  With regulation, therefore, potential supply is not observable individual by
individual, though it is possible to estimate it for a
population and assign values to individuals.

If a woman's reproductive life is viewed
prospectively, the model states that she will continue to
have children until the number living reaches the number
desired.  From that point on, assuming that the desired
number remains fixed, she will be motivated to control
her fertility by some means.  Thus the model assumes that
all fertility regulation behavior will be for the purpose
of limiting rather than spacing births.  (There are of
course many reasons for spacing not recognized in the
model.)  When a cross section is examined, so that there
are women at each stage of the reproductive process, the
problem of relating supply to demand and measuring motivation is more difficult since a woman may have already
used a method of fertility control.  These problems and
limitations will be taken up more fully below.

Fourth, although it is possible in principle to estimate the entire structural model, a number of studies,
including this one, focus on selected parts.  Some studies
(like the preceding chapters in these volumes) concentrate
on the determinants of supply and demand.  Others analyze
the relationship between fertility regulation and fertility.  One example is Bongaarts' (1982) analysis of the
proximate determinants of aggregate variation in fertility.  Other studies include attempts to estimate fertility
rates as a function of contraceptive prevalence (Nortman
and Hofstatter, 1980; Bongaarts and Kirmeyer, 1982) and
analyses that emphasize the effect of family planning
program acceptance on fertility.  Other evaluations of

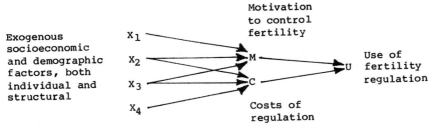

FIGURE 2   Basic Model of Factors Affecting Fertility
Regulation

family planning investigate the chain from socioeconomic
structure to regulation costs to fertility regulation, or
the relationship between program inputs (an aspect of
costs) and level of fertility regulation. Some of these
evaluation studies are reviewed in a later section. It
is also possible to concentrate on reduced forms, that
is, to study the relationship between a given endogenous
variable and the exogenous or predetermined variables.
Examples would be investigations into the social structural and individual determinants of contraceptive use,
breastfeeding, and so on. However, even when only a
portion of the model is being estimated, attention to the
whole model is useful in selecting and operationalizing
variables and in choosing the appropriate estimation
technique.

The portion of the model to be emphasized here is
sketched in Figure 2. Interest will center on studies
that examine how motivation to control and regulation
costs combine to determine the level and means of fertility regulation, as well as on the exogenous variables
(individual and structural) that determine the levels of
motivation and costs.

Fifth, the model portrayed by Figures 1 and 2 is from
the standpoint of the individual or couple, but it
includes social-structural or aggregate variables as one
set of exogenous factors. Many of these have implications for individual-level characteristics. For example,
the number and location of family planning clinics, an
aggregate variable, will largely determine the accessibility of services to the individual. Whether this
aspect of cost is best measured from an individual or
aggregate viewpoint, however, is a question to be taken
up below.

Although the issues posed by an individual model may also be addressed at the aggregate level, an aggregate model is likely to be quite different in character. At the aggregate level there is not the same type of supply-demand equilibration as that posited for the family level. Rather, what is observable are levels and trends in vital rates and other key demographic measures (e.g., birth rates, death rates, growth rates, age structure, migration patterns, unemployment levels), and a host of economic and development indices such as rates of capital investment and social service expenditures. These are the inputs into policies and programs. The actions taken will affect family demographic behavior to some degree, but may coincide either poorly or well with the economic and demographic circumstances of most families. A clear example is the decision to launch a family planning program: insofar as that decision arises from consideration of aggregate demographic factors, concordance with family-level motivation is an open question. From this viewpoint, policymakers may decide to launch a family planning program after there is considerable popular motivation for fertility control (possibly relying on survey estimates of the level of individual motivation in designing the program), or program initiation may precede the development of significant motivation. The point here is that data and models exist at both levels, and it is important to be clear about the referent to ensure proper analysis and inference.

The remainder of this paper is organized as follows. The next section reviews data on the prevalence of contraception and other means of fertility regulation. The following section addresses motivation to control and discusses various issues in motivation analysis; the next section treats regulation costs in a parallel fashion. This is followed by discussion of a series of issues connected with estimating the model in Figure 2, and an examination of the choice of means of fertility regulation. Special attention is then given to the family planning programs and their evaluation, and some new lines of attack are discussed. The final section presents major points and conclusions.

## LEVELS OF THE USE OF FERTILITY REGULATION

This section briefly outlines the patterns and trends in fertility regulation, sketching the broad contours and directing the reader to sources of additional detail. Contraceptive prevalence--the proportion of married women of reproductive age practicing contraception at some point in time--can be estimated from appropriate surveys or from program service statistics in combination with census data. Though the concept is straightforward, there can be various comparability problems in measures because of the contraceptive methods included, the definition of the base population, and the estimation techniques (see Nortman and Hofstatter [1980:90-93] for a succinct discussion of these problems). In general, care must be exercised in comparing estimates from service statistics with survey data, particularly if a significant portion of use arises from the private sector or through traditional methods of contraception. With the advent of the World Fertility Survey (WFS) and the Contraceptive Prevalence Surveys (Lewis and Novak, 1982), which provide high-quality and generally comparable data, greater reliance has been placed on surveys for prevalence estimates. Figure 3 presents data by type of method on the proportion of currently married women who are using contraception, as established through 20 WFS surveys covering the period 1974-78. These data reveal a considerable range in prevalence--from 2 percent in Nepal to 64 percent in Costa Rica. More extensive tables for developing countries, combining estimates of prevalence from various sources, are presented by Larson (1981) and Nortman and Hofstatter (1980:Table 21). Those studies also provide comparisons with a number of developed countries. Several developing societies have prevalence rates well above 50 percent, at par with the European countries at the lower end of the developed-country distribution. At the same time, rates below 10 percent are still found in a sizeable number of developing countries. Nortman and Hofstatter (1980) also provide statistics over time for many countries. These reveal very rapid increases in prevalence in less than a decade for a number of countries, including Colombia, Hong Kong, Malaysia, Mauritius, Mexico, the Philippines, Taiwan, Thailand, and Singapore.[2] It should be noted that most of the data now available pertain to the mid to late 1970s, and there may have been significant gains since then in a number of countries.[3]

From the method distributions shown in Figure 3 and other sources (see Larson, 1981; Nortman and Hofstatter, 1980), several generalizations emerge:

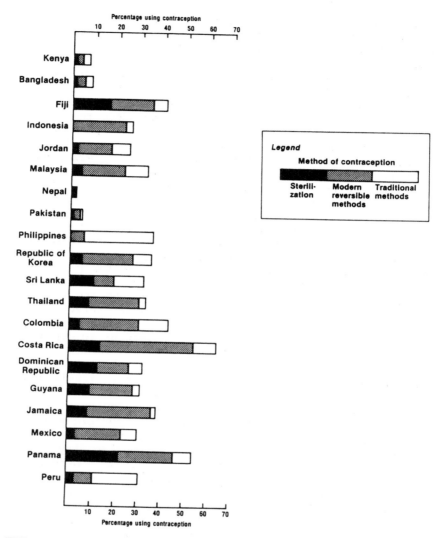

**FIGURE 3  Percent of Currently Married Women Using Contraception, by Type of Method, 1974–78:  20 WFS Countries**

Note:  Modern reversible methods include chemical and mechanical means of contraception; traditional methods include rhythm, withdrawal, abstinence, douche, and "folk" methods.

Source:  United Nations (1981:Figure 1).

- In many countries, a high proportion of users rely on modern means. In 15 of the 20 countries in Figure 3, two-thirds of users were using such means (sterilization or modern reversible methods).

- Generally, increases in contraceptive prevalence have been accompanied by shifts to more modern techniques. In this connection, the rapid rise in the use of female sterilization in some countries is noteworthy (see Population Reports [1978] for a detailed review and bibliography).

- Despite these trends and patterns, there is very little correlation between the overall prevalence rate and the proportion of users relying on traditional methods. Stated otherwise, there are countries at different levels of prevalence that show heavy reliance on traditional methods, just as there are countries at different levels of prevalence that show heavy reliance on modern methods.[4] The implications of these patterns will be pursued in a later section.

Data on the incidence of abortion are generally available only for those legally performed, and countries maintaining statistics are only a subset of those in which such abortions take place. Data for 27 countries over time are presented in Tietze (1981:Table 2). Some speculative estimates of worldwide and country-specific levels have attempted to incorporate the large number of illegal abortions (e.g., People, 1978:18); these studies are reviewed by David (in these volumes).[5]

The degree to which breastfeeding is used to regulate fertility will be taken up in a later section. On the prevalence of breastfeeding, comparative data from WFS studies are given in Ferry (1981b) and Population Reports (1981). These data show that a very high proportion of children (above 80 percent) are breastfed in nearly all the countries, with the likelihood and duration of breast-feeding generally higher in Asia and Africa than in Latin America and the Caribbean.

MOTIVATION TO CONTROL FERTILITY

This section addresses motivation for fertility regulation: its measurement, its interrelations with contraceptive use and with various socioeconomic and demographic characteristics, and its use as an independent variable and a dependent variable in multivariate analyses.

## Measurement of Motivation to Control

Measuring motivation to control requires measures of demand and supply. The most common approach to measuring demand is through respondent reports (McClelland, in these volumes). Two alternative techniques for measuring motivation are frequently used:

1. Obtaining a direct answer to a question of the form, "Do you want another child sometime?" Though the answer reflects future demand, it also taps whether supply has reached or exceeded demand. For this reason, the response has often been used as a direct measure of motivation to control.

2. Obtaining the number of children that is desired or ideal, in answer to a question like, "If you could choose exactly the number of children to have in your whole life, how many would that be?"[6] This number may be compared with the actual number of living children or another indicator of supply. If the actual number of living children equals or exceeds the desired number, motivation to control fertility may be presumed; if the desired number exceeds the actual, motivation is presumed to be absent.

Much of the early analysis of these questions addressed contentions that women in developing countries could not meaningfully express their preferences or motivations (Hauser, 1967; Knodel and Prachuabmoh, 1973; McClelland, in these volumes). To this end, such analyses compared the two measures of motivation discussed above, and systematically related them to contraceptive use or fertility. The comparisons generally showed good consistency between the two measures. Hermalin et al. (1979:77) show that, in Taiwan, 90 and 86.5 percent of responses were consistent in 1967 and 1970, respectively. Palmore and Concepcion (1981) present a consistency range of 73 to 91 percent for the two measures for 10 WFS countries.

Relating the measures to behavior also demonstrated they were meaningful. Freedman et al. (1975), using longitudinal data for Taiwan, showed that a live birth occurred within three years to only 13.5 percent of those who said they wanted no more children in 1967, and to 75 percent of those who said they wanted more. This was true despite the fact that 45 percent of those who did not want more children were not using contraception in 1967. The low fertility among those wishing to cease childbearing was achieved in part by a high level of

abortion (33 per 100 pregnancies between 1967 and 1970
were aborted) and by subsequent adoption of contraception.  Of those who wanted no more children but were not
using contraception in 1967, 45 percent were using
contraception by 1970.  When the same sample was studied
in 1974, only 22 percent of those who wanted no more
children in 1967 had had a live birth, as contrasted with
85 percent for those who wanted more (Hermalin et al.,
1979).  This degree of consistency between intentions and
outcomes is comparable to that observed in the United
States at the same time (Hermalin et al., 1979:Table 10;
Westoff and Ryder, 1977; see also McClelland, in these
volumes; Pullum, in these volumes).

The concept of desired number of children, one component of motivation, has been further refined by a model
in which each woman has an underlying preference function
that associates some utility with each possible number of
children (Terhune and Kaufman, 1973).  A question on
desired family size may elicit the modal value of this
function (Pullum, 1980:10).  However, if this preference
function is flat or nearly so in the vicinity of the mode
(indicating relative indifference across this range),
this important characteristic will not be revealed in an
attempt to elicit a single number for desired children
(Pullum, 1980).

Theory and measurement issues related to preference
functions have been most extensively developed by Coombs
et al. (1975), who hypothesize separate single-peaked
utility functions for number of children and for sex
preference (defined as preferred number of boys minus
preferred number of girls).  They operationalize these
functions through rankings of family sizes and sex compositions, paying attention not only to first but also to
subsequent choices.  The scale values produced by the
method--which can be incorporated into a typical fertility questionnaire--have been shown to be highly
predictive (see, e.g., Coombs, 1979, for Taiwan).[7]
These scales are essentially refined measures of the
demand for children (McClelland, in these volumes).  They
can be used as an adjunct in studies that explore the
role of motivation to control, but they cannot be combined directly with values for supply of children to
produce a single measure of this motivation.

Less attention has been paid to measures of supply or
potential family size.  One approach is that of Easterlin
and Crimmins (1981).  To obtain a measure of a household's
natural fertility, they first regress children ever born

on a fertility control variable and a series of other
proximate determinants of fertility. Then they use the
equation to estimate natural fertility with the fertility
control variable set to zero. Finally, this estimate is
multiplied by the household's ratio of living children to
children ever born to produce the estimate of potential
family size.

Easterlin and Crimmins use this measure of supply,
together with desired family size as a measure of demand,
to predict fertility control. Unfortunately, their
measure of fertility control--years since first use of
contraception or abortion--is the same measure used in
the equation for natural fertility, introducing some
circularity. An alternate approach to estimating
potential family size is presented by Boulier and Mankiw
(1980), who use the natural-fertility schedule developed
by Coale and Trussell (1974) to estimate the supply of
births. This approach would avoid circularity, but at
present produces the same value for all women of a given
age.

Proper temporal ordering between the measures of
motivation and fertility control must be observed.
Indications of motivation based on wanting more children
or the comparison of actual and desired numbers of
children are as of the time of the survey and thus should
be predictive of current or future use of deliberate
control methods. (The effect of prior use on actual
number of children, however, must be considered, as
discussed below.) One would not expect these measures to
be closely associated with the number of years since
control was adopted, for example, because they do not
take into account the effectiveness with which control
methods have been exercised. Among couples who adopted
at the same time in the past, some will greatly exceed
their desired number because of ineffective practice,
while others will be at their desired number because of
efficient use. The current difference between actual and
desired numbers cannot distinguish the fact that these
couples had equal motivation in the past.


## Interrelation between Socioeconomic and Demographic
## Variables and Contraceptive Use

Given the very recent development and continuing limitations of household-level measures of supply, most of the
work that can be cited on the correlates of motivation to

control actually involves only measures of wanting more children or comparison of actual and desired numbers. Concepcion (1981) has analyzed the relationship between desire for more children and a number of socioeconomic and demographic characteristics. For 18 WFS countries, she shows that the proportion wanting no more children is positively related to age, family size, and marital duration. There is a less clear-cut pattern of desire for more children with education and urban-rural residence among women 25 to 34 (Concepcion, 1981:Tables 10 and 11). In many countries, those with less education are more likely to want no more children; in a few countries the relationship was the reverse; and occasionally the pattern was curvilinear. In most countries, urban women were more likely than rural to want no more children, although this pattern was reversed in several countries. This mixture of patterns can probably be traced to differentials in age at marriage among socioeconomic and residence groups in the different countries, and consequent differences in stage of family building among the women in this age group.

A number of studies have examined the relationship of desire for more children to contraceptive use, though relatively few have examined the relationship to other forms of fertility control. The WFS data facilitate comparisons across countries. Table 1, taken from a United Nations (1981b) report, presents the percentage of exposed women currently using contraception by education and by whether they want more children for 17 countries (see also Concepcion, 1981:Table 20). A number of patterns emerge:

- In each of the countries, current use of contraception is higher among exposed women who want no more children than among those who want more.
- The range in use across countries among those wanting no more is considerable, from a low of 8 percent in Nepal to a high of 84 percent in Costa Rica. There is also considerable intercountry variation in use among those wanting more. The proportion using contraception for spacing (i.e., those who want more children) tends to be higher in countries where use among limiters is higher.[8]
- Differentials in use between those who do and do not want more children persist within educational categories in each of the countries. At the same time, contraceptive use increases with education, both among

women who want more children and among those who do
not.  In 10 of the 17 countries, more than 3 out of 4
women who want no more children and have 10 or more
years of schooling are using contraception, and in
four others the proportion is between 60 and 75
percent.

## Estimating the Effect of Motivation

Multivariate analyses involving motivation to control
have often been carried out without sufficient attention
to an underlying model, thereby generating confusion
about the relationship between motivation and fertility
regulation.  This section attempts to clarify the issues
involved in using motivation as both a dependent and an
independent variable.

Figures 1 and 2 indicate that socioeconomic, demographic, and other factors do not directly affect fertility regulation.  Instead they affect motivation and costs,
and their relation to fertility regulation depends on
these links.  That is, the correlation between one such
variable, $X_1$, and use of fertility regulation will be a
function of the effects (i.e., path or standardized
regression coefficients) of motivation and costs on use
and the correlations of $X_1$ with motivation and costs.
Symbolically, the <u>observed</u> correlation between $X_1$ and
use should be

$$p_{UM} r_{X_1M} + p_{UC} r_{X_1C} \tag{1}$$

where $p_{UM}$ and $p_{UC}$ are the path coefficients to use
from motivation and costs, respectively, and $r_{X_1M}$ and $r_{X_1C}$
are zero-order correlations.

The model in Figure 2 can be tested by comparing the
actual or observed correlations between the $X_1$ variables
and use against those expected from expression (1).  The
absence of reasonable correspondence would signify (a)
deficient measurement of the motivation and cost variables; (b) relatedly, the failure of the M and C measures
to capture aspects of motivation or cost embedded in the
$X_i$ variables; or (c) deficiencies in the model.  Of
course, it is never easy to disentangle these competing
possibilities, and several different tests are rarely
sufficient to dispose of the issue.

In fact, direct empirical tests of Figure 2 have not been attempted. A common approach is a hierarchical decomposition of the explained variance, in which socioeconomic and demographic variables are entered first and motivation (e.g., desire for more children) entered next, and the percentage of additional variance explained by motivation compared with that explained by the other variables (United Nations, 1981b:Table 24; Johnson-Acsadi and Weinberger, 1982:Table 3; Palmore and Concepcion, 1981:Table 1; Cleland et al., 1979[9]). This is not an appropriate test. One such study shows, for example, that across 11 WFS countries, the desire for more children, when entered after six other variables, explains only 1 to 3 percent of the variance in current contraceptive use, although it explains 1 to 10 percent of the variance when entered alone (Palmore and Concepcion, 1981). This type of result is not surprising. Insofar as the variables entered first in a hierarchical analysis largely determine motivation or costs (like the $X_i$ variables of Figure 2), one would expect them to overlap considerably with motivation or costs in the variance they explain. Hence there may be little net contribution from the motivation variable if it is entered later. Using analysis of covariance, however, Palmore and Concepcion also show that multivariate adjustment for the six variables does not affect the differentials in contraceptive use between those who do and do not want more children. These results tend to confirm the model: taken together they show that a number of demographic and socioeconomic factors appear closely related to desire for more children, but in addition, <u>within each category</u> of these factors, those who want no more children use contraception more frequently than those who want more. Table 1, which shows differentials in use within education categories, illustrates the second part of this statement.

## Studying the Determinants of Motivation

To this point, the discussion has focused on motivation as an independent variable. To explore issues relating to the study of the determinants of motivation, it is convenient to use a series of regression equations. For simplicity, a linear additive form is assumed, though this will not always be the optimum specification, and error terms are omitted.

TABLE 1  Percent of Exposed Women Currently Using
Contraception, by Education and Desire for More Children:
Selected WFS Countries

| Country and Desire for More Children | Total | Years of Education Completed | | | | |
|---|---|---|---|---|---|---|
| | | 0 | 1-3 | 4-6 | 7-9 | 10 |
| **Africa** | | | | | | |
| Kenya | | | | | | |
| Wants more[a] | 7 | 4 | 5 | 9 | 12 | 19 |
| Wants no more | 21 | 15 | 18 | 25 | 38 | (48) |
| **Asia and Oceania** | | | | | | |
| Bangladesh | | | | | | |
| Wants more | 3 | 2 | 3 | 4 | 9 | |
| Wants no more | 14 | 10 | 18 | 21 | 44 | |
| Fiji | | | | | | |
| Wants more | 35 | 27 | 31 | 33 | 35 | 40 |
| Wants no more | 69 | 70 | 74 | 69 | 64 | 77 |
| Indonesia | | | | | | |
| Wants more | 26 | 21 | 29 | 29 | 35 | 46 |
| Wants no more | 53 | 48 | 55 | 62 | 75 | 89 |
| Jordan | | | | | | |
| Wants more | 22 | 8 | 15 | 25 | 33 | 61 |
| Wants no more | 59 | 41 | 69 | 73 | 78 | 84 |
| Korea, Republic of[b] | | | | | | |
| Wants more | 17 | 10 | 11 | 13 | 19 | 28 |
| Wants no more | 56 | 49 | 51 | 54 | 61 | 69 |
| Malaysia | | | | | | |
| Wants more | 34 | 17 | 29 | 39 | 44 | 55 |
| Wants no more | 52 | 41 | 54 | 58 | 73 | 82 |
| Nepal | | | | | | |
| Wants more | -- | -- | | 4 | | 13 |
| Wants no more | 8 | 8 | | (24) | | (30) |
| Pakistan | | | | | | |
| Wants more | 1 | 1 | -- | 5 | (12) | (15) |
| Wants no more | 15 | 13 | (29) | 26 | (38) | (61) |
| Sri Lanka | | | | | | |
| Wants more | 13 | 5 | 11 | 20 | 27 | 35 |
| Wants no more | 54 | 38 | 47 | 55 | 64 | 73 |
| Thailand | | | | | | |
| Wants more | 29 | 22 | (18) | 29 | (27) | 49 |
| Wants no more | 56 | 46 | 55 | 57 | (73) | (82) |
| **Latin America** | | | | | | |
| Colombia | | | | | | |
| Wants more | 45 | 18 | 30 | 52 | 71 | 73 |
| Wants no more | 56 | 33 | 49 | 67 | 79 | 86 |
| Costa Rica | | | | | | |
| Wants more | 71 | (44) | 61 | 73 | 76 | 76 |
| Wants no more | 84 | 71 | 80 | 88 | 89 | 94 |
| Dominican Republic | | | | | | |
| Wants more | 25 | 8 | 13 | 27 | 46 | 59 |
| Wants no more | 57 | 36 | 52 | 63 | 77 | (85) |

TABLE 1 (continued)

| Country and Desire for More Children | Total | Years of Education Completed | | | | |
|---|---|---|---|---|---|---|
| | | 0 | 1-3 | 4-6 | 7-9 | 10 |
| Guyana[c] | | | | | | |
|   Wants more | 29 | (19) | 18 | 23 | 27 | 63 |
|   Wants no more | 45 | 40 | 46 | 46 | 44 | (67) |
| Panama | | | | | | |
|   Wants more | 50 | (24) | 29 | 47 | 64 | 61 |
|   Wants no more | 74 | 51 | 59 | 75 | 84 | 85 |
| Peru | | | | | | |
|   Want more | 33 | 7 | 20 | 41 | 58 | 63 |
|   Wants no more | 46 | 21 | 38 | 62 | 72 | 82 |

Note: Figures in parentheses are based on 20 to 49 cases. Dashes indicate still fewer cases.

[a]Including undecided.
[b]Education categories are none, less than primary, primary graduate, secondary graduate, and above.
[c]Women who attended secondary school or higher but for whom the number of years completed was not stated are included in the 7-9 category.

Source: United Nations (1981b:Table 20).

Because potential supply of children is so difficult to measure, the actual number of children is often used instead; the measure of motivation would then be actual minus desired number of children (treated as an interval scale). This creates certain problems, however, as will now be shown.

As sume that actual number of children (A) is a function of education ($X_1$, reflecting health and nutritional factors) and marital duration ($X_2$), whereas desired number of children (D) is affected by education and husband's occupation ($X_3$). This model is not meant to be complete or fully realistic; the aim is merely to illustrate the range of variables that could affect motivation (for a detailed discussion of variables affecting desired number of children, see Pullum, in these volumes).

$$A = a_1 + b_1 X_1 + b_2 X_2 \qquad (2)$$

$$D = a_2 + c_1 X_1 + c_2 X_3 \qquad (3)$$

Then motivation to control, measured by A − D, would be

$$A - D = (a_1 - a_2) + (b_1 - c_1)X_1 + b_2X_2 - c_2X_3 \qquad (4)$$

This last equation is of the nature of a reduced form, omitting the intervening demand and supply variables.

It is not unusual for analysts to overlook the underlying model represented in equations (2) and (3) and include actual number of children as a determinant of motivation in equation (4). This produces an equation of the form

$$A - D = a + d_1X_1 + d_2X_2 + d_3X_3 + d_4A \qquad (5)$$

A appears on both sides of the equation, and A − D necessarily increases with A. Thus, when motivation to control, as measured in this manner, is regressed on actual number of children, a strong positive effect is expected. Furthermore, it has been assumed that the $X_i$ variables include the determinants of A (see equation 2) and that explicitly including this variable is redundant and could produce meaningless results. If one assumes that demand and potential supply are fixed early in the marriage and are invariant thereafter, there is no reason to introduce actual fertility on the right-hand side of equation (5). For example, economists often make this assumption, and their models of demand focus on relatively time-invariant socioeconomic characteristics of a couple (see, e.g., Boulier and Mankiw, 1980, and references they provide). The alternative sequential view—that demand and potential supply change over the reproductive life cycle (Namboodiri, 1972; in these volumes)—is more complex. Desired number of children would be a function of actual fertility, and actual fertility a function of desired numbers. This might be the case, for instance, if couples did attempt to achieve their goals, but also adjusted these goals or rationalized them if they failed.[10] In such cases, either several measures of desired numbers over time or a simultaneous equations model would be needed. This further complicates the equation for motivation to control, as represented by A − D.

A primary conclusion to be drawn from the discussion in this section is that the independent variables chosen as determinants of motivation to control must be selected with clear attention to the framework of Figure 1. The independent variables should be those which determine

demand and supply.  If A - D is used as a measure of
motivation, actual fertility should not be included as a
determinant.  If A - D is used and a sequential model of
preferences is assumed, the reciprocal influence between
desires and actual fertility will have to be taken into
account.  Longitudinal data or a simultaneous equations
model may be needed.  Other implications of the sequential framework for studying the determinants of motivation do not appear well developed at present.  The
problems of simultaneity or reciprocal effects and model
identification are even more troublesome when one considers the determinants of fertility regulation, pointing
up the need for better measures of motivation.  Since
this aspect of the model involves measures of regulation
costs as well as motivation, further discussion of this
issue will be postponed to a later section.


### COSTS OF FERTILITY REGULATION

This section focuses on the costs of fertility control,
which together with motivation comprise the primary
determinants of the adoption of fertility regulation.
The following subsections classify the elements of the
concept of costs and illustrate their measurement, and
then provide a critical assessment of measurement and
analytic issues.


### Conceptualization and Classification of Costs

A useful preliminary distinction can be made between
measurable costs and costs that might be considered
infinite or almost infinite, or constraints.  In an
influential article, Coale (1973) has posited three
prerequisites for a sustained decline in marital
fertility:

1.  Fertility must be within the calculus of conscious
    choice . . . .
2.  Reduced fertility must be advantageous . . . .
3.  Effective techniques of fertility reduction must
    be available . . . .  Procedures that will in fact
    prevent births must be known.

The third prerequisite suggests that a method of fertility regulation must exist and be available to some

degree within a society before it is meaningful to consider measuring its costs. For example, the absence of a
reversible coitus-free male method of contraception is a
constraint or an absolute barrier to this means of fertility regulation; similarly, the absence of female
sterilization from a country might be properly considered
a constraint.[11]

Potentially measurable costs might be broadly classified into economic, health, and subjective costs. Economic costs include the monetary and time costs of
gaining information about and access to a method of
fertility regulation. Health costs include major as well
as minor side effects of methods. Subjective costs
encompass cultural, social, personal, perceived health,
and psychic factors. Figure 4 elaborates on this typology. Some of the cost elements listed have been studied
systematically (Schearer, in these volumes), but many
have not, particularly the subjective ones. Bogue (in
these volumes) reviews some of the literature relevant to
each of the subjective costs and uses a 1980 Egyptian
survey to assess the saliency of each one. On the basis
of both their prevalence and impact, Bogue concludes that
the most important subjective costs are social disapproval, difficulties of communication between spouses,
the need for "inner control," changes in self-perception
and one's family role, temporary discomfort, fears of
permanent health damage, and anxiety over possible contraceptive failure.

The aspect of cost that has received the most systematic and longstanding attention is the level and
distribution of knowledge of contraceptive methods,
representing the net result of expenditures by individuals
and public and private providers of services. Knowledge
of contraceptive methods was a standard topic in family
planning KAP (knowledge, attitude, and practice) surveys
and was incorporated into the WFS. Table 2 shows the
percentages of ever-married women in 20 WFS countries who
had heard of specific contraceptive methods. Comparisons
with earlier KAP surveys for selected countries generally
show substantial increases, suggesting that there has
been a major change in a relatively short span of time.
The relative uniformity in knowledge across these countries can be contrasted with the differentials in
prevalence of contraceptive use (shown in Figure 3 for
the same countries). Such a comparison indicates that
knowledge can explain only a small part of the variation
in prevalence.[12] Thus, although knowledge can be

FIGURE 4   Classification of Costs of Fertility Regulation

---

Economic Costs
   Monetary costs of obtaining information and using a technique
   Time costs of obtaining information and using a technique

Health Costs
   Major side effects
   Minor side effects

Subjective Costs
   Threats to cultural norms
      Nonconformity with religious and moral beliefs
      Social disapproval and fear of sanctions
   Threats to social adjustment
      Disharmony in the extended family
      Unconventional communication about sex between spouses
      Discord between spouses
      Undermining family status or security
   Threats to personal adjustment
      Adoption of "inner control" or "efficacy"
      Change in self-perception and family role
      Loss of enjoyment of children
      Threat to sexual adjustment
   Psychic threats to physical and mental health
      Temporary discomfort (i.e., side effects)
      Fear of permanent damage to health
      Fear of infant death
      Shyness toward gynecological examination
      Anxiety over contraceptive failure
   Psychologistics:  Perceived accessibility of contraceptive services

---

Sources:  Easterlin (1975); Schearer (in these volumes); Bogue (in these volumes).

viewed as setting an upper bound on prevalence, it is not a good predictor of actual levels of use.

Whether a woman has heard of a specific method is only one aspect of the cost of information; recognition of its name need not imply that the woman knows what the method looks like, how to use it, what it costs, or where to obtain it.  There has been increased concern with questions like these, including knowledge of an outlet for contraceptive services and various characteristics of that outlet, such as perceived distance, travel time, means of transportation, and degree of contact.  This line of research seeks to capture more of the economic cost elements involved in obtaining contraceptive information (Lewis and Novak, 1982; Rodriguez, 1977).[13]

United Nations (1981b:Table 3) data for nine WFS countries show several countries where a high proportion of women who know of a method also know of an outlet, but

TABLE 2  Percent of Ever-Married Women Who Had Heard of Specific Contraceptive Methods:  Selected WFS Countries

| Country | Number of Women[a] | Any Method | Any Modern Method[b] | Any Traditional Method[b] | Female Sterilization | Male Sterilization | Pill | Injection | IUD | Condom | Foam, Diaphragm, etc. | Rhythm | Withdrawal | Abstinence | Douche | Other |
|---|---|---|---|---|---|---|---|---|---|---|---|---|---|---|---|---|
| **Africa** | | | | | | | | | | | | | | | | |
| Kenya[c] | 8,100 | 88 | 84 | 70 | 54 | 14 | 74 | 55 | 49 | 40 | 20 | 50 | 25 | 45 | 12 | 2 |
| **Asia and Oceania** | | | | | | | | | | | | | | | | |
| Bangladesh | 6,515 | 82 | 80 | 49 | 53 | 51 | 64 | -- | 40 | 21 | 10 | 28 | 15 | 12 | 31 | 5 |
| Fiji | 4,928 | 100 | 100 | 87 | 96 | 40 | 98 | 50 | 97 | 83 | 41[d] | 57 | 56 | 57 | --[d] | 5 |
| Indonesia | 9,155 | 77 | 75 | 34 | 11 | 8 | 71 | 17 | 50 | 41 | 5 | 12 | 7 | 13 | 3 | 28 |
| Jordan | 3,611 | 97 | 97 | 81 | 79 | 19 | 96 | -- | 76 | 51 | 21 | 50 | 54 | 33 | 20 | 55 |
| Korea, Rep. of | 5,430 | 97 | 97 | 68 | 66 | 84 | 94 | 5 | 91 | 75 | 5 | 58 | 37 | 25 | 27 | 2 |
| Malaysia | 6,318 | 92 | 90 | 61 | 73 | 34 | 87 | 48 | 40 | 52 | 26 | 38 | 30 | 30 | -- | 21 |
| Nepal | 5,940 | 23 | 22 | 6 | 13 | 16 | 12 | 0 | 6 | 5 | 0 | 0 | 0 | 5 | 0 | 1 |
| Pakistan | 4,952 | 75 | 75 | 4 | 7 | 2 | 63 | 13 | 48 | 14 | 7 | 0 | 0 | 2 | 0 | 1 |
| Philippines | 9,268 | 94 | 94 | 79 | 75 | 70 | 90 | -- | 86 | 88 | 40 | 66 | 65 | 36 | 21 | 4 |
| Sri Lanka | 6,808 | 91 | 90 | 56 | 82 | 38 | 79 | 43 | 62 | 51 | 11 | 44 | 20 | 31 | 9 | 3 |
| Thailand | 3,820 | 97 | 96 | 55 | 87 | 70 | 92 | 71 | 86 | 48 | 22 | 32 | 22 | 36 | 17 | 1 |
| **Latin America** | | | | | | | | | | | | | | | | |
| Colombia | 3,302 | 96 | 95 | 74 | 72 | 38 | 90 | 71 | 82 | 60 | 56 | 56 | 47 | 28 | 41 | 9 |
| Costa Rica[e] | 3,037 | 100 | 100 | 91 | 94 | 67 | 98 | 88 | 91 | 91 | 71 | 81 | 67 | 31 | 60 | 7 |
| Dominican Republic | 2,256 | 98 | 98 | 75 | 95 | 30 | 91 | 68 | 78 | 72 | 60 | 43 | 56 | -- | 47 | 12 |
| Guyana | 3,616 | 95 | 95 | 71 | 79 | 22 | 78 | 38 | 79 | 73 | 45 | 46 | 48 | 32 | 36 | 10 |
| Jamaica | 2,765 | 98 | 98 | 78 | 88 | 40 | 95 | 87 | 84 | 90 | 67 | 39 | 59 | 38 | 43 | 3 |
| Mexico | 6,255 | 90 | 89 | 63 | 68 | 38 | 83 | 68 | 75 | 42 | 28 | 48 | 47 | --[f] | 38 | 4 |
| Panama[e] | 3,203 | 99 | 98 | 86 | 93 | 65 | 95 | 26 | 89 | 76 | 56 | 66 | 61 | 35 | 62 | 4 |
| Peru | 5,639 | 82 | 78 | 69 | 60 | 19 | 63 | 61 | 42 | 40 | 31 | 55 | 40 | 24 | 47 | 11 |

[a] Unless otherwise indicated, women are under 50 or 15-49, ever-married or in a union.
[b] Modern methods include sterilization, the pill, injection, the IUD, the condom, and female vaginal methods (diaphragm, foam, other spermicides).  Other methods are counted as traditional.
[c] Based on all women aged 15-50.
[d] Douche included with foam.
[e] Based on women aged 20-49.
[f] Included with "other."

Source:  United Nations (1981:Table 2), citing Vaessen (1980:16) and standard recode tapes.  Data obtained spontaneously and by direct probes, but not all methods were probed in all countries, and no probes were used in Pakistan (Vaessen, 1980).

in other countries this is not the case. There is much
greater variation in knowledge of an outlet than in
knowledge of a method across these nine countries.
Rodriguez's (1978) analysis of individual accessibility
in five countries (Colombia, Costa Rica, Korea, Malaysia,
and Nepal) shows that current use of efficient contraception tends to rise with increased perceived availability (measured as time to an outlet) in four out of five
cases; however, this relationship is weakened when controls are introduced for demographic and socioeconomic
characteristics. Most of the reduction is due to controlling urban-rural residence, reflecting the strong
relationship between perceived accessibility and place of
residence. Rodriguez also shows the reverse effect:
differentials in contraceptive use by place of residence
and education are reduced after controlling for perceived
availability. Thus his analysis suggests some independent effect of perceived availability on use. Lewis and
Novak (1982), on the other hand, find few differences
between users and nonusers of contraception in Thailand
and Costa Rica as regards perceived availability:
knowledge of a source, travel time, or travel mode.
Perceived availability among nonusers alone does vary as
expected by residence and education, being generally high
in urban areas and among the more educated. Though this
analysis suggests little effect of perceived availability
on use in these two countries, a more detailed analysis
is needed to establish this finding conclusively.[14]

Availability, as well as other costs, involve a wide
array of market and nonmarket factors. There is no
common denominator for combining these cost factors; only
a few can be expressed in monetary or time units. In
addition, it should be clear that some elements of cost
(such as price, and time and distance to an outlet) can
vary with the specific method considered, whereas others
(such as social climate, family considerations, and other
subjective costs) may be common to all methods. A number
of other critical issues in the measurement and analysis
of costs are pursued in the next subsection.

Issues in the Measurement and Analysis of Costs

This section presents three related assertions about the
measurement and analysis of costs:

1.  There is an inherent simultaneity of effects
    between most elements of costs, as usually
    measured, and contraceptive use; this simultaneity
    confounds analysis of the relationships involved
    and limits program or policy inferences.
2.  Many elements of costs, though by no means all,
    can be viewed as functions of program or macro
    characteristics, rather than of individuals.
3.  The inference to be drawn from assertions (1) and
    (2) is that multilevel analysis involving both
    individual (i.e., micro) and program or macro
    variables can produce useful insights into the
    relationships between costs and contraceptive
    use.  This type of analysis can also provide
    policymakers with direct guidance on future
    program directions.

The question of simultaneity between survey measures
of costs and contraceptive use arises because contraceptive use affects reported knowledge and attitudes,
which are in turn taken to affect current use.  Since
earlier knowledge and attitudes cannot be established
from a cross-sectional survey, the inherent simultaneity
cannot be unraveled in this way.  This means that
analyses incorporating current knowledge and attitudes as
determinants of use are likely to produce biased and
misleading conclusions.  The problem is well stated by
Easterlin and Crimmins (1981:20) in their analysis of the
effect of motivation and costs on fertility regulation.
They use as a measure of regulation costs the "number of
methods of fertility control known to the respondent and
reported without special prompting," but point up the
problem in using this measure as a determinant of
regulation:

One would like data that . . . antedate the actual
decision on fertility regulation, because one
consequence of a decision to use control is likely to
be a positive shift in users relative to nonusers with
regard to both knowledge of methods and favorableness
of attitudes.

Their subsequent finding that methods known predicts to
years since adoption of contraception may then be
explained by the reverse effect they describe.  This
latter direction of influence seems plausible given
Immerwahr's (1981:Table 10) analysis for Sri Lanka (one

of the two countries used by Easterlin and Crimmins),
which shows a considerable degree of shifting from the
first method adopted to other methods. Similarly, the
relationships identified by Bogue (in these volumes)
between attitudes and use could be due as much to the
effect of use on reported attitudes as to the reverse.

One solution to this problem is to carry out
individual-level longitudinal analysis in which knowledge, attitudes, and other aspects of costs, as well as
contraception behavior, can be traced over time. This
type of design is very costly and not without problems of
maintaining the panel, avoiding contaminated responses,
and the like. However, in settings where there is
ongoing contact with users, such as in clinic-provided
services or in integrated maternal and child health/
family planning programs, it may be possible to conduct
baseline surveys of adopters to establish their knowledge
and relevant attitudes, and then provide mechanisms for
gathering follow-up information on continuation and
pregnancy.

A more satisfactory and feasible approach stems from
the second assertion presented above: that many elements
of cost can be viewed as characteristics of communities
or areas. In describing market costs, Szykman (1982:322)
states that

> the effective cost of fertility regulation is deter-
> mined primarily by the availability of contraceptive
> information, of contraceptive services, of contra-
> ceptive method mix, of access to outlets in terms of
> time, distance, transportation, frequency, etc., of
> medical follow-up, and of course, by the price of
> individual contraceptive methods.

These are essentially program or macro characteristics
for which the same value could be assigned to each
community or small geographic cluster. The same may be
done for the social and cultural factors included under
subjective costs in Figure 4: social norms and values
can be treated as characteristics of aggregates.

How might these macro variables be measured to avoid
the problem of simultaneity? Contraceptive availability
may be taken as an example. Individual perceptions of
availability are usually obtained from survey questions,
but macro-level measures of actual availability can be
derived by counting the number of outlets serving a
community, measuring the distance from some central spot

to each outlet, and the like.  Of course, there are interrelationships between perceived and actual availability:  perceived availability helps translate the macro characteristic of actual availability into the micro behavioral response of contraceptive use; actual availability, individual attributes, and prior experience with birth control methods will all influence perceived availability.  Nevertheless, both actual and perceived availability can be separately measured, and measures of community availability are not determined by individual contraceptive use.

Analyzing actual community availability has an additional advantage:  program administrators derive more guidance from actual rather than perceived availability. Low community availability may signal to program admini- strators the need for more outlets.  Low perceived availability may do the same, but only if this perception accords with reality; otherwise, the appropriate policy response is probably more publicity and outreach.

As an example, Entwisle et al. (1982a) derived a mea- sure of actual availability from the distance between a rural village and the nearest health center, obtained by field supervisors as part of the second round of the Thailand Contraceptive Prevalence Survey.  They used this, rather than perceived availability, in predicting contraceptive use.  The authors hypothesize positive relationships between the probability of contraceptive use and education, the desire for no more children, and actual availability.  An additional feature of their analysis was that the strength of micro relationships, such as the effects of desire for more children and education on use, was hypothesized to depend on the level of community availability.  Such interactions are dis- cussed further in a later section.  It might be noted here, however, that the results of their analysis were generally in conformity with the hypotheses.

The logic of this framework, and the analysis of community-level  costs, might be extended to include other factors such as method mix, price levels, type of services provided, and related items, insofar as these vary from community to community.  The type of data needed may already exist in the records of the family planning program and private providers, or they might have to be obtained by a special effort.  The cost of the latter should not be great since the data are needed only for the communities that are sampled as part of the fertility survey.  It is also possible in some cases to aggregate individual survey data to obtain measures of social norms and values that are part of the regulation cost structure. This potential is illustrated by Casterline's (1981) WFS analysis, which uses the level of contraceptive use in a community as an aggregate variable to predict intention to use in the future among never users. Casterline argues that the community's level of use reflects its norms about contraception and will therefore affect expressions of future intentions. His findings confirm this expectation in some countries but not in others. This logic can be extended to other cost elements; for example, one can test whether the intentions of never users are a function of the proportion of users reporting side effects, perceived conflicts of family planning with norms or religious beliefs, and so on.

## ESTIMATING THE BASIC MODEL

The framework for fertility regulation shown in Figure 2 involves a simple three-variable problem; as just discussed, however, measurement of motivation to limit and regulation costs introduces complications.

The Easterlin and Crimmins (1981) study discussed above comes closest to using the three-variable model. The regression of their fertility-control variable—years since first use—on the motivation and costs measures shows the expected pattern: motivation is positively related to fertility control, whereas cost is negatively related (i.e., greater knowledge, signifying lower costs, has a positive effect on control). As to magnitude, the standardized coefficients indicate greater explanatory power for motivation, even though the costs coefficient may be biased upward due to its ex post character.

Few other studies have used the three-variable model directly. In the absence of direct measures of costs, it is common to regress a measure of fertility regulation (e.g., current use or nonuse of contraception) on motivation and a series of socioeconomic and demographic variables. The measure of motivation frequently used is the difference between actual and desired number of children. This common approach may be represented as

$$U = a_3 + e_1 (A - D) + e_2 A + e_3 X_1 + e_4 X_2 \tag{6}$$

where U is a measure of regulation use; $X_1$ and $X_2$ are socioeconomic or demographic characteristics, say, marital duration and education; and A and D are as previously defined.

Following Figure 2, it may be argued that any independent variable included in addition to motivation to limit must be justified as a proxy for cost.[15] For example, education might be justified on the grounds that better-educated women are likely to have more knowledge of contraception and lower psychic and monetary costs than less-educated women. Though actual fertility (A) is often included separately on the right-hand side, there seems to be little justification for this, since it is already embedded in the motivation variable.

The most serious problem associated with the equation is that it ignores the reciprocal influence of contraceptive use on actual fertility: past contraceptive use affects current actual fertility at the same time that actual fertility affects current use. Thus, among other difficulties, the coefficient of motivation estimated from a single equation like this will be biased because actual fertility is part of the motivation variable.

A better model of contraceptive use would involve an improved measure of motivation using potential supply instead of actual fertility, as well as an explicit measure of costs. The supply and demand measures may be entered separately, as in

$$U = a_4 + g_1PS + g_2D + g_3C \tag{7}$$

or combined into a single motivational variable, as in

$$U = a_5 + g_4(PS-D) + g_5C \tag{8}$$

When A is used in place of PS, the coefficients should be different unless actual fertility is equal to potential supply. This might be so, to a close approximation, only in a country where contraceptive use is relatively recent, so that most users adopted for the first time in the open interval. In this case, if adoption is indeed recent, actual fertility at the time of the survey will be little affected by prior contraceptive use, but will be determined directly by supply, i.e., by a couple's natural fertility and experience with child mortality. However, this criterion may be difficult to satisfy. Tables 3 and 4 show that more ever users adopted since the last birth in Taiwan (two-thirds of ever users) than

TABLE 3   Percent of Ever Users Adopting After Last
Birth, 1972:   Taiwan

| Current Parity | No. of Married Women | Percent Ever Users | Percent of Ever Users Adopting After Last Birth | | | | |
|---|---|---|---|---|---|---|---|
| | | | Total | Years Married | | | |
| | | | | 0-4 | 5-9 | 10-14 | 15+ |
| One | 545 | 34 | 82 | -- | -- | -- | -- |
| Two | 935 | 62 | 74 | -- | -- | -- | -- |
| Three | 1,288 | 81 | 67 | 52 | 63 | 73 | 80 |
| Four | 1,076 | 87 | 67 | -- | 53 | 63 | 81 |
| Five | 620 | 88 | 66 | -- | 50 | 60 | 73 |
| Six | 275 | 87 | 60 | -- | -- | 44 | 70 |
| Seven+[a] | 169 | 83 | 60 | -- | -- | -- | -- |
| Total | 5,133[b] | 72[b] | 68 | | | | |

Note:   Dashes indicate few or no cases in the cell.

[a]Approximated by proportion of women with seven or more births who
first used after six births.
[b]Includes data for 225 nulliparous women.

Source:   Adapted from Siddiqui (1979:Tables III-2 and III-5).

in Sri Lanka (one-half), despite the latter program being
more recent and producing much lower prevalence. The
difference appears to be due in large part to the relatively widespread use of rhythm in Sri Lanka, reported
quite frequently at low parities (Immerwahr, 1981:Table
9). In both countries, there also appears to be a trend
toward adoption earlier in the reproductive cycle (Table
3 and Immerwahr, 1981:Tables 7 and 8), which would make
actual fertility diverge even more from potential supply
as younger cohorts enter reproductive age. Thus, even
where there is close correspondence between actual
fertility and supply at one point in time, they may
diverge rapidly; with more widespread adoption of
contraception, the assumption of equality will therefore
become less tenable. This means that continued use of
actual fertility in place of potential supply will produce increasingly biased coefficients. On the other
hand, the difficulties of estimating supply have already
been noted.

TABLE 4   Percent of Ever Users Adopting
After Last Birth, by Age, 1975:   Sri
Lanka

| Age | No. of Ever Users | Percent |
|-----|-------------------|---------|
| Under 25 | 337 | 67 |
| 25-29 | 563 | 52 |
| 30-34 | 626 | 51 |
| 35-39 | 569 | 50 |
| 40-44 | 384 | 52 |
| 45-49 | 311 | 42 |
| Total | 2,790 | 52 |

Note:  Percentage was determined by
tabulating number of living children
when contraception was first used by
current number of living children.
Cases in which the former variable
equalled or exceeded the latter were
assumed to adopt after the last birth.

Source:  Tabulated from WFS standard
recode tape.

The model of fertility control assumes that couples
adopt contraception to limit family size; insofar as
there is widespread use for spacing, one would not expect
motivation to limit to distinguish users from nonusers.
Table 1 shows that in 10 of 17 countries, one-quarter or
more of the women who want more children are using
contraception, presumably for spacing.  To the extent
that this use expands, the power of the model to distinguish users from nonusers will diminish, and new
models incorporating the determinants of adoption for
spacing will be needed.  Of course, it may be argued
that, as contraceptive use becomes sufficiently
widespread, interest in predicting use will disappear;
most likely, the problem will be reconceptualized to
focus on other facets of use, such as when contraception

is adopted, the specific methods adopted, and the effectiveness of use.


## CHOICE OF MEANS OF FERTILITY REGULATION

The simple model of fertility control explored here has for the most part assumed that some form of contraception (including sterilization) will be chosen as the regulating mechanism. This need not be the case. Couples may attempt to influence any of the following:

- Factors affecting exposure to intercourse
  Voluntary abstinence
  Coital frequency
- Factors affecting exposure to conception
  (Contraception and sterilization)
  Duration of breastfeeding
- Factors affecting gestation
  Voluntary abortion

Omitted from this list are the formation and dissolution of unions, since decisions about these are generally not expected to be influenced by the desire to regulate fertility (cf. Bongaarts and Menken, in these volumes).[16]

Of the factors in the list, voluntary abstinence in its various forms (nonsystematized, calendar rhythm, etc.) is generally treated as a traditional and behavioral means of contraception and will be similarly treated here. (Postpartum abstinence, in particular, is an important factor in childspacing in some parts of Africa [Page and Lesthaeghe, 1981].)

Relatively little is known about coital frequency and the extent to which it is systematically varied to control childbearing. Data from the United States (Westoff, 1974) show higher coital frequency among couples using highly effective means of contraception, and, among contraceptive users, higher frequency for those intending to delay than for those wishing to prevent a birth. These data also reveal that, among nonusers not wishing to have another child at the moment, coital frequency is much lower among women intending no more children than among those intending to have more. This suggests some reduction in frequency among those desiring to reduce the probability of conception. Similar data and analyses for developing countries do not appear to be available.[17]

There is growing evidence that women do prolong their
duration of breastfeeding to increase the length of the
birth interval.  This evidence is based on an observed
inverse relationship between use of contraception and
duration of breastfeeding that suggests these two
behaviors are partial substitutes for each other (Jain
and Bongaarts, 1981; Millman, 1982; Johnson-Acsadi and
Szykman, 1981).  By introducing controls available from
WFS data, Jain and Bongaarts (1981) show that this
relationship is not spurious (see also Millman, 1982).
They argue, however, that breastfeeding is used mainly to
regulate birth intervals rather than to help limit family
size, because duration of breastfeeding was not systematically related to parity in the eight countries.  This may
not be a conclusive test:  other things being equal, women
who breastfeed for a shorter period will have higher
parity, thereby masking any trend to lengthen breastfeeding at higher parities.  Millman (1982) treats this
issue by directly introducing a motivation variable into
her analysis for Taiwan, and finds generally that, after
controlling for contraceptive use, those who wished to
stop childbearing breastfed longer than those who
intended future births.  Of course, the hypothesis that
women alter their breastfeeding behavior to regulate
fertility can only be sustained if women are aware of
breastfeeding's fertility-inhibiting effects.  Aside from
numerous subjective reports, systematic data on this
point are scarce, with few surveys attempting measures of
women's awareness.[18]  A more sensitive line of ques-
tioning on this topic and replication across countries
are needed.  Also needed is more research on the extent
to which breastfeeding contributes to the lack of contraceptive use among a portion of women wanting more
children.[19]

Abortion has been an important and widespread means of
fertility regulation in both developed and developing
societies.  Legal  restrictions in many places and the
social stigma associated with its practice have greatly
limited the range and accuracy of both aggregate and
individual-level data.  As a result, it is difficult to
mount careful comparative studies of the interrelationships between contraception and abortion.  Studies
cited by David (in these volumes) indicate that women
highly motivated to limit family size use both contraception and abortion, and that experience with one type of
fertility regulation contributes to experimentation with
the other (see also Freedman et al., 1975).  David's

review of trends in Chile reveals a case in which, under
an intensive family planning program, contraceptive use
increased sharply and abortion decreased.

In addition to the means of fertility regulation
listed above, there is a wide choice among contraceptive
methods. As noted earlier, modern methods predominate
among 20 WFS countries; moreover, in countries for which
time-series data exist, modern methods represent an
increasing proportion of total use (United Nations,
1981b:26). Nevertheless, there is little correlation
between the overall prevalence rate and the proportion of
users relying on traditional methods. It is interesting
to note that, in a number of developed countries, traditional methods account for a higher proportion of total
use than in most of the developing countries shown in
Figure 3 (Larson, 1981:Table 2); at the same time, there
were substantial shifts toward modern methods among the
developed countries in the 1965-75 period (Leridon,
1981:Table 8). Among couples in the developed countries,
the safety, convenience, and effectiveness of modern
methods were attractive alternatives to the traditional
methods they had been using; to many couples in the
developing countries, these features were probably
necessary for them to initiate fertility regulation. The
availability, and in many places the promotion, of modern
methods appear instrumental in reducing costs to the
point where significant gains in prevalence can occur.

THE ROLE OF FAMILY PLANNING PROGRAMS AND COMMUNITY
CHARACTERISTICS IN FERTILITY REGULATION

The present analysis has focused on fertility regulation
largely from the viewpoint of the individual woman or
couple. However, the model set forth in Figure 1 assigns
a role to various community or societal mechanisms, and
it was argued above that many components of costs are
usefully viewed as macro characteristics. This section
focuses on the role of the macro variables--family
planning programs and community characteristics--in
fertility regulation.

Family planning programs represent the major social
innovation designed to accelerate contraceptive use and
reduce fertility in developing countries. On the scope
and nature of programs, major sources of comparative data
have been the various editions of Population and Family
Planning Programs (e.g., Nortman and Hofstatter, 1980).

Topics covered include governmental positions on population growth and family planning; legal and de facto regulations related to family planning methods; indicators of
inputs into family planning programs, covering data on
funds, personnel, and facilities; and indicators of
program output, including data on acceptors by method,
characteristics of acceptors, and estimates of prevalence
by private and public sectors. Another important source
of information on governmental policy in relation to fertility and family planning, as well as other demographic
factors, has been the monitoring reports of the United
Nations, initiated after the 1974 U.N. World Population
Conference in Bucharest (United Nations, 1980, 1981a).
These reveal, for example, that, as of 1978, 73 percent
of the 116 countries surveyed supported (directly or
indirectly) access to modern methods of birth control
(United Nations, 1980:Table 19). Nortman and Hofstatter
(1980:Table 5) indicate that over 90 percent of the
developing world's population resides in countries that
support family planning to reduce population growth or
promote health. Family planning delivery systems have
been undergoing rapid change in recent years with the
greater promotion of commercial retail sales, the
integration of family planning services with primary
health care and development programs, and the increased
emphasis on community-based distribution systems. These
and other trends are reviewed in the report of the
International Conference on Family Planning in the 1980s
(1981:Annex).

The present discussion examines various approaches for
evaluating family planning programs, with the goal of
ascertaining how to analyze their role in the model (see
also Ross, in these volumes; Mauldin, in these volumes;
Retherford and Palmore, in these volumes). Programs may
facilitate the adoption of fertility regulation both by
strengthening motivation to limit and by reducing regulation costs. The latter influence is the more obvious
and has received more attention, particularly in the
earlier phases of many programs. By providing information about contraception, opening up convenient service
points, subsidizing purchase of various methods, and
legitimizing their use, programs reduce a number of the
monetary and psychic costs described earlier. Programs
may also strengthen motivation by promoting lower family-
size norms, thus furthering an interest in fertility
regulation at earlier stages of reproduction, or encouraging those undecided about stopping at a given parity to
do so (Freedman, 1979; Knodel and Debavalya, 1978).

When the effects of a program are evaluated, there is usually no attempt made to identify its relative contribution to reducing costs and strengthening motivation; interest tends to center on a program's ultimate contribution to reducing fertility. Concern with this issue has led to the development of a number of evaluation techniques (Chandrasekaran and Hermalin, 1975; United Nations, 1978, 1979b); the eight major ones are listed in Table 5, by type of effect and type of data required (Hermalin, 1982a). The middle four techniques estimate only fertility reduction deriving directly from supplies and services provided by the program, basically through accounting procedures that start with the number of couples served by the program; make use of the length and effectiveness of contraceptive use; and take account of a number of other factors, such as a woman's age, the risks of secondary sterility and marital dissolution, overlap between postpartum amenorrhea and contraceptive use, and potential fertility (the fertility that acceptors would have in the absence of the program). These four methods do not take into account the role of socioeconomic development in heightening motivation or in reducing costs.

Other methods incorporate this factor, and several attempt to separate program from nonprogram effects or to estimate the total effect from all sources. Two of these--standardization and trend analysis--rely on demographic data. The former attempts to disentangle the role of marital fertility from the roles of age structure and marital status in fertility changes. Since a program affects only marital fertility, standardization sets a limit on the fertility change arising from it. Trend analysis also relies on demographic data, but by using time series and some strong assumptions, provides an estimate of both program and nonprogram effects. The essential method is to project fertility trends prior to the start of a program, and to contrast this with the actual trend after the program started. The first trend is assumed to capture underlying socioeconomic processes, and the difference between the two trends provides an implicit measure of the added effect of the program.

Both nonprogram and program effects can be measured explicitly by the last two techniques in Table 5, experimental design and multivariate areal analysis. The basic idea of the former is to assign family planning programs randomly to administrative areas within a country. After several years, the difference in fertility between program

TABLE 5 Techniques for Measuring Family Planning Program Effects, Cross-Classified by Type of Effect and Type of Data

| Technique | Type of Effect Analyzed | | | Type of Data Employed | | | |
|---|---|---|---|---|---|---|---|
| | Program Effect | Non-program Effect | Total Effect | Program Vari-ables | Nonprogram Variables | | |
| | | | | | Socio-economic | Demo-graphic | Bio-logical |
| Standardization | - | - | X | - | O | X | - |
| Trend Analysis | I | X | X | - | - | X | - |
| (Standard) Couple Years of Protection | X | - | - | X | - | X | O |
| Analysis of Reproductive Process | X | - | - | X | - | X | X |
| Component Projection | X | - | - | X | - | X | O |
| Simulation | X | - | - | X | - | X | X |
| Experimental Design and Matching Studies | X | X | X | X | O | O | - |
| Multivariate Areal Analysis | X | X | X | X | X | X | O |

Note:

X = Effect or data explicitly involved.

I = Effect obtained implicitly.

O = Data of this type occasionally employed or potentially employable.

- = Effect or data not generally part of technique.

Source: Hermalin (1982a).

and nonprogram areas should indicate the program effect; if initial fertility levels are known, an estimate of nonprogram effects can also be derived. Practical problems, such as contamination between test and control areas and the need to distinguish short- from long-term effects, come into play in carrying out a specific design (Cuca and Pierce, 1977; Phillips et al.,1982; Stinson et al., 1982). In areal multivariate analysis, data are needed for administrative areas on both program inputs and nonprogram factors thought to influence fertility. The effect of the program is tested by determining the relationship between program factors and fertility across the areal units, after taking into account the socioeconomic factors involved. Typically, regression analysis will be used to estimate the effects of each independent variable in the model, thus providing measures of program and specific nonprogram effects (Hermalin, 1979).

The use of these different techniques has spurred theoretical and empirical research on reconciling their results. An important distinction should be made between gross and net program effects. When gross effects are assessed, a program receives credit for all acceptors from the public sector, including those who switched from a private source and, hypothetically, those who might have used a private source if a public source were not available; at the same time, those who were motivated by the program to adopt contraception but who choose a private source are not included (this is often referred to as the catalytic impact of a program). Net program effect seeks to isolate more precisely the program's contribution to fertility regulation through its enhancement of motivation and reduction of costs. Of the techniques considered, trend analysis, multivariate areal analysis, and experimental design can produce estimates of net effect, while the remaining methods yield gross estimates (see also Bongaarts, forthcoming). Empirical research on cross-method variance has consisted of applying the different techniques to the same setting to determine whether they yield similar inferences about program impact (United Nations, 1978, 1982; Potter, 1981; Hermalin, 1982b). These studies indicate that a major source of variation across methods (connected in part to the distinction between gross and net effects) is the level of potential fertility used explicitly or implicitly by each technique. Continuing research should eventually establish reasonably narrow bounds for program effects.

These techniques were developed to evaluate family planning programs within specific countries. A number of analyses have also looked at program effects cross-culturally. The major approach is a modification of areal multivariate analysis, with countries as the units of analysis; measures of program strength[20] and indices of socioeconomic development as the independent variables; and a measure of fertility or fertility change as the dependent variable (Mauldin and Berelson, 1978; Hernandez, 1981; Cutright and Kelly, 1981). These studies show a distinct effect of family planning programs on fertility, but variation in magnitude. In describing the limitations of such areal analyses, Hermalin (1979) notes that results are likely to be sensitive to differences in conceptual models, operational definitions, and techniques of estimation. Thus, establishing narrow bounds for program effects cross-culturally remains elusive.

The availability of comparable fertility data for many countries in the World Fertility Survey and the Contraceptive Prevalence Surveys has presented some new possibilities for measuring program effects. One of these has been the development of a prevalence model for estimating gross program effect. Bongaarts and Kirmeyer (1982) and Bongaarts (forthcoming) regress nationwide fertility measures, such as total fertility and total marital fertility rates, on prevalence of contraceptive use. These equations, together with Bongaarts' modeling of fertility according to proximate determinants, permit the derivation of gross program effects and births averted from the prevalence of program contraception, the prevalence of contraception from nonprogram sources, the crude birth rate, and population size. Bongaarts has also extended this model to provide age-specific and method-specific results.

The availability of comparable surveys also permits the use of multilevel analysis, combining data on individuals with that on communities or countries. This is a general strategy with a large number of possible applications. Although this section has focused on ultimate effects on fertility, many of the immediate and intermediate goals of a country's program can be profitably investigated.[21] As noted earlier, multilevel analysis can be used to determine the effect of contraceptive availability and other dimensions of costs on contraceptive use. A similar strategy can be used to explore a program's effect on demand for children and hence on motivation, using a design along the lines shown

FIGURE 5   Outline of Multilevel Model for Studying Effects of Family
Planning Programs on Desired Number of Children

| | |
|---|---|
| Dependent variable<br>(individual-level) | Desired number of children |
| Independent variables<br>(individual-level) | Wife's education<br>Husband's occupation<br>Wife's labor force status<br>Childhood residence<br>Age |
| Independent variables<br>(community-level) | Program inputs (IEC efforts, or personnel<br>  and facilities)<br>Modernization (electricity, educational<br>  facilities, health facilities, etc.)<br>Communication (movies, television, etc.)<br>Distance to nearest city<br>Region |
| Major interactions | Program input x education<br>Program input x labor force status<br>Modernization x education<br>Communications x education |

in Figure 5.   The analysis is carried out by regressing
the dependent variable on the individual- and community-
level independent variables and hypothesized interactions
between the two.   Coefficients of the interaction terms
would be of particular interest.   One might hypothesize,
for example, that the relationship between education and
desired number of children will differ in communities
with high versus low information-education-communication
(IEC) efforts:   successful IEC might reduce the desired
number of children to a greater extent among the less-
educated than among the more-educated.

Another illustration of this technique suitable for
cross-country analysis might be given.   Assume a
simplified model in which contraceptive use depends on
motivation and education (as a proxy for costs), and in
which the system is affected by two global variables--
family planning program effort and socioeconomic development.   Table 6 presents hypotheses about the relationship among education, motivation, and use at
different levels of the macro-variables.   For example,
given the role of family planning programs in

TABLE 6  Hypothesized Relationship Between Family Planning Program Effort and Socioeconomic Development on Micro Relationships

| Micro Relationship | Family Planning Program Effort | | | Socioeconomic Development | | | |
|---|---|---|---|---|---|---|---|
| | Weak | Strong | Corre-lation[a] | Low | Moderate | High | Corre-lation[a] |
| Effect of Education on Motivation | Strong Positive | Weak Positive | Negative | Weak Positive | Strong Positive | Weak Positive | Negative[b] |
| Effect of Education on Use | Strong Positive | Weak Positive | Negative | Moderate Positive | Strong Positive | Weak Positive | Negative[b] |
| Effect of Motivation on Use | Weak Positive | Strong Positive | Positive | Weak Positive | Moderate Positive | Strong Positive | Positive |

[a]predicted correlation between macro characteristic and micro relationship.
[b]Assumes that most countries will be at moderate to high levels of socioeconomic development.

strengthening motivation and reducing costs, countries
with a strong program could be expected to show a greater
effect of motivation on use and a weaker effect of education.  Similarly, level of development, which strengthens
motivation to limit and makes contraceptives more widely
available, can be expected to have the same effects.  A
curvilinear effect of development on the education-
motivation relationship is hypothesized:  at low levels
of development, few people in any educational strata will
be motivated to restrict childbearing; with more development, clear socioeconomic differentials will occur,
attenuated as development proceeds further.  Preliminary
tests with 15 WFS countries and a set of earlier KAP data
(derived from Freedman and Coombs, 1974) generally support
these hypotheses.[22]

A particular strength of multilevel analysis, therefore, is that it encourages the formulation of hypotheses
about interactions like these.  It thus helps operationalize some of the ideas presented by Retherford and Palmore
(in these volumes) on the way regression coefficients
might be expected to change with the diffusion of fertility regulation.  It also provides ideas to test with the
clustered samples that Potter (in these volumes) recommends for investigating social and community mechanisms.
This form of analysis can also provide important insights
for family planning program administrators in determining
the efficacy of specific program procedures.


CONCLUSION

This review has chosen a rather narrow framework from
which to explore the question of fertility regulation.
Rather than touch on the multitude of studies that address
one or another part of the regulation process, it has
exploited a rather simple paradigm.  This paradigm is
widely recognized, but is frequently ignored in the
actual execution of research.  This contributes to a
state of disarray within the field and a lack of systematic progress.  The present investigation of the
paradigm connecting regulation costs and motivation to
limit with the use of fertility regulation has detected a
number of areas where improvements are needed.  These
include methods of measuring motivation that avoid
introducing simultaneities with contraceptive use;
improved conceptualization and measurement of costs,
recognizing that many of the components are global or

macro in character; and modes of analysis that incorporate both individual and community (or country) variables.

The potential utility of the model presented here should not obscure its weaknesses. The model is likely to become increasingly dated with the growing availability and use of effective contraception in developing countries. The increasing practice of spacing will attenuate the relation between desire for more children and contraceptive use; interest will center more on when couples decide to limit childbearing than on whether those who want no more children are using contraception. One might therefore expect that increasing attention will be focused on the study of childspacing, and on the determinants of the total number of children desired.

## NOTES

1. The term community is used throughout to refer to both limited geographical areas within which a major share of people's activities and meaningful inter-actions take place, and larger aggregations such as regions and nations whose policies may influence individual behavior. Where necessary, the specific level of aggregation will be noted.

2. This list does not attempt to be exhaustive. A thorough analysis would reveal other examples of sharp increases. Overall, it appears that some 15 countries have increased their prevalence rates by 20 points or more in a decade or less.

3. Data on contraceptive prevalence for earlier time points are presented in Watson and Lapham (1975), for circa 1973; Freedman and Coombs (1974), for 1966-71; and United Nations (1979a), for 1963-71.

4. A number of studies provide basic data derived from the World Fertility Survey on the relationship between contraceptive use and various demographic and socio-economic characteristics (Sadik, 1981; United Nations, 1981b; Lightbourne, 1980; Carrasco, 1981). A compila-tion of data for developing and developed countries on one traditional method, periodic abstinence, including estimates over time, is presented in Population Reports (1981a:Table 4).

5. The legal status of abortion in each country as of mid-1980 is given in Tietze (1981:Table 1). This review indicates that 9 percent of the world's popula-tion lived in countries where abortion was prohibited

without exception, 19 percent where it was permitted
only to save a woman's life, 10 percent where it was
permitted on broader medical grounds, 24 percent
where social and economic factors could be taken into
account, and 38 percent where abortion was available
on request. Between 1976 and 1980, about 40 jurisdictions extended the grounds for abortion, while 6
made legal access more restrictive.

6.  This is the form basically employed by the WFS (Singh,
1980). Alternative wordings are given in Population
Council (1970). See also Knodel and Prachuabmoh
(1973) and Szykman (1982) for discussions of alternate
concepts such as ideal and expected number of children
and relevant references. Pullum (1980) also contains
a useful bibliography on this topic.

7.  The method is based on psychological unfolding theory.
The independence and additivity of the scales can be
established, justifying the use of conjoint measurement. Responses are generally meaningful and
consistent.

8.  United Nations (1981b:52) reports a correlation of
over 0.8 between proportions using among those
wanting more and among those wanting no more.

9.  The Cleland et al. (1979) analysis does not involve
the motivation variable but describes in detail the
hierarchical approach.

10. Pullum presents data for Sri Lanka showing that the
number of children women report as ideal rises
directly with their actual number. He argues that
this association is due to rationalization as well as
to implementation of preferences, therefore justifying an analysis in the form of equation (5).
Jejeebhoy (1981), on the other hand, shows that when
cohorts in Taiwan are traced across successive
surveys, there is a surprisingly high persistence of
stated preferences, indicating for these women a
minimum of rationalization. The degree to which
desired numbers are adjusted or rationalized in the
course of family building cannot be determined
conclusively from a single cross-sectional survey.
Pullum (1980) advocates resorting to ancillary as
well as survey data. For example, he suggests that
heavy rationalization is plausible if stated preferences rise with actual number of children, if final
fertility is in excess of the number desired, and if
the country's fertility rates suggest natural fertility or there is little efficient contraception.

He advocates including actual fertility as a determinant of desired number in such cases; this would be used as a control or intervening variable, as illustrated in equation (4), so that the effects of the other variables would be net of this bias. For cases where it cannot be determined whether there is heavy rationalization or implementation of preferences, Pullum suggests restricting the analysis to women of short marital duration; for these women, little rationalization would have occurred, and preferences can therefore be treated solely as a function of socioeconomic variables and appropriate demographic controls.

11. Technically, measurable costs could be involved in such a case if the wealthy few could travel elsewhere to obtain this method.

12. It would be more correct to contrast knowledge with ever use of contraception rather than with current use; however, since these two measures of use are highly correlated, the overall relationship would not change much. The lack of relationship between knowledge and use on the aggregate level does not, of course, preclude a relationship at the individual level. Nevertheless, where the overall knowledge in a country is very high, one would not expect much relationship, as confirmed by Sadik (1981).

13. Terminology in this area appears to be evolving. Rodriguez uses "availability" for knowledge of a source, and "accessibility" for time, distance, and means of transport to that source. Lewis and Novak define "availability" as including both effective knowledge of a source (whether couples have sufficient knowledge about a source to obtain contraception if they so desire) and proximity (travel time, travel mode, and convenience). They regard availability as one aspect of general accessibility, which also includes such factors as costs, quality of services, availability of medical personnel, and adequacy of supplies.

14. It is interesting that in the one country studied by both Rodriguez and Lewis and Novak—Costa Rica—Rodriguez finds no effects of accessibility on use. Additional analysis can be found in Brackett (1981).

15. Given weak measures of motivation, some of the independent variables must be justified as reducing measurement error, explaining systematic variation, or capturing the intensity of motivation, if the latter were a concept in the model.

16. Infanticide, though not a method of fertility control, has been used to regulate the consequences of fertility in a number of societies at certain stages of development (see Scrimshaw, in these volumes).

17. Muangman et al. (1973) report data for a suburb of Thailand showing very similar distributions of coital frequency between those using and not using contraception; however, these tabulations do not control for age or other factors. Questions on coital frequency have been included in surveys done in several African countries, as well as in Colombia and the Philippines, but results are not yet available.

18. In a 1967-68 Taiwan survey, women were asked, "Can a woman get pregnant while breastfeeding?" The 22 percent of married women answering "No" provide a minimum estimate of those who might use breastfeeding to influence fertility, since many others who answered "Yes" are likely to be aware that breastfeeding lessens the likelihood of contraception without affording absolute protection. In the Fiji World Fertility Survey (Fiji, Bureau of Statistics, 1976:514), a question on the efficacy of breastfeeding was included among those on knowledge and use of contraceptive methods. Among ever-married women, 50 percent reported hearing of this method, but less than 7 percent reported ever using it. Lactation was also included as a method of contraception in the Paraguay Contraceptive Prevalence Survey (Morris et al., 1978). Butz and Habicht (1976:215) cite a Guatemalan study indicating that three-quarters of mothers believed lactation postpones a new conception. Questions on knowledge of the effect of breastfeeding were also included in the Malaysian Family Life Survey (Butz and DaVanzo, 1978).

19. The substitution of breastfeeding for contraception may help explain why a significant portion of women who say they want no more children are not using contraception—the so-called unmet need for birth control, of considerable current interest (Westoff, 1978). However, Szykman's (1982) analysis suggests that breastfeeding may account for only a small portion of the unmet need. For an unidentified WFS country, he shows that 58 percent of women who wanted no more children and were not using contraception were breastfeeding, but only half of them intended to contracept in the future. He interprets this as indicating that many of the motivated breastfeeding

women did not associate their breastfeeding with
fertility regulation.

20. An index of program strength or effort was developed
by Lapham and Mauldin (1972) using 15 programmatic
criteria. This index has been widely used, most
notably by Mauldin and Berelson (1978), who provide
values for 94 countries circa 1970. Despite the
availability of such an index, however, there are
many facets of family planning program inputs that
are not well measured (Mauldin and Lapham, 1982).

21. Ross (in these volumes) describes the gains possible
by improving contraceptive continuation—one intermediate goal. A general review of program objectives
is given by Chandrasekaran and Freymann (1965).

22. Some evidence that program effort and socioeconomic
development interact in their effect on these micro
relationships has been found in a large-scale comparative analysis of WFS data (Entwisle et al.,
1982b).

## BIBLIOGRAPHY

Bongaarts, J. (1982)  The fertility inhibiting effects of
the intermediate variables. Studies in Family
Planning 13:179-189.

Bongaarts, J. (forthcoming)  The concept of potential
fertility in the evaluation of the fertility impact
of family planning programs. In Proceedings of the
Third Expert Group Meeting on Methods of Measuring
the Impact of Family Planning Programmes on
Fertility, Geneva. New York:  United Nations.

Bongaarts, J., and S. Kirmeyer (1982)  Estimating the
impact of contraceptive prevalence on fertility:
Aggregate and age-specific versions of a model. In
A. I. Hermalin and B. Entwisle, eds., The Role of
Surveys in the Analysis of Family Planning Programs.
Liege:  Ordina.

Boulier, B. L., and N. G. Mankiw (1980)  An Econometric
Model of the Demand, Supply, and Regulation of
Fertility. Paper presented at the annual meeting of
the Population Association of America, Denver.

Brackett, J. W. (1981)  The role of family planning
availability and accessibility in family planning use
in developing countries. Pp. 19-49 in World
Fertility Survey Conference 1980, Record of
Proceedings, Vol. 2. Voorburg:  International
Statistical Institute.

Butz, W. P., and J. DaVanzo (1978)  The Malaysian Family Life Survey:  Summary Report.  R-2351-AID.  Santa Monica, Calif.:  Rand Corporation.

Butz, W. P., and J.-P. Habicht (1976)  The effects of nutrition and health on fertility:  Hypotheses, evidence, and interventions.  In R. G. Ridker, ed., Population and Development.  Baltimore, Md.:  The Johns Hopkins University Press.

Carrasco, E. (1981)  Contraceptive Practice.  WFS Comparative Studies, No. 9.  London:  World Fertility Survey.

Casterline, J. B. (1981)  Community Effects on Fertility Intentions:  The Effect of Aggregate Levels of Contraceptive Use on Individual Intentions to Use. WFS Technical Papers 1703.  London:  World Fertility Survey.

Chandrasekaran, C., and M. W. Freymann (1965)  Evaluating community family planning programs.  In M. C. Sheps and J. C. Ridley, eds., Public Health and Population Change.  Pittsburgh, Pa.:  University of Pittsburgh Press.

Chandrasekaran, C., and A. I. Hermalin, eds. (1975) Measuring the Effect of Family Planning Programs on Fertility.  Liege:  Ordina.

Cleland, J. G., R. J. A. Little, and P. Pitaktepsombati (1979)  Illustrative Analysis:  Socio-Economic Determinants of Contraceptive Use in Thailand.  WFS Scientific Reports, No. 5.  London:  World Fertility Survey.

Coale, A. J. (1973)  The demographic transition.  Pp. 53-72 in International Population Conference, Liege 1973.  Liege:  International Union for the Scientific Study of Population.

Coale, A. J., and T. J. Trussell (1974)  Model fertility schedules:  Variations in the age structure of childbearing in human populations.  Population Index 40:185-257.

Concepcion, M. B. (1981)  Family formation and contraception in selected developing countries: Policy implications of WFS findings.  Pp. 197-260 in World Fertility Survey Conference 1980, Vol. 1. London:  World Fertility Survey.

Coombs, C. H., L. C. Coombs, and G. H. McClelland (1975) Preference scales for number and sex of children. Population Studies 29:273-298.

Coombs, L. C. (1979)  Prospective fertility and underlying preferences:  A longitudinal study in Taiwan.  Population Studies 33:447-455.

Cuca, R., and C. S. Pierce (1977) Experiments in Family Planning: Lessons from the Developing World. Baltimore, Md.: The Johns Hopkins University Press.

Cutright, P., and W. R. Kelly (1981) The role of family planning programs in fertility declines in less developed countries, 1958-1977. International Family Planning Perspectives 7:145-151.

Easterlin, R. A. (1978) The economics and sociology of fertility: A synthesis. In C. Tilly, ed., Historical Studies of Changing Fertility. Princeton, N.J.: Princeton University Press.

Easterlin, R. A., and E. M. Crimmins (1982) An Exploratory Study of the 'Synthesis Framework' of Fertility Determination with WFS Core Questionnaire Data. Paper prepared for the International Union for the Scientific Study of Population International Population Conference, Manila.

Entwisle, B., A. I. Hermalin, P. Kamnuansilpa, and A. Chamratrithirong (1982a) A Multilevel Model of Family Planning Availability and Contraceptive Use in Rural Thailand. Population Studies Center Research Report. Ann Arbor, Mich.: University of Michigan.

Entwisle, B., A. I. Hermalin, and W. Mason (1982b) Socioeconomic Determinants of Fertility Behavior in Developing Nations: Theory and Initial Results. Washington, D.C.: National Academy Press.

Ferry, B. (1981) Breastfeeding. WFS Comparative Studies, No. 13. London: World Fertility Survey.

Fiji, Bureau of Statistics (1976) Fiji Fertility Survey 1974, Principal Report. London: World Fertility Survey.

Freedman, R. (1975) The Sociology of Fertility. New York: Irvington Publishers.

Freedman, R. (1979) Theories of fertility decline: A reappraisal. Social Forces 58:1-17.

Freedman, R., and L. Coombs (1974) Cross-Cultural Comparisons: Data on Two Factors in Fertility Behavior. New York: Population Council.

Freedman, R., A. I. Hermalin, and M.-C. Chang (1975) Do statements about desired family size predict fertility? The case of Taiwan, 1967-1970. Demography 12:407-416.

Hauser, P. (1967) Family planning and population programs--a book review article. Demography 4:397-414.

Hermalin, A. I. (1979) Multivariate areal analysis. Pp. 99-111 in The Methodology of Measuring the Impact of

Family Planning Programmes on Fertility, Manual IX.
   New York:  United Nations.
Hermalin, A. I. (1982a)  Techniques for measuring family
   planning program effects on fertility.  In J. Ross,
   ed., International Encyclopedia of Population.  New
   York:  The Free Press.
Hermalin, A. I. (1982b)  Issues in the comparative
   analysis of techniques for evaluating family planning
   programmes.  In Evaluation of the Impact of Family
   Planning Programs on Fertility:  Sources of
   Variance.  New York:  United Nations.
Hermalin, A. I., R. F. Freedman, T.-H. Sun, and M.-C.
   Chang (1979)  Do intentions predict fertility?  The
   experience in Taiwan, 1967-74.  Studies in Family
   Planning 10:75-95.
Hernandez, D. J. (1981)  A note on measuring the
   independent impact of family planning programs on
   fertility declines.  Demography 18:627-634.
Immerwahr, G. (1981)  Contraceptive Use in Sri Lanka.
   WFS Scientific Reports, No. 18.  London:  World
   Fertility Survey.
International Conference on Family Planning in the 1980s
   (1981)  Family Planning in the 1980s.  New York:
   United Nations Fund for Population Activities,
   International Planned Parenthood Federation, and
   Population Council.
Jain, A. K., and J. Bongaarts (1981)  Socio-biological
   factors in exposure to childbearing:  Breastfeeding
   and its fertility effects.  Pp. 255-302 in World
   Fertility Survey Conference 1980, Record of
   Proceedings, Vol. 2.  Voorburg:  International
   Statistical Institute.
Jejeebhoy, S. J. (1981)  Cohort consistency in family
   size preference:  Taiwan, 1965-73.  Studies in Family
   Planning 12:229-232.
Johnson-Acsadi, G. G., and M. Szykman (1981)  Selected
   Characteristics of Exposed Women Wanting No More
   Children and Not Using Contraceptives.  Paper
   prepared for the International Union for the
   Scientific Study of Population Seminar on the
   Analysis of the WFS Family Planning Module, Genting
   Highlands, Malaysia.
Johnson-Acsadi, G. G., and M. B. Weinberger (1982)
   Factors affecting use and non-use of contraception.
   Pp. 51-84 in A. I. Hermalin and B. Entwisle, eds.,
   The Role of Surveys in the Analysis of Family
   Planning Programs.  Liege:  Ordina.

Knodel, J., and N. Debavalya (1978)  Thailand's reproductive revolution.  International Family Planning Perspectives and Digest 4:34-49.

Knodel, J., and V. Prachuabmoh (1973)  Desired family size in Thailand:  Are the responses meaningful? Demography 10:619-637.

Lapham, R. J., and W. P. Mauldin (1972)  National family planning programs:  Review and evaluation.  Studies in Family Planning 3(3).

Larson, A. (1981)  Patterns of Contraceptive Use Around the World.  Washington, D.C.:  Population Reference Bureau.

Leridon, H. (1981)  Fertility and contraception in 12 developed countries.  Family Planning Perspectives 13:93-102.

Lesthaeghe, R. (1980)  On the social control of human reproduction.  Population and Development Review 4:527-538.

Lewis, G. L., and J. A. Novak (1982)  An approach to the measurement of availability of family planning services.  Pp. 241-278 in A. I. Hermalin and B. Entwisle, eds., The Role of Surveys in the Analysis of Family Planning Programs.  Liege:  Ordina.

Lightbourne, R. E. (1980)  Urban-Rural Differentials in Contraceptive Use.  WFS Comparative Studies, No. 10. London:  World Fertility Survey.

Mauldin, W. P., and B. Berelson (1978)  Conditions of fertility decline in developing countries.  Studies in Family Planning 9:89-147.

Mauldin, W. P., and R. J. Lapham (1982)  Measuring the input of family planning programs.  In A. I. Hermalin and B. Entwisle, eds., The Role of Surveys in the Analysis of Family Planning Programs.  Liege:  Ordina.

Millman, S. (1982)  Breastfeeding in Taiwan:  A Study of Change.  Unpublished Ph.D. dissertation.  University of Michigan, Ann Arbor, Michigan.

Morris, L., J. E. Anderson, R. S. Monteith, R. Kriskovich, J. Shoemaker, and O. Frutos (1978)  Contraceptive prevalence in Paraguay.  Studies in Family Planning 9:272-279.

Muangman, D., R. G. Burnight, and P. J. Donaldson (1973) Contraception and coital frequency.  Asian Journal of Medicine 9:127-128.

Namboodiri, N. K. (1972)  Some observations on the economic framework for fertility analysis.  Population Studies 26:108-206.

Nortman, D., and Hofstatter, E. (1980) *Population and Family Planning Programs*, 10th ed. New York: Population Council.

Page, H. J., and R. Lesthaeghe, eds. (1981) *Child-Spacing in Tropical Africa: Traditions and Change*. London: Academic Press.

Palmore, J. A., and M. B. Concepcion (1981) Desired family size and contraceptive use. Pp. 513–542 in *World Fertility Survey Conference 1980*, Vol. 2. London: World Fertility Survey.

*People* (1978) Abortion. *People* 5:4–21.

Phillips, J. F., W. S. Stinson, S. Bhatia, M. Rahman, and J. Chakraborty (1982) The demographic impact of the family planning: Health services project in Matlab, Bangladesh. *Studies in Family Planning* 13:131–140.

Population Council (1970) *A Manual for Surveys of Fertility and Family Planning: Knowledge, Attitudes, and Practice*. New York: Population Council.

Population Reports (1978) Voluntary sterilization: World's leading contraceptive method. *Population Reports*, Series M, Number 2.

Population Reports (1981a) Periodic abstinence: How well do new approaches work? *Population Reports*, Series I, Number 3.

Population Reports (1981b) Breastfeeding, fertility, and family planning. *Population Reports*, Series J, Number 24.

Potter, R. G. (1981) The Analysis of Cross-Method Variance in Assessing Family Planning Programme Effects on Fertility. Paper prepared for the International Union for the Scientific Study of Population, International Population Conference, Manila.

Pullum, T. W. (1980) *Illustrative Analysis: Fertility Preferences in Sri Lanka*. WFS Scientific Reports, No. 9. London: World Fertility Survey.

Rodriguez, G. (1977) *Assessing the Availability of Fertility Regulation Methods: Report on a Methodological Study*. WFS Scientific Reports, No. 1. London: World Fertility Survey.

Rodriguez, G. (1978) Family planning availability and contraceptive practice. *International Family Planning Perspectives and Digest* 4:100–115.

Sadik, N. (1981) Use of family planning services. Pp. 565–595 in *World Fertility Survey Conference 1980*, Vol. 2. London: World Fertility Survey.

Siddiqui, M. K. (1979)  The Initiation of Contraception
in Taiwan. Unpublished Ph.D. dissertation.
University of Michigan, Ann Arbor, Michigan.

Singh, S. (1980)  Comparability of Questionnaires. WFS
Comparative Studies, No. 2. London:  World Fertility
Survey.

Stinson, W. S., J. F. Phillips, M. Rahman, and J.
Chakraborty (1982)  The demographic impact of the
contraceptive distribution project in Matlab,
Bangladesh. Studies in Family Planning 13:141-148.

Szykman, M. (1982)  The concept of demand for family
planning and its measurement. Pp. 313-337 in A. I.
Hermalin and B. Entwisle, eds., The Role of Surveys
in the Analysis of Family Planning Programs. Liege:
Ordina.

Terhune, K. W., and S. Kaufman (1973)  The family size
utility function. Demography 10:559-618.

Tietze, C. (1981)  Induced Abortion, A World Review, 4th
ed. New York:  Population Council.

United Nations (1978)  Methods of Measuring the Impact of
Family Planning Programmes on Fertility:  Problems
and Issues. New York:  United Nations.

United Nations (1979a)  Factors Affecting the Use and
Non-Use of Contraception. Population Studies No.
69,ST/ESA/SER.A/69. New York:  United Nations.

United Nations (1979b)  The Methodology of Measuring the
Impact of Family Planning Programmes on Fertility,
Manual IX. New York:  United Nations.

United Nations (1980)  World Population Trends and
Policies 1979 Monitoring Report, Volume II,
ST/ESA/SER.A/70/Add.1. New York:  United Nations.

United Nations (1981a)  Report on Monitoring of
Population Policies. ESA/P/WP.69. New York:  United
Nations.

United Nations (1981b)  Variations in the Incidence of
Knowledge and Use of Contraception:  A Comparative
Analysis of World Fertility Survey Results for Twenty
Developing Countries. New York:  United Nations.

United Nations (1982)  Evaluation of the Impact of Family
Planning Programs on Fertility:  Sources of
Variance. New York:  United Nations.

Vaessen, M. (1980)  Knowledge of Contraceptive Methods.
WFS Comparative Studies, No. 8. London:  World
Fertility Survey.

Watson, W. B., and R. J. Lapham (1975)  Family planning
programs:  World review 1974. Studies in Family
Planning 6:205-322.

Westoff, C. F. (1974)   Coital frequency and contraception. Family Planning Perspectives 6:136-141.

Westoff, C. F. (1978)   The unmet need for birth control in five Asian countries. International Family Planning Perspectives and Digest 4:9-18.

Westoff, C. F., and N. B. Ryder (1977)   The predictive validity of reproductive intentions. Demography 1:431-453.

World Fertility Survey (1978)   Sri Lanka 1975, First Report. Department of Census and Statistics, Ministry of Plan Implementation. London:  World Fertility Survey.

Chapter 2

# Birth Control Methods and Their Effects on Fertility

JOHN A. ROSS

Among fertility determinants, none has a more direct effect on individual fertility than the use of birth control. Moreover, none has undergone a greater transformation over the past two decades: the de facto practice of birth control has increased dramatically in many developing countries, and this has itself resulted in changed traditional attitudes and new legitimated behavior.

Birth control covers contraception, including sterilization, and abortion. The prevalence of these methods is examined below, followed by a discussion of the relationship between their prevalence and patterns of acceptance and continuation. Next is an analysis of the use-effectiveness of the various methods, and a general discussion of the links between birth control and fertility. Finally, some propositions are presented relating to birth control and fertility change and to technological concerns.

## PREVALENCE OF BIRTH CONTROL METHODS

### Contraception

Levels

Recent summaries (Nortman, 1980; forthcoming) give data on the prevalence of contraceptive use for 31 countries (Table 1): in 23 of these countries, the level of use falls above 20 percent; among these, the level in 19 falls above 30 percent.

The eight largest developing countries, which together make up two-thirds of the developing world, show a spread

in contraceptive use, with Bangladesh, Pakistan, and
probably Nigeria at the low end, at 12 percent or below;
Brazil perhaps next in line; India between 20 and 30
percent; and Mexico, Indonesia,[1] and probably China
above 30 percent.

The smaller developing countries are very much
scattered in their prevalence levels.  A clear pattern
can be discerned only by region:  sub-Saharan Africa is
far below Asia and Latin America; the Middle East and
North Africa are also below, though Tunisia, Egypt, and
Turkey are modest exceptions.  Within Asia, Burma
(besides the large countries of Bangladesh and Pakistan)
is very low; within Latin America, Bolivia and Ecuador
are similarly low.  There are no special patterns by size
of country, religion, or political type, although the
Mauldin and Berelson (1978) analysis does show a regular
increase in prevalence with more advanced social setting,
as well as with greater program strength.


Age and Family Size

This section briefly discusses data on age produced
recently for a relatively large set of countries by a
common calculation procedure based chiefly on World
Fertility Survey (WFS) data (Bongaarts and Kirmeyer,
1980; see their Appendix for a description of data
imputation procedures and sources other than WFS).  This
study yields a model schedule of the proportions using
contraception, with each figure representing an average
of the values for that age in 26 countries (Table 2).
The shape of this schedule was found to parallel the
average shape in both high- and low-use countries; that
is, as Nortman (1980:19) also observes on WFS data for 8
countries, the pattern by age seems insensitive to the
overall level of prevalence.

Family size, on the other hand, is different:  lower-
parity women stand at relatively higher levels of use in
countries with high overall prevalence (Nortman, 1980;
Carrasco, 1980).  A similar pattern would have been
expected to emerge in the age data:  younger couples
should have higher levels of use in countries with higher
overall prevalence.  This pattern is in fact supported by
Carrasco's (1980:18, Fig. 5) analysis of WFS data.  It is
possible that the age data are simply complicated by
differences in age at marriage and birth intervals.

TABLE 1   Contraceptive Prevalence in Developing Countries:
Percentage of MWRA Practicing Contraception, by Source of
Supply, for Latest Year with Available Data

| Prevalence Range, Country, and Year | Both Sectors | Public Sector | Private Sector |
|---|---|---|---|
| **Below 10 Percent** | | | |
| Ghana, 1978 | 4 | 4 | 0 |
| Pakistan, 1980 | 6 | u | u |
| Kenya, 1975 | 7 | u | u |
| 1979 | u | 7 | u |
| **10 to 19 Percent** | | | |
| Bangladesh, 1977 | 9 | u | u |
| 1980 | 12 | u | u |
| Zimbabwe, 1978 | 14 | u | u |
| Paraguay, 1977 | 16 | 8 | 8 |
| Guatemala, 1978 | 18 | u | u |
| Egypt, 1979 | 17 | u | u |
| 1981 | 19 | 10 | 9 |
| **20 to 29 Percent** | | | |
| Tunisia, 1977 | 20 | 17 | 3 |
| El Salvador, 1976 | 22 | 7 | 15 |
| 1978 | 20 | u | u |
| India, 1975 | u | 16 | u |
| 1979 | u | 23 | u |
| 1981 | u | 23 | u |
| Jordan, 1976 | 24 | u | u |
| **30 to 49 Percent** | | | |
| Peru, 1977 | 31 | u | u |
| Guyana, 1975 | 32 | u | u |
| Indonesia, 1976 | 26 | u | u |
| 1979 | 29 | 24 | 5 |
| 1981 | u | 36 | u |
| Malaysia, 1974 | 33 | u | u |
| 1979 | 36 | 17 | 19 |
| 1981 | 42 | 26 | 16 |
| Dominican Republic, 1976 | 24 | 13 | 11 |
| 1977 | 31 | 10 | 21 |
| 1978 | 38 | 13 | 25[a] |
| Fiji, 1978 | 38 | 34 | 4 |
| Turkey, 1978 | 38 | u | u |

TABLE 1 (continued)

| Prevalence Range, Country, and Year | Both Sectors | Public Sector | Private Sector |
|---|---|---|---|
| Thailand, 1975 | 27 | 19 | 8 |
| 1979 | 39 | 34 | 5 |
| 1981 | u | 52 | u |
| Mexico, 1973 | 13 | 1 | 12 |
| 1978 | 40 | 19 | 21 |
| 1979 | 38 | 20 | 18 |
| Sri Lanka, 1975 | 30 | u | u |
| 1977 | 41 | u | u |
| Colombia, 1974 | 31 | u | u |
| 1978 | 46 | u | u |
| Philippines, 1974 | 15 | u | u |
| 1979 | 37 | 16 | 21 |
| 1981 | 48 | 27 | 21 |
| 50 Percent or More | | | |
| Mauritius, 1975 | 56 | 52 | 4 |
| 1979 | 53 | 50 | 3 |
| 1981 | 51 | 39 | 11 |
| Panama, 1976 | 54 | u | u |
| Korea, 1975 | 34 | 27 | 7 |
| 1978 | 49 | 25 | 24 |
| 1980 | 55 | 30 | 25 |
| Costa Rica, 1976 | 34 | u | u |
| 1978 | 64 | 26 | 38 |
| 1981 | 65 | 25 | 41 |
| Taiwan, 1974 | 55 | 21 | 34 |
| 1979 | 66 | 35 | 31 |
| 1981 | 70 | 47 | 23 |
| Singapore, 1974 | 60 | u | u |
| 1978 | 71 | 53 | 18 |
| Hong Kong, 1975 | 57 | 29 | 28 |
| 1979 | 79 | 46 | 33 |

Note:   MWRA is an acronym for married women of reproductive age, generally 15–44; u indicates unavailable.

[a]Private-sector figure extrapolated from 21 percent estimate for 1977.

Source:   Nortman (1980, forthcoming).

TABLE 2   Model Schedules of Age-
Specific Contraceptive Use Rates

| Age | Proportion Using Contraception | Index |
|-----|-------------------------------|-------|
| 15-19 | .194 | 60 |
| 20-24 | .295 | 92 |
| 25-29 | .375 | 116 |
| 30-34 | .423 | 131 |
| 35-39 | .418 | 130 |
| 40-44 | .335 | 104 |
| 45-49 | .211 | 66 |
| Mean | .322 | 100 |

There is an almost universal tendency for both the
average age and family size of program acceptors to
decline over time (Ross, 1979). This occurs regardless
of contraceptive method examined (including sterilization), program strength, program duration, chronological
period examined, or geographic region. This trend cannot
be explained by saturation of the upper age and parity
groups due either to their higher acceptance and continuation rates, or to graduation of younger users into
those groups (Ross and Potter, 1980). A likely hypothesis
is that, over time, younger couples with fewer children
have developed much greater interest in contraception and
hence have accepted at higher rates, raising their
proportion of the total.


Method and Sector

It is clear that few developed or developing countries
achieve a high prevalence level without heavy reliance on
the pill (Table 3). Japan is an interesting exception;
the pill is also conspicuously absent in India and Sri
Lanka, and minor in the Philippines, Taiwan, and Peru.
After the pill, sterilization has the highest prevalence
in a surprising number of countries, often outranking the
IUD.

Nothing very definitive is known about differences in prevalence between the private and public sectors, although in Table 1, the private sector leads in three countries and the public sector in twelve. However, in fourteen countries the relative levels are unknown and in two are equal. The factors controlling the private-public division are thought to be quite diverse, including in particular variations among countries in methods offered by the two sectors. Moreover, the private sector might more accurately be termed the "nonprogram" sector, since it covers such dissimilar components as small shops, pharmacies, midwives, and doctors. This of course adds to the difficulties of gathering reliable data and analyzing use patterns.

General Trends

In a number of countries, a substantial rise in contraceptive prevalence can be traced over time. Although survey documentation is available only at irregular intervals, the proportion of couples using modern contraceptive methods has risen sharply from minimal levels in the early 1960s. In some countries, repeat surveys show a continuation of this trend over the past few years. In addition, China is thought to have rapidly increased its prevalence of use (though comprehensive figures are not available), a trend that the present drive toward the one-child family must be reinforcing. Thus, from a historical standpoint, a 15- to 20-year period has seen a fundamental and far-reaching transformation in much of Asia and Latin America.

On the other hand, it must be remembered that a number of individual countries, many of them small, located in Africa, and lacking in data, are as yet at low prevalence levels and show little upward movement; in addition, among the eight largest developing countries, Pakistan, Bangladesh, and Nigeria remain at low levels. Overall, however, 70 percent of the developing world is above 10 percent prevalence, with a large proportion well above that. Although absolute levels are significant, perhaps more so is the rapidity of change in such major populations as China, Indonesia, and others of important size such as Mexico, Colombia, Korea, and Thailand. Equally significant is the fact that essentially all this change has occurred within a two-decade period, and much of it within one decade.

TABLE 3   Percentage of MWRA Using Specified Contraceptive
Method, for Countries with Available Data

| Country and Year | All Methods | IUDs | Orals | Sterilization | Other |
|---|---|---|---|---|---|
| **Africa** | | | | | |
| Egypt, 1975 | 21 | 9 | 11 | 0 | 1 |
| Mauritius, 1978 | 53 | 2 | 34 | 0 | 17 |
| 1981 | 51 | 3 | 30 | 0 | 18 |
| Tunisia, 1971 | 12 | 5 | 3 | 1 | 3 |
| 1977 | 17[a] | 6 | 5 | 6 | 1 |
| Zimbabwe, 1979 | 14 | 0 | 11 | 0 | 3 |
| **Asia** | | | | | |
| Fiji, 1974 | 40 | 4 | 8 | 16 | 12 |
| 1978 | 38 | 5 | 10 | 17 | 6 |
| Hong Kong, 1976 | 72 | 3 | 25 | 19 | 25 |
| 1981 | 80 | 2 | 32 | 19 | 27 |
| India, 1976[a] | 17 | 1 | -- | 13 | 3 |
| 1979 | 23 | 1 | 1 | 20 | 1 |
| 1981[a] | 23 | 1 | -- | 20 | 2 |
| Indonesia, 1979 | 24 | 7 | 15 | 1 | 1 |
| 1981[a] | 36 | 10 | 23 | 1 | 2 |
| Jordan, 1976 | 24 | 2 | 11 | 2 | 9 |
| Korea, Rep. of, 1978 | 49 | 10 | 7 | 17 | 15 |
| 1980 | 55 | 10 | 8 | 20 | 17 |
| Malaysia, 1979 | 36 | 1 | 24 | 6 | 5 |
| 1981 | 42 | 1 | 17 | 5 | 19 |
| Philippines, 1979 | 37 | 2 | 6 | 4 | 25 |
| 1981 | 48 | 4 | 16 | 3 | 24 |
| Singapore, 1970 | 45 | 2 | 38 | 0 | 5 |
| 1978 | 71 | 3 | 17 | 22 | 29 |
| Sri Lanka, 1975 | 33 | 5 | 2 | 10 | 16 |
| 1977 | 41 | 5 | 3 | 18 | 15 |
| Taiwan, 1979 | 66 | 27 | 7 | 16 | 16 |
| 1981 | 70 | 25 | 6 | 20 | 19 |
| Thailand, 1979 | 39 | 5 | 23 | 11 | 0 |
| 1981[a] | 52 | 5 | 31 | 16 | -- |
| Turkey, 1978 | 38 | 3 | 6 | 0 | 29 |
| **Latin America** | | | | | |
| Colombia, 1976 | 42.6 | 8.5 | 13.3 | 4.2 | 16.6 |
| 1978 | 46 | 8 | 17 | 8 | 13 |
| Costa Rica, 1978 | 64 | 5 | 25 | 15 | 19 |
| 1981 | 65 | 6 | 23 | 19 | 19 |
| Dominican Rep., 1975 | 31 | 3 | 8 | 12 | 8 |
| 1977 | 31 | 3 | 8 | 12 | 8 |
| El Salvador, 1976 | 22 | 2 | 7 | 10 | 3 |
| 1978 | 34 | 3 | 9 | 18 | 4 |
| 1980 | 20 | 2 | 4 | 14 | 0 |
| Guatemala, 1978 | 18 | 1 | 6 | 6 | 5 |
| Jamaica, 1975 | 38 | 2 | 18 | 8 | 10 |

TABLE 3 (continued)

| Country and Year | All Methods | IUDs | Orals | Sterilization | Other |
|---|---|---|---|---|---|
| Mexico, 1978 | 40 | 6 | 17 | 7 | 10 |
| 1979 | 38 | 6 | 15 | 9 | 8 |
| Panama, 1976 | 53.9 | 3.7 | 17.0 | 21.6 | 11.6 |
| Paraguay, 1977 | 16 | 2 | 7 | 2 | 5 |
| Peru, 1977 | 30.7 | 1.3 | 4.1 | 2.9 | 22.4 |
| Developed Countries | | | | | |
| Belgium, 1975–76 | 87 | 3 | 32 | 6 | 46 |
| France, 1972 | 64 | 1 | 11 | 0 | 52[b] |
| 1978 | 79 | 9 | 31 | 5 | 34[b] |
| Hungary, 1977 | 73[c] | 9 | 36 | 0 | 28[b] |
| Japan, 1975 | 61 | 5 | 2 | 3 | 51[d] |
| Netherlands, 1975 | 75 | 4 | 50 | 5 | 16 |
| Poland, 1972 | 57 | 1 | 2 | 0 | 54[b] |
| U.S.A., 1973 | 70 | 7 | 25 | 16 | 22 |
| 1976 | 68 | 6 | 22 | 19 | 21 |

Note:  Dash indicates unknown.

[a]Public sector only.
[b]Predominantly withdrawal.
[c]The base is married women aged 15–39.
[d]Predominantly condom users.

Source:  Nortman (forthcoming).


## Sterilization

Sterilization has undergone a rapid increase to substantial levels in a number of countries (Ross and Huber,
1982).  One study (Henry et al., 1980) of worldwide
prevalence estimates about 62 million currently sterilized women; of these, 50 million are in the developing
regions, with 46 million in Asia (including China).
Another review (Lubell and Frischer, 1980) estimates 90
million couples sterilized for contraceptive purposes as
of 1978, with China contributing 36 million, India 22
million, and the United States 12 million.  Although such
figures necessarily contain an element of guesswork, they
may be taken as the best efforts of knowledgeable
observers to combine judgment with the available data.

A surprising number of countries approach or exceed
one-fifth of couples of reproductive age sterilized.
Various compilations of country estimates have been made
(Nortman and Hofstatter, 1980; forthcoming; Klinger,
1979; Rochat et al., 1979; Ross and Huber, 1982).  Table
3 shows the share of all contraception that belongs to
sterilization, while Table 4 gives age detail; both tables
give estimates of the overall proportion sterilized.  The
two tables reflect different sources and dates.  Using
the later (higher) figure where the tables disagree,
countries in the 15-22 percent range include Costa Rica,
El Salvador, Panama (and Sao Paulo, Brazil, not shown) in
Latin America, and India, Korea, Sri Lanka, Taiwan,
Thailand, Fiji, Singapore, and Hong Kong in Asia.  The
figure for China given above of 36 million represents
roughly 22 percent of married women of reproductive age
(MWRA) in that country.

Table 4 also documents the greater frequency of female
than male sterilization:  an average of 86 percent of all
cases are female in the nine Asian and Latin American
countries showing information.  Another review (Sardon,
1979) looks specifically at this sex division (as of
1976) and finds the same high female proportions in most
countries except in India (25 percent).  (Bangladesh at
29 percent and Nepal at 33 percent are also low, but few
couples are sterilized in those countries.)  Factors
contributing to this pattern include improvements in the
simplicity, effectiveness, and cost of female sterilization techniques.  Of course, vasectomy is the lowest-cost
and simplest technique of all; however, public access to
it is often limited because of national program decisions,
which may in turn reflect real or perceived cultural
concerns.

Again, age and family-size patterns are only incidental
to the present discussion.  However, some data in Table 4
are relevant.  In most countries reviewed, the proportion
sterilized by age peaks in the range 35-44 and then falls
at 45-49.  However, for the number of living children
(not shown), the proportion rises regularly with few
exceptions, reaching especially high levels in the 5+
group, although whether this figure would decline within
this open-ended category is not clear.


Abortion


Though abortion is quite prevalent, it is probably not
fruitful to estimate its overall ranking relative to such

TABLE 4   Percentage of Currently Married Women (or Their Husbands) Contraceptively Sterilized, by Age of the Woman

| Country and Year | Age of Woman Under 24 | 25-34 | 35-44 | 45-49 | All Ages | Wife Sterilized | Husband Sterilized |
|---|---|---|---|---|---|---|---|
| **Asia and Oceania** | | | | | | | |
| Bangladesh, 1975 | 0.4 | 0.7 | 1.9 | 0.3 | 0.7 | -- | -- |
| Fiji, 1974[a] | 0.6 | 9.4[b] | 23.6[c] | 21.8[d] | 14.9 | 14.9 | 0.0 |
| Indonesia, 1976 | 0.0 | 0.2 | 0.5 | 0.3 | 0.2 | -- | -- |
| Rep. of Korea, 1974[e] | 0.2 | 3.8 | 7.3 | 4.6 | 4.7[e] | 1.6 | 3.1 |
| Malaysia, 1974 | 0.3 | 2.9 | 6.2 | 3.1 | 3.5 | 3.1 | 0.4 |
| Nepal, 1976 | 0.2 | 2.1 | 2.4 | 1.2 | 1.5 | 1.5 | 0.1 |
| Pakistan, 1975[a] | 0.0 | 0.5 | 1.9 | 2.6 | 0.9 | -- | -- |
| Sri Lanka, 1975 | 1.6 | 10.4 | 12.3 | 5.6 | 8.9 | 8.4 | 0.5 |
| Thailand, 1975 | 1.7 | 8.7 | 11.4 | 5.3 | 7.6 | 5.6 | 2.0 |
| **Latin America** | | | | | | | |
| Colombia, 1976 | 0.6 | 4.0 | 6.2 | 2.2 | 3.6 | 3.4 | 0.2 |
| Dominican Rep., 1975 | 2.2 | 14.0 | 15.3 | 7.6 | 9.9 | 9.8 | 0.1 |
| Costa Rica, 1976 | -- | 4.3[f] | 16.9[c] | 15.6[d] | 11.7 | 10.9 | 0.8 |
| Panama, 1976 | -- | 6.9[f] | 12.6[c] | 29.2[d] | 18.3 | -- | -- |
| Mexico, 1976 | 0.7 | 2.4 | 4.9 | 2.8 | 2.6 | -- | -- |
| **Europe** | | | | | | | |
| Belgium, 1976 | 0.5 | 2.2 | 4.6 | -- | 2.7 | 2.3 | 0.4 |
| France, 1978 | 0.9 | 2.8 | 7.5 | -- | 4.4 | 4.3 | 0.1 |
| Great Britain, 1976 | 3.0 | 14.0 | 22.0 | 7.0 | 14.0 | 7.0 | 7.0 |
| Hungary, 1977 | 0.4 | 1.1 | 1.7[g] | -- | 1.0 | 1.0 | 0.0 |
| Netherlands, 1975 | 0.5 | 4.4 | 8.6 | 5.2 | 4.2 | 2.0 | 2.2 |
| Norway, 1977[a] | 0.2 | 4.0 | 11.9 | -- | 6.3 | 4.0 | 2.3 |
| **North America** | | | | | | | |
| United States, 1976 | 3.7 | 16.4 | 23.5 | -- | 16.1[h] | -- | -- |

Note:  Dash indicates unavailable.

[a]Includes those sterilized for medical reasons.
[b]For women aged 25-29.
[c]For women aged 30-39.
[d]For women aged 40-49.
[e]The 1980 survey indicates that the prevalence of sterilization has increased to 20 percent since 1974.  See Table 3.
[f]For women aged 20-29.
[g]For women aged 35-39.
[h]Inconsistent with Table 3, but retained here to accompany the age-specific information.

Source:  Klinger (1979).

methods as the pill or withdrawal.  Such rankings change
sharply from country to country; moreover, where abortion
is illegal, it may still be important without close
estimates being possible, and where it is legal, it is
usually quite important but may nevertheless be
underreported.

Abortion is now legal in much of the developed world
and, because legalized in China and India, in much of the
developing world as well, although it is prohibited in
many individual countries (David, in these volumes;
Tietze, 1979:7-17).  In general, however, it can seldom
be ignored, and in numerous countries it is important for
fertility reduction.  Two kinds of data are available on
the prevalence of abortion.  First, abortion levels and
trends, limited to relatively reliable country-specific
data, are compiled in Tietze (1981; forthcoming); data
for countries of particular interest are reprinted here
in Table 5.  Second, Huber (1974:57), using relaxed
reporting criteria, estimated comprehensive worldwide
abortion figures for 1971.  This study, prepared for the
International Planned Parenthood Foundation (IPPF), is
based on questionnaire replies from country informants,
as well as on available ancillary information.  The
resulting world total of 55 million abortions is a
relatively high estimate; indeed, it equals something
like half of all births.  Klinger's (1969) estimate of 30
million is a more conservative world figure.  It must be
reiterated that data on abortions are notoriously difficult to obtain, and that the officially reported number
of legal abortions worldwide (chiefly in developed
countries) is only about four million.  Comprehensive
estimates are based on judgmental extrapolation from
these and other, softer figures.  Although the resulting
picture is necessarily speculative, the official figures
are obviously far from the mark; for example, they omit
the USSR and China.

Based on the original IPPF study and the Tietze compilation, the general picture is as follows.  The greatest
prevalence of abortion appears to be in China, in Japan,
and in both Eastern and Western Europe.  Among other
large countries, the USSR probably has high abortion
prevalence and the United States has experienced a large
apparent increase in abortions since the Supreme Court
decision of 1973, although it is unclear to what extent
this represents a substitution for previously illegal
abortions.  India has increased from a tiny reported
base; the abortion ratio is still very low.  For the

other large countries--Indonesia, Bangladesh, Pakistan, Brazil, Nigeria, and Mexico--either there has been little increase, or little is known.  (For a detailed discussion of country-specific abortion data, see David, in these volumes.)

## ACCEPTANCE AND CONTINUATION

In general, the prevalence of use (P) of the various birth control methods is simply the product of the acceptance rate (A) and the mean continuation (C):  P = AC.  For example, if 10 percent of couples accept each year, and mean continuation is two years, then 20 percent will be using at any one time, once the program has settled down into a "steady state."  Thus prevalence rises in direct proportion either to the acceptance rate or to mean continuation.

However, continuation is usually not measured as a mean, but as the life table proportion still using at one or two years.  This is a distribution measure and is related to prevalence quite differently.  Under the usual formula $R = ae^{-rt}$, a is the proportion not terminating immediately, e is the natural logarithm base 2.718, r is the annual termination risk, t is the number of years, and $R_1$ is, for example, the proportion continuing at one year.  The mean duration of continuation C is simply a/r.  Recalling that P = AC and rearranging the formula[2], Aa/(ln a - ln $R_1$).  Prevalence still rises in direct proportion to the acceptance rate A, but it rises exponentially with $R_1$.  When $R_1$ improves five points, from .50 to .55 (letting a = .95), mean continuation rises from 1.48 to 1.74 years, and prevalence improves by only 17 percent; however, when $R_1$ moves from .80 to .85, continuation rises from 5.53 years to 8.54 years, and prevalence jumps by 55 percent.  These prevalence gains with improvements in life table continuation are not usually appreciated, nor is the disproportion in the gains at stake in the upper range.

The actual country improvements in prevalence noted above are due variously to increases in both acceptance and continuation and in both private and public sectors.  Direct documentation for increased acceptance is provided by Nortman and Hofstatter (1980).  As they have shown, annual acceptance in the stronger programs has risen to well above 10 percent of couples, and has been sustained year after year at that level.  Continuation has also

TABLE 5    Number of Legal Abortions, Abortion Rates, and Abortion Ratios:    Selected Areas, Years, and Characteristics

| Area, Year, and Characteristics | Number of Abortions[a] | Abortion Rate per 1,000 | | Abortion Ratio per 100 | |
|---|---|---|---|---|---|
| | | Total Population | Women 15-44 | Live Births[b] | Known Pregnancies[c] |
| China[d,e] | | | | | |
| 1971 | 3,910,100 | 4.7 | 21.6 | 12.8 | 11.3 |
| 1972 | 4,813,500 | 5.6 | 25.8 | 19.3 | 16.2 |
| 1973 | 5,110,400 | 5.8 | 26.6 | 20.9 | 17.3 |
| 1974 | 4,984,600 | 5.6 | 25.1 | 21.2 | 17.5 |
| 1975 | 5,084,300 | 5.6 | 24.9 | 24.2 | 19.5 |
| 1976 | 6,570,300 | 7.1 | 31.2 | 36.1 | 26.5 |
| 1977 | 5,229,000 | 5.6 | 24.2 | 32.3 | 24.4 |
| 1978 | 5,528,000 | 5.5 | 24.8 | 31.8 | 24.1 |
| Cuba | | | | | |
| 1968 | 28,500 | 3.4 | 16.7 | 11.7 | 10.5 |
| 1969 | 46,100 | 5.5 | 26.6 | 19.2 | 16.1 |
| 1970 | 70,500 | 8.2 | 40.2 | 28.3 | 22.1 |
| 1971 | 84,800 | 9.8 | 47.4 | 33.6 | 25.2 |
| 1972 | 100,000 | 11.3 | 54.9 | 42.2 | 29.7 |
| 1973 | 112,100 | 12.4 | 60.3 | 52.3 | 34.3 |
| 1974 | 131,500 | 14.3 | 69.5 | 66.4 | 39.9 |
| 1975 | 126,100 | 13.5 | 65.3 | 66.2 | 39.8 |
| 1976 | 121,400 | 12.8 | 61.0 | 68.1 | 40.5 |
| 1977 | 114,800 | 12.0 | 55.9 | 72.4 | 42.0 |
| 1978 | 110,400 | 11.3 | 52.1 | 75.7 | 43.1 |
| 1979 | 106,500 | 10.9 | 48.8 | 76.0 | 43.2 |
| 1980 | 104,000 | 10.7 | 47.1 | 76.1 | 43.2 |
| Hong Kong | | | | | |
| 1973 | 200 | 0.05 | 0.2 | 0.2 | 0.2 |
| 1974 | 600 | 0.14 | 0.6 | 0.7 | 0.7 |
| 1975 | 1,000 | 0.24 | 1.1 | 1.3 | 1.3 |
| 1976 | 2,200 | 0.49 | 2.3 | 2.7 | 2.6 |
| 1977 | 3,800 | 0.84 | 3.9 | 4.8 | 4.6 |
| 1978 | 5,500 | 1.2 | 5.4 | 6.7 | 6.3 |
| 1979 | 7,000 | 1.5 | 6.7 | 8.4 | 7.7 |
| 1980 | 9,400 | 1.9 | 8.6 | 10.4 | 9.8 |
| 1981 | 10,600 | 2.1 | 9.5 | 12.0[f] | 10.7 |

TABLE 5 (continued)

| Area, Year, and Characteristics | Number of Abortions[a] | Abortion Rate per 1,000 | | Abortion Ratio per 100 | |
|---|---|---|---|---|---|
| | | Total Population | Women 15-44 | Live Births[b] | Known Pregnancies[c] |
| India[g,h,i] | | | | | |
| 1973 | 24,300 | 0.04 | 0.2 | 0.1 | 0.1 |
| 1974 | 44,800 | 0.08 | 0.4 | 0.2 | 0.2 |
| 1975 | 97,800 | 0.16 | 0.8 | 0.4 | 0.4 |
| 1976 | 214,200 | 0.35 | 1.7 | 0.9 | 0.9 |
| 1977 | 278,900 | 0.44 | 2.1 | 1.3 | 1.3 |
| 1978 | 247,000 | 0.38 | 1.8 | 1.2 | 1.2 |
| 1979 | 317,700 | 0.48 | 2.2 | 1.5 | 1.5 |
| 1980 | 358,000 | 0.53 | 2.5 | 1.7 | 1.7 |
| Japan[g] | | | | | |
| 1950-54 | 827,400 | 9.7 | 40.7 | 41.4 | 29.3 |
| 1955-59 | 1,135,800 | 12.5 | 52.2 | 69.5 | 41.0 |
| 1960-64 | 983,600 | 10.4 | 41.9 | 59.8 | 37.4 |
| 1965-69 | 780,200 | 7.8 | 30.3 | 43.3 | 30.0 |
| 1970 | 732,000 | 7.1 | 28.0 | 37.5 | 27.3 |
| 1971 | 739,700 | 7.1 | 28.2 | 36.4 | 26.7 |
| 1972 | 732,600 | 6.8 | 27.6 | 35.3 | 26.1 |
| 1973 | 700,500 | 6.4 | 26.3 | 34.0 | 25.4 |
| 1974 | 679,800 | 6.2 | 25.5 | 34.6 | 25.7 |
| 1975 | 671,000 | 6.0 | 25.2 | 35.3 | 26.1 |
| 1976 | 664,100 | 5.9 | 24.9 | 37.2 | 27.1 |
| 1977 | 641,200 | 5.6 | 24.1 | 35.4 | 26.1 |
| 1978 | 618,000 | 5.4 | 23.3 | 36.8 | 26.9 |
| 1979 | 613,700 | 5.3 | 23.1 | 37.8 | 27.4 |
| 1980 | 598,100 | 5.1 | 22.5 | 37.7[f] | 27.4 |
| Japan (adjusted)[j] | | | | | |
| 1955 | 2,790,000 | 31.1 | 131.9 | 164.3 | 62.2 |
| 1960 | 3,150,000 | 33.5 | 138.1 | 197.2 | 66.3 |
| 1965 | 2,750,000 | 27.8 | 108.6 | 174.7 | 63.6 |
| 1970 | 2,780,000 | 26.6 | 104.9 | 142.5 | 58.8 |
| 1975 | 2,250,000 | 20.1 | 84.2 | 120.5 | 54.7 |

TABLE 5 (continued)

| Area, Year, and Charac- teristics | Number of Abortions[a] | Abortion Rate per 1,000 | | Abortion Ratio per 100 | |
|---|---|---|---|---|---|
| | | Total Population | Women 15-44 | Live Births[b] | Known Preg- nancies[c] |
| **Korea, Republic of** | | | | | |
| 1961 | 104,000 | 4.1 | 19.5 | 10.5 | 9.5 |
| 1962 | 127,000 | 4.9 | 23.3 | 13.1 | 11.6 |
| 1963 | 152,000 | 5.7 | 27.2 | 16.1 | 13.9 |
| 1964 | 191,000 | 7.0 | 33.3 | 20.8 | 17.3 |
| 1965 | 223,000 | 7.9 | 37.9 | 24.8 | 19.9 |
| 1966 | 252,000 | 8.8 | 41.9 | 29.3 | 22.7 |
| 1967 | 264,000 | 9.0 | 42.9 | 29.8 | 23.0 |
| 1968 | 293,000 | 9.8 | 46.4 | 33.9 | 25.3 |
| 1969 | 315,000 | 10.3 | 48.8 | 35.8 | 26.3 |
| 1970 | 331,000 | 10.6 | 50.1 | 37.0 | 27.0 |
| Seoul, 1969-71 | 93,000 | -- | 64.1 | 64.3 | 39.1 |
| Other Urban, 1969-71 | 124,300 | -- | 70.0 | 59.2 | 37.2 |
| Rural, 1969-71 | 127,100 | -- | 37.2 | 23.2 | 18.8 |
| Seoul, 1977-78 | 480,000 | -- | 235.0 | 330.0 | 76.7 |
| **Singapore[g,k]** | | | | | |
| 1970 | 1,900 | 0.9 | 4.1 | 4.2 | 4.1 |
| 1971 | 3,400 | 1.6 | 7.2 | 6.9 | 6.5 |
| 1972 | 3,800 | 1.8 | 7.7 | 7.5 | 7.0 |
| 1973 | 5,300 | 2.4 | 10.4 | 11.5 | 10.3 |
| 1974 | 7,200 | 3.2 | 13.6 | 17.2 | 14.6 |
| 1975 | 12,900 | 5.7 | 23.5 | 31.9 | 24.2 |
| 1976 | 15,500 | 6.8 | 27.5 | 37.7 | 27.4 |
| 1977 | 16,400 | 7.1 | 28.3 | 42.8 | 30.0 |
| 1978 | 17,200 | 7.4 | 28.9 | 42.8 | 30.0 |
| 1979 | 17,000 | 7.2 | 27.7 | 41.8 | 29.5 |
| 1980 | 18,200 | 7.5 | 28.4 | -- | -- |
| **Tunisia[l]** | | | | | |
| 1966 | 1,400 | 0.3 | 1.5 | 0.6 | 0.6 |
| 1967 | 1,300 | 0.3 | 1.4 | 0.6 | 0.6 |

TABLE 5 (continued)

| Area, Year, and Characteristics | Number of Abortions[a] | Abortion Rate per 1,000 | | Abortion Ratio per 100 | |
|---|---|---|---|---|---|
| | | Total Population | Women 15-44 | Live Births[b] | Known Pregnancies[c] |
| 1968 | 2,200 | 0.5 | 2.4 | 1.1 | 1.1 |
| 1969 | 2,900 | 0.6 | 2.9 | 1.5 | 1.5 |
| 1970 | 2,700 | 0.5 | 2.7 | 1.4 | 1.4 |
| 1971 | 3,200 | 0.6 | 3.0 | 1.7 | 1.7 |
| 1972 | 4,600 | 0.8 | 4.2 | 2.2 | 2.1 |
| 1973 | 6,500 | 1.2 | 6.0 | 3.4 | 3.3 |
| 1974 | 12,400 | 2.2 | 10.9 | 6.3 | 5.9 |
| 1975 | 16,000 | 2.8 | 13.7 | 7.8 | 7.2 |
| 1976 | 20,300 | 3.5 | 17.1 | 9.8 | 9.0 |
| 1977 | 21,200 | 3.6 | 17.2 | 10.3 | 9.4 |
| 1978 | 21,000 | 3.5 | 16.5 | 10.3[f] | 9.4 |
| 1979 | 19,200 | 3.1 | 14.6 | -- | -- |

Note:  Dash indicates unavailable.  Some figures have fewer decimal places because of differences in the original data sources.

[a]All numbers rounded.  Because of rounding, components may not add to totals.  Data for most recent periods may be subject to revision.
[b]Six months later.
[c]Live births plus legal abortions.
[d]Chen (1982).
[e]Completeness of reporting of abortions and of births not determined.
[f]Ratio computed per 100 births in same calendar year(s), not six months later.
[g]Reporting incomplete.
[h]Abortions performed under the National Family Planning Program.
[i]Fiscal years ending 31 March.
[j]Estimates adjusted for underreporting by Muramatsu (in Tietze, 1981:13; forthcoming).
[k]Including the private sector.
[l]"Social" abortions performed under the National Family Planning Program.

Source:  Tietze (1981; forthcoming), except for Korea, which is from Tietze (1979).  See these sources for full references to original data sources.

increased, although this is due chiefly to a better method mix rather than to improvements in the continuation of each method. Prevalence has risen more quickly for the efficient methods than for the traditional inefficient ones; this reflects in part the success of several national programs with sterilization, as well as some sterilization increases in the private sectors.

Continuation rates vary greatly by method and by country, as well as by local and personal characteristics. They rise regularly by age and number of living children. They are also higher for rural women, and for those terminating childbearing rather than spacing births. Different clinics show different continuation rates (Snowden, 1972). Finally, continuation of any particular method seems shorter where alternatives are easily available, as in urban settings and among the better educated.

A few other broad conclusions about continuation can be drawn. First, the ranking of methods by continuation is sterilization, IUD, and pill: within any one country and acceptor subgroup, the IUD is superior to the pill in continuation (although the pill has better acceptance), even when stated motivation (spacing or stopping) is the same (Sivin, 1974). An overview of IUD and pill continuation rates (Table 6) documents both the broad trends across countries and the IUD advantage. The latter rests on its fewer side effects and the fewer personal or other reasons given for discontinuation; this reflects in turn the IUD's asset of automatic continuation during ambivalent motivation.

It must be stressed that, apart from sterilization, no single method of contraception has more than an average continuation of 1-3 years. However, there are two factors to consider here. Around a low mean of continuation for a particular method, there is still a substantial proportion on the high side, and appreciable numbers of acceptors of each method do find it satisfactory and use it for a long time. Second, given the availability of several methods, couples will try more than one; thus couple continuation is superior to method continuation. In combination, these two features are highly significant: each method tends to find its own market, and the more methods offered, the higher the overall proportion protected.

On the other hand, method-specific continuation must not be neglected. A program's administrative costs rise greatly for methods requiring constant resupply or reservicing. For example, when mean continuation is one year

TABLE 6   Oral Contraceptive and IUD Discontinuation Rates
by Reason, for Selected Developing Countries:   Median
Percentages

| Reason | Oral Contraceptives | | IUDs | |
|---|---|---|---|---|
| | 12 months | 24 months | 12 months | 24 months |
| Pregnancy | 3.5(9) | 5.3(5) | 2.3(20) | 3.6(13) |
| Expulsion | -- | -- | 8.3(19) | 10.4(12) |
| Planned pregnancy | 5.2(8) | 6.6(5) | 1.1(8) | 2.6(6) |
| Medical and side effects | 30.6(8) | 35.9(4) | 18.3(19) | 19.3(8) |
| Personal or Other | 18.7(10) | 19.2(4) | 2.9(12) | 4.6(8) |
| All reasons | 54.7(10) | 71.3(5) | 33.8(20) | 43.5(13) |

Note:   Each figure is a median across studies with relevant data.
Number of studies is given in parentheses.

Source:   Abstracted by Mauldin (1978) from Kreager (1977).

rather than four, a program must recruit four times the
number of acceptors each year to maintain the same
prevalence level.  Thus as continuation rises above the
low range, there are vast administrative gains.

However, no mass program is known to have succeeded in
raising its method-specific continuation rates.  Although
continuation appears to improve when acceptors receive
early reassurance (Chan, 1971), this is not easily accomplished:  the costs of arranging mass home visits for
this purpose are prohibitive, and one experiment indicates that calling acceptors back to the clinic for an
early check up (at one or two weeks) and reassurance can
actually generate more removals (Bang, 1971).  Most large
programs can affect mean continuation only by shifting
acceptors to the IUD and sterilization, although a counter tendency occurs as acceptors come from progressively
younger age groups and smaller families.

A danger is that strong pressures for high acceptance
rates can damage continuation rates.  This involves a
trade-off as regards couple years of protection, which
rise with higher acceptance rates but fall with lower
continuation rates.  In the early Korean program, rapidly
rising targets hurt continuation rates for the acceptor

cohorts of 1966 and 1967; however, the additional accep-
tances were numerous enough to produce a net gain in use
time. The pill may be especially sensitive to the
"quality" of acceptance. In the 1973 Indonesian program,
intensive recruitment campaigns were used toward the end
of the fiscal year to meet targets. Follow-up surveys
showed little deterioration in the IUD continuation rate
for campaign acceptors, but substantial damage to the
pill rate (Sullivan et al., 1974), reflecting the pill's
easy start-easy stop character. Indonesia, incidentally,
shows overall continuation rates that are probably the
highest of any major program (Suyono, 1977; Nurhajati et
al., 1977); these appear to be related to the very powerful community support mechanisms in much of Java.

Overall acceptance and prevalence both appear to rise
when there are more method choices. It seems clear that
with the differences among principal methods, each tends
to find its own subgroup of satisfied users. If sterilization were the only method available, few younger couples
would use it; if only the pill were available, many women
who found it unsuitable would try the IUD if they could.
Each method adds a further layer of users, at least
within some overall limit set by other determinants such
as the dispersion of program service points or broader
social factors.

## USE-EFFECTIVENESS

The use-effectiveness of a birth control method is defined
as the proportionate reduction it achieves in the monthly
chance of conception. As an example, the normal monthly
risk of conceiving for a healthy cohabiting couple is
generally given as about 20 percent; if the IUD has a
use-effectiveness of .95, it will reduce this monthly
risk to 1 percent.

In practice, only two items are empirically measured,
and rarely on the same couples. First, the monthly chance
of conception is estimated from the delay to pregnancy
experienced by newly married couples in societies where
they are considered to start intercourse only after marriage; sometimes it is measured for couples just terminating
contraception deliberately in order to have a desired
pregnancy. Both groups are free of lactation effects,
but both may contain a few who at the start of the study
are unknowingly sterile. Second, the failure rate, the
actual proportion of method users who become pregnant

during use, is observed in a different group of women.
These rates may reflect extraneous factors like coital
frequency, which decreases with age.  Use-effectiveness
is then estimated from these two sets of data from
separate samples.

Most literature on use-effectiveness concerns the
United States and Britain.  Vaughan et al. (1977, 1980)
and Trussell and Menken (1980) discuss methodology and
give recent estimates (see also Table 1 in Bongaarts,
1978).  Hatcher (1982) references much of the better
literature and gives both theoretical and typical failure
rates, also based mainly on Western data, for an extensive
list of contraceptive methods.

Some developing country data are provided in Bongaarts
and Kirmeyer (1980).  They drew upon Philippine data for
direct use-effectiveness estimates, comparing the pregnancy rates reported by users of each method to the standard of pregnancy rates reported for comparable nonusers.
Although this method corrects for many confounding
variables, it is of course subject to the self-selection
process that affects the particular method used, including no method.  The values turn out as follows:
sterilization, 1.00; IUD, 0.95; pill, 0.90; and other
methods, 0.70.  Overall values of use-effectiveness for
22 countries were then calculated by weighting these
figures by the proportions using each method (Table 7).
Rates for most countries are in the eighties, the precise
level reflecting only the method mix in that country.  It
should be noted that the Philippine figure for the pill,
0.90, is below the 0.99 usually quoted; this reflects the
behavioral component in regularity and strictness of
use.  The same observation applies to the "other methods"
category, which includes methods that can theoretically
give nearly complete protection but in actual practice do
not.

The relation of use-effectiveness to fertility reduction is complex.  Of two methods that are otherwise
equivalent, the one with superior use-effectiveness will
of course prevent more births, and there are probably
disproportionate gains as use-effectiveness enters the
upper range.  Nevertheless, calculation of the difference
is not straightforward (Bongaarts and Kirmeyer, 1980).
As a guide to the development of new contraceptive technology, it can be argued (Berelson, 1976, 1978) that
present methods (including sterilization, the IUD, the
pill, and the injectable) already have such high use-
effectiveness that further gains will be small.  On the

TABLE 7   Estimates of Use-Effectiveness of Contraception
for 22 Developing Countries

| Country | Year | Use-Effectiveness | Country | Year | Use-Effectiveness |
|---------|------|-------------------|---------|------|-------------------|
| Bangladesh | 1975 | .82 | Malaysia | 1974 | .85 |
| Colombia | 1976 | .84 | Mexico | 1976 | .86 |
| Costa Rica | 1976 | .86 | Nepal | 1976 | .94 |
| Dominican Republic | 1975 | .89 | Pakistan | 1975 | .83 |
| Guatemala[a] | 1972 | .87 | Panama | 1976 | .90 |
| Hong Kong | 1978 | .86 | Peru | 1977 | .78 |
| Indonesia | 1976 | .87 | Philippines | 1976 | .78 |
| Jamaica | 1976 | .84 | Sri Lanka | 1975 | .84 |
| Jordan | 1976 | .84 | Syria | 1973 | .87 |
| Kenya | 1976 | .75 | Thailand | 1975 | .91 |
| Lebanon[a] | 1976 | .83 | Turkey | 1968 | .80 |

[a]Refers to subnational unit.

Source: Bongaarts and Kirmeyer (1980).

other hand, the final contribution of any new method will
depend heavily upon its use-effectiveness, which besides
contributing to its fertility effect also determines the
need for abortion backup.

## LINKS TO FERTILITY

Clearly, many forces and conditions affect fertility
levels and trends.  Moreover, proximate causes are in
turn always affected by other, secondary causes.  Thus
although contraception, abortion, lactation, and marriage
age are the primary fertility determinants (Bongaarts,
1978),[3] the forces controlling each of these must in
turn be examined.  As these secondary forces recede from
the proximate determinants, they approach the more remote
social and economic matrix, and analysts differ considerably as to which part of these claims they prefer to
examine.  Logically, it is possible to cut through the
resultant methodological difficulties by examining the
potential effect on fertility of removing a particular
set of factors.  Thus one might ask what would have
happened to fertility in the developing world without
modern birth control methods and without the implementing
programs that they made possible.  To restate the ques-

tion, what would the course of fertility have been with
the cumbersome contraceptive technology of 1960, and
without the distribution systems, both public and private, that modern contraception inspired (such as rural
distribution of the pill by nonmedical personnel)?
Although such hypothetical questions cannot be finally
answered, reasonable conclusions must be drawn as a basis
for ongoing administrative decisions and the allocation
of large resources. The principal conclusions about
linkages between fertility control methods and fertility
rates are traced below.

Since the early 1960s, a large body of literature has
been concerned with the fertility effects of contraception, sterilization, and abortion. Some of this literature is at the individual level, focusing on how birth
control interferes with the reproductive process and
modifies the normal probabilities of childbearing. Some
of the literature assesses the actual reduction of
fertility among acceptors in a family planning program.
Finally, some assesses program effect upon fertility of
the general population; however, because investigators'
aims and methods vary widely, no single typology is
altogether satisfactory. (The problem of disentangling
program from nonprogram effects is treated by Mauldin, in
these volumes.)

This section focuses primarily upon the general effects
of contraceptive prevalence on fertility reduction. General reviews of this literature, including summaries of
results, are found in Ross et al. (1972), Forrest and
Ross (1978), Ross and Forrest (1978), and United Nations
(1978, 1979, 1982). The U.N. references reflect collaborative work over a period of several years between
the U.N. Population Division and the IUSSP Committee for
the Analysis of Family Planning Programs (and its
predecessor Committee on Demographic Aspects of Family
Planning Programs); the last source contains major
country case studies, each of which applies several
methods of analysis. Table 8 presents the chief methods
that are possible and describes their principal characteristics. Also, Ross (1975) describes the approaches
used in estimating the future fertility effects of
programs in a number of actual national plans.

Much, although by no means all, of this literature
rests on (a) counts of acceptors and (b) their continuation rates, projected to give (c) the number using
contraception at various points in the future (according
to calendar year, by time elapsed since acceptance, or

TABLE 8 Methods for Studying the Effect of Family Planning Programs on Birth Rates

| Method Characteristics | Decomposition of Crude Birth Rate Change | Correspondence Between Program Activity and Fertility Change | Matching Studies | Experimental and Control Areas | Multiple Regression Across Areal Units | National Effects of Births Averted among Acceptors | Simulation |
|---|---|---|---|---|---|---|---|
| Subjects | Total population or subgroup. | Total population or subgroup. | Total population (matched areas) or acceptors (matched individuals). | Total population or subgroup. | Total population or subgroup. | Total population, subgroup, or acceptors. | Total population, or acceptors. |
| Use of controls | No | No | Post hoc matching may approximate controls. | Yes | Only statistical controls. | No | Not applicable |
| Separate estimates for roles of other factors | Yes: age distribution, nuptiality, program vs. private contraceptive source. | No | No | No | Yes: both demographic and socioeconomic factors. | No | Yes: demographic factors. |
| Data requirements | Age distribution of women of childbearing age; percent married by age; marital age-specific fertility rates; contraceptive use by supply source. | Fertility and program data for time periods, geographical areas, or population subgroups. | Measures for matching variables; fertility measures. | Measures to establish initial similarity; fertility and program measures. | Extensive: program strength; fertility measures; other demographic and socioeconomic measures by area. | Fertility or pregnancy measures for acceptor and comparison experience; methods accepted; reproductive process measures. | Extensive |

| Complexity of design | Simple | Simple | Intermediate | Simple | Complex | Complex | Complex |
|---|---|---|---|---|---|---|---|
| Advantages | Simple calculations. Good first step. Isolates effect of marital fertility change. | Few statistical assumptions. | Uses independent comparison group. Controls many confounding variables. | Independent comparison group. Areal basis. Controls many confounding variables. | Can separate program effect from socioeconomic factors. Covers both direct and indirect effects. | Subjects available through program. Links acceptance and continuation to fertility. Estimates program effect on whole country. | Useful exploratory tool. Full population component framework. |
| Limitations | No direct link between program activity and fertility change. Data by age groups often unavailable. Program-private division may not reflect true relative contributions. | Hard to rule out competing explanations. | Unavailability of data for matching. Contamination dangers. Hard to control for motivation, leadership. Lack of nonprogram match areas in national programs. | Contamination dangers. Small numbers of areas. Equivalence of areas hard to achieve. Political and practical problems in execution. | Poor data availability. Complexity of data manipulation and interpretation. Unclear temporal implications of cross-sectional data. Small numbers of units. | Often omits indirect program effects. Uncertainty in estimation of "expected" acceptor fertility. | Extensive data needs and data manipulation requirements. Numerous assumptions for unavailable data. |

Source: Forrest and Ross (1978). Illustrative applications and references for each method are given in the source.

simply by the mean period of use per acceptor). Corrections are entered to the projected use time to allow for periods not at risk of conception, and potential fertility rates are applied. However, dissatisfaction with this methodology has grown because of measurement problems and conceptual difficulties with acceptors, continuation, potential fertility, and other quantities. Moreover, with time, certain imponderable factors emerge in national programs that offer several contraceptive methods, often in competition with the private sector. Many acceptors circulate in and out of the user group, switch methods, and experience intervening pregnancies and births, all of which undercuts assumptions in the methodology described.

As a result, an alternative approach has received increasing attention. This approach works directly from prevalence levels, without asking what acceptance schedules and continuation rates stand behind those levels. This approach has gained impetus from the growth of surveys, notably the increasing cross-national standardization of data from the World Fertility Survey series and the series of contraceptive prevalence surveys of the Centers for Disease Control and the Westinghouse organization. Of course, these survey estimates of prevalence have their own methodological problems.

Summarized here is that part of the prevalence-based literature which has carried the analytic approach farthest. First, Berelson (1974) discovered a very close correlation between contraceptive prevalence and crude birth rates (CBR) over a number of countries. With the most recent international data (32 countries; see Nortman and Hofstatter, 1980), the relationship can be represented as $CBR = 46.9 - 42U$, where $U$ is the proportion of married women of reproductive age using contraception. Thus if there are no users, the CBR averages 46.9; if half are using, it falls to 25.9, a 45 percent decline. There is remarkably small scatter about the least squares line, reflected in the $R^2$ value of 0.91.

Recognizing that the CBR responds not just to contraceptive use but also to other factors, Bongaarts and Kirmeyer (1980) developed refined correlations to eliminate the confounding effects of the age distribution, the proportions married, and the duration of lactation. Abortion was assumed absent since the 22 developing countries studied were believed to have only minimal abortion rates. For these countries, the relation of the total fertility rate (TFR), which frees the picture of age-structure

effects, is TFR = 7.30 - 6.42U. Thus, with no users, the
rate is 7.30 (natural fertility); if half use, the TFR is
4.09, a reduction of 44 percent ($R^2$ of 0.72).

A comparable equation was developed for the total
marital fertility rate (TMFR)[4], with other refinements
introduced to remove the effect of lactation. The result
is an "adjusted total marital fertility rate": TMFRA =
15.25 - 13.71U. This calculation estimates that natural
fertility would be 15.25 with marriage at age 15, no
lactation, and no abortion. As before, the result is
that if half are using contraception, the rate will fall
by 45 percent. These calculations are repeated for each
age group separately.

Although the CBR and TFR equations can be used to
estimate a country's fertility level directly, a more
precise approach is given for estimating not fertility
levels, but rather the proportionate decline in a fertility rate of interest as prevalence rises. Three cases
are treated. First, if only prevalence changes (not
marriage pattern or lactation), the fertility decline
remains proportionate to the rise in prevalence,
discounted for imperfect use-effectiveness. The new
fertility rate will then equal the old rate multiplied by
the ratio $(1 - .899\ U_2)/(1 - .899\ U_1)$, where $U_1$ is
the initial proportion of users and $U_2$ the later proportion. Separate equations are given for the various
age groups. Second, if both prevalence and use-effectiveness change, but nothing else does, the ratio of the two
fertility rates (at time 1 and time 2) is now as follows:

$$\frac{1 - e_2 U_2/0.927}{1 - e_1 U_1/0.927}$$

Third, more complex procedures are used in the case where
lactation and marriage patterns also change, although the
first case above can often be used because the effects of
these changes tend to cancel one another out over the
countries examined. Again, all of these procedures are
treated on an age-specific basis. This work breaks new
ground, and is both empirically based and analytically
imaginative. Although the question of the potential
fertility of users is treated only implicitly, that is
perhaps an acceptable trade-off for the special advantages
provided by these methods.

An especially noteworthy study (Mauldin and Berelson,
1978) focuses specifically on program effect. Its methodology is rich, and it is the most recent and comprehensive

in country coverage. Data for 94 developing countries are subjected to not one but several multivariate techniques, giving results that closely parallel the trends visible in simple cross-tabulations. Countries with stronger social settings (i.e., that are more developed) have experienced sharper fertility declines than countries with weaker social settings; those with stronger family planning programs have experienced sharper declines than those with weaker or no programs; and those fortunate enough to have been strong on both have experienced by far the sharpest declines (Mauldin, in these volumes, Table 4). Direct fertility reduction over the short term is more easily achieved by manipulating the program variables than the social setting, which tends to be rather intractable to the direct influence of population specialists within a country.

## PROPOSITIONS

The propositions below are grouped in two general areas: the influence of birth control methods on fertility levels, and potential effects of technological developments on future fertility reduction.

### Influence of Birth Control on Fertility

1. Existing birth control methods do not achieve full potential in fertility reduction. No current method has both high acceptability and long continuation; moreover, younger couples, having the highest potential fertility, tend to choose methods with shorter continuation, while older couples, with lower potential fertility, tend to chose methods with longer continuation, such as the IUD or sterilization. Because no current method offers both high acceptability and long continuation to all couples, existing motivation to control fertility is not fully translated into action.

2. In spite of these limitations, a good deal of evidence has accumulated on the response of fertility levels to the use of birth control. Empirically and theoretically, the relationship between increased prevalence of use and decreased fertility has been established. This relationship is independent of the influence of age structure, abortion, lactation, and marriage pattern, and holds over a range of developing countries.

3.  A distinction is properly made between method and program effects:  a program can try to change motivation as well as offer implementing methods.  On the other hand, in practice, the working propositions behind much of the research have concerned the combined effects of both.  Moreover, the breakthroughs in methods generated those in programs; both occurred in the early to mid-1960s, when the IUD appeared and the cost of the pill fell enough to permit mass distribution.  In fact, method and program effects cannot be separated:  the methods do not work in a vacuum, and the programs could not exist without the methods.  Some propositions related to these effects are given below, based in part on Ross et al. (1972).

3.1.  Multiple regression analyses and other multivariate techniques indicate that areas with stronger program activity or higher acceptance rates tend to have larger decreases in fertility.  These results appear across small areas, such as in Taiwan, and across larger units such as Indian states and entire countries.

3.2.  Comparisons between program and nonprogram areas of roughly equivalent character have shown larger fertility declines in the program areas.  The two kinds of areas are not strictly matched, so that the role of uncontrolled influences must be considered; nevertheless, the results suggest program effects.  Similar effects are indicated by formal matching of areas as units, as well as by other studies in which correspondence is found between the timing of program activity and unusual fertility declines.  Further program effects have been found in designs using experimental and control areas.

3.3.  At the individual level, fertility declines among program acceptors have been greater than among nonacceptors matched for other characteristics; acceptors also experience lower fertility after acceptance than before, and persist in these lower levels.  It should be noted that in some programs, acceptors who terminate the initial method or become pregnant while using it resort to supplementary contraception or abortion to keep their postacceptance fertility low.  Some of this contraception is program-provided, and some is not.  This supplementary birth control is not included in a number of studies which calculate that a first segment of IUD or pill use averts less than one birth, and that sterilization generally averts more than two.

4.  In national data, the high proportions of couples using contraception, together with the large role of

marital fertility declines in changing crude birth rates, suggest that contraceptive use (often largely program-provided) has been an important cause of fertility decline in a number of countries. Moreover, age patterns correspond: age groups with higher acceptance and prevalence rates have shown greater fertility declines.

## Potential Effects of Technological Developments on Fertility

The revolution in contraceptive technology over the past 20 years has fundamentally changed the field. Among the older methods, the condom and vasectomy remain important; however, even they have been generally eclipsed by the pill, the IUD, simplified female sterilization, and simplified early abortion. The injectable method is also important in selected locations and in parts of the private sector. In addition to the new technology, a vast body of research in reproductive physiology and contraceptive development has appeared since 1960. Thus permanent gains have been made, and while attention is often fixed upon the unfortunate shortcomings of the available methods, in a historical perspective it is their revolutionary strengths that stand out. The propositions below address some of the most important aspects of technological developments in birth control methods, present and future.

5. The pill is clearly in first place in acceptability, and sterilization in continuation; the IUD is intermediate in both categories. All three are high in use-effectiveness. Abortion is important both as a backup for contraceptive failure and as a primary birth control method. The condom and other traditional methods are sometimes used as the preferred choice, but more often as a fall-back in lieu of something more suitable. It is worth noting that, in countries where all major methods are readily available, each attracts a substantial group of users. This probably reflects the fact that no perfect method exists, and that, despite the new technology, different people in different circumstances must continue to search for a least unsatisfactory method.

6. As regards future advances, the focus should be on the demographic, not just the biomedical, aspects of contraceptive technology. The propositions below, condensed from two treatments by Berelson (1976, 1978), address some guidelines for such a focus.

6.1.  It has been demonstrated by several family planning programs that the introduction of a new contraceptive method does not merely substitute for current methods, but adds a new layer of users.  Thus improved technology can have a significant impact by attracting those to whom available choices are somehow unacceptable.

6.2.  Several innovations in contraception are being explored; these include implants, vaccines, once-a-month pills, biochemical sperm suppression, and preidentification of ovulation, as well as improvements in current methods.  However, such innovations take quite some time before being ready for mass use:  usually 5-10 years for methods like those now being clinically investigated, approximately double that for those in the laboratory development stage, and still longer for those undergoing basic research.

6.3.  Once developed, some innovations will not work; those that do can still be expected to present certain problems, just as current methods do.  These problems may be not only medical, but also religious, cultural, and political.

6.4.  Contraceptive technology can have demographic impact in three basic areas:  effectiveness, or fewer failures in use; acceptability, or more initial users; and continuation, or longer duration of use.  Of these, the latter two are especially significant, particularly in light of the high effectiveness already attained by current methods.  As an example, an increase in continuation of 10 percent could have an impact equal to doubling the low acceptance rates in several developing countries with large populations.

6.5.  Two current methods--sterilization and abortion-- have recently undergone significant improvement.  Fuller use of these improved methods in current family planning programs could have greater demographic impact than most new or improved methods now being developed.

6.6.  Given current technology and program efforts, many developing countries are likely to reach a crude birth rate of 20 by the year 2000.  However, many others lack the technology, programs, and social conditions to make this possible.  In such countries as Bangladesh, Pakistan, Nigeria, and other large Moslem and Black African nations, improved technology, if properly adapted to cultural conditions, might make a critical contribution.

## NOTES

1. Indonesia is at 36 percent as of early 1981 as estimated from program service statistics.
2. The general formula is $C = a/r = at/(\ln a - \ln R_t)$. This simplifies to $C = a/(\ln a - \ln R_1)$ when t is one year. If a can be assumed to be 1.0, then $C = 1/r = t/(-\ln R_t)$.
3. It may be noted in passing that in the more developed countries, fertility within marriage is largely controlled by contraception and abortion, not by breast-feeding. In general, age at marriage is somewhat earlier in the developing countries.
4. This is the sum of the age-specific marital fertility rates from age 15 to 49, and in concept is realized only for women married during that entire period. The rate at 15-19 is difficult to measure accurately; therefore the value for each country was set at .75 times the 20-24 rate.

## BIBLIOGRAPHY

Altman, D. L., and P. T. Piotrow (1980)  Social marketing:  Does it work?  Population Reports, Series J, No. 21.

Baer, E. C., and B. Winikoff, eds. (1981)  Breast-feeding:  Program, policy, and research issues. Studies in Family Planning 12:123-206.

Bang, S. (1971)  Korea:  The relationship between IUD retention and check-up visits.  Studies in Family Planning 2:110-112.

Berelson, B. (1974)  World Population:  Status Report 1974.  Reports on Population/Family Planning 15.

Berelson, B. (1976)  The Impact of New Technology.  In The Royal Society, Contraceptives of the Future.  A Royal Society Discussion organized by R. V. Short and D. T. Baird.  (Also appears in Proceedings Royal Society of London, Series B 195:25-35.

Berelson, B. (1978)  Demographic Requirements of Fertility Control Technology:  15 Propositions.  A PIACT Paper.  Program for the Introduction and Adaptation of Contraceptive Technology, Seattle, Washington.

Berelson, B., W. P. Mauldin, and S. J. Segal (1980) Population:  Current status and policy options. Social Science and Medicine 14C:71-97.

Bongaarts, J. (1978)  A framework for analyzing the proximate determinants of fertility. Population and Development Review 4:105-132.

Bongaarts, J., and S. Kirmeyer (1980)  Estimating the Impact of Contraceptive Prevalence on Fertility: Aggregate and Age-Specific Versions of a Model. Center for Policy Studies Working Paper No. 63.  New York:  Population Council.

Buchanan, R. (1975)  Breastfeeding:  Aid to infant health and fertility control. Population Reports, Series J., No. 4.

Campbell, A., and B. Berelson (1971)  Contraceptive specifications:  Report on a workshop. Studies in Family Planning 2:14-19.

Carrasco, E. (1980)  Contraceptive Practice. WFS Comparative Studies, Cross National Summaries No. 9. London:  World Fertility Survey.

Chan, K. C. (1971)  Hong Kong:  Report of the IUD reassurance project. Studies in Family Planning 2:225-233.

Chen, P. C. (1982)  Evolution of China's birth planning policy. Pp. 205-219 in World Population and Fertility Planning Technologies. Washington, D.C.:  Office of Technology Assessment.

Coleman, S. J. (1978)  Induced Abortion and Contraceptive Method Choice among Urban Japanese Marrieds. Unpublished PhD dissertation.  Columbia University, New York.

Conservation Foundation (1953)  The Physiological Approach to Fertility Control:  Report of the Conservation Foundation Working Group on Fertility Control. New York:  Conservation Foundation.

Foreit, J. R., M. E. Gorosh, D. G. Gillespie, and C. G. Merritt (1978)  Community-based and commercial contraceptive distribution:  An inventory and appraisal. Population Reports, Series J, No. 19.

Forrest, J. D., and J. A. Ross (1978)  Fertility effects of family planning programs:  A methodological review. Social Biology 25:145-163.

Freedman, R., and B. Berelson (1976)  The record of family planning programs. Studies in Family Planning 7:1-40.

Greep, R. O., M. A. Koblinsky, and F. S. Jaffe (1976) Reproduction and Human Welfare:  A Challenge to Research. Cambridge, Mass.:  MIT Press.

Hatcher, R. A., G. Stewart, F. Stewart, F. Guest, N. Josephs, and J. Dale (1982)  Contraceptive Technology 1982-1983, 11th ed. New York:  Irvington Publishers.

Henry, A., W. Rinehart, and P. Piotrow (1980)   Reversing
    female sterilization. Population Reports, Series C,
    No. 8.
Huber, S. C. (1974)   World survey of family planning
    services and practice.   In Survey of World Needs in
    Population.   London:   International Planned Parenthood
    Federation.
Klinger, A. (1969)   Demographic aspects of abortion.   Pp.
    1153-1164 in International Population Conference,
    London.   London:   International Union for the
    Scientific Study of Population.
Klinger, A. (1979)   International comparative data on
    sterilization, infertility, sterility.   Summarized in
    S. E. Khoo, The Prevalence and Demographic Analysis of
    Sterilization.   IUSSP Papers No. 17.   Liege:
    International Union for the Scientific Study of
    Population.
Kreager, P. (1977)   Family Planning Drop-outs
    Reconsidered:   A Critical Review of Research and
    Research Findings.   Research for Action No. 3.
    London:   International Planned Parenthood Federation.
Lubell, I., and R. Frischer (1980)   The international
    status of voluntary surgical contraception and its
    implications for national health programs.   In M. E.
    Schima and I. Lubell, eds., Voluntary Sterilization:
    A Decade of Achievement.   New York:   Association for
    Voluntary Sterilization.
Mauldin, W. P. (1978)   Experience with Contraceptive
    Methods in Less Developed Countries.   Paper presented
    at the National Academy of Sciences' Symposium on
    Contraceptive Technology, Washington, D.C.   (Also a
    Working Paper of the Population Council, Center for
    Policy Studies, New York.)
Mauldin, W. P., and B. Berelson (1978)   Conditions of
    fertility decline in developing countries, 1965-75.
    Studies in Family Planning 9:89-147.
Nortman, D. (1980)   Empirical Patterns of Contraceptive
    Use:   A Review of the Nature and Sources of Data and
    Recent Findings.   Paper prepared for an IUSSP Seminar
    on The Use of Surveys for the Analysis of Family
    Planning Programmes, Bogota.
Nortman, D., and E. Hofstatter (1980)   Population and
    Family Planning Programs:   A Compendium of Data
    through 1978, 10th ed.   New York:   Population
    Council.
Nurhajati, J. Teachman, and J. Parsons (1977)   Sources of
    Bias in the Indonesian Quarterly Acceptor Survey and

<u>Their Adjustment</u>. Monograph No. 18. Jakarta: National Family Planning Coordinating Board.

Polgar, S., and J. F. Marshall (1976) The search for culturally acceptable fertility regulating methods. In <u>Culture, Natality, and Family Planning</u>. Monograph 21. Chapel Hill, N.C.: Carolina Population Center, University of North Carolina.

Rochat, R., L. Morris, and J. E. Anderson (1979) Using contraceptive prevalence surveys to study the demographic impact of contraceptive sterilization in Latin America. Summarized in S. E. Khoo, <u>The Prevalence and Demographic Analysis of Sterilization</u>. IUSSP Papers No. 17. Liege: International Union for the Scientific Study of Population.

Ross, J. A. (1975) Acceptor targets. Pp. 55-91 in C. Chandrasekaran and A. I. Hermalin, eds., <u>Measuring the Effect of Family Planning Programs on Fertility</u>. Dolhain, Belgium: Ordina Editions.

Ross, J. A. (1979) Declines in the age and family size of family planning programme acceptors: International trends. <u>Studies in Family Planning</u> 10:290-299.

Ross, J. A., and J. D. Forrest (1978) The demographic assessment of family planning programs: A bibliographic essay. <u>Population Index</u> 44:8-27.

Ross, J. A., and D. Huber (1982) Vasectomy: Acceptance and Prevalance in Developing Countries. Paper prepared for the conference on Vasectomy, cosponsored by the Ministry of Plan Implementation and the World Federation of Health Agencies for the Advancement of Voluntary Surgical Contraception, Colombo, Sri Lanka.

Ross, J. A., and R. Potter (1980) Changes in acceptors' and users' ages: A test of an explanatory mechanism. <u>Population Studies</u> 34:367-380.

Ross, J. A., A. Germain, J. Forrest, and J. Van Ginneken (1972) Findings from family planning research. <u>Reports on Population/Family Planning</u> No. 12.

Sardon, J. P. (1979) World patterns of sterilization. Summarized in S. E. Khoo, <u>The Prevalence and Demographic Analysis of Sterilization</u>. IUSSP Papers No. 17. Liege: International Union for the Scientific Study of Population.

Sivin, I. (1974) <u>Contraception and Fertility Change in the International Postpartum Program</u>. New York: Population Council.

Snowden, R. (1972) Social and personal factors involved in the use-effectiveness of the IUD. Pp. 74-81 in A. Goldsmith and R. Snowden, eds., <u>Family Planning</u>

Research Conference:  A Multidisciplinary Approach. Amsterdam:  Excerpta Medica.

Sullivan, J., W. Bahrawi, H. Suyono, and A. Hartoadi (1974)  Contraceptive Use-Effectiveness in Mojokerto Regency, East Java. Monograph No. 9.  Jakarta: National Family Planning Coordinating Board.

Suyono, H. (1977)  Some Preliminary Calculations on Contraceptive Use Rates in Indonesia. Monograph No. 17.  Jakarta:  National Family Planning Coordinating Board.

Tietze, C. (1979)  Induced Abortion:  1979, 3rd ed.  A Population Council Fact Book. New York:  Population Council.

Tietze, C. (1981)  Induced Abortion:  A World Review, 1981, 4th ed.  A Population Council Fact Book.  New York:  Population Council.

Trussell, J., and J. Menken (1980)  Life Table Analysis of Contraceptive Use-Effectiveness.  Paper prepared for an IUSSP Seminar on The Use of Surveys for the Analysis of Family Planning Programmes, Bogota.

United Nations (1978)  Methods of Measuring the Impact of Family Planning Programmes on Fertility:  Problems and Issues.  Population Division, Population Studies No. 61, ST/ESA/SER.A/61.  New York:  United Nations.

United Nations (1979)  The Methodology of Measuring the Impact of Family Planning Programmes on Fertility, Manual IX.  Population Division, Population Studies No. 66, ST/ESA/SER.A/66.  New York:  United Nations.

United Nations (1982)  Sources of Variance in Family Planning Evaluation Methodology.  U.N. Publication ST/ESA/SER.A/76.  Forthcoming.

Vaughan, B., J. Trussell, J. Menken, and E. Jones (1977) Contraceptive failure among married women in the United States, 1970-1973.  Family Planning Perspectives 9:251-258.

Vaughan, B., J. Trussell, J. Menken, E. Jones, and W. Grady (1980)  Contraceptive efficacy among married women aged 15-44 years.  Vital and Health Statistics, Series 23, No. 5.

# Chapter 3

# Monetary and Health Costs of Contraception

S. BRUCE SCHEARER

## INTRODUCTION

This paper reviews current knowledge about the costs of contraceptive use.[1] These fall into two broad categories: monetary and health costs. For purposes of this review, contraceptive methods are classified according to 14 basic categories, as shown in Figure 1. Included within these categories are nearly 100 contraceptive drugs and devices marketed under more than 600 brand names (Kestelman and Kleinman, 1976).[2] The discussion below focuses first on monetary and then on health costs, surveying the available data, examining the relationship between these costs and contraceptive use, and suggesting areas for further research.

## MONETARY COSTS OF CONTRACEPTION

The relationship between monetary costs and contraceptive use is difficult to define empirically because of the complexities involved. First, there are basically four components of these costs: costs of production (generally including development costs), of related services required for use, of distribution of products and services, and of gaining access. Second, it is often difficult to distinguish who pays these costs, and thus to determine how they vary among different settings and socioeconomic groups. The subsections below review the nature of the various costs, who pays them, and how they affect contraceptive use.[3]

FIGURE 1  Principal Categories of Contraceptive Methods

---

Behavioral Methods

Withdrawal and related techniques
Abstinence (unsytematized; calendar rhythm; temperature rhythm;
   cervical mucus methods; symptothermal rhythm)
Prolonged breastfeeding
Postcoital douching

Drugs and Devices

Oral contraceptives (standard dosage; low-dose regimens)
Progestin-only minipill oral contraceptives
Injectable contraceptives (monthly; 2-monthly; 3-monthly; implants)
Postcoital pills
Intrauterine devices (inert; drug-releasing)
Vaginal spermicides (foams; creams; jellies; tablets; suppositories)
Vaginal barrier devices (diaphragms; cervical caps)
Condoms

Sterilization

Vasectomy
Female sterilization (laparotomy; minilaparotomy; laparoscopy;
   culdoscopy)

---

## Nature of Monetary Costs

Most contraceptive methods require the use of some con-
sumable product; among the techniques listed in Figure 1,
only withdrawal, unsystematized abstinence, and prolonged
breastfeeding do not.  Production costs will depend on a
number of components:  materials used, the actual production process and related overhead, added charges to provide a profit, added charges to compensate those having
rights to the technology involved, and charges added to
recover research and development costs.  Those components
will vary considerably depending on the particular
product; in general, however, the latter three components
are frequently greater than costs of materials and
production.

Many birth control methods require related services,
such as formal instruction required for use of one of the
systematized versions of abstinence or of the vaginal
diaphragm.  Many methods require medical services, such
as insertion of an IUD, screening of a potential oral

contraceptive user, or surgery to perform a sterilization. The costs of these services vary widely depending
on the particular techniques employed, the nature of the
provider, and the type of health or other service delivery
system involved.

Costs of providing related services are often closely
associated with those of maintaining sources of supply,
or distribution costs. These costs generally include
promotional, informational, or marketing activities;
maintenance of facilities and staff; personnel training;
and costs of mananging and planning the program, including
program research and evaluation. In general, there are
two sources of supply: the private and the public sectors. The former includes profit-making individuals,
institutions, and organizations; the latter includes
those engaged in not-for-profit activities, both governmental and voluntary agencies. When the source of supply
is private, distribution costs are added to production
and service costs and charged to the user. In fact,
these can comprise the better part of the user's total
cost (Sollins and Belsky, 1970; Westinghouse Population
Center, 1974; Black 1973; Farley and Tokarski, 1975).
When the source of supply is public-sector health and
family planning programs, these costs at most comprise a
nominal cost to the user (Nortman and Hofstatter, 1980).

Finally, the costs of gaining access to sources of
supply include travel to these sources and opportunity
costs such as loss of income. Such costs to users vary
inversely with the availability of products and services.
When availability is limited, the relationship is negative: the more limited the supply of products and
services, the higher the cost of locating, reaching, and
waiting to receive services from a source; when availability is high, the cost of access decreases until it reaches
constant minimum.

Magnitude of Costs in the Private and Public Sectors

The monetary costs of contraceptive use will be borne
differently depending on the source of the products and
services. When the source is private, most costs are
paid by the user. When the source is public, on the
other hand, the majority of these costs are paid through
funds obtained from government revenues, foreign aid, and
private philanthropic contributions.[4] These two
categories of cost-bearing are discussed below.

Private-Sector Costs

Costs to users for contraceptive products and services
provided through private-sector channels in twenty
developing countries in 1980 are shown in Table 1 and
Appendix Tables 1 and 2.  Although there is some substantial variation, generally these costs are remarkably
similar in most developing countries.  Ignoring extreme
cases, yearly costs are also comparable for different
methods, ranging from $23.00 to $34.00 for the four most
popular methods (the pill, the IUD, the condom, and female
sterilization).  These prices can be substantial compared
to local per capita income levels in some countries.  As
indicated in Table 2, the cost of a year's supply (or its
equivalent) varies from a low of 0.3 percent of average
annual per capita income for oral contraceptives in Mexico
to a high of 28.1 percent for spermicides in Zaire, but
averages in most developing countries from 1 to 5 percent
of annual per capita income.

From the data in Table 1 and Appendix Table 1, it is
possible to estimate the cost of providing a population
with contraceptive products and services exclusively
through private channels.  A typical proportional use of
different methods is assumed.  For example, if the method
mix were assumed to be 50 percent pill, 10 percent IUD,
10 percent condom, 5 percent spermicide, 5 percent injection, 8 percent female sterilization, 2 percent vasectomy,
and 10 percent other nonpharmacologic methods, then the
yearly average per capita cost of contraception at current
prices would amount to $22.17 (Farley and Tokarski, 1975;
Westinghouse Population Center, 1974; Sollins and Belsky,
1970).

These costs reflect nearly all of the charges users
pay for these methods.  However, in the case of oral and
injectable contraceptives, any fees charged for examinations, prescriptions, or injections are not included.
Service-related costs for these and other methods appear
in Appendix Table 2.

It must be stressed that none of these cost data
reflect the cost of gaining access to supplies and
services.  These costs will be negligible for users with
ready access to private sources of supplies and services.  In fact, however, this is not the case for many
people living in developing countries.  In these
countries, legal and cultural restrictions often limit
private-sector provision of contraception (Farley and
Tokarski, 1975; Westinghouse Population Center, 1974;

TABLE 1 Yearly Cost of Contraception Obtained Through Private-Sector Channels
(1980 U.S. dollars)

| Country | Oral Contraceptives[a] | IUDs[b] | Condoms[c] | Spermicides[d] | Injectables[e] | Female Sterilization[f] | Vasectomy[f] |
|---|---|---|---|---|---|---|---|
| Bangladesh | 16.64 | -- | -- | -- | -- | 6.59 | 2.03 |
| Brazil | 8.19 | 49.00 | 27.60 | 14.40 | 20.64 | 151.61 | 68.75 |
| Colombia | 10.40 | 18.45 | 27.60 | -- | 8.64 | 24.11 | 17.68 |
| Dominican Rep. | 33.15 | 26.10 | 34.80 | 27.60 | 27.48 | 28.57 | 35.71 |
| Egypt | 5.98 | 20.16 | 22.80 | 8.40 | -- | 20.71 | 25.93 |
| El Salvador | 46.80 | 18.60 | -- | -- | 62.40 | 33.14 | 20.00 |
| Guatemala | 29.25 | 14.00 | 39.60 | 16.80 | 16.92 | 25.00 | 14.29 |
| Indonesia | 17.94 | 12.64 | 14.40 | -- | 14.04 | 17.14 | 3.47 |
| Jamaica | 22.62 | 15.00 | -- | 26.40 | 48.00 | 26.86 | 24.86 |
| Jordan | 15.99 | 39.12 | 40.80 | 31.20 | 34.32 | 57.74 | 43.00 |
| Kenya | 46.02 | 18.45 | 42.00 | 39.60 | 45.48 | -- | -- |
| Korea, South | 13.26 | 18.56 | 12.60 | 16.80 | -- | 10.13 | 10.13 |
| Madagascar | 26.39 | -- | 57.60 | 27.60 | 33.72 | -- | -- |
| Mexico | 5.33 | -- | 19.20 | 13.20 | -- | -- | -- |
| Morocco | 32.50 | 25.16 | 20.40 | -- | -- | -- | -- |
| Nigeria | 90.74 | 29.68 | 97.20 | 57.60 | 151.32 | -- | -- |
| Panama | 25.74 | 14.00 | 30.00 | 57.60 | 72.00 | 42.86 | 25.00 |
| Philippines | 15.60 | 9.79 | 22.20 | 30.00 | 18.72 | -- | -- |
| Thailand | 16.25 | -- | -- | 8.40 | -- | 22.14 | 12.86 |
| Zaire | 46.15 | 35.50 | 32.40 | 13.20 | 35.52 | 12.68 | -- |
| Average, all countries | 26.19 | 22.76 | 33.82 | 29.86 | 42.09 | 34.23 | 23.36 |

[a]Cost of supplies only; any prescription fees or medical examination costs not included.
[b]Includes cost of device, insertion, and (except for Nigeria), one follow-up visit and assumes an average use of 2.5 years.
[c]Cost of supplies only; assumes use of 120 pieces per year.
[d]Cost of supplies only; diaphragm not included; assumes use of 120 applications per year.
[e]Cost of supplies only; includes both monthly and 3-monthly regimens; any prescription fees, medical examination costs or fees for injection not included.
[f]Includes all costs; assumes an average use of 7.0 years.

Source:  This table is based on a study described in Note 3.  Costs in this table are 12-month costs based on the price data in Appendix Table 1.

93

TABLE 2 Percentage of Income Required to Obtain One-Year's Supply of Contraceptives from Private-Sector Channels

| Country | Average Annual Per Capita Income, 1979 (U.S. dollars) | Oral Contraceptives | IUDs | Condoms | Spermicides | Injectables | Female Sterilization | Vasectomy |
|---|---|---|---|---|---|---|---|---|
| Bangladesh | 100 | 16.6 | -- | -- | -- | -- | 6.5 | 2.0 |
| Brazil | 1,690 | 4.8 | 2.8 | 1.6 | 0.8 | 1.2 | 8.9 | 4.0 |
| Colombia | 1,010 | 1.0 | 1.8 | 2.7 | -- | 0.8 | 2.3 | 1.7 |
| Dominican Rep. | 990 | 3.3 | 2.6 | 3.5 | 2.7 | 2.7 | 2.8 | 3.6 |
| Egypt | 460 | 1.3 | 4.3 | 4.9 | 1.8 | -- | 4.5 | 5.6 |
| El Salvador | 670 | 6.9 | 2.7 | -- | -- | 9.3 | 4.9 | 2.9 |
| Guatemala | 1,020 | 2.8 | 1.3 | 3.8 | 1.6 | 1.6 | 2.4 | 1.4 |
| Indonesia | 380 | 4.7 | 3.3 | 3.7 | -- | 3.6 | 4.5 | 0.9 |
| Jamaica | 1,240 | 1.8 | 1.2 | -- | 2.1 | 3.8 | 2.1 | 2.0 |
| Jordan | 1,180 | 1.3 | 1.5 | 3.4 | 2.6 | 2.9 | 4.8 | 3.6 |
| Kenya | 380 | 12.1 | 4.8 | 11.0 | 10.4 | 11.9 | -- | -- |
| Korea, South | 1,130 | 1.1 | 1.6 | 1.1 | 1.4 | -- | 0.8 | 0.8 |
| Madagascar | 290 | 9.1 | -- | 19.8 | 9.5 | 11.6 | -- | -- |
| Mexico | 1,590 | 0.3 | -- | 1.2 | 0.8 | -- | -- | -- |
| Morocco | 740 | 4.3 | 3.4 | 2.7 | -- | -- | -- | -- |
| Nigeria | 670 | 13.5 | 4.4 | 14.5 | 8.5 | 22.5 | -- | -- |
| Panama | 1,350 | 1.9 | 1.0 | 2.2 | 4.2 | 5.3 | 3.1 | 1.8 |
| Philippines | 600 | 2.6 | 1.6 | 3.6 | 5.0 | 3.1 | -- | -- |
| Thailand | 590 | 2.7 | -- | -- | 1.4 | -- | 3.7 | 2.1 |
| Zaire | 260 | 17.7 | 13.6 | 12.4 | 28.1 | 13.6 | 4.8 | -- |

Note: The cost of a one-year supply of each method is taken from Table 1. See footnotes to Table 1 to determine which costs are included.

94

Sollins and Belsky, 1970; UNFPA, 1976). Moreover, the
commercial infrastructure in rural areas is often weak,
and physicians and public health care facilities often
sparse. Thus private-sector supplies and services are
often quite limited in rural areas and urban slums in
most developing nations; this is particularly true for
methods requiring medical procedures, such as IUD insertion or sterilization. As a result, users often incur
substantial additional costs of locating, traveling to,
and obtaining access to private sources of supply, as
discussed below.

In general, the various monetary costs of contraceptives obtained in the private sector appear not to have
risen significantly over time (Sollins and Belsky, 1970;
Farley and Tokarski, 1975; see Table 1 and Appendix Table
1). Only modest increases have occurred over the past
decade, and these have been more than offset by inflation
and rising income levels.[5]

Public-Sector Costs

The overall cost of providing contraceptives through
public family planning programs is generally calculated
by dividing total yearly program costs by one of two
measures: the annual number of all clients served by the
program, or the calculated number of clients that receive
a full year's use of contraceptive services and supplies
from the program (see Tables 3 and 4). This latter measure, usually referred to as couple-years-of-protection,
is the most comprehensive, and is the most comparable with
the costs discussed above for private-sector channels.
However, as noted above, numerous methodological problems
make it difficult to quantify the monetary costs of public
family planning programs.[6] For example, the budgeted
cost of family planning programs usually does not include
significant resources supplied by external sources
(Simmons, 1973; Reardon et al., 1974; Nortman, 1981).
Consequently, exhaustive analysis of cost components is
generally required to obtain accurate estimates of total
program costs.

Because of these methodological problems, estimates of
costs vary widely. The data in Table 3, along with the
findings reviewed by Gillespie et al. (1981) and Robinson
(1979), indicate that it costs most public family planning
programs in developing countries between 10 and 30 1980
U.S. dollars to provide a year's worth of contraceptive

TABLE 3   Monetary Costs of Contraception Provided by Public-Sector Family Planning Programs (U.S. dollars in year indicated)

| Country (Region) | Reference | Date of Findings | Cost of Supplies and Services for All Methods Combined | |
|---|---|---|---|---|
| | | | Per New Acceptor | Per Couple-Year of Protection |
| Indonesia | Rahardgo and Resse (1972) | 1968 | 80.90 | 48.51 |
| | | 1970 | 25.61 | 17.85 |
| | | 1972 | 9.59 | 4.48 |
| Thailand (Chiang Mai) | Baldwin (1978) | 1977 | -- | 7.15 |
| Thailand | Chen (1981) | 1979 | -- | 14.39[a] |
| Colombia | Bailey and Correa (1975) | 1973 | 6.28 | 10.84 |
| | Ojeda et al. (1981) (clinic program) | 1977 | -- | 8.24 |
| | | 1978 | -- | 10.68 |
| | | 1979 | -- | 14.42 |
| | | 1980 | -- | 15.27 |
| India (Narangual) | Reinke (1981) | 1974 | 17.73 | 29.91[b] |
| Haiti | Bordes et al. (1981) | 1980 | 24.73 | 40.72 |
| Zaire | Blumenfeld (1981) | 1973-76 | 37.26[b] | 20.84[c] |
| United States | Correa et al. (1972) | 1968 | -- | 42.03 |
| | Reardon et al. (1974) | 1972 | 89.80 | 78.40 |

Note:  The table provides costs for all methods combined.  Correa et al. (1972) provide these costs per couple-year of protection for particular methods in the United States:  oral contraceptives, 49.81; IUD, 36.11; and spermicides, 41.27.  Reardon et al. (1974) give these costs:  oral contraceptives, 72.70; IUD, 97.40; diaphragm, 71.00; female sterilization, 224.70; and vasectomy, 48.40.  Similar costs for England, 1972, are provided by Trussell (1974):  oral contraceptives, 15.78; IUD, 15.05; condoms, 14.75; diaphragm, 17.19; spermicides, 20.44; and vasectomy, 32.86.

[a]Total costs, calculated from Table 1, plus commodity costs from Chen (1981).
[b]Calculated using data and method provided in Reinke (1981:13).
[c]Average cost for those areas cited in Blumenfeld (1981: Table 3), couple-years of protection calculated as 12 times the cost per contraception-month.

**TABLE 4**  Cost of Contraceptives from Public-Sector Family Planning Programs[a] (1980 U.S. dollars)

| Country | Oral Contraceptives[b] (per cycle) | IUDs[b] (device and insertion) | Condoms (per piece) | Diaphragms (device and initial fit) | Spermicides (per application) | Injectables[b] (per month) | Female Sterilization[b] | Vasectomy |
|---|---|---|---|---|---|---|---|---|
| Bangladesh | Free | .00–7.10 | .00–.01 | Not available | .00–.02 | Free | Free | Free |
| Brazil | Free | Unknown | Free | Free (limited availability) | Unknown | Unknown | Free (limited availability) | Free (limited availability) |
| China, P. R. | Free | Free | Free | Unknown | Free | Free | Free | Unknown |
| Colombia | .04–.30 | .00–3.38 | .09 | Not available | Not available | Not available | 4.50–11.25 | 4.50–11.25 |
| Dominican Rep. | Free | Free | Free | Not available | Free | Not available | 5.15 | 1.00–45.00[c] |
| Egypt | .07–.26 | .00–3.00 | .05–.07 | Not available | .02 | Not available | Free | Free |
| El Salvador | .00–.40 | .00–3.00 | .00–.04 | 2.00 | Unknown | .00–1.20 | Free | Free |
| Guatemala | .25 | 1.00–5.00 | .02 | Unknown | .02–.04 | 1.25 | .00–30.00 | .00–10.00 |
| Indonesia | Free | Free | Free | Unknown | Unknown | Free | 8.00[d] | Unknown |
| Jamaica | Free | Free | .00–.05 | Free | Free | Free | Free | Free |
| Jordan | .00–.34 | .00–3.44 | .09 | Free | Not available | Not available | 51.60 | Unknown |
| Kenya | Free | Free | Free | Free | Free | Unknown | Free | Unknown |
| Korea, South | .16–.24 | .00–2.83 | .02–.04 | Unknown | Unknown | Unknown | 22.50 | 15.00 |
| Madagascar | 1.20 | Not available | Free | 2.43 | .09 | 1.06 | Unknown | Not available |
| Mexico | .00–.28 | Unknown | .10 | Unknown | .05–.09 | Unknown | Unknown | Unknown |
| Morocco | Free | Free | Free | Free | Free | Not available | Free | Not available |
| Nepal | Free | Free | .00–.01 | Not available | Free | Free | Free | Free |
| Nigeria | .58 | 1.55 | .06 | Not available | .09 | 1.96 | Unknown | Unknown |
| Panama | .00–1.00 | .00–5.00 | .00–.08 | Free | .09 | 5.25 | 25.00 | Unknown |
| Philippines | Free | Free | Free | Unknown | Unknown | Not available | Free | Not available |
| Thailand | .00–.45 | 1.00 | .02–.10 | Not available | .06 | .25 | .00–7.50 | .00–2.50 |
| Vietnam | Free | Free | Free | Not available | Not available | Unknown | 4.00–4.50 | 4.00 |
| Zaire | Free[e] | Free[e] | Free | Free[e] | Free | Free[e] | 42.25 | Unknown |

[a]Including publicly subsidized commercial retail sales programs.
[b]Prices may vary by brand, type of product, type of device, or type of procedure.
[c]Price depends on ability of client to pay.
[d]Not officially a program method, but government subsidizes privately performed procedures for some low income women.
[e]A fee of 3.55 is charged for a clinic visit.

Source: The study upon which this table is based is described in Note 3.

supplies and services to one client. (Costs are higher in the United States and England.) Although this is a very rough estimate, it does suggest that the monetary costs of contraception provided by public-sector family planning programs do not differ markedly from those of private-sector sources.

It should be noted that most family planning programs do not seek to defray these costs by charging fees to clients. Table 4 shows the fees charged to clients by family planning programs in 23 developing countries in 1980. Even where fees are charged, in almost all instances except for sterilization and contraceptive injections, prices are very low compared to the private-sector retail prices listed in Table 2 and Appendix Table 1.


Components of Costs in the Public and Private Sectors

The monetary costs to users can be broken down into the four basic components described above. Although these general categories are the same for contraceptives in both the private and public sectors, there are some important differences in emphasis.

Cost data for the manufacture of contraceptive products by private companies are generally proprietary information. However, some estimates of these costs can be made by examining the lowest prices for which products are sold when most or all of the costs associated with distribution and promotion are excluded. (The data in Table 1 cannot be used because they include distribution costs.) This is generally the case when private companies sell bulk contraceptives under a competitive bidding system to a public-sector procurement agency, such as the Agency for International Development of the U.S. Government or the United Nations Fund for Population Activities. Under these circumstances, the "ex-factory" price of one month's supply of oral contraceptives, including packaging, can be as little as $0.15 to $0.25 (Newman, 1980; Badham, 1978). IUDs range from $0.10 to about $1.00, depending on the particular type (Population Council, 1979; Badham, 1978). The basic manufactured cost of most types of vaginal spermicides and condoms ranges from $0.01 to $0.05 per application or device (Newman, 1980; Badham, 1978). Although costs of some types of specialized sterilization equipment, such as a fiber-optic laparo-scope, can be in the thousands of dollars, this type of

equipment is reused for many years, not only for sterilizations, but also for other medical procedures; thus the
cost per procedure is small. Therefore, although there
may be some exceptions, the basic manufactured cost of
contraceptive products is generally low. When only the
basic cost of manufacturing is considered, a year's supply
or equivalent use ranges from a few cents to under $2.00
for most available products.

Appendix Table 2 provides data on the prices of contraceptive services provided by the private sector in
developing countries. These price data include not only
the direct cost of the service itself, but also charges
arising from the operation and maintenance of the service
delivery system. These include staff time, profit for
the service, and the general costs of maintaining the
service.

As noted above, costs arising from distribution,
including marketing, account for the better part of the
total price of most contraceptive products sold in the
private sector.[7] It is possible to estimate these
costs by subtracting the manufacturing cost from the
total price of the product. Using the above estimates
for manufacturing costs and the data in Appendix Table 1
and Table 1, distribution costs for oral contraceptives
can be estimated to comprise about 90 percent of their
total average retail cost.[8] As Appendix Table 1
indicates, the overall prices of contraceptives obtained
in the private sector are remarkably uniform from country
to country. Since manufacturing costs do not vary widely,
it can be assumed that there is a common basic cost
structure for these private services among developing
countries, although there does appear to be some
depression of costs in the lowest-income countries.

As noted above, the costs of gaining access to supplies
from retail outlets can be substantial; however, the
actual monetary value of these costs is not well documented (Rodriguez, 1977, 1978; Brackett, 1980; Foreit and
Gorosh, 1978; Morris et al., 1981). One study indicated
that many people living in rural areas of India, Panama,
and Turkey must pay over $1.00 U.S. to travel to and from
a retail source (Rodriguez, 1977); for methods such as
the pill requiring regular resupply, annual travel costs
could therefore total $10 or more. For many rural people,
substantial cost is involved in the time required to
travel to and from the nearest source.[9] Moreover, these
trips sometimes prove in vain: outlets can be out of
stock when customers arrive to purchase their supplies

(Farley and Tokarski, 1975). Additional costs are associated with learning about sources in places where supplies are only sparsely available; in some areas of Bangladesh and Korea, for example, as many as three-quarters of the people do not know where they can obtain supplies and services (Foreit and Gorosh, 1978).

Relationship of Monetary Costs to
Contraceptive Use and Fertility

The negative relationship between contraceptive prevalence and fertility levels is well established, both empirically and theoretically (Nortman amd Hofstatter 1980; Morris et al., 1981; Anderson and Morris, 1981; Ross, in these volumes). The theoretical analyses demonstrate that the effect of contraceptive use on fertility varies according to the mix of methods employed: the effect is greater in populations using higher proportions of more effective methods--oral contraceptives, injectables, IUDs, and sterilization--than in those using less effective methods (Bongaarts and Kirmeyer, 1980). Consequently, two issues are raised that determine the impact of the monetary costs of contraception on fertility: the extent to which these costs influence overall levels of use, and the extent to which they influence the mix of methods used by different populations. These two issues are discussed below for developed and developing countries.

Effects of Monetary Costs in Developed Countries

In developed countries, where the majority of contraceptive products and services are obtained from private sources, the monetary cost of contraception amounts to a relatively small fraction of per capita income. At prevailing price levels, overall use in most of these countries stands at nearly the maximum level consistent with very low levels of fertility (Menken et al., 1979; Dunnell, 1979; Leridon, 1981). Although price differences may influence selection of methods or particular brands of products, cost appears to have virtually no impact on overall levels of contraceptive use.

The impact of cost on the mix of methods also seems minimal in these countries. The most costly method, female sterilization, has been rapidly increasing in popularity despite the high fees involved (Family Planning

Perspectives, 1980a; Dunnell, 1979). The new copper-
bearing intrauterine devices, which cost about double the
price of older polyethylene models, have rapidly attained
major shares of the IUD market in North America and
Europe (Power, 1981). In short, other factors that
determine choice of method (such as effectiveness,
convenience, safety, and acceptability to one's partner)
seem to be far more important than monetary cost.[10]
    Since monetary costs have little or no impact either
on overall levels of use or on the mix of methods, their
influence on fertility in developed countries can be
assumed to be negligible.


Effect of Monetary Costs in Developing Countries

It is clear that there is some negative effect of monetary
costs on both levels of contraceptive use and the mix of
methods in developing countries.
    The largest effect is an indirect one:  in contrast to
developed countries, private-sector distribution channels
for contraceptives do not reach the bulk of the population in most developing countries.  Private-sector sources
have little interest in establishing marketing and distribution channels in areas where they believe their

volume of sales is likely to be low, such as rural areas
and the poor, marginal areas of cities (Business International, 1978; Westinghouse Population Center, 1974;
Folch-Lyon et al., 1981; Chen, 1981).  As a result,
private sources of supply serve only part, sometimes only
a small part, of the population in Third World countries
(Business International, 1978; Sollins and Belsky, 1970;
Morris et al., 1981).  While this limitation is offset in
those countries with active family planning programs, in
most developing nations the high costs of these public
programs have limited the extent of their coverage, as
well as the range of methods they can afford to provide.
As a result, because of cost, restricted access still
constitutes a substantial barrier to the use of contraceptives in most developing nations (Rodriguez, 1978;
Schearer and Fincancioglu, 1981; Morris et al., 1981;
Anderson and Morris, 1981).  This results in increased
levels of fertility in many developing nations (Kendall,
1979; Rodriguez, 1978; Morris et al., 1981; Anderson and
Morris, 1981; Westoff, 1981).
    The second way in which monetary costs influence con-
traceptive usage in developing countries is by directly

discouraging use of methods, even where they are available, because of their high costs to the potential users. Unfortunately, little is known about the extent of this direct effect of costs. On the one hand, some economists have claimed that the monetary costs of contraception constitute real barriers to contraceptive use for many individuals in developing countries (Enke and Hickman, 1976; Correa, 1975; Mertaugh, 1980). Prices charged by the private sector for nearly all products and associated services appear to be well in excess of what the poorest laborers and subsistence farmers can afford in developing countries.

On the other hand, there is evidence that prevailing commercial prices may not be a substantial deterrent to contraceptive use among very large segments of the population in many Third World countries. It appears that, at prevailing price levels, many couples in developing countries may regard the direct monetary costs of contraception as negligible in comparison with other, more basic factors related to social and economic aspirations and family size. The fraction of the population that obtains supplies from private sources even when public programs offer alternative free or low-cost supplies is quite large in many developing nations (Nakamura and Fonesca, 1979; Morris et al., 1981). Few people cite the cost of contraception as a barrier to use (Nakamura and Fonesca, 1979; Folch-Lyon et al., 1981; Morris et al., 1981); in a number of experimental programs, price has not proved to be an important determinant of contraceptive use (Wang, 1974; Folch-Lyon et al., 1981; Committee on Family Planning, 1973; Cross River Study, Ministry of Health, 1981). Social marketing programs indicate a substantial purchasing capacity even among low-income groups in rural areas (Altman and Piotrow, 1980); in some market tests, it has been demonstrated that even low-income groups often prefer to purchase contraceptive products rather than receive them free of charge (Reddy and Murthy, 1977; Talwar, 1980; Folch-Lyon et al., 1981).

This issue is a matter of some importance: if people's ability to pay for contraception is higher than is generally believed, private sources of supply may be capable of serving much larger segments of the population than they now do. Also, public family planning programs may be able to effect savings through charging for services and by reducing overlap of services in areas where private sources are available. Additional research is therefore urgently needed, especially in view of increasing financial pressures on these public programs.

HEALTH COSTS OF CONTRACEPTION

As a consequence of extensive epidemiological research
over the past decade, much is now known about the nature
and incidence of both minor and long-term adverse health
effects of contraceptive drugs and devices, and sterilization and abortion procedures. Although most of the
available methods of birth control cause some risk to
health, all confer at least partial protection against
pregnancy, which of course carries its own risks (see
Tietze, 1979; Chen et al., 1979; Tomkinson et al., 1979;
Hatcher et al., 1980; Office of Technology Assessment,
1982; Bruce and Schearer, 1979).[11] Assessing the costs
of contraception involves the complex task of weighing
risks against benefits. The following section of this
paper focuses exclusively on health costs of contraception (and, in the case of a few methods, direct health
benefits unrelated to fertility); the effects of these
costs on contraceptive use and fertility are then
examined.


Nature and Magnitude of Health Costs

Although there is generally no clearcut biological
separation between minor and more lasting adverse health
effects of contraception, the following descriptions of
the health costs of various birth control methods distinguishes minor side effects, serious health effects,
and potential hazards for purposes of discussion. Methods
are discussed in the order listed in Figure 1, excluding
the three little-used methods noted earlier.

Withdrawal and Related Techniques  No adverse health
effects are known to be associated with male or female
orgasm with the penis outside the vagina, either in
conjunction with withdrawal of the penis during intercourse just prior to male orgasm (coitus interruptus) or
in conjunction with oral, anal, or masturbatory sexual
practices. Historically, a wide variety of gynecological,
urological, neurological, and psychiatric disorders have
been attributed to the practice of withdrawal; however,
no objective data exist to justify these claims. Masters
and Johnson have demonstrated that a progression of
complex physiological changes from early excitation
through plateau and orgasm to final resolution occurs in
the female during normal coitus (Masters and Johnson,

1964). These findings have led to new speculation that
coitus interruptus on a regular basis might result in
observable physiological consequences in women (Calderone,
1970:437-438); thus far, however, these speculations
remain unstudied and undocumented.

Abstinence   No adverse health effects are known to be
associated with sexual abstinence, including systematized
forms of sexual abstinence (the latter includes calendar
rhythm, temperature rhythm, mucus method, and symptothermal rhythm, which is a combination of the first three).
However, psychological stress is common.  Some evidence
points to a possible health risk to the children of
couples practicing rhythm, especially versions that
permit intercourse only after ovulation has occurred.
One study found an elevated incidence of congenital
abnormalities in children accidentally conceived during
practice of the strict version of temperature rhythm
(Jongbloet, 1971).  Animal studies suggest that "overripe"
eggs fertilized at extended periods after ovulation do
exhibit an abnormally high frequency of chromosomal
abberations (Orgebin-Crist, 1973; O'Ferrall, 1973).
However, data on this potential side effect are too
limited to be conclusive.

Prolonged Breastfeeding   Prolonged breastfeeding in
malnourished women may cause health problems arising from
nutritional depletion.  It is possible that trauma to the
mother's nipple can occur after the infant's teeth emerge.
If breastfeeding provides the sole source of food beyond
infancy, malnutrition of the child can result.

Postcoital Douching   This ineffective folk method of
contraception can cause minor and, in extreme cases,
serious irritation of vaginal tissues, depending on the
solution used.  (See the section below on vaginal
spermicides for pertinent discussion of douching with
these substances.)

Oral Contraceptives   The most popular reversible
method of birth control, oral contraceptives, is believed
also to be the most extensively studied medication ever
marketed.  As summarized in Figure 2 and Table 5, oral
contraceptives have been associated with a wide variety
of minor side effects, as well as a number of serious
health hazards.  For many of these, data are sufficient
to demonstrate a direct causal relationship with oral

FIGURE 2  Minor Side Effects Reported to be Associated
with Oral Contraceptive Use

| Side Effects | Sources |
|---|---|
| Nausea | a,b,c,d,e,f,g |
| Weight change (usually gain, but in some cases loss) | c,h,i |
| Breast tenderness and other signs of fluid retention | c,f,h,i |
| Spotty darkening of skin (sometimes permanent) | a,b |
| Rashes and itching | a,i,j |
| Breakthrough menstrual bleeding and spotting | b,d,e,f,j,i,k,l |
| Decreases in menstrual flow | a,b,d,e,g,i,j |
| Menstrual cramping | c,i |
| Acne (usually reduced, but stimulated in some women) | a,b |
| Fatigue, mood changes, depression, nervousness | a,d,e,g,h,i,m |
| Headaches | a,d,e,f,g,h,i,j,n |
| Change in sex drive (usually increased, but decreased in some women) | a,d,h,i |
| Abdominal swelling and cramping | a |
| Vaginal yeast infections, itching, and discharge | a,i,o,p |
| Chronic ulcerations of the cervix | a,b,j |
| Hayfever and related allergies | a,j |
| Urinary tract infections (usually without symptoms) | a,j,q |
| Sensitivity of skin to light | a |
| Delay in return of menstruation following cessation of use | a,j,m,r |
| Delay in return of fertility following cessation of use | a,j,m,r |

Sources:
[a] Royal College of General Practitioners (1974)
[b] Sanhueza et al. (1979)
[c] Talwar and Berger (1977)
[d] Brat (1976)
[e] Ingemanson et al. (1976)
[f] Rudel et al. (1978)
[g] WHO (1980a)
[h] Hunton (1976)
[i] Briggs (1977)
[j] Vessey et al. (1976)
[k] Talwar et al. (1977)
[l] Bounds et al. (1979)
[m] Huggins (1977)
[n] Bourdais (1977)
[o] Spellacy et al. (1971)
[p] Soepari (1978)
[q] Takahashi and Loveland (1976)
[r] Vessey et al. (1978)

contraceptive use.  Just to what extent these adverse
health effects are due to biased reporting and to what
extent they are due to the medication is uncertain, since
women who use oral contraceptives may be more concerned
about their health and may notice and report general
health problems more frequently than nonusers.  The
serious side effects listed in Table 5 are less susceptible to biased reporting than are minor side effects,
but are difficult to measure and establish because of

TABLE 5   Serious Side Effects Associated with the Use of
Combined Oral Contraceptives

| Side Effect | Excess Morbidity or Mortality per Year per 100,000 Users | | |
| --- | --- | --- | --- |
| | Diagnosis | Hospitalizations | Deaths |
| Stroke | 31[a] | 35[b] | 9.7[c] |
| Deep-vein thrombosis or pulmonary embolism | 91[a] | 70[b] | 3.4[c] |
| Superficial or un-specified thrombosis | 125[a] | | |
| Heart attack and other non-rheumatic heart disease | 17[c] | 17[c] | 8.0[c] |
| Gallbladder disease (surgically confirmed) | 79[d] | 79[b,d] | -- |
| Kidney infection | 383[a] | -- | -- |
| Benign liver tumor | 1[e,f] | 1[e,f] | 0.1[e] |
| Hypertension | 406[a] | -- | 1.7[e] |
| Total | 1,133 | 202 | 22.9 |

Sources:
[a]Royal College of General Practitioners (1974).
[b]Vessey (1978).
[c]Royal College of General Practitioners (1981b).
[d]Boston Collaborative Drug Surveillance Program (1973).
[e]Rooks (1979a, 1979b).
[f]Nissen et al. (1979a, 1979b).

their infrequent occurrence.  Six serious adverse health
effects have been conclusively connected to the use of
oral contraceptives--stroke, heart attack, deep vein
thromboses and pulmonary embolism, supervicial thromboses,
hypertension, and benign tumors of the liver (Vessey,
1980; Slone et al., 1981; see references in Figure 2);
two other serious effects have been the subject of conflicting findings--gallbladder disease and kidney infection.  Studies cited in Table 5 indicate that about 1 of
500 (0.2 percent) of users in Western countries is likely
to experience one of the potentially life-threatening
side effects each year; an additional 0.9 percent is
likely to develop hypertension, kidney infections, or
superficial or unspecific thromboses.  An estimated 2 out
of every 1,000 oral contraceptive users are hospitalized
annually as a result of these side effects (see Table 5;
Ramcharan et al., 1976, 1980; Vessey, 1978), while about
2 out of every 10,000 users die (see Table 5; Royal
College of General Practitioners, 1981b).

The morbidity and mortality rates associated with serious side effects are overall averages applicable to white, Western women. Incidences of serious health problems vary widely among this group, depending on age, smoking habits, degree of inherent biological risk for cardiovascular disease, and, for some side effects, length of use. Among older women, heavy smokers, and those susceptible to vascular diseases, much higher rates of adverse health effects occur (Royal College of General Practitioners, 1981b). The incidence of many of the minor side effects associated with oral contraceptives decreases after the first several months of use; the risk of some of the serious side effects, however, increases with length of use, and in some cases produces irreversible damage to health (Nissen et al., 1979a, 1979b; Rooks et al., 1979a, 1979b; Royal College of General Practitioners, 1981b; Slone et al., 1981).

Biological susceptibility to adverse health effects of oral contraceptives has led to wide-scale screening of potential users. Obesity, high blood pressure, high cholesterol or triglyceride concentrations in the blood, and previous history of vascular disease are among the factors believed to increase the risk of circulatory system side effects. (Mann and Inman, 1975; Royal College of General Practitioners, 1974, 1981b; Vessey and Mann, 1978; Krueger et al., 1980; Mann 1978; Mann et al., 1976; Ory, 1977; Stolley, 1977; Vessey, 1980; Shapiro et al., 1979).

Most of the side effects associated with oral contraceptives have been shown to be dose-related (Royal College of General Practitioners, 1974, 1981b; Inman et al., 1970; Stolley et al., 1975). Increased use of low-dose combined oral preparations should lower the incidence of side effects somewhat. Studies have shown that a reduction in the estrogen component of 25-60 percent reduces the incidence of various estrogen-related side effects by a roughly equivalent amount (Royal College of General Practitioners, 1974; Inman et al., 1970, Stolley et al., 1975). The amount of progestin also needs to be reduced to lower the incidence of some vascular side effects (Kay, 1980; Meade et al., 1980). Additional epidemiological data will be required to evaluate the long-term health effects of the new low-dose combined oral contraceptive preparations.[12]

A number of potential hazards of oral contraceptives have been ruled out in recent years as a result of ongoing investigations. These include diabetes, infertility fol-

lowing extensive periods of use, and increased incidence
of birth abnormalities following discontinuation of use[13]
(Wingrave et al., 1979, 1980; Vessey et al., 1978, 1979b;
Hull et al., 1981; Huggins, 1977; Coulam et al., 1979;
Ramcharan et al., 1980; Rothman and Louk, 1979; Royal
College of General Practitioners, 1974, 1976). However,
a number of potential health effects remain to be determined. These include various forms of cancers, abnormalities of vision, effects on the immune system and on
resistance to some types of infectious disease, and
effects on nursing infants. Cancer, in particular, is of
concern. A recent report from one of the two major
British studies indicates a possible though uncertain
association of breast cancer with use of oral contraceptives (Royal College of General Practitioners, 1981a);
two recent small-scale case-controlled studies have shown
a higher risk of breast cancer among two types of
populations using this method (Jick et al., 1981b; Pike
et al., 1981). Recent findings from the second major
British study and the only comparable U.S. study indicate
a possible direct association between long-term oral
contraceptive use and cancer of the cervix (Harris et
al., 1980; Swan and Brown, 1980).

It must be stressed that the serious side effects
reviewed above emerge from studies conducted among Western
women, and their applicability to women in developing
countries is uncertain. Susceptibility to a disease
varies markedly with social and economic setting, climate,
nutrition, genetic constitution, and a variety of other
factors. Diseases involving blood clotting or arterio-
sclerotic disorders are rare in developing countries,
while many parasitic and infectious diseases endemic to
these settings are virtually absent in developed countries. Without controlled epidemiological studies
conducted in developing countries, informed judgments
about the long-term health consequences of oral contraceptive use in these settings cannot be made (Nordberg and
Atkinson, 1979; Ratnam and Prasad, 1979; Toppozada, 1979;
WHO, 1980a).

A number of studies have identified health benefits of
oral contraceptive use. These include reduction in breast
cysts and benign breast disease (Royal College of General
Practitioners, 1974; Vessey, 1978, 1979; Vessey et al.,
1976; Ory et al., 1974, 1976); reduction in both benign
and malignant cysts and tumors of the ovaries (Royal
College of General Practitioners, 1974; Vessey, 1979;
Vessey et al., 1976; Newhouse et al., 1977; McGowan et

al., 1979; Casagrande et al., 1979; Ramcharan et al.,
1980); reduction in rheumatoid arthritis (Royal College
of General Practitioners, 1974, 1978); reduction in
menstrual disorders (Royal College of General Practitioners, 1974; Vessey et al., 1976); and reduction in
iron deficiency anemia (Royal College of General Practitioners, 1974). The savings in morbidity and hospitalization for these health problems is substantial; the
reduction in iron deficiency anemia, which results from
less menstrual blood loss among oral contraceptive users,
is a potentially significant benefit for those women whose
diets are inadequate. In addition, as yet inconclusive
evidence points to important health benefits of oral
contraceptives in two other areas: a reduction in endometrial cancer (Weiss and Sayvetz, 1980; Kaufman et al.,
1980a; Ramcharan et al., 1980) and a reduction in the
incidence of pelvic inflammatory disease (Royal College
of General Practitioners, 1974; Vessey et al., 1976;
Vessey, 1978; Senanayake and Kramer, 1980; Eschenbach et
al., 1977; Ryden et al., 1979; Osser et al., 1980).

Intrauterine Devices   Like oral contraceptives, intrauterine devices have undergone extensive study during the
past two decades. More than 100 IUDs have been developed
and tested, and at least a dozen different types are being
used in different settings today; all share similar minor
and serious side effects. In addition, recently introduced devices that release small quantities of drugs
within the uterus have some actual and potential side
effects of their own related to the medication they
release. In the United States, it has been estimated
that a total of 2 to 10 deaths per million users per year
are associated with IUDs (Vessey, 1978; Kahn and Tyler,
1975c); overall hospitalization rates are estimated to be
roughly 1,000 times higher (Vessey, 1978; Kahn and Tyler,
1975a; Jennings, 1974).

The three most common side effects of all IUDs are
spontaneous expulsion of the device by the uterus, pain
in the pelvic area, and excessive menstrual or intermen-
strual bleeding. Expulsion has no direct adverse effect,
but may result in an accidental pregnancy if it goes
unnoticed. Almost all women fitted with an IUD experience
increased bleeding and pain immediately following the
insertion of the device. Although these effects in most
users subside within a month or two, increased menstrual
flow, often at double normal levels, remains a permanent
feature of this mode of contraception for as many as

10-25 percent of all users (Edelman et al., 1979; Guillebaud et al., 1976; Liedholm et al., 1975; WHO, 1980a). This side effect is regarded only as an annoyance by many IUD users; however, it does cause a higher incidence of anemia in women using this method (Vessey et al., 1976; WHO, 1980a; Guillebaud, 1979). It has been estimated that, depending on the type of IUD, between 1 and 10 out of every 1,000 IUD users annually require hospitalization to treat excessive bleeding (Tietze, 1970; Vessey et al., 1976; Kahn and Tyler, 1975a).

In addition to these three common side effects, a number of relatively rare but potentially more serious effects have been documented. These include perforation of the uterus; pelvic inflammatory disease (PID), sometimes associated with subsequent infertility; ectopic pregnancy; and other complications of pregnancy. Of these, the most prevalent is PID (see Table 6). Nearly one-third of all IUD-related hospitalizations involve some pelvic infection (Kahn and Tyler, 1975a; Jennings, 1974), and half of all deaths connected with IUD use in the United States since 1966 have been related to this kind of infection (Kahn and Tyler, 1975c; Jennings, 1974; Dreishpoon, 1975; Cates et al., 1976). Since oral contraceptives, the diaphragm, and the condom protect against PID, the relative risk for IUD users is much higher.

Although the rates of PID associated with IUD use are relatively high, mortality rates associated with infection and IUDs in developed countries are very low--in the range of 3 deaths per million IUD users per year (Kahn and Tyler, 1975c; Jennings, 1974). Studies comparable to those in Table 6 are not available from developing countries; however, in standard clinical trials of IUDs, the observed rates of PID are not markedly different in developed and developing countries.

The data in Table 6 indicate that young, nulliparous women who use an IUD have a much higher risk of contracting PID than do older or parous IUD users. However, this may not be due to a differential effect of the IUD on these two populations, but rather to the much greater incidence of multiple sexual partners among the high-risk group, a factor that is known to greatly increase PID risk. Because of this observed higher risk, however, health authorities in many countries are advising against the use of the IUD in young women who have not yet had children, not only because of the risk of infection

TABLE 6   Summary of Major Epidemiological Studies of IUDs
and Pelvic Infection

| Study | Type of Investigation | Risk of Hospitalization for Pelvic Inflammatory Disease | |
| | | Relative Risk | Excess Incidence Per 1,000 Users |
|---|---|---|---|
| Burkman et al. (1980) | case control | 1.6 fold | -- |
| Eschenbach et al. (1977) | case control | 4.4 fold (9.0 fold in nullipara) | -- |
| Falkner and Ory (1976) | case control | 5.1 fold | -- |
| Gray (1976) | reassessment of 1976 Westrom data | 7 to 8 fold in nullipara; 0.0 in others | -- |
| Jahn and Tyler (1975a) | cross-sectional survey | -- | 0.4-2.8 per 1,000 |
| Kaufman et al. (1980b) | case control | 7.9 fold | -- |
| Lippes (1975) | case control | 1.9 fold | -- |
| Targum and Wright (1974) | case control | 9.3 fold | -- |
| Vhaler et al. (1978) | case control | 3.3 fold | -- |
| Vessey et al. (1981c) | prospective cohort | 5.5 fold (10.5 fold for acute PID; 2.5 fold for chronic PID) | 1.68 per 1,000 |
| Westrom et al. (1976) | case control | 3.0 fold (7.0 fold in young nullipara) | -- |
| Wright and Laemmle (1968) | retrospective cohort | 6.9 fold | 56.6 per 1,000 |

itself, which can give rise to chronic pelvic pain and subsequent ectopic pregnancies, but especially because of the risk of consequent infertility (Physicians' Desk Reference, 1980; Guillebaud, 1979; Gray, in these volumes).

Although the risk of developing most forms of PID as a result of IUD use appears not to rise with increasing duration of use, one very rare form of infection does seem to increase with extended use. Recent research indicates that actinomyces-related PID may be caused by calcium build-up, especially on non-copper bearing plastic IUDs, after long periods of use (Boon et al., 1981; Gonzalez, 1981; Sparks, 1981; Duguid et al., 1980; Family Planning Perspectives, 1980b; Contraceptive Technology Update, 1981a).

Another rare type of infection is associated with IUD use: acute infection during pregnancy with an IUD in place, accompanied by abortion and sepsis. The observed incidence of this complication is very low, with mortality estimated at less than 3 deaths per million IUD users per year (Kahn and Tyler, 1975c; Jennings, 1974; Cates et al., 1976). Moreover, the incidence for IUDs currently in use is even lower, since a high proportion of the cases of this infection are known to have occurred with one particular IUD, the Dalkon Shield, which is no longer being marketed (Jennings, 1974; Cates et al., 1976; Edelman et al., 1979). Also, since the condition only occurs when an IUD is in place during pregnancy, both physicians and users are now removing the device in instances of accidental pregnancy.

Other complications of pregnancy are more frequent when an IUD is in utero during gestation. In addition to the elevated incidence of infected spontaneous abortions, the rate of common spontaneous abortions is about three times greater for IUD-bearing women than for pregnant women with no IUD (Kahn and Tyler, 1975a; Vessey et al., 1976; Edelman et al., 1979). There is also a higher incidence of premature labor, premature rupture of the amniotic membranes, and hemorrhage when an IUD is present during pregnancy (Kahn and Tyler, 1975a; Dreishpoon, 1975; Vessey et al., 1979b). Removal of the device increases the risk of spontaneous abortion, but greatly reduces the other risks (Dreishpoon, 1975; Edelman et al., 1979; Vessey et al., 1979b).

One other potential complication associated with pregnancies resulting from IUD contraceptive failure has been documented. It is known that the IUD is more effective in preventing normal uterine pregnancies than

the rare pathological pregnancies that sometimes occur in
the Fallopian tubes, ovaries, or abdomen (Tietze, 1970;
Ory, 1981; Vessey et al., 1979a; Edelman et al., 1979).
As a result, the proportion of these ectopic pregnancies
is high among IUD contraceptive failures, and the risk
increases to very high levels--about 1 in 10--for long-
term users (Tietze, 1970; Vessey et al., 1979a; Ory,
1981; Edelman et al., 1979).

Injectable Contraceptives    Controlled epidemiological
studies have not been carried out for injectable contraceptives.  Injectables contain high doses of one of the
two drugs used in oral contraceptives.  Such relatively
minor side effects as headache, nausea, dizziness,
nervousness, depression, menstrual pain, breast discomfort, acne, and others listed in Figure 2 for oral
contraceptives are reported by 2 to 4 out of every 10
women using injectable contraceptives (Nash, 1975; Fraser
and Weisberg, 1981; WHO, 1981), and the incidence of each
of these minor side effects and the extent of their
association with the medication are uncertain; however,
these effects have not been clearly documented as they
have for oral contraceptives.  It is clear that these
types of contraceptives give rise to menstrual bleeding
irregularities in the vast majority of users and cause
appreciable weight gain among a small proportion of users
(Nash, 1975; Fraser and Weisberg, 1981; WHO, 1981a, 1981b;
Gray, 1979, 1980).  About 1 out of every 200 women using
injectable contraceptives experiences very heavy menstrual
bleeding that can place her at risk of developing anemia.
In 1 to 5 out of every 1,000 users, bleeding is sufficiently severe to require hospitalization and surgical
treatment (Report to USAID, 1980; IPPF Medical Bulletin,
1980; Fraser and Weisberg, 1981; Parveen et al., 1977).
On the other hand, reduced menstrual bleeding is experienced by a large proportion of users (Report to USAID,
1980).
    It is known that the return of both menstruation and
fertility is delayed after cessation of use of this method
in a large proportion of women using the most popular
injectable contraceptive, Depo-Provera.  These delays are
much longer and more frequent than those observed among
past oral contraceptive users.  Fertility appears to be
recovered eventually in virtually all users, but data on
this issue are not conclusive (Fraser and Weisberg, 1981;
Nash, 1975; Pardthaison et al., 1980).  If injectable
contraceptives are accidentally given to pregnant women

or if pregnancy occurs during use, there is concern that
abnormalities in fetal development could result (Fraser
and Weisberg, 1981).

Beyond this effect, little is known about the serious
hazards and comparative safety of injectable contraceptives. Among the side effects that might be expected are
effects on liver function, blood pressure, and cardiovascular disease. As with oral contraceptives, carcinogen-
icity is of potential concern, since the drugs employed
in injectable contraceptives have been shown to stimulate
the formation of cancer in animals. Although there is no
evidence of this effect in humans (Greenspan et al., 1980;
Fraser and Weisberg, 1981), it remains of particular concern for the monthly and three-monthly varieties, which
use different types of progestins that exhibit strong
tumorogenic action (Fraser and Weisberg, 1981; Hearings
Before the Select Committee on Population, 1978; Report
to USAID, 1980; IPPF Medical Bulletin, 1980).

Again as in the case of oral contraceptives, injectable
contraceptives provide some significant health benefits
to users. Among the large proportion of users who experience decreased menstrual bleeding, the risk of anemia is
reduced (Report to USAID, 1980). Preliminary evidence
also suggests some reduction in the incidence of vaginal
infections among users (Toppozada et al., 1979).

Vaginal Spermicides, Vaginal Barrier Devices, and
Condoms  Barrier contraceptives--spermicides, the
diaphragm and cervical cap, and the condom--cause no
known disease or mortality. The principal minor adverse
health effect associated with these methods is vaginal or
cervical erosion in users of vaginal barrier devices
arising from mechanical abrasion. This effect is generally rare and mild among diaphragm users, but more
frequent and severe among those using the cervical cap
(Patanelli, 1981). There are also rare instances of
allergic reactions to the rubber or dusting powder used
in condoms and diaphragms, and the chemicals present in
spermicides and diaphragms (Belsky, 1975; Wortman, 1976b;
Coleman and Piotrow, 1979; Lalu, 1957). Some types of
spermicides cause a sensation of warmth in the vagina as
they are dissolving, but this is not associated with any
adverse effect on vaginal tissues. Recently, it has been
realized that some of the chemicals in spermicides are
likely to be absorbed through penile or vaginal tissues
into the bloodstream (Connell, 1979; Chvapil et al.,
1980; Food and Drug Administration, 1980). However,

little is known about the toxicity of these chemicals, and they are used only intermittently, so that significant health hazards do not seem highly likely. In the case of spermicidal jellies and creams used in conjunction with the diaphragm, actual clinical data over seven years of observation have revealed no associated illness or disease (Vessey et al., 1976). Spermicidal agents could also have an adverse effect on fetal development either in women who become pregnant while using them or among ex-users (Jick et al., 1981a); however, studies to date have not provided conclusive evidence on this question.

Like oral and injectable contraceptives, barrier contraceptives also offer some health benefits. Diaphragm users have a reduced incidence of pelvic inflammatory disease and, possibly, cervical cancer (Vessey et al., 1976; Vessey et al., 1981c; Wright et al., 1978). Condom users are partially protected against venereal diseases (Cutler, 1975; Ledger, 1974; Berger et al., 1975), a protective effect that can also reduce the risk of pelvic inflammatory disease and subsequent infertility.

Vasectomy   Few side effects, minor or serious, have been shown to be caused by vasectomy. Adverse effects associated with the surgical procedure are generally minor and infrequent. The rate of surgical complications, both major and minor, associated with vasectomies ranges widely from less than 1 per 1,000 procedures to over 122 per 1,000; an average for nearly 25,000 vasectomies of 47 complications per 1,000 procedures has been reported (Wortman, 1975; Pichai et al., 1981). Hematoma, infection, and epididymitis make up the bulk of these complications (Wortman, 1975; Schmidt, 1975; Davis, 1980); most can be treated without hospitalization.

It has been well established that different classes of antibodies against sperm are produced as a result of vasectomy in about 50 percent of cases, probably as a result of sperm granulosa formation following the procedure (Berendes and Crozier, 1975; Ansbacher et al., 1975). More recently, it has been shown that men also develop autoimmune antibodies to tissue antigens other than sperm (Mathews et al., 1976). It has also been found that vasectomy gives rise to autoimmune diseases and related secondary effects, including heart disease, in some species of animals (Alexander et al., 1974; Alexander and Clarkson, 1978; Clarkson and Alexander, 1979). However, despite very extensive and careful

study, no disease or pathology of any kind has been found
to date in men who have been vasectomized for up to
several years (Mathews et al., 1976; Goldacre et al.,
1978; Berendes and Crozier, 1975; Ansbacher et al.,
1975). Longer-term follow-up studies are continuing in
both the United States and Great Britain.

   Female Sterilization  In contrast to vasectomy, which
entails an extremely simple surgical procedure, female
sterilization has traditionally been associated with a
significant risk of injury and death because it requires
a major surgical procedure. This is true of the newer
endoscopic and minilaparatory methods, as well as tubal
ligation either by laparotomy or the vaginal approach.
   Major and minor side effects associated with abdominal
tubal ligation vary significantly depending on when in
pregnancy the procedure is carried out. Data from developed countries indicate that postoperative complications
and morbidity are very high when sterilization is undertaken in conjunction with delivery by Cesarean section
(Shepard, 1974), and may be even more frequent when
sterilization is carried out at the time of induced
abortion. Both postpartum and interval abdominal tubal
ligation are associated with much lower incidences of
surgical morbidity and postoperative complications
(Shepard, 1974; Dusitsin et al., 1980). The most common
complications following such surgery include postoperative hematoma, vaginal bleeding, other hemorrhage,
thrombophlebitis and thromboembolism, transient excess
blood loss, and a variety of local and systemic infections and abscesses. The reported incidence of morbidity
and/or complications following vaginal tubal ligation is
about the same as that for abdominal tubal ligation;
however, a greater proportion of the complications
associated with vaginal tubal ligation are of a more
serious nature (Shepard, 1974). Conventional laparotomy
coupled with tubal ligation is associated with a significant risk of death--in the range of 2.5 deaths per
10,000 procedures (Presser, 1970). Both laparoscopic
sterilization and sterilization by minilaparotomy are
associated with much lower rates of complications and
morbidity, as well as much lower mortality (Shepard,
1974; Phillips, 1980; McCann, 1978; Wortman, 1976a;
Mumford et al., 1980; McCann and Cole, 1980; WHO, 1980;
Vitoon, 1976). Although these rates may be slightly
higher when the procedure is performed in outlying areas
in developing countries or when tubal rings are used,

minilap complications are generally less severe than those associated with laparoscopy and less dependent on the skill of the operator. Two other endoscopic techniques, hysteroscopy and culdoscopy, are associated with much higher rates of complication and are consequently little used (Darabi et al., 1978; WHO, 1980a).

Little is known about long-term complications or side effects that might result after surgery. The only serious complication of concern is the possibility of ectopic pregnancy in instances where the sterilization procedure has not been fully effective. There is evidence that menstrual bleeding disorders occur more frequently following sterilization; however, the severity and extent of this side effect is not well documented (Shepard, 1974; Rioux, 1980; Noble, 1978).

### Effects of Health Costs
### on Contraceptive Use and Fertility

Like monetary costs, health costs affect fertility in two ways: through their effect on overall levels of contraceptive use, and through their effect on the mix of methods used. These effects are discussed below for developed and developing countries.

### Effect of Health Costs in Developed Countries

The overall level of contraceptive use in developed nations is little affected by the fact that some methods can cause both minor and serious health problems. It is possible, however, that contraceptive use might fall and fertility rise accordingly if the hazards of a major contraceptive method such as the pill, female sterilization, or vasectomy were to become widespread and serious enough to discourage its use in a country where it is extremely popular.

Many of the most widely used contraceptive methods cause actual or potential serious health problems in substantial numbers, although small proportions, of users. Awareness of this among people of childbearing age, health workers, and policymakers does decrease the use of particular contraceptive methods and thereby influence the prevailing mix of methods in a number of ways.

First, occurrence of a side effect can cause discontinuation of use.  On the other hand, since serious side
effects occur at worst among only about 1.0 to 0.001
percent of users annually, the impact of direct discontinuation on overall levels of use is small.  Method
switching also allows contraceptive use to remain high
despite side effects.

Second, serious side effects can reduce the use of
particular methods if they cause regulatory authorities
to restrict their availability.  Although the health
risks of contraceptives are appreciably outweighed by the
risks of pregnancy for most women, in the case of oral
contraceptives, this calculus of costs versus benefits
has become increasingly unfavorable for older women and
those who smoke (Tietze and Lewit, 1980; Ory, 1979;
Vessey, 1978).  Similarly, the tradeoff between the cost
of potential infertility at older ages and the benefit of
effective contraception at younger ages has become increasingly unfavorable for the IUD in recent years.  At
both the formal level of national health regulations and
the informal level of medical practice, such restrictions
substantially curtail the use of oral contraceptives,
IUDs, and injectable contraceptives in Western countries
(see prescription information for oral contraceptives and
IUD products in the Physicians' Desk Reference, 1981; see
also Contraceptive Technology Update, 1981b; Guillebaud,
1979).  Quantitative estimates of this reduction in
potential use, however, have not been made.

Third, serious side effects can discourage initial use
of a particular contraceptive method by altering perceptions of its benefits and costs.  In developed countries,
especially the United States, this effect has increased
in recent years as public knowledge about the hazards of
different types of contraceptives has risen (Blake, 1977;
Jones et al., 1980; Bruce and Schearer, 1979).  This has
reduced the use of more hazardous methods--oral contraceptives, IUDs, and injectable contraceptives--while
increasing the use of less hazardous ones--sterilization,
the diaphragm, spermicides, and condoms.  Although the
extent of these changes is not known quantitatively,
sales data, market surveys, and other limited surveys do
indicate a substantial shift in usage in these directions
(Colen, 1978; Family Planning Perspectives, 1980a, 1980b;
Torres et al., 1981; Aved, 1981; Power, 1981).[14]

Of course, fully objective knowledge about the health
hazards of contraceptives does not exist; thus the perceptions of both individuals and policymakers play a

large role in their assessments of these costs. These
perceptions are sometimes unrelated to scientific knowledge. Several studies have shown that press reports and
other publicity focusing on serious health hazards of
contraceptives have resulted in sharp, though sometimes
temporary, declines in the use of particular methods
(Jones et al., 1980; Badarocco et al., 1973).

As for minor side effects, the way these influence
selection and continuing use of particular methods is not
well understood. Evidence does suggest that, on the
whole, women in developed countries have a high tolerance
for minor side effects. Although, as noted above, there
has been a trend toward discontinuation of oral and
injectable contraceptives and the IUD, this seems to be
due to concern not about short-term side effects, but
about long-term health hazards (Potts et al., 1975).
Thus, although minor side effects clearly influence the
selection and continued use of different methods, they do
not appear in themselves to be major determinants of
contraceptive use in developed nations.[15]

It is not yet known whether the shift away from more
hazardous methods now being observed in developed countries will affect fertility. However, two factors
strongly suggest that any effect will be negligible.
First, much of the shift away from the highly effective
oral contraceptive and IUD methods has been toward a
still more effective method--sterilization (Family
Planning Perspectives, 1980a; Dunnell, 1979). Second,
the use of abortion has been increasing in developed
nations during recent years (Tietze, 1979, 1981).

However, the fact remains that major shifts in the mix
of contraceptive methods can occur as a result of health
hazards. If very serious new adverse findings about
major methods such as oral contraceptives, intrauterine
devices, or sterilization were to emerge and cause
elimination of two or more of these methods (especially
if coupled with restrictions on the availability of
abortion), the result could be appreciable rises in
fertility, at least until new technology became available. In view of current uncertainties about the
long-term effects of oral contraceptives on cancer, IUDs
on fertility, and vasectomy on autoimmune disease, as
well as the current political climate in many countries
regarding abortion, these possibilities cannot be
disregarded.

## Effect of Health Costs in Developing Countries

In contrast to developed countries, where objective knowledge about the serious side effects of contraceptives appears to exert a strong influence on the mix of methods, evidence suggests that such knowledge exerts only a weak influence on method selection and, indirectly, on the overall prevalence of contraceptive use in developing countries.

Serious health hazards strongly restrict the levels of use of particular methods in Western nations through drug regulatory policies and related screening requirements. Although some limitations of this kind also occur in developing countries, the effect is much weaker. Many developing countries do adopt the same screening and prescription requirements to minimize the serious risks of contraceptives; however, they generally lack adequate medical resources to implement these requirements. In many countries, prescription and screening requirements have been relaxed in recent years, greater use is being made of paramedical personnel for such screening, public health services are expanding, and contraceptives are readily available without screening or authorization despite legal prescription requirements.

In addition, drug regulation is usually less formalized and rigorous in developing than in developed countries, and contraceptive products are more easily approved. For example, injectable contraceptives, which have not yet been approved for general use in most Western countries, are registered and marketed in well over 70 developing countries (Fraser and Weisberg, 1981). In part, this easier approval results from a lack of the technical capacity and data required for comprehensive review of these products (Cook et al., 1981). However, it also reflects the widely held perception of health authorities that the health costs of contraceptive use observed in developed nations may not apply to developing country populations, and that, in any case, such costs are offset by the benefits of controlling fertility and avoiding the high health risks associated with childbearing in these settings (Potts et al., 1978; Atkinson et al., 1974; Kahn and Huber, 1978; Rochat et al., 1978; Fathalla, 1977).

In addition to these differences, the effect of objective knowledge of serious side effects on individual decisions about contraceptive use appears very limited in developing countries. In most Third World nations, levels of knowledge about science, health, and family planning are very low among the majority of people. Information about the serious health hazards of different contraceptives is much less widely publicized and much less widely emphasized in either private medical services or public family planning programs (see e.g., WHO, 1980b).

On the other hand, although objective information about serious health hazards may not play a large role in contraceptive use, fears about serious health problems undoubtedly do. These fears are widespread and often in direct conflict with objective knowledge about such effects. In Mexico, for example, many men and women believe oral contraceptives cause cancer in users and birth defects in children conceived after the method has been stopped (Folch-Lyon et al., 1981). Due to misconceptions about reproductive anatomy, illiterate women sometimes fear that IUDs can become lost within the body (Shedlin and Hollerbach, 1981; Hollerbach, 1980). These fears, rather than knowledge of actual hazards, reduce both the overall practice of contraception and the selection of particular methods in developing countries (Folch-Lyon et al., 1981; Shedlin and Hollerbach, 1981; Hollerbach, 1980).

These fears can also intensify the impact of minor side effects on levels of contraceptive use. For methods that cause numerous minor side effects--oral contraceptives, IUDs, and injectable contraceptives--many more users abandon the method in developing than in developed countries. Discontinuation-of-use rates for these three methods range from 20 to 80 percent per year in developing countries, with mean rates of about 40 percent for oral contraceptives and 30 percent for IUDs; roughly one-third of those stopping use say they are doing so because of minor side effects (Kreager, 1977; Mauldin, 1979). The impact of minor side effects on use is intensely subjective. With strong family planning counseling, client support, and community endorsement of birth control methods, minor side effects may not be a major obstacle to contraceptive use (Tsu, 1980). In most developing country settings, however, these ideal conditions are not present. Although survey research has not extensively examined this issue, limited data indicate that substantial numbers of women in developing countries who want no more children avoid contraceptives because of fear of side effects (see Table 7). This impact of fear of side effects on contraceptive use can have a significant effect on fertility. The extent of this impact varies considerably from country to country and within countries,

TABLE 7   Percentage of All Married Women of Reproductive
Age Who Are Not Using Contraception Mainly Because of
Fear of Side Effects

| Country and Region | Year | Percent | Country and Region | Year | Percent |
|---|---|---|---|---|---|
| Brazil | | | Guatemala | 1978 | 19 |
| Piaui State | 1979 | 36 | Korea, South | 1979 | 11 |
| Sao Paulo State | 1978 | 31 | Mexico | 1978 | 9 |
| Colombia | 1978 | 11 | Panama | 1979 | 31 |
| Costa Rica | 1978 | 27 | Thailand | 1978 | 60 |
| El Salvador | 1978 | 24 | Tunisia (Jendouba) | 1979 | 28 |

Source:  Morris et al. (1981).

depending on the proportion not using contraception and
not wishing to have more children.[16]

As family planning programs are extended more widely
in developing countries and as levels of contraceptive
use increase, it is likely that fears of side effects
will be attenuated.  Indeed, the effect of greater
knowledge and experience on reducing fears of contraception may be a major reason for the very rapid increase in
levels of use in most developing nations over the past
decade (Kendall, 1979; Morris et al., 1981).  On the
other hand, it is also likely that this diffusion of
information and services will ultimately exert a negative
impact on usage, at least for those methods known to
cause serious health problems.  Thus, it appears likely
that over the short term, very substantial increases in
contraceptive use will result from a decline in subjective fears and the associated impact of minor side
effects.  Over the long run, however, the importance of
serious objective health hazards is likely to increase,
both at the individual and at the national drug-regulating
and policymaking levels, creating a situation closely
analogous to that which exists now in developed countries.


PROPOSITIONS

The following propositions summarize the major points
raised in the above discussion.
1.   There are basically four components of the monetary
costs of contraception:  costs of development and production, of related services required for use, of distribution of products and services, and of gaining access.

2. The monetary costs of contraceptive use will be borne differently depending on the source of the products and services. When the source is private, most costs are paid by the user. When the source is public (e.g., health clinics and family planning programs), most costs are paid through funds obtained from government revenues, foreign aid, and philanthropic contributions.

2.1. Costs arising from distribution, including marketing, account for the better part of the total price of most contraceptive products sold in the private sector.

2.2. The overall monetary costs of contraceptives obtained in the private sector are remarkably uniform from country to country. Since manufacturing costs do not vary widely, it can be assumed that there is a common basic structure for distribution costs among developing countries.

2.3. In general, the monetary costs of contraceptives obtained in the private sector appear not to have risen significantly over time.

2.4. In general, the monetary costs of contraception provided by private and public sources do not differ markedly, although they are borne differently.

3. The negative effect of contraceptive use on fertility is well documented. The precise nature of this effect varies with the mix of methods used—whether more or less effective. Thus the monetary costs of contraception will affect fertility through both overall levels of use and method mix.

3.1. In developed countries, the effect of monetary costs on both overall use and method mix is apparently minimal. Therefore, the impact of these costs on fertility levels in these countries is also minimal.

3.2. Monetary costs have a greater effect in developing countries. The apparent inability of significant numbers of people to afford contraceptives discourages private firms from extending their marketing and distribution activities beyond higher-income to rural areas and the marginal areas of cities, where income is typically lower. This greatly limits availability of contraceptives through private channels.

3.3. The relatively low availability of contraceptives from private sources in developing countries in turn requires large expenditures of public funds to provide contraception through family planning programs. In many countries, however, the coverage of these programs is limited, in significant measure because of insufficient public revenue to cover their costs. Thus,

except in those countries with very active family
planning programs, contraceptive use is decreased and
fertility increased because the monetary costs of
contraception substantially reduce the availability of
supplies and services.

3.4.   However, people's ability to pay for contraceptives may be higher than is generally believed.  Evidence
indicates a substantial price elasticity for contraceptives among all but the poorest segments of society in
many developing countries.  Further study is needed on
this issue, since private sources of supply may be capable
of serving much larger portions of the population than
they now do.  Also, savings may be possible by reducing
the overlap of services that result when full-scale
family planning programs are established in areas where
private services are available because it is believed
that high private costs will discourage use.

4.   All birth control methods provide at least partial
protection against pregnancy.  However, these benefits
(in the form of reduced personal fertility and avoidance
of the potential adverse effects of pregnancy and childbirth, especially in developing countries) must be
weighed against the minor side effects and major health
hazards of most contraceptive methods.

5.   Like monetary costs, health costs of contraception
affect fertility through both overall levels of use and
mix of methods.

5.1.   In developed countries, awareness of potential
serious health effects influences the mix of methods by
reducing use of those with the most severe effects (oral
and injectable contraceptives and the IUD).  Short-term
side effects do not appear to have a significant
influence on patterns of use.

5.2.   The effect of these shifts away from more hazardous methods on fertility levels in developed countries
is probably negligible:  much of the shift has been toward
an even more effective method--sterilization--and the use
of abortion has been increasing in these countries.

5.3.   In developing countries, knowledge of the serious
health hazards of contraceptives has a much weaker effect
on both overall use and mix of methods.  On the other
hand, fears about these effects do have a significant
negative impact.  These fears both prevent initial use of
methods and intensify the impact of minor side effects on
discontinuation of use.

5.4.   The impact of such fears of contraceptive use on
fertility levels varies from country to country and

within countries, depending on the proportion not using
contraception and not wishing to have more children.
Diffusion of knowledge and experience through increased
use of contraception in a society and through provision
of information and supportive services by family planning
programs can substantially reduce these fears. However,
over the long term, this greater knowledge will eventually have a negative effect on the use of those methods
known to have serious health effects, as has occurred in
developed countries.

## NOTES

1.  Abortion techniques, which are the subject of another
    paper, will not be included in this analysis (see
    David, in these volumes).
2.  Since the prevalence of use of methods in three of
    these categories--postcoital douching, minipill oral
    contraceptives, and postcoital contraceptives--is
    extremely limited, these categories will not be
    discussed in detail in this paper.
3.  In 1980, the author conducted a questionnaire of 99
    professional staff members of the Population Council,
    the United Nations Fund for Population Activities,
    the Ford Foundation, and the United States Agency for
    International Development located in 46 developing
    countries. Respondents were asked to provide data on
    the prices charged to consumers for contraceptive
    products and services; these data were obtained
    directly from local pharmacies, physicians, and
    family planning service outlets. By June 1981,
    responses had been received from 29 respondents in 23
    developing countries. After clarification of
    ambiguous responses by telephone and letter, these
    data were used as the basis for Tables 1-3 and
    Appendix Tables 1 and 2.
4.  On the average, about 40 percent of the total
    monetary costs of contraception provided through
    public-sector channels in developing countries is
    borne by the developing country governments them-
    selves, about 50 percent is borne by foreign aid from
    developed nations, and about 10 percent is borne by
    private charitable contributions, mainly from
    foundations located in the United States. These
    proportions differ widely from country to country, as
    do the proportions of total local governmental

revenues devoted to public family planning programs (Office of Technology Assessment, in press).

5. Although survey data are not available, reports from those familiar with family planning programs suggest that the price of IUDs may have risen much more significantly during the last decade. Major new technical innovations in this method, adding significantly to its manufacturing costs, could help to explain these cost increases; however, market factors appear responsible for a major share.

6. These problems have been reviewed recently in depth at an International Workshop on Cost Effectiveness Analysis and Cost Benefit Analysis in Family Planning Programs held on August 17-20, 1981 at The Johns Hopkins University. The reader is referred to papers prepared for presentation at this workshop, as well as to Kelly, 1971; Simmons, 1971, 1973; Agarwala, 1971; Correa et al., 1972; Lawrence et al., 1973; Reardon et al., 1974; Trussell, 1974; Haran, 1979; Chamie and Henshaw, 1981; Nortman, 1981.

7. It should be noted that the yearly average costs described include few if any expenditures for public information, education, or promotional activities. In contrast to public family planning programs, private sources avoid direct public contact and instead concentrate their marketing and advertising on the medical professionals, pharmacists, and others involved in drug distribution (Farley and Tokarski, 1975; Black, 1973; Business International, 1978).

8. In seven countries, this figure is as low as 50-65 percent for some brands of pills; in a few it is much higher, rising to as much as 97 percent in Nigeria. Although there has been some study of the cause for these variations in range, much more detailed empirical analysis of the pertinent market conditions is needed to explain them.

9. More than one-half hour of travel time is required for 26 percent of rural Thai users, 46 percent of rural Indian users, 27 percent of rural Panamanian users, 34 percent of rural users in Sao Paulo State, Brazil, and 44 percent of rural Turkish users (Rodriguez, 1977; Foreit and Gorosh, 1978; Nakamura and Fonesca, 1979).

10. Although monetary costs associated with private-sector sources of supply may affect contraceptive decision making for some of the poorest segments of the population in some developed countries, this

impact is cushioned by social welfare programs in most instances.

11. In addition to direct deleterious health effects, adverse effects of pregnancies arising as a consequence of a method's incomplete effectiveness can also be considered (see Hatcher et al., 1980; Office of Technology Assessment, 1982, Bruce and Schearer, 1979). However, the present discussion will not address this risk.

12. Their short-term effects have been extensively studied, revealing an increase in the incidence of menstrual bleeding irregularities, but decreases in other minor side effects (Sanhueza et al., 1979; Talwar and Berger, 1977; Talwar et al., 1977; Brat, 1976; Rudel et al., 1978; Ingemanson et al., 1976).

13. There is inconclusive evidence, however, that birth abnormalities may be increased if conception occurs during or within the first few weeks after cessation of use of oral contraceptives (Kasan and Andrews, 1980; Harlap et al., 1979).

14. Although it is difficult to demonstrate conclusively that this shift results from serious health costs and the public's perception of them, the body of evidence cited above indicates that health costs play a major role. It should also be noted, however, that numerous other factors enter into personal assessments of the risks and benefits of contraceptive use in a highly complex, individualized manner, and that, for many individuals, some of these other factors appear to have greater weight than health risks (Kee and Darroch, 1981; Hollerbach, 1980; Miller, 1979; Folch-Lyon et al., 1981).

15. The strength of placebo effects observed for contraceptives and the difficulty of disentangling both the objective and perceived threat of serious health hazards from the occurrence of minor side effects suggests that minor side effects can have some impact on use. When anxiety about serious health effects is high, minor side effects can trigger a decision to discontinue use or avoid a particular method.

16. In Thailand, for example, although 47 percent of the married, reproductive-age women are not using contraception, only about one third of these are sexually active, fecund, and want no more children.

Of this group, those who directly state they use no method because of fear of side effects amount to 9 percent of the overall reproductive-age, married population.  Assuming that 10 percentage points in contraceptive practice results in roughly one less live birth per women on the average, fears about the health effects of contraception in Thailand increase the total fertility rate by at least one (Morris et al., 1981).

## BIBLIOGRAPHY

Agarwala, S. (1971)  The measurement of costs and benefits of different methods of family planning.  Pp. 41-51 in Aspects of Population Policy in India.  New Delhi:  Council for Social Development.

Alexander, N., and T. Clarkson (1978)  Vasectomy increases the severity of diet-induced atherosclerosis.  Macaca Fascicularis Science 201:538-541.

Alexander, N., B. Wilson, and G. Patterson (1974)  Vasectomy:  Immunological effects on Rhesus monkeys and men.  Fertility and Sterility 25:149-156.

Altman, D., and P. Piotrow (1980)  Social marketing--does it work?  Population Reports, Series J:393-436.

Anderson, J., and L. Morris (1981)  Fertility differences and the need for family planning services in five Latin American countries.  International Family Planning Perspectives 7:16-21.

Andolsek, L. (1975)  The Ljublijana IUD experience:  Ten years.  Pp. 205-216 in F. Hefnawi and S. Segal, eds., Analysis of Intrauterine Contraception.  New York: North Holland/American Elsevier.

Ansbacher, R., B. Williams, and D. Mumford (1975)  Vas ligation:  Sperm antibodies.  Pp. 189-195 in J. J. Sciarra, C. Markland, and J. J. Speidel, eds., Control of Male Fertility.  New York:  Harper and Row.

Atkinson, L., R. Castadot, A. Cuadros, and A. Rosenfield (1974)  Oral contraceptives:  Considerations of safety in non-clinical distribution.  Studies in Family Planning 5:242-249.

Aved, B. (1981)  Trends in contraceptive method of use by California family planning clinic clients aged 10-55, 1976-1979.  American Journal of Public Health 71:1162-1164.

Badarocco, M., M. Vessey, and P. Wiggins (1973) The effect of the statement by the Committee on Safety of Drugs Concerning Oral Contraceptives Containing Oestrogens on the contraceptive practices of women attending two family planning clinics. Journal of Obstetrics and Gynecology of the British Commonwealth 80:353-356.

Badham, D. (1978) Quantities and Dollar Values of Contraceptives Purchased by WHO, 1976-78. Personal communication, March 28.

Bailey, J., and J. Correa (1975) Evaluation of the Profamilia rural family planning program. Studies in Family Planning 6:148-155.

Baldwin, B. (1978) The McCormick family planning program in Chiang Mai, Thailand. Studies in Family Planning 9:300-313.

Belsky, R. (1975) Vaginal contraceptives--a time for reappraisal? Population Reports, Series H:37-75.

Berendes, H., and R. Crozier (1975) Vasectomy research program of the Center for Population Research. Pp. 164-168 in J. J. Sciarra, C. Markland, and J. J. Speidel, eds., Control of Male Fertility. New York: Harper and Row.

Berger, G., L. Keith, and W. Moss (1975) Prevalence of gonorrhea among women using various methods of contraception. British Journal of Venereal Diseases 51:307.

Black, T. (1973) Rationale for the involvement of private sector marketing institutions in family planning in Africa. Studies in Family Planning 4:25-32.

Blake, J. (1977) The pill and the rising costs of fertility control. Social Biology 24:267-280.

Blumenfeld, S. (1981) Cost Analysis of the Danfa (Ghana) Project Family Planning Component. Paper prepared for International Workshop on Cost-Effectiveness Analysis and Cost-Benefit Analysis in Family Planning Programs, The John Hopkins University, Baltimore, Md.

Bongaarts, J. (1978) A framework for analyzing the proximate determinants of fertility. Population and Development Review 4:105-132.

Bongaarts, J., and S. Kirmeyer (1980) Estimating the Impact of Contraceptive Prevalence on Fertility, Aggregate and Age-Specific Versions of a Model. Paper presented at the IUSSP Seminar on Use of Surveys for Analysis of Family Planning Programmes, Bogota, Colombia.

Boon, M., R. Kirk, and G. de Graaff (1981) Psammoma bodies and some opportunistic infections detected in cervical smears of women fitted with an IUD. Contraceptive Delivery Systems 2:231–236.

Bordes, A., J. Allman, J. Revson, and A. Verly (1981) Household Distribution of Contraceptives in Rural Haiti: The Results and Costs of the Division of Family Hygiene's Experimental Project. Paper prepared for the International Workshop on Cost-Effectiveness Analysis and Cost-Benefit Analysis in Family Planning Programs, The John Hopkins University, Baltimore, Md.

Boston Collaborative Drug Surveillance Program (1973) Contraceptives and venous thromboembolic disease, surgically confirmed gallbladder disease and breast tumors. Lancet 1:1399–1404.

Bounds, W., M. Vessey, and P. Wiggins (1979) A randomized double-blind trial of two low dose combined oral contraceptives. British Journal of Obstetrics and Gynecology 86:325–329.

Bourdais, J. P., P. Delavierre, O. Bourdais-Varenne, and J. Hureau (1977) Headache and the O.C. Seminaires Hospitaliare de Paris 53:425–432.

Brackett, J. (1980) The Role of Family Planning Availability and Accessibility in Family Planning Use in Developing Countries. Paper presented at World Fertility Survey Conference, London.

Brat, T. (1976) Four years overall experience with a new low estrogen low progestin O.C. Acta Obstetrica Gynecologica Scandanavia Supplement 54:67–70.

Briggs, M. H. (1977) Combined oral contraceptives. Pp. 253–282 in E. Dizfalusy, ed., Regulation of Human Fertility. Copenhagen: Scriptor.

Bruce, J., and S. B. Schearer (1979) Contraceptives and Common Sense: Conventional Methods Reconsidered. New York: Population Council.

Burkman, R., and the Women's Health Study (1980) Association between intrauterine device and pelvic inflammatory disease. Obstetrics and Gynecology 57:269–276.

Business International (1978) International Factfinding Study: Private Sector Marketing of Contraceptives in Eight Developing Countries. Study prepared for the Population Council. New York: Business International.

Calderone, M. (1970) Editor's note on coitus interruptus. Pp. 437–438 in M. S. Calderone, ed., Manual of Family Planning and Contraceptive Practice. Baltimore, Md.: The Williams and Wilkins Co.

Casagrande, J. T., E. W. Louie, M. C. Pike, and S. Roy (1979)  Incessant ovulation and ovarian cancer. Lancet 11:170-173.

Cates, W., Jr., H. Ory, R. Rochat, and C. Tyler (1976) The intrauterine device and deaths from spontaneous abortion. New England Journal of Medicine 295:1155-1159.

Chamie, M., and S. Henshaw (1981)  The costs and benefits of government expenditures for family planning programs. Family Planning Perspectives 13:117-124.

Chen, K. M. (1981)  The Cost-Effectiveness of a Community-Based Social Marketing Project in Thailand: The Family Planning Health and Hygiene Project.  Paper prepared for the International Workshop on Cost-Effectiveness Analysis and Cost-Benefit Analysis in Family Planning Programs, The John Hopkins University, Baltimore, Md.

Chen, L., M. Gesche, S. Ahmed, A. Chowdhury, and W. Mosley (1979)  Maternal mortality in rural Bangladesh. Studies in Family Planning 5:334-341.

Chvapil, M., C. Eskelson, V. Stiffel, J. Owen, and W. Droegemueller (1980)  Studies on nonoxynol-9.  II. Intravaginal absorption, distribution metabolism, and excretion in rats. Contraception 22:325-339.

Clarkson, T., and N. Alexander (1979)  Effect of long-term vasectomy on the occurrence and extent of arteriosclerosis in rhesus monkeys fed monkey chow. Federation Proceedings 38(part 2):1346.

Coleman, S., and P. Piotrow (1979)  Spermicides-- Simplicity and safety are major assets. Population Reports, Series H:77-120.

Colen, G. (1978)  Article in The Washington Post, January 25.

Committee on Family Planning (1973)  Taiwan Population Studies Summaries.  Study No. 55 and unnumbered study, "Free Offer."  Taichung, Taiwan:  Taiwan Provincial Department of Health.

Connell, E. (1979)  Vaginal contraception:  Current FDA status.  Pp. 221-223 in G. Zatuchni, A. Sobrero, J. Speidel, and J. Sciarra, eds., Vaginal Contraception, New Developments.  New York:  Harper and Row.

Contraceptive Technology Update (1981a)  Actinomyces in IUD users:  Management, prevention sparks controversy. Contraceptive Technology Update 2:29-32.

Contraceptive Technology Update (1981b)  Updated contra-indications to combined Ocs. Contraceptive Technology Update 2:39.

Cook, R., J. Strand, and S. B. Schearer (1981) Contraceptives and Drug Regulation: An International Perspective. PIACT Paper, Program for the Introduction and Adaptation of Contraceptive Technology, Seattle, Wash.

Correa, H. (1975) Population, Health, Nutrition and Development. Lexington, Mass: Lexington Books.

Correa, H., V. Parrish, and J. Beasley (1972) A three-year longitudinal evaluation of the costs of a family planning program. American Journal of Public Health 62:1647-1657.

Coulam, C. B., J. F. Annegers, C. F. Abboud, E. R. Laws, and L. T. Kurland (1979) Pituitary adenoma and oral contraceptives: A case-control study. Fertility and Sterility 31:25-28.

Cross River Study, Ministry of Health (1981) The Calabar Rural Maternal and Child Health Family Planning Project 1975-1980 Final Report. Calabar, Nigeria: Cross River State Ministry of Health.

Cullberg, G., and B. Larsson (1979) Some adverse effects of copper IUDs. Acta Obstetrica Gynecologica Scandanavia 58:87.

Cutler, J. (1975) Prevention of V.D.--Returning to the birth control devices of the past. Medical Opinion October:4-10.

Darabi, K., K. Roy, and R. Richart (1978) Collaborative study on hysteroscopic sterilization procedures: Final report. Pp. 81-101 in J. Sciarra, G. Zatuchni, and J. Speidel, eds., Risks, Benefits, and Controversies in Fertility Control. New York: Harper and Row.

Davis, J. (1980) Risks and benefits of vasectomy. Pp. 260-266 in L. Koth, ed., The Safety of Fertility Control. New York: Springer Publishing.

Davis, K., and J. Blake (1956) Social structure and fertility: An analytic framework. Economic Development and Cultural Change 4:211.

Dreishpoon, I. H. (1975) Complications of pregnancy with an intrauterine contraceptive device in Situ. American Journal of Obstetrics and Gynecology 121:412-413.

Duguid, H., D. Parratt, and R. Traynor (1980) Actinomyces-like organisms in cervical smears from women using intrauterine contraceptive devices. British Medical Journal 281:534.

Dunnell, I. K. (1979) Family Formation, 1976. Office of Population Censuses and Surveys, Social Survey

Division, Her Majesty's Stationery Office (HMSO),
    London.

Dusitsin, N., S. Varakamin, P. Ningsanen, S. Chalapati,
    and B. Boonsiri (1980) Postpartum tubal ligation by
    nurse-midwives and doctors in Thailand. Lancet
    1:638-639.

Edelman, D., G. Berger, and L. Keith (1979) Intrauterine
    Devices and Their Complications. Boston: G. Kitall.

Enke, S., and B. Hickman (1976) Offering bonuses to
    reduce fertility. Pp. 191-210 in M. Keely, ed.,
    Population, Public Policy and Economic Development.
    New York: Praeger.

Eschenbach, D. A., J. P. Harnisch, and K. K. Holmes
    (1977) Pathogenesis of acute pelvic inflammatory
    disease: Role of contraception and other risk
    factors. American Journal of Obstetrics and
    Gynecology 128:838-850.

Falkner, W., and Ory, H. (1976) Intrauterine devices and
    acute pelvic inflammatory disease. Journal of the
    American Medical Association 235:1851-1853.

Family Planning Perspectives (1980a) 1.1 million
    sterilizations were performed in 1978; Six in ten were
    to women. Family Planning Perspectives 12:113.

Family Planning Perspectives (1980b) Bacterial infection
    from actinomyces, though rare, is found to be a
    problem among some IUD users. Family Planning
    Perspectives 12:306-307.

Farley, J., and S. Tokarski (1975) Legal restrictions on
    the distribution of contraceptives in the developing
    nations: Some suggestions for determining priorities
    and estimating impact of change. Columbia Human
    Rights Law Review 6:415-446.

Fathalla, M. (1977) Safety of the Pill. Paper presented
    at 2nd Regional Conference on Village and Household
    Availability of Contraceptives, Tunis, Tunisia.

Folch-Lyon, E., L. de la Macorra, and S. B. Schearer
    (1981) Focus group and survey research on family
    planning in Mexico. Studies in Family Planning
    12:409-432.

Food and Drug Administration, Department of Health and
    Human Services (1980) Part V. Vaginal contraceptive
    drug products for over the counter human use;
    establishment of a monograph; proposed rulemaking.
    Federal Register 45(242):82014-82049.

Foreit, J., and M. Gorosh (1978) Community-based and
    commercial contraceptives distribution: An inventory
    and appraisal. Population Reports, Series J:1-29.

Fraser, I., and E. Weisberg (1981)  A comprehensive review of injectable contraception with special emphasis on depot medroxyprogesterone acetate.  The Medical Journal of Australia, Special Supplement, Vol. 1, No. 1.

Gillespie, D., M. Mamlouk, and K. M. Chen (1981) Cost-Effectiveness of Family Planning:  Overview of the Literature.  Working Draft.  Paper prepared for International Workshop on Cost-Effectiveness Analysis and Cost Benefit Analysis in Family Planning Programs, The John Hopkins University, Baltimore, Md.

Goldacre, M., M. Vessey, J. Clarke, and M. Heasman (1978)  Record linkage study of morbidity following vasectomy.  Pp 567-579 in F. Lepou and H. Crozier, eds., Vasectomy:  Immunologic and Pathophysiologic Effects in Animals and Man.  New York:  Academic Press.

Goldzieher, J., L. Moses, E. Averkin, C. Scheel, and B. Tabler (1971)  A placebo controlled doubleblind crossover investigation of side effects attributed to oral contraceptives.  Fertility and Sterility 22:609-623.

Gonzalez, E. (1981)  Calcium deposits on IUDs and infection.  Journal of the American Medical Association 245:1625.

Gray, R. (1976)  Pelvic inflammatory disease and intrauterine contraceptive devices.  Lancet 2:521.

Gray, R. (1979)  Norethisterone oenanthate as an injectable contraceptive.  British Medical Journal 1:343.

Gray, R. (1980)  Patterns of bleeding associated with the use of hormonal contraceptives.  Pp. 14-19 in E. Diczfalusy, I. Fraser, and F. Webb, eds., Endometrial Bleeding and Steroidal Contraception.  England: Pitman Press.

Greenspan, A., R. Hatcher, M. Moore, M. Rosenberg, and H. Ory (1980)  The association of depomedroxyprogesterone acetate and breast cancer.  Contraception 21:563:569.

Guillebaud, J. (1979)  The safety of intrauterine devices.  Studies in Family Planning 10:174-177.

Guillebaud, J., J. Bonnar, J. Morehead, and A. Mathews (1976)  Menstrual blood loss with intrauterine devices.  Lancet 1:21-24.

Haran, E. (1979)  An optimization model for the allocation of resources in family planning programs. Socioeconomic Planning Sciences 13:13-20.

Harlap, S., P. Shiono, F. Pellegrin, M. Golbus, R. Bachman, J. Mann, L. Schmidt, and J. Lewis (1979)

Chromosome abnormalities in oral contraceptive breakthrough pregnancies. Lancet 8130:1342-1343.

Harris, I. R. W. C., L. A. Brinton, R. H. Cowdell, D. C. G. Skegg, P. G. Smith, M. P. Vessey, and R. Doll (1980) Characteristics of women with dysplasia or carcinoma in situ of the cervix uteri. British Journal of Cancer 42:359.

Hatcher, R., G. Stewart, F. Steward, R. Guest, D. Schwartz, and S. Jones (1980) Contraceptive Technology: 1980-1981. New York: Irvington Publishers.

Hearings Before the Select Committee on Population (1978) The Depo-Provera Debate. U.S. House of Representatives. Washington, D.C.: U.S. Government Printing Office.

Hollerbach, P. (1980) Factors That Determine the Appropriateness of New Technologies to Consumer Needs. Paper prepared for the Office of Technology Assessment of the U.S. Congress. Population Council, New York.

Huggins, G. R. (1977) Contraceptive use and subsequent fertility. Fertility and Sterility 28:603-612.

Hull, M., D. Brownham, P. Savage, and J. Jackson (1981) Normal fertility in women with post-pill amenorrhea. Lancet 8234:1329-1332.

Hunton, M. (1976) A retrospective survey of over 1,000 patients on O.C. in a group practice. Journal of the Royal College of General Practitioners 26:538-546.

Ingemanson, C. A., M. Jagerhorn, J. Zizala, B. Nilsson, and G. Zader (1976) Preliminary results from a Swedish multicenter trial of a new low dose comined O.C. Acta Obstetrica Gynecologica Scandanavia Supplement 54:71-75.

Inman, W. H. W., M. P. Vessey, B. Westerholm, and A. Engelund (1970) Thromboembolic disease and the steroid content of oral contraceptives. A report to the Committee on Safety of Drugs. British Medical Journal 2:203-209.

International Planned Parenthood Federation Medical Bulletin (1980) IPPF International Medical Advisory Panel Meeting - October 1980; Injectable Contraception. IPPF Medical Bulletin 14:1-3.

Jennings, J. (1974) Report of Safety and Efficacy of the Dalkon Shield and other IUDs. Mimeo prepared by the ad hoc Obstetric-Gynecology Advisory Committee (to the U.S. Food and Drug Administration).

Jick, H., A. Walker, K. Rothman, J. Hunter, L. Holmes, R. Watkins, D. D'Ewart, A. Danford, and S. Madsen (1981a) Vaginal spermicides and congenital disorders. Journal of the American Medical Association 245:1329-1332.

Jick, H., A. Walker, R. Watkins, D. D'Ewart, J. Hunter, A. Danford, S. Madsen, B. Dinan, and K. Rothman (1981b) Oral contraceptives and breast cancer. American Journal of Epidemiology 112:577.

Jones, E., J. Beniger, and C. Westoff (1980) Pill and IUD discontinuation in the United States, 1970-1975: The influence of the media. Family Planning Perspectives 12:293-300.

Jongbloet, P. (1971) Month of Birth and Gametopathy. Pp. 62-79 in Mental and Physical Handicaps in Connection with Overripeness Ovopathy. Leiden: H.E. Stenfert Kroese, N.V.

Kahn, A., and D. Huber (1978) Safety of Contraceptive Practice as Compared to Non-Contraception. FRP Technical Report No. 7. Bangladesh Fertility Research Programme, Dacca, Bangladesh.

Kahn, H., and C. Tyler (1975a) IUD related hospitalizations, United States and Puerto Rico, 1973. Journal of the American Medical Association 234:53-56.

Kahn, H., and C. Tyler (1975b) IUD insertion practices in the United States and Puerto Rico. Family Planning Perspectives 7:209-212.

Kahn, H., and C. Tyler (1975c) Mortality associated with the use of IUDs. Journal of the American Medical Association 234:57-59.

Kasan, P., and J. Andrews (1980) Oral contraception and congenital abnormalities. British Journal of Obstetrics and Gynecology 87:548.

Kaufman, D., S. Shapiro, D. Slone, L. Rosenberg, O. Meittinen, P. Stolley, R. Knapp, T. Leavitt, Jr., W. Watring, N. Rosenchein, J. Lewis, Jr., D. Schottenfeld, and R. Engle (1980a) Decreased risk of endometrial cancer among oral contraceptive users. New England Journal of Medicine 303:1045-1047.

Kaufman, D., S. Shapiro, L. Rosenberg, R. Monson, O. Mettinen, P. Stolley, and D. Sloane (1980b) Intrauterine contraceptive device use and pelvic inflammatory disease. American Journal of Obstetrics and Gynecology 136:159-162.

Kay, C. R. (1980) The happiness pill? Journal of the Royal College of General Practitioners 30:8-19.

Kee, P. K., and R. Darroch (1981) Perception of methods of contraception: A semantic differential study. Journal of Biosocial Sciences 13:209-218.

Kelly, W. (1971) A Cost-Effectiveness Study of Clinical Methods of Birth Control: With Special Reference to Puerto Rico. New York: Praeger.

Kendall, M. (1979) The world fertility survey: Current status and findings. Population Reports, Series M:73-104.

Kestelman, P., and R. Kleinman, eds. (1976) Directory of Contraceptives. London: International Planned Parenthood Federation.

Kreager, P. (1977) Family Planning Drop-Outs Reconsidered. London: International Planned Parenthood Federation.

Krueger, D., S. Ellenberg, S. Bloom, B. Calkins, C. Maliza, D. Nolan, R. Phillips, J. C. Rios, I. Rosin, R. B. Shekelle, K. Spector, V. Stadel, P. Stolley, and M. Terris (1980) Fatal myocardial infarction and the role of oral contraceptives. American Journal of Epidemiology 111:655-674.

Lalu, P. (1957) Une glossite. Maroc Medical 36:487.

Lawrence, C., A. Mundigo, and C. Revelle (1973) Analysis of allocation of resources in family planning programs. Management Science 20:520-531.

Ledger, W. (1974) Relationship of pelvic infection to various types of contraception. Clinical Obstetrics and Gynecology 17:79-81.

Leridon, H. (1981) Fertility and contraception in 12 developed countries. International Family Planning Perspectives 7:70-78.

Liedholm P., G. Rybo, N. O. Sjoberg, and L. Solvell (1975) Copper IUD influence on menstrual blood loss and iron deficiency. Contraception 12:317.

Lippes, J. (1975) Infection and the IUD: A Preliminary Report. Contraception 12:103.

Luukkainen, T., N. Nielson, K. G. Nygren, T. Pyorala, and A. Kosenen (1979) Randomized comparison of clinical performance of two copper releasing IUDs, Nova-T and Copper-T 200, in Denmark, Finland, and Sweden. Contraception 19:1-9.

Mann, J. (1978) Oral contraception and myocardial infarction in younger women: Data from countries other than the United States. In J. Sciarra, G. Zatuchni, and T. Speidel, eds., Risks, Benefits, and Controversies in Fertility Control. New York: Harper and Row.

Mann, J., and W. Inman (1975) Oral contraceptives and death from myocardial infarction. British Medical Journal 2:245-248.

Mann, J. I., R. Doll, M. Thorogood, M. P. Vessey, and W. E. Waters (1976)  Risk factors for myocardial infarction in young women. British Journal of Preventive and Social Medicine 30:94-100.

Masters, W., and V. Johnson (1964)  Sexual response: Anatomy and physiology. Pp. 460-473 in C. W. Lloyd, ed., Human Reproduction and Sexual Behavior. Philadelphia: Lea and Febiger.

Mathews, J., D. Shegg, M. Vessey, M. Konice, E. Holborow, and J. Guillebaud (1976)  Weak autoantibody reactions to antigens other than sperm after vasectomy. British Medical Journal 2:1359-1360.

Mauldin, W. P. (1979)  Experience with contraceptive methods in developing countries. Pp. 50-104 in Contraception: Science, Technology, and Application. Washington, D.C.: National Academy of Sciences.

McCann, M. (1978)  Laparoscopy versus minilaparotomy. Pp. 68-80 in J. Sciarra, G. Zatuchni, and J. Speidel, eds., Risks, Benefits, and Controversies in Fertility Control. New York: Harper and Row.

McCann, M., and L. Cole (1980)  Laparoscopy and minilaparotomy:  Two major advances in female sterilization. Studies in Family Planning 11:119-127.

McGowan, L., L. Parent, W. Lednar, and H. Norris (1979) The woman at risk for developing ovarian cancer. Gynecological Oncology 7:325-344.

Meade, T., G. Greenberg, and S. Thompson (1980) Progestogens and cardiovascular reactions associated with oral contraceptives and a comparison of the safety of 50 and 30$\mu$ g oestrogen preparations. British Medical Journal 280:1157-1161.

Menken, J., J. Trussell, K. Ford, and W. Pratt (1979) Experience with contraceptive methods in developed countries. Pp. 24-44 in Contraception: Science, Technology, and Application. Washington, D.C.: National Academy of Sciences.

Mertaugh, M. (1980)  Factors Influencing the Demand for Children and Their Relationships to Contraceptive Use. Paper prepared for the Office of Technology Assessment of the U.S. Congress. Population Council, New York.

Miller, W. (1979)  Psychosocial aspects of contraception. In Contraception: Science, Technology, and Application. Washington, D.C.: National Academy of Sciences.

Mishell, D., Jr. (1975)  The clinic factor in evaluating IUDs. Pp. 27-36 in F. Hefnawi and S. Segal, eds.,

Analysis of Intrauterine Contraception. North Holland, The Netherlands: American Elsevier.

Morris, L., G. Lewis, D. Powell, J. Anderson, A. Way, J. Cushing, and G. Lawless (1981) Contraceptive prevalence surveys: A new source of family planning data. Population Reports, Series M:161-200.

Mumford, S., P. Bhiwandiwala, and F. Chi (1980) Laparoscopic and minilaparotomy female sterilization compared in 15,167 cases. Lancet 2:1066.

Nakamura, M., and J. Fonesca (1979) Sao Paulo State Contraceptive Prevalence Survey. Final Report. Pontifica Universidade Catolica de Campanas. Campinas, Brazil.

Nash, H. (1975) Depo-provera: A review. Contraception 12:377-393.

Newhouse, M., R. Pearson, J. Fullerton, E. Boeson, and H. Shannon (1977) A case control study of carcinoma of the ovary. British Journal of Preventive and Social Medicine 31:148-153.

Newman, D. (1980) Personal communication.

Nissen, E., S. Nissen, and D. R. Kent (1979a) Liver neoplasia and oral contraceptives. Pp. 176-184 in J. Sciarra, G. Zatuchni, and J. Speidel, eds., Risks, Benefits, and Controversies in Fertility Control. New York: Harper and Row.

Nissen, E., D. Kent, and S. Nissen (1979b) Role of oral contraceptive agents in the pathogenesis of liver tumors. Journal of Toxicological and Environmental Health 5:231-254.

Noble, A. (1978) Female sterilization: Long term effects. Pp. 102-107 in J. Sciarra, G. Zatuchni, and J. Speidel, eds., Risks, Benefits, and Controversies in Fertility Control. New York: Harper and Row.

Nordberg, O., and L. Atkinson (1979) Evaluation of the Safety of Modern Contraceptives in Developing Countries. PIACT Paper, Seattle, Wash.

Nortman, D. (1981) Measurement of Family Planning Program Inputs in Different Program Structures. Center for Policy Studies Working Paper. Population Council, New York.

Nortman, D., and E. Hofstatter (1980) Population and Family Planning Programs, 10th ed. New York: Population Council.

O'Ferrall, G. (1973) Effect of varying the time of artificial insemination in relation to ovulation or conception and prenatal losses in the rabbit. Biology of Reproduction 9:338-342.

Office of Technology Assessment (1982)  <u>World Population</u> <u>and Fertility Planning Technologies:  The Next 20</u> <u>Years</u>. Washington, D.C.:  U.S. Government Printing Office.

Ojeda, G., J. Anedeo, and A. Monroy (1981)  Cost Per Couple-Year-of-Protection:  The Case of Profamilia, 1977-1980.  Paper prepared for Internatonal Workshop on Cost-Effectiveness Analysis and Cost-Benefit Analysis in Family Planning Programs, The Johns Hopkins University, Baltimore, Md.

Orgebin-Crist, M. (1973)  Sperm age:  Effects on zygote development.  Pp. 85-93 in W. A. Uricchio and M. K. Williams, eds., <u>Natural Family Planning</u>. Washington, D.C.:  The Human Life Foundation.

Ory, H. (1977)  Association between oral contraceptives and myocardial infarction:  A review.  <u>Journal of the</u> <u>American Medical Association</u> 237:2619-2622.

Ory, H. (1979)  The risks and benefits of fertility control.  Pp. 110-121 in <u>Contraception:  Science,</u> <u>Technology and Application</u>. Washington, D.C.: National Academy of Sciences.

Ory, H. (1981)  Ectopic pregnancy and intrauterine contraceptive devices:  New perspectives. <u>Obstetrics</u> <u>and Gynecology</u> 57:137-144.

Ory, H., and the Boston Collaborative Drug Surveillance Program (1974)  Functional ovarian cysts and oral contraceptives:  Negative association confirmed surgically.  <u>Journal of the American Medical</u> <u>Association</u> 228:68.

Ory, H., P. Cole, B. MacMahon, and R. Hoover (1976)  Oral contraceptives and reduced risk of benign breast diseases.  <u>New England Journal of Medicine</u> 249:419-422.

Osser, S., B. Gullberg, P. Liedholm, and N. Sjoberg (1980)  Risk of pelvic inflammatory disease among intrauterine-device users irrespective of previous pregnancy.  <u>Lancet</u> 1:386-388.

Pardthaison, T., R. Gray, and E. McDaniel (1980)  Return of fertility after discontinuation of depot medroxyprogesterone acetate and intrauterine devices in Northern Thailand.  <u>Lancet</u> 1:509-511.

Parveen, L., A. Chowdhury, and Z. Choudhury (1977)  Injectable contraception (medroxyprogesterone acetate) in rural Bangladesh.  <u>Lancet</u> 5:946-948.

Patanelli, D. (1981)  Personal communication based on data obtained in studies funded by the National Institute for Child Health and Human Development.

Paulson, N., and M. Kao (1977)  Cervical perforation by
  the copper-7 intrauterine device.  Obstetrics and
  Gynecology 50:621.
Phillips, J. (1980)  Complications in laparoscopy.  Pp.
  247-259 in L. Koth, ed., The Safety of Fertility
  Control.  New York:  Springer Publishing.
Physicians' Desk Reference (1981)  Oradell, N.J.:
  Medical Economics Company.
Pichai, B., R. Banterng, D. Visit, K. Bhankasame, T.
  Wiset, S. Yod, W. Somsak, and D. Nikorn (1981)
  Comparison of vasectomy performed by medical students
  and surgeons in Thailand.  Studies in Family Planning
  12:316-317.
Pike, M., B. Henderson, J. Casagrande, I. Rosario, and G.
  Grady (1981)  Oral contraceptive use and early
  abortion as risk factors for breast cancer in young
  women.  British Journal of Cancer 43:72-76.
Piotrow, P., and C. Lee (1974)  Oral contraceptives:  50
  million users.  Population Reports, Series A:1-28.
Piotrow, P., W. Rinehart, and J. Schmidt (1979)
  IUDs--Update on safety, effectiveness, and research.
  Population Reports, Series B:49-100.
Population Council (1979)  Five Intrauterine Devices for
  Public Programs.  New York:  Population Council.
Potts, M., T. Van der Vlugt, P. Piotrow, L. Gail, and S.
  Huber (1975)  Advantages of orals outweigh
  disadvantages.  Population Reports, Series A:29-52.
Potts, M., J. Speidel, and E. Kessel (1978)  Relative
  risks of various means of fertility control when used
  in less developed countries.  Pp. 28-51 in J. Sciarra,
  G. Zatuchni, and J. Speidel, eds., Risks, Benefits,
  and Controversies in Fertility Control.  New York:
  Harper and Row.
Power, R. G. (1981)  Personal communication.
Presser, H. (1970)  Voluntary sterilization:  A world
  view.  Reports on Population/Family Planning 5:1-36.
Rahardgo, P., and T. Reese (1972)  A cost-effectiveness
  analysis.  Technical Report Series, Monograph No. 3.
  National Family Planning Coordinating Board, Jakarta,
  Indonesia.
Ramcharan, S., F. Pellegrin, and E. Hoag (1976)  The
  occurrence and course of hypertensive disease in users
  and nonusers of oral contraceptive drugs.  Pp. 1-15 in
  The Walnut Creek Study, Vol. II.  U.S. Department of
  Health, Education, and Welfare Public No. (NIH)
  76-563.  Washington, D.C.:  U.S. Department of Health
  Education, and Welfare.

Ramcharan, S., F. Pellegrin, R. Ray, and J. Hsu (1980)
    The Walnut Creek Contraceptive Drug Study, Vol. III.
    U.S. Department of Health, Education and Welfare
    Public No. (NIH) 76-563. Washington, D.C.: U.S.
    Department of Health, Education, and Welfare.
Ratnam, S., and R. Prasad (1979) Clinically important
    factors in safety and health hazards of fertility
    regulating agents in the developing world. Singapore
    Journal of Obstetrics and Gynecology 9:17-24.
Reardon, M., S. Deeds, N. Dresner, J. Diksa, and W.
    Robinson (1974) Real costs of delivering family
    planning services. American Journal of Public Health
    64:860-868.
Reddy, P., and C. Murthy (1977) Social marketing of
    Nirodh: An interim assessment of an experiment.
    Population Centre Bangalore Newsletter 3:1-14.
Reinke, W. (1981) Cost-Effectiveness with Equity: A
    Review of Narangwal Project Experience. Paper
    prepared for the International Workshop on
    Cost-Effectiveness Analysis and Cost-Benefit Analysis
    in Family Planning Programs, The Johns Hopkins
    University, Baltimore, Md.
Report to USAID (1980) Report to USAID of the Ad Hoc
    Consultative Panel on Depot Medroxyprogesterone
    Acetate. Office of Population, U.S. Agency for
    International Development.
Rioux, J. (1980) Uterine bleeding following tubal
    occlusion in gynecology. Pp. 267-280 in L. Koth, ed.,
    The Safety of Fertility Control. New York: Springer
    Publishing.
Robinson, W. (1979) The cost per unit of family planning
    services. Journal of Biosocial Science 11:93-103.
Rochat, R., H. Ory, and K. Schulz (1978) Methods for
    measuring safety and health hazards of presently
    available fertility regulating agents in the
    developing world. Singapore Journal of Obstetrics and
    Gynecology 9:1-16.
Rodriguez, G. (1977) Assessing the Availability of
    Fertility Regulation Methods: Report on a
    Methodological Study. WFS Scientific Reports No. 1.
    London: World Fertility Survey.
Rodriguez, G. (1978) Family planning availability and
    contraceptive practice. International Family Planning
    Perspectives and Digest 4:100-115.
Rooks, J., H. Ory, K. Ishak, L. Strauss, J. Greenspan, A.
    P. Hill, and C. W. Tyler (1979a) Epidemiology of
    hepatocellular ademona: The role of oral contra-

ceptive use. Journal of the American Medical Association 242:644-648.

Rooks, J., H. Ory, K. Ishak, L. Strauss, J. Greenspan, A. P. Hill, and C. W. Tyler (1979b)  Pp. 131-146 in Institut National de la Sante et de la Recherche Medicale, Conseil Superior de l'Information Sexuelle. Paris: INSERM.

Rothman, K., and C. Louk (1979)  Oral contraceptives and birth defects. New England Journal of Medicine 299:522.

Royal College of General Practitioners (1974)  Oral Contraceptives and Health. London: Pitman Medical.

Royal College of General Practitioners (1976)  Oral contraception study:  The outcome of pregnancy in former oral contraceptive users. British Journal of Obstetrics and Gynecology 83:608-616.

Royal College of General Practitioners (1978)  Oral contraception study:  Reduction in incidence of rheumatoid arthritis associated with oral contraceptives. Lancet 1:569-571.

Royal College of General Practitioners (1981a)  Breast cancer and oral contraceptives:  Findings in Royal College of General Practitioners' Study. British Medical Journal 282:2089-2093.

Royal College of General Practitioners (1981b)  Oral contraceptive study:  Further analysis of mortality in oral contraceptive users. Lancet 1:541-546.

Rudel, H., M. Maqueo, J. Calderone, and J. Manatou (1978)  Safety and effectiveness of a new low dose oral contraceptive:  A three-year study of 1,000 women. Journal of Reproductive Biology 21:79-88.

Ryden, G., L. Fahraeus, L. Molin, and K. Ahman (1979)  Do contraceptives influence the incidence of acute pelvic inflammatory disease in women with gonorrhea? Contraception 20:149-157.

Sanhueza, H., I. Sivin, S. Kumar, M. Kessler, A. Carrasco, and J. Yee (1979)  A randomized double blind study of two oral contraceptives. Contraception 20:29-48.

Schearer, S. B. (1977)  The status of technology for contraception. Pp. 581-604 in J. Money and Y. Muspah, eds., Handbook of Sexology. New York: Excerpta Medica.

Schearer, S. B., and N. Fincancioglu (1981)  Family Planning in the 1980's:  Challenges and Opportunities. Basic Background Document for the International Conference on Family Planning in the 1980s. New York: Population Council.

Schmidt, S. (1975) Complication of vas surgery. Pp. 78-88 in J. J. Sciarra, C. Markland, and J. J. Speidel, eds., Control of Male Fertility. New York: Harper and Row.

Senanayake, P., and D. Kramer (1980) Contraception and the Etiology of PID: New Perspectives. Paper presented at the International Symposium on Pelvic Inflammatory Disease, Atlanta, Ga.

Shapiro, S., O. Slone, and C. Rosenberg (1979) Dual contraceptive use in relation to myocardial infarction. Lancet 1:743-747.

Shedlin, M., and P. Hollerbach (1981) Modern and traditional fertility regulation in a Mexican community: The process of decision-making. Studies in Family Planning 12:278-296.

Shepard, M. (1974) Female contraceptive sterilization. Obstetrical and Gynecological Survey 29:739-787.

Simmons, G. (1971) The Indian Investment in Family Planning. New York: Population Council.

Simmons, G. (1973) Public Expenditure Analysis and Family Planning Programs. Population Planning Working Paper No. 2. University of Michigan, Ann Arbor, Mich.

Sivin, I., and J. Stern (1979) Long-acting and more effective copper-T devices. Studies in Family Planning 10:263-281.

Slone, D., S. Shapiro, D. Kaufman, L. Rosenberg, O. Miettinen, and P. Stolley (1981) Risk of myocardial infarction in relation to current and discontinued use of oral contraceptives. New England Journal of Medicine 305:420-424.

Soepari, S. (1978) Some observations on safety and health hazards of contraceptives in Indonesia. Singapore Journal of Obstetrics and Gynecology 9:91-95.

Sollins, A., and R. Belsky, (1970) Commercial production and distribution of contraceptives. Reports on Population/Family Planning 4:1-23.

Sparks, R. (1981) Bacterial colonization of uterine cavity. British Medical Journal 282:1189.

Spellacy, W., N. Zaias, W. Buhi, and S. A. Birk (1971) Vaginal yeast growth and contraceptive practices. Obstetrics and Gynecology 38:343.

Stolley, P. (1977) A review of data from the United States concerning the relationship of thromboembolic disease to oral contraceptives. Pp. 122-126 in J. J. Sciarra, G. Zatuchni, and J. J. Speidel, eds., Risks, Benefits and Controversies in Fertility Control. Hagerstown, Md.: Harper and Row.

Stolley, P., J. Tonascia, M. Tockman, P. Sartwell, A.
    Rutledge, and M. Jacobs (1975)  Thrombosis with
    low-estrogen oral contraceptives. American Journal of
    Obstetrics and Gynecology 102:197.
Swan, S. H., and W. L. Brown (1980)  Oral contraceptive
    use, sexual activity and cervical carcinoma. American
    Journal of Obstetrics and Gynecology 129:52.
Takahashi, M., and D. B. Loveland (1976)  Bacteriuria and
    oral contraceptives:  Routine health examinations of
    12,076 middle class women.  Pp. 95-103 in S.
    Ramcharan, ed., The Walnut Creek Study, Vol. II.  U.S.
    Department of Health, Education, and Welfare Public
    No. (NIH) 76-563.  Washington, D.C.:  U.S. Department
    of Health, Education, and Welfare.
Talwar, P. (1980)  Distribution effectiveness of Nirodh:
    Free vs. commercial channels.  Population Center
    Luchow Newsletter 5:1-6.
Talwar, P., and G. Berger (1977)  The relation of body
    weight to side effects associated with O.C.  British
    Medical Journal 1:1637-1638.
Talwar, P., J. Dingfelder, and R. Ravenholt (1977)
    Increased risk of breakthrough bleeding when one O.C.
    tablet is missed.  New England Medical Journal
    296:1236-1237.
Targum, S., and N. Wright (1974)  Association of the
    intrauterine device and pelvic inflammatory disease:
    A retrospective pilot study.  American Journal of
    Epidemiology 262-271.
Thaler, I., E. Paldi, and D. Steiner (1978)  Intrauterine
    device and pelvic inflammatory disease.  International
    Journal of Fertility 23:69.
Tietze, C. (1970)  Evaluation of intrauterine devices:
    Ninth progress report of the cooperative statistical
    program.  Studies in Family Planning 1:1-40.
Tietze, C. (1979)  Induced Abortion:  1979, 3rd ed.  New
    York:  Population Council.
Tietze, C. (1980)  Maternal mortality excluding abortion
    mortality.  World Health Statistics Report 30:312-338.
Tietze, C. (1981)  Induced Abortion:  A World Review,
    1981, 4th ed.  New York:  Population Council.
Tietze, C., and S. Lewit (1980)  Mortality associated
    with reversible methods of fertility regulation.  Pp.
    42-48 in L. Koth, ed., The Safety of Fertility
    Control.  New York:  Springer Publishing.
Tomkinson, J., A. Turnbull, G. Robson, E. Cloake, A.
    Adelstein, and J. Weatherall (1979)  Report on
    Confidential Enquiries into Maternal Deaths in England

and Wales, 1973-1975. Department of Health and Social
Security, Report on Health and Social Subjects 14, Her
Majesty's Stationery Office, London.

Toppozada, M. (1979) Safety and hazards of oral
contraceptives and prostaglandins with special
reference to the developing world. Singapore Journal
of Obstetrics and Gynecology 9:37-41.

Toppozada, M., F. Onsy, and E. Fares (1979) The
protective influence of progestin-only contraception
against moniliasis. Contraception 20:99.

Torres, A., J. Forrest, and S. Eisman (1981) Family
planning services in the United States, 1978-1979.
Family Planning Perspectives 13:132-141.

Trussell, J. (1974) Cost versus effectiveness of
different birth control methods. Population Studies
28:85-106.

Tsu, V. (1980) Underutilization of health centers in
rural Mexico: A qualitative approach to evaluation
and planning. Studies in Family Planning 11:145-153.

United Nations Fund for Population Activities (1976)
Survey of Contraceptive Laws: Country Profiles,
Checklists, and Summaries. New York: UNFPA.

U.S. Food and Drug Administration Advisory Committee on
Obstetrics and Gynecology (1968) Report on
Intrauterine Contraceptive Devices. Washington,
D.C.: U.S. Government Printing Office.

Vessey, M. P. (1978) Contraceptive methods: Risks and
benefits. British Medical Journal 2:721-722.

Vessey, M. P. (1979) Oral contraception and neoplasia.
British Journal of Family Planning 4:69-71.

Vessey, M. P. (1980) Female hormones and vascular
disease: An epidemiological overview. British
Journal of Family Planning 6(Supplement):1-12.

Vessey, M. P., and J. I. Mann (1978) Female sex hormones
and thrombosis. British Medical Bulletin 34:157-162.

Vessey, M. P., R. Doll, R. Peto, B. Johnson, and P.
Wiggins (1976) A long-term follow-up study of women
using different methods of contraception: An interim
report. Journal of Biosocial Science 8:375-427.

Vessey, M. P., K. McPherson, and B. Johnson (1977a)
Mortality among women participating in the
Oxford-Family Planning Association Contraceptive
Study. Lancet 2:731-733.

Vessey, M. P., C. R. Kay, J. A. Baldwin, J. A. Clarke,
and J. MacLeod (1977b) Oral contraceptives and benign
liver tumors. British Medical Journal 1:1064-1065.

Vessey, M. P., N. H. Wright, K. McPherson, and P. Wiggins (1978) Fertility after stopping different methods of contraception. British Medical Journal 1:265-267.

Vessey, M. P., D. Yeates, and R. Flavel (1979a) Risk of ectopic pregnancy and duration of use of an intrauterine device. Lancet 2:501-502.

Vessey, M. P., L. Meisler, R. Flavel, and D. Yeates (1979b) Outcome of pregnancy in women using different methods of contraception. British Journal of Obstetrics and Gynecology 86:548-556.

Vessey, M. P., K. McPherson, and D. Yeates (1981a) Mortality in oral contraceptive users. Lancet 1:549.

Vessey, M. P., K. McPherson, and R. Doll (1981b) Breast cancer and oral contraceptives: Finding in Oxford-Family Planning Association Study. British Medical Journal 282:2093-2094.

Vessey, M. P., D. Yeates, R. Flavel, and K. McPherson (1981c) Pelvic inflammatory disease and the intrauterine device: Findings in a large cohort study. British Medical Journal 282:855.

Vitoon, O. (1976) Minilaparotomy for interval female sterilization. Pp. 112-119 in J. Sciarra, W. Droegemueller, and J. Speidel, eds., Advances in Female Sterilization Techniques. New York: Harper and Row.

Wang, C. (1974) Voluntary sterilization in Taiwan area. Pp. 447-453 in M. Schima, et al., eds., Advances in Voluntary Sterilization. New York: American Elsevier.

Weiss, N. S., and T. A. Sayvetz (1980) Incidence of endometrial cancer in relation to the use of oral contraceptives. New England Journal of Medicine 302:551-554.

Westinghouse Population Center (1974) Contraceptive Distribution in the Commercial Sector of Selected Developing Countries: Summary Report. Columbia, Md.: Westinghouse Population Center.

Westoff, C. (1981) Unwanted fertility in six developing countries. International Family Planning Perspectives 7:43-52.

Westoff, C., and N. Ryder (1968) Duration of use of oral contraception in the United States, 1960-1965. Public Health Reports 83:277-287.

Westrom, L. (1975) Effect of acute pelvic inflammatory disease on fertility. American Journal of Obstetrics and Gynecology 121:707-713.

Westrom, L., L. Bengstsson, and P. Mardh (1976) The risk of pelvic inflammatory disease in women using intrauterine contraceptive devices as compared to non-users. _Lancet_ 2:221.

Wingrave, S., C. Kay, and M. Vessey (1979) Oral contraceptives and diabetes mellitus. _British Medical Journal_ 1:23.

Wingrave, S., C. Kay, and M. Vessey (1980) Oral contraceptives and pituitary adenomas. _British Medical Journal_ 8:685-686.

World Health Organization (1980) _Ninth Annual Report, Special Program of Research Development and Research Training in Human Reproduction._ Geneva: WHO.

World Health Organization (1981) Report from the Special Programme for Research, Development and Research Training in Human Reproduction's Task Force on Long-Acting Systemic Agents for the Regulation of Fertility. _British Journal of Obstetrics and Gynecology_ 88:317-321.

World Health Organization, Task Force on Psychosocial Research in Family Planning and Task Force on Service Research in Family Planning (1980b) User preference for contraceptive methods in India, Korea, the Philippines, and Turkey. _Studies in Family Planning_ 11:267-273.

Wortman, J. (1975) Sterilization: Vasectomy--what are the problems? _Population Reports_, Series D, No. 15.

Wortman, J. (1976a) A review of the complications of laparoscopic sterilization. Pp. 37-47 in J. Sciarra, W. Droegemueller, and J. Speidel, eds., _Advances in Female Sterilization Techniques._ New York: Harper and Row.

Wortman, J. (1976b) The diaphragm and other intravaginal barriers--A review. _Population Reports_, Series H:57-76.

Wright, N., and P. Laemmle (1968) Acute pelvic inflammatory disease in an indigent population. _American Journal of Obstetrics and Gynecology_ 101:979.

Wright, N., M. P. Vessey, B. Kenward, K. McPherson, and R. Doll (1978) Neoplasia and dysplasia of the cervix uteri and contraception. _British Journal of Cancer_ 38:273-279.

APPENDIX TABLE 1  Retail Prices of Contraceptive Products from Private-Sector Outlets (1980 U.S. dollars)

| Country | Average Monthly per Capita Income | Oral Contraceptives (per cycle) | IUD (device only) | Condom (per piece) | Diaphragm (device only) | Spermicides (per application[a]) | Injectables (per month's supply[b]) |
|---|---|---|---|---|---|---|---|
| Bangladesh | 7.75 | 1.28 | -- | -- | -- | -- | -- |
| Brazil | 123.50 | 0.56-0.70 | 35.00-70.00 | .14-.33 | 14.70-17.50 | .07-.17 | 1.44-2.00 |
| Colombia | 64.50 | 0.56-1.04 | 2.25-22.50 | .23 | -- | -- | 0.72 |
| Dominican Rep. | 74.75 | 1.65-3.45 | 8.00-12.50 | .25-.33 | 6.50-15.00 | .14-.33 | 1.63-2.95 |
| Egypt | 40.41 | 0.46 | 6.89 | .19 | -- | .04-.09 | -- |
| El Salvador | 51.25 | 1.20-6.00 | 3.00-10.00 | -- | 2.00-10.00 | -- | 1.20-9.20 |
| Guatemala | 72.41 | 2.25 | 15.00 | .33 | -- | .06-.22 | 1.25-1.58 |
| Indonesia | 26.66 | 1.13-1.62 | 12.80-15.00 | .08-.16 | 2.23 | -- | 1.17 |
| Jamaica | 130.00 | 1.04-2.44 | -- | -- | 12.04 | .22 | 4.00 |
| Jordan | -- | 1.19-1.27 | 10.32-17.20 | .23-.46 | 13.73-14.30 | .06-.46 | 2.86 |
| Kenya | 25.75 | 3.00-4.08 | 12.01-17.88 | .31-.40 | -- | .16-.51 | 3.79 |
| Korea, South | 79.16 | 0.78-1.26 | 0.78-1.26 | .08-.13 | -- | .12-.15 | -- |
| Madagascar | 18.20 | 1.74-2.32 | -- | .48 | -- | .23 | 2.59-3.04 |
| Mexico | 96.66 | 0.41 | -- | .16 | -- | -- | -- |
| Morocco | 47.50 | 2.50 | 8.00-12.00 | .17 | -- | .08-.13 | -- |
| Nepal | 8.83 | 0.58-1.12 | -- | -- | 12.05-23.28 | -- | -- |
| Nigeria | 33.25 | 6.98 | 9.80-23.28 | .81 | 3.30-11.94 | .48 | 12.61 |
| Panama | 104.16 | 1.98 | 10.00 | .25 | -- | .47-.49 | 6.00 |
| Philippines | 38.25 | 0.42-2.00 | 13.60 | .07-.30 | -- | .15-.34 | 1.56 |
| Thailand | 34.33 | 0.50-2.00 | -- | -- | -- | .05-.10 | -- |
| Zaire | 12.33 | 3.55 | 3.55-53.25 | .18-.36 | -- | .61 | 2.96 |
| Mean, all countries | 54.48 | 1.96 | 18.38 | .27 | 3.93 | .24 | 2.93 |

Note: Excludes publicly subsidized products.  Prices vary by brand of product and type of outlet.

[a] Defined as one foaming tablet or liquefying suppository, 6.4 g. of contraceptive jelly or cream, or 1.3 g. of contraceptive foam.
[b] One month's supply is calculated on the basis of three months' effective action.

Source: The study upon which this table is based is described in Note 3.

149

APPENDIX TABLE 2  Prices Charged for Contraceptive Services by Private Physicians, Clinics, and Hospitals (1980 U.S. dollars)

| Country | IUD | | Diaphragm | | Female Sterilization | Vasectomy |
|---|---|---|---|---|---|---|
| | Insertion | Follow-up Visit | Initial Fitting | Follow-up Visit | | |
| Bangladesh | -- | -- | -- | -- | 35.50-56.80 | 7.10-21.30 |
| Brazil | 50.00-500.00[a] | -- | 52.40 | 17.50 | 122.50-2,000.00 | 262.50-700.00 |
| Colombia | 6.75-22.50 | 6.75-22.50 | -- | -- | 112.50-225.00 | 67.50-180.00 |
| Dominican Rep. | 30.00-60.00 | 10.00 | 15.00-20.00 | 10.00 | 100.00-300.00 | 200.00-300.00 |
| Egypt | 14.50-72.50[a] | -- | -- | -- | 73.00-218.00 | 145.00-218.00 |
| El Salvador | 20.00-40.00 | 10.00 | 10.00-14.00 | 10.00 | 184.00-280.00 | 120.00-160.00 |
| Guatemala | 10.00-24.00 | 10.00 | -- | -- | 150.00-200.00 | 120.00-160.00 |
| Indonesia | 12.00 | 4.80 | -- | -- | 120.00 | 100.00 |
| Jamaica | 11.60-37.30 | 8.70 | 5.80-21.00 | -- | 174.00-203.00 | 24.30 |
| Jordan | 51.60-130.20 | 6.88-10.32 | 17.20 | -- | 120.40-688.00 | 174.00 |
| Kenya | 21.45 | 10.72-14.30 | 21.45 | 10.72-14.30 | -- | 258.00-344.00 |
| Korea, South | 19.20-27.20 | 1.60-3.20 | -- | -- | 47.25-94.50 | -- |
| Morocco | 12.13 | 2.91 | -- | -- | -- | 47.25-94.50 |
| Nigeria | 48.50 | -- | 29.10 | -- | -- | -- |
| Panama | 25.00[a] | -- | -- | -- | 200.00-400.00 | 100.00-250.00 |
| Philippines | -- | 5.44 | -- | -- | -- | -- |
| Thailand | 25.00 | -- | -- | -- | 60.00-250.00 | 30.00-150.00 |
| Zaire | 35.50 | 28.40 | -- | -- | 88.75 | -- |
| Mean, all countries | 30.79 | 9.87 | 23.31 | 11.38 | 239.71 | 163.53 |

Note:  Data provided only for products not subsidized by publicly funded commercial retail sales programs. Prices vary depending upon brand of product and type of outlet.

[a]Including follow-up.
Source:  The study upon which this table is based is described in Note 3.

150

Chapter 4

# Normative and Psychic Costs of Contraception

DONALD J. BOGUE

## CONTRACEPTION AS DISJUNCTION WITH THE INDIVIDUAL'S PAST

Contraception is a goal-oriented, voluntary behavior, each episode of which is the result of conscious volition. It is motivated by one particular need--to have sex without conception and thereby to avoid the potential negative consequences of pregnancy.

Explaining contraceptive behavior is a complex theoretical effort. There is a major disjunction, at the level of the individual and the couple, between noncontrol of fertility and the use of fertility-control practices. Learning, motivation, intention formation, and experimentation--all in a cultural and social context--are involved in this disjuncture; a new mode of behavior (adoption of an innovation) must be initiated and reinforced, and become habitual. Because this new behavior is intimately linked to culture, religion, and one's perception of self and one's role in the family, the neighborhood, and the community, this adaptation is of major significance. This may be especially true for people in developing countries, who may have to abandon a former behavior pattern and substitute a new one; in developed societies, in contrast, little more than the initiation of new generations into conventional adult behavior may be involved. Fertility decline has a causal pattern more complex than simply the weakening or relaxing of factors that formerly resulted in high fertility. The determinants of fertility-regulation behavior are not necessarily the obverse of the determinants of noncontrol of fertility; contraception may be a new way of achieving some of the society's oldest and most treasured goals. In fact, what appears at the aggregate level to be a smooth "demographic transition" is actually the increasing prevalence of couples making a distinctive behavior change, based on unique and complex combinations of social and psychological forces. Research on fertility must therefore address contraceptive behavior in its most disaggregated form--the individual and the couple. This in turn requires the study of the adoption of contraception from a social-psychological perspective.

The transition to use of contraception involves a cost/benefit analysis by one or both members of a couple, in which the perceived net benefits of having another child (Fawcett, in these volumes) are compared with the perceived net costs of practicing contraception (Schearer, in these volumes). The focus of the present discussion is the nonmaterial "normative and psychic" costs of contraceptive behavior: the attitudes and beliefs that imply a negative evaluation of contraceptive use, or the cultural, social, and psychological forces that influence individuals and couples not to begin contraceptive practice or to abandon it after a brief trial. For purposes of this discussion, it is assumed that the individuals or couples involved are at least partially informed about family planning, are motivated to practice it, and are in the process of making the cost/benefit calculation. In Asia, Latin America, and North Africa, a substantial proportion of couples with two living children fall into this category--more than 50 percent in many nations; in sub-Saharan Africa, such couples are a much smaller minority, but their proportion appears to be increasing thanks to a quarter century of worldwide discussion of "the population crisis." Mass awareness that contraception is possible and is practiced widely in the "modernized" nations has been aroused in even the more remote parts of all continents.

This paper first catalogues the various normative and psychic costs of the adoption of contraception, and then provides a brief review of theory and research related to each. Finally, it synthesizes these findings to indicate trends, identify topics for essential further research, and suggest which approaches may be most useful to family planning programs.

## A CATALOG OF THE NORMATIVE AND PSYCHIC COSTS OF CONTRACEPTION

There are numerous possible normative and psychic costs of practicing contraception. In the context of the

present discussion, all of these are beliefs or attitudes
learned or formed by communication and interaction with
others or by first-hand experience; they may or may not
be "valid" as judged by scientists. These costs can be
grouped into six major categories:

- <u>Contraception as a threat to cultural values and norms</u>
    - As nonconformity with religious and moral beliefs
    - As socially illegitimate behavior
- <u>Contraception as a challenge to social institutions</u>
  <u>and group values and norms</u>
    - As disharmony with the extended family system
    - As requiring communication about sex between
      spouses
    - As provoking discord between spouses
    - As undermining family security and status
- <u>Contraception as foregoing perceived benefits of</u>
  <u>childbearing</u>
    - As a threat to self-fulfillment and security in
      the family role
    - As a loss of enjoyment of children
    - As making the family vulnerable to infant mortality
- <u>Contraception as behavior inconsistent with personal</u>
  <u>values and norms</u>
    - As implying "inner control" or "efficacy"
    - As a threat to sex roles and sexual adjustment
    - As violating modesty and privacy in sexual matters
- <u>Anxiety costs of practicing contraception</u>
    - Anxiety about temporary side effects
    - Fears of permanent damage to health
    - Anxiety about contraceptive failure
- <u>Psychologistics: Perceived acessibility of</u>
  <u>contraceptive services</u>

This classification is only one of several possible.
It is organized according to the source and nature of the
costs, progressing simultaneously from society to the
individual, from the religious to the secular, from the
abstract to the specific, and from contemplation to
action. This classification places contraception in a
context that makes it easy to apply a broad range of
social science perspectives, theory, and research. The
classification itself has a theoretical infrastructure:
it is intended to be applicable to a number of different
social development innovations, with contraception being
only an unusually important instance; it is also intended
to be equally valid for developing and developed nations,

since there should be a single coherent theory of fertility decline. Consistent with the principles underlying
the classification, some of the values attached to having
children (Fawcett, in these volumes) are included in this
list. Such values can be seen as primarily affecting the
demand for children rather than regulation costs. However, since they are often expressed by survey respondents as reasons for not contracepting, they are also
treated briefly here.

It should be noted that, although all of the constraints listed are expressed in psychological or
social-psychological terms in keeping with the present
focus on individuals and couples, none deals with
personality traits. The Whelpton and Kiser studies of
Indianapolis (1946 to 1958) and the Westoff et al.
Princeton Studies (1961, 1963) showed no relationship
between such personality traits as anxiety level, com-
pulsiveness, tolerance of ambiguity, need-achievement,
and need for nurturance, and desired family size and the
practice of contraception. Although psychologists and
psychiatrists continue to speculate about personality
traits in Third World countries, this is assumed here to
be somewhat of a blind alley in research.

The costs or constraints listed above have been
collected from fertility and family planning reports
(both research and administrative). They have been
formulated by anthropologists; sociologists; educators;
psychologists and psychiatrists; physicians, nurses, and
paramedical workers; field workers for family planning;
social workers; and others. The importance of each in
limiting contraception depends upon two factors:

- Prevalence--the proportion of the population of
  reproductive age that experiences the particular cost
- Impact--how closely the cost (when it occurs) is
  correlated with use or nonuse of contraception

Both of these parameters can vary from population to
population; they can also change over time for a
particular population. Unhappily, empirical data about
both the prevalence and impact of these costs are more
scarce than data about most other aspects of fertility.
Most of these variables were not included in the World
Fertility Survey or in other demographic or social
surveys involving fertility. Although frequently cited
in the literature, the evidence provided is often
anecdotal, conjectural, circumstantial, or little more

than opinionated assertions.  The analysis presented
below attempts to provide an overview and synthesis of
what is known about these costs.

As illustration for some of the costs, data from a
recent survey of 2,000 Egyptian households are presented;
this survey was jointly conducted in 1980 by the State
Information Service (Population I-E-C Unit), of the Arab
Republic of Egypt and the Social Development Center.  It
should be noted that contraceptive prevalence rates in
this survey are higher than rates for Egypt from other
sources.  These data are not meant to represent other
Third World countries, but to demonstrate the possibilities for research into psychic and normative costs.


CONTRACEPTION AS A THREAT TO CULTURAL VALUES AND NORMS

This category includes challenges to sacred or deeply
held cultural and social values that are widely shared
and recognized as principles of "right" or "good" conduct.


### Contraception as Nonconformity with Religious and Moral Beliefs

Many couples who wish to practice contraception find that
it is condemned as immoral by their religion; as a consequence, those followers who contracept may experience
feelings of moral guilt and sinfulness.  The Roman
Catholic position illustrates this problem.  In many
Third World nations, leading Christian, Moslem, Buddhist,
Hindu, Confucian, and other theologians take a liberal
view of contraception, but local religious leaders in the
villages often vehemently oppose it.  Such opposition
appears to be greatest among the more conservative or
fundamentalist branches of many religions.

Nevertheless, research has indicated that religious
beliefs and moral codes are far less of an obstacle to
contraceptive use than might be expected.  On the basis
of his own studies and those of others, Stycos (1968)
reported that the position of the Catholic Church does
not constitute a major obstacle to family planning in
Latin America.  No consistent differences were found
between Catholic and non-Catholic women in attitudes,
contraceptive practice, or fertility.  He concludes, "If
Catholicism is having little impact on fertility, it may
be partly because the average woman is not very

'Catholic'" (Stycos, 1968:183).  In rural Guatemala,
Bertrand et al. (1978) found that nearly one-half of
those surveyed believed family planning to be against
God's will.  However, closer analysis traced this
attitude not to membership in a specific church but to
degree of religiosity:  those who considered themselves
very religious (whether Catholic or Protestant) were less
likely to approve of or use contraception than those who
were only "somewhat religious."  In Indonesia, Sujono
(1974) found that Moslems were more resistant to family
planning than Hindus, Buddhists, Protestants, Catholics,
or Confucians; however, this greater resistance seems to
have been based on more limited information about family
planning rather than upon theological considerations.
Sinquefield (1974) found that, in rural Alabama, women
who disapproved of contraception tended to say that it
was against God's will; nevertheless, of those women who
had achieved their ideal family size, substantial numbers
were practicing family planning anyway.

Table 1 provides some data on this subject for Egypt.
The left-hand column shows the prevalence of the normative or psychic cost, while the right-hand column shows
its impact through its relationship to contraceptive
use.  In Egypt, there is an undercurrent of "moral
uneasiness" and perhaps some guilt about contraceptive
use, but this is definitely a minority view.  Among the
minority that believe religion to be against family
planning, use is significantly lower than among those who
see no conflict; however, an impressive proportion of the
former group who want no more children are nevertheless
users.

Recent major declines in fertility in such developing
nations as Indonesia (Muslim), Thailand (Buddhist),
Colombia, the Philippines, Chile, Mexico, Brazil
(Catholic), India (Hindu, Muslim), China (Confucian),
Tunisia (Muslim), Malaysia (Muslim, Confucian, Hindu),
South Korea (Confucian), and Turkey (Muslim) provide
additional indirect evidence that religion poses less of
a psychological barrier to the adoption of contraception
than had been previously anticipated.  Certainly, the
prevalence of replacement-level fertility among the Roman
Catholic populations of Europe and North America supports
this view.

On the basis of this evidence, it can be tentatively
concluded that, although deep conservative religiosity
does generate psychological costs to contraception in the
Third World as a whole, intense feelings of inconsistency

TABLE 1    Threats to Moral and Religious Beliefs as
Normative or Psychic Costs of Contraception:
Illustrative Data from Egypt, 1980

| Question | Prevalence (Percent distribution) | Impact (Percent using contraception) |
|---|---|---|
| How much would it be against your religious beliefs to practice family planning? | 100 | 56 |
| No response, undecided, don't know | 15 | 49 |
| Very much against | 16 | 45 |
| Somewhat against | 10 | 53 |
| No conflict with beliefs | 59 | 60 |
| (Chi square = 21.4 with 3 d.f., sig. at .0001) | | |
| Do you think the local khateeb or priest would approve, disapprove, or not care if he learned you were practicing family planning? | 100 | 56 |
| Would approve | 47 | 60 |
| Would not care either way | 17 | 64 |
| Don't know | 25 | 41 |
| Would disapprove | 11 | 56 |
| (Chi square = 35.1 with 3 d.f., sig. at .0001) | | |

Note:  The left-hand column of this table reports data for all 2,001
cases in the sample to show the prevalence of the belief or attitude.
The right-hand column, however, is confined to 1,280 cases who
reported that they want to have no more children.  This permits an
assessment of the impact of psychic and normative costs among couples
who are already motivated and hence are in a position to make a
cost/benefit analysis of contraception.

Source:   State Information Service (Population I-E-C Unit), Arab
Republic of Egypt, and the Social Development Center, Chicago.

between religion and family planning are felt by a
minority in most of these countries.  Among that minority
(which is likely to consist of rural peasants and an
urban proletariat), this cost constrains contraceptive
use.  Roman Catholicism and Islam undoubtedly generate
varying degrees of ambivalence toward use among a
majority of their followers; when these followers are
sufficiently motivated on other grounds, this ambivalence
may impede, but does not prevent, contraceptive use.

## Contraception as Socially Illegitimate Behavior

Where high fertility is customary and large families are regarded as a virtue, couples who deliberately restrict births to a number substantially below the norm may suffer popular criticism until the practice of family planning becomes socially acceptable or "legitimate." This can pose a major normative cost to potential users.

A strong theoretical and research formulation for the importance of social pressures has been advanced by Fishbein and Jaccard (1973). They see a person's intention to behave (which leads to behavior) as a function of two factors: beliefs about family planning, together with a "normative component"--the perception that close friends, spouse, or parents want the person to have additional children, weighted by the person's propensity to comply with these perceived wishes. In empirical testing of this conception by Davidson and Jaccard (1976), the normative component was found to be highly predictive of future intentions to practice or not to practice family planning.

Leibenstein (1974) asserts that each couple is exposed to a particular social influence group (SIG), which tends to set standards for the legitimacy of family planning. He emphasizes that these pressures not only vary according to the socioeconomic and other characteristics of the SIG, but also differ for each birth order: pressures to have a first or second child may be vastly different from pressures to have a fourth. Bertrand et al. (1978:31-32) found that, in Guatemala, "the more disapproval a person perceives from 'significant others' the less will be his/her approval of family planning," and "those people who perceive more disapproval of family planning (by peers) are less likely to be using contraceptives." Sujono (1974:96) concluded from analysis of Indonesian data that "the more an individual who personally approves of family planning perceives that it is socially approved, the higher the probability is that he will adopt it." Shevasunt and Hogan (1979) found in northern Thailand that acceptance of family planning was strongly correlated with the perception that the practice was approved by a majority of one's peers. Of course, social legitimacy can also foster contraceptive use, as shown by Freedman and Takeshita (1969:356) for Taiwan:

The belief that other people who were trusted-- friends, relatives, and neighbors--were accepting

birth control in large numbers was important in
encouraging acceptance.  Legitimation in various ways
appeared to be important in a situation of considerable ambivalence where new birth control practices
conflicted with traditional family values.

Data on the social legitimacy of family planning in
Egypt provided in Table 2 show very little evidence that
contraception is perceived as illegitimate.  Only about 4
to 6 percent of respondents indicated fear of being
ostracized or subjected to social criticism if they were
to become contraceptors.  Nevertheless, fear of being in
a minority does appear to be a strong factor:  the right-
hand column of Table 2 shows that there is less contraceptive use among those who believe that family planning is
disapproved by many than among those who believe it is
disapproved by only a few.
Recent data from the World Fertility Survey (Lightbourne et al., 1982) and other samples have shown that a
majority of the public in several developing nations
either approves of contraception or else reports that no
more children are desired.  This may be accepted as
additional evidence that the social illegitimacy of
contraception may rapidly be becoming a minority rather
than a majority view.  Nevertheless, the evidence is
quite clear that, among those who perceive that the
people nearest to them want them to have more children,
the practice of contraception would have major social
legitimacy costs that would repress contraceptive
behavior.


## CONTRACEPTION AS A CHALLENGE TO SOCIAL INSTITUTIONS
## AND GROUP VALUES AND NORMS

Somewhat less general, abstract, and sacred than culture
and religion is the realm of "social organization" and
"customary behavior."  Because these are rooted in a
long-term adjustment to the environment, they exert
considerable influence over the behavior of individuals,
and to challenge them can involve high costs.


### Contraception as Disharmony
### with the Extended Family System

In developing countries, the behavior of adults is
influenced by parents, in-laws, siblings, aunts and

160    Donald J. Bogue

TABLE 2   Social Disapproval as a Normative or Psychic
Cost of Contraception:   Illustrative Data from Egypt, 1980

| Question | Prevalence (Percent distribution) | Impact (Percent using contraception) |
|---|---|---|
| Of the women who live in this town (city), how many of them do you think approve of family planning?  Would you say: | 100 | 56 |
|   Less than 3/4 | 63 | 50 |
|   About 3/4 or more | 37 | 65 |
|     (Chi square = 27.4 with 1 d.f., sig. at .001) | | |
| Of the men who live in this town (city), how many of them do you think approve of family planning?  Would you say: | 100 | 56 |
|   Less than 3/4 | 63 | 50 |
|   About 3/4 or more | 37 | 65 |
|     (Chi square = 26.4 with 1 d.f., sig. at .001) | | |
| Do you think your best friend would approve, disapprove, or would not care either way if she (he) found you were using family planning? | 100 | 56 |
|   Would not disapprove | 94 | 57 |
|   Would disapprove | 6 | 34 |
|     (Chi square = 11.5 with 1 d.f., sig. at .001) | | |

Note:   See note to Table 1.

Source:   State Information Service (Population I-E-C Unit), Arab Republic of Egypt, and the Social Development Center, Chicago.

uncles, and more distant relatives, even when there is more than one household involved.  When the attitudes of these kin are strongly pronatalist, the practice of contraception may threaten the harmony in the extended family (see Beckman, in these volumes).  Lee (1974:5) has eloquently expressed the dominance of the extended family over the individual in developing societies, and its pronatalist influence:

In addition to the very basic functions of reproduction and companionship, the (extended) family is the most essential organization of economic

production and consumption, the main educational agent
for transmitting technical skills and moral values
from generation to generation, the centre for
controlling and regulating social behavior, the
fundamental unit of worship and religio-ritual
observance and the major source of welfare and health
care. . . . Rare is any individual who does not
depend on the family or the wider kin groups for his
social, political, and economic security.    A
consequence of the high dependence on the family and
kinship system is the development of a collective
orientation.    This collective orientation is conducive
to high fertility motivation. . . .

Several years ago, when family planning was a new idea
in Third World countries, it is probable that the older
members of the extended family had much more negative
attitudes toward contraception than did younger couples,
who may therefore have hesitated to practice family
planning.    Although this situation may persist in many
cultures today, it is probably declining in most countries.    As noted above, general public opinion is
becoming more favorable toward family planning, and the
majority favor it in many places.    The climate of opinion
in extended families is shifting accordingly.    Consistent
with this, Stoeckel (1970) found that joint and nuclear
families did not differ significantly in their knowledge
and practice of family planning in East Pakistan.

Caldwell (1976) has given a strong description of the
pervasive pronatal social pressures imposed by the family
system and the extended kin/clan network of traditional,
particularly African, villages.    He believes this family
system may be undergoing an inexorable change toward the
nuclear family form due to "Westernization," quite
independently of shifts in family planning from
illegitimate to legitimate.    He concludes that "fertility
decline is more likely to precede industrialization (than
to follow it) and to help bring it about" (p. 12).

Table 3 summarizes attitudes of extended family
members in Egypt.    An overwhelming majority of
respondents reported that their relatives either would
approve outright or would not care if they practiced
family planning.    (This was not true for grandparents
only because many respondents did not know their
grandparents' opinions.)    Only 6-18 percent reported that
their close relatives would have objections.    The lower
panel of Table 3 shows how objections by family members

TABLE 3   Disharmony in the Extended Family as a Normative
or Psychic Cost of Contraception:   Illustrative Data from
Egypt, 1980

| Relative[a] | | Prevalence (Percent distribution) | | | |
|---|---|---|---|---|---|
| | | Approve | Not care | Dis- approve | Don't know |

Would _____ approve, disapprove
or not care if they were to learn
you were using family planning?

| Relative[a] | | Approve | Not care | Dis- approve | Don't know |
|---|---|---|---|---|---|
| Father | Mother | 55 | 11 | 12 | 22 |
| Uncle (paternal) | Aunt (paternal) | 51 | 19 | 11 | 19 |
| Uncle (maternal) | Aunt (maternal) | 50 | 19 | 11 | 20 |
| Brother | Sister | 67 | 13 | 6 | 14 |
| Father-in-law | Mother-in-law | 45 | 13 | 19 | 23 |
| Grandfather | Grandmother | 28 | 12 | 13 | 47 |

| Relative | | Impact (Percent using contraception) | | |
|---|---|---|---|---|
| | | Relative dis- approves | Relative approves | Signifi- cance |
| Father | Mother | 58 | 56 | Not sig. |
| Uncle (father) | Aunt (father) | 59 | 56 | Not sig. |
| Uncle (mother) | Aunt (mother) | 59 | 59 | Not sig. |
| Brother | Sister | 37 | 62 | Sig. |
| Father-in-law | Mother-in-law | 53 | 61 | Sig. |
| Grandfather | Grandmother | 60 | 63 | Not sig. |

Note:  See note to Table 1.

[a]Male respondents were asked about the perceived approval or
disapproval only of male relatives.  Female respondents were asked
only about female relatives.

Source:  State Information Service (Population I-E-C Unit), Arab
Republic of Egypt, and the Social Development Center, Chicago.

correlate with contraceptive use.   Only where it is
believed that a brother or sister (6 percent of
respondents) or father- or mother-in-law would object (18
percent) is there a lower rate of use; for all other
relatives, there is no significant difference.
  It may thus be hypothesized that the trend in
developing countries is toward approval of contraception

by members of the extended family, perhaps lagging
somewhat below the degree of approval in the general
public. In many Third World nations today, having a few
disapproving relatives appears to exert little influence
on use or nonuse of contraception, and the trend is for
this to become more common; sub-Saharan Africa appears to
be some decades behind Asia and Latin America in this
process.

### Contraception as Requiring Communication about Sex between Spouses

For many Third World cultures, it is reported that most
couples almost never talk about sex, and that wives are
extremely shy about mentioning it to their husbands.
Because the effective and sustained use of contraception
requires such communication, couples incur the psychic
cost of violating these taboos (see Beckman, in these
volumes). A few empirical examples will illustrate this
point.

In rural Guatemala, Bertrand et al. (1978:40) found
that "the less husband-wife communication there is, the
less likely one is to approve of family planning," and
that "those people who have less communication with their
spouses are less likely to be using contraceptives than
those with more communication." Sinquefield (1974) also
verified this empirically in rural Alabama, with the
surprising finding that 60 percent of adopters (and 80
percent of nonadopters) had never discussed family
planning with their spouses; apparently, secret use of
oral pills and IUDs was common. In a study in Dacca,
Figa-Talamanca et al. (1974) found that a much higher
proportion of contraceptive users than nonusers had
discussed both sexual matters and family planning with
their spouses. Keller (1973) found that lack of
communication between spouses is related to early
discontinuation of contraception. In citing issues on
which psychologists can make major contributions to
family planning, Palmore (1976) gives first priority to
the need to know more about the interaction between
husband and wife as it relates to reproduction.

Table 4 presents recent data on this subject for
Egypt. One-third of the couples of reproductive age
reported never having discussed contraception; among this
group, the proportion practicing contraception was only
40 percent that of couples that had held such discussions.

Table 4   Need for Communication Between Spouses as a
Normative or Psychic Cost of Contraception:   Illustrative
Data from Egypt, 1980

| Question | Prevalence (Percent distribution) | Impact (Percent using contraception) |
|---|---|---|
| Have you and your spouse ever talked about using some method of family planning? | 100 | 56 |
| Yes | 67 | 66 |
| No | 33 | 26 |
| (Chi square = 145.2 with 1 d.f., sig. at .001) | | |
| In general, do you feel that a husband and wife can talk to each other about family planning without feeling embarrassed? | 100 | 57 |
| Most can | 91 | 59 |
| About one-half can | 4 | 40 |
| Most cannot | 4 | 23 |
| Don't know | 1 | 12 |
| (Chi square = 26.0 with 3 d.f., sig. at .001) | | |

Note:  See note to Table 1.

Source:  State Information Service (Population I-E-C Unit), Arab
Republic of Egypt, and the Social Development Center, Chicago.

Despite the high proportion of couples who had not
discussed contraception, only 4 percent said that most
people cannot have such discussions; among this small
group, use of contraception was extremely low.

Overcoming shyness or cultural taboos against discussing contraception with one's spouse are still major
psychic costs for significant numbers of couples in Third
World countries.  It is possible that this is less so in
many modernizing countries, however, and that it is
continuing to diminish.


Contraception as Provoking Discord Between Spouses

If one spouse wishes to practice contraception and the
other wishes to have more children, this represents a
major disagreement.  It is commonly believed that wives
are more likely to favor family planning than their

husbands. In male-dominated societies, women are reluctant to challenge their husband's authority; physical as well as verbal abuse may result. Hence, having an uncooperative spouse may result in the surreptitious practice of contraception and in major psychic costs. However, the uncooperative male is a stereotype. Although it is true that women have an earlier and stronger motivation for family planning, the lag in husbands' attitudes is generally very slight. As "breadwinners," men can equally appreciate the benefits of childspacing and limiting family size, a fact that emerged early in the empirical literature. Bogue (1962) discussed it for India; it was verified by CELADE and CFSC (1972:78-79) in a survey of seven Latin American metropolises; and it has been reported regularly since. Nevertheless, the stereotype persists, perhaps because of the periodic appearance of dramatic cases to the contrary. Even where spouses do not talk to each other about family planning, each is independently exposed to the mass media, to discussions with peers, and to contact with family planning programs. By the time the second or third child is born, both spouses tend to arrive at a similar attitude toward contraception, and open disagreement over whether or not contraception should be practiced occurs only in a minor percentage of cases.

Recent data from Egypt about husband-wife agreement over contraception illustrate this point. Respondents were asked whether or not their spouses approved of family planning. This was cross-tabulated against the respondent's own attitude toward family planning, to yield the results shown in Table 5. Only about 6 percent of the couples reported themselves to be fully discordant over the issue of family planning; an additional 5 percent did not know the spouse's attitude. Thus, in about 90 percent of the cases, there was apparently a consensus that family planning is a good thing, or at least tolerance by one spouse of the other's approval. Unwillingness of husbands to permit their spouses to use contraception is reported today most frequently for nations of sub-Saharan Africa, and less for Asia and Latin America, where campaigns on "responsible parenthood" have focused attention on the male.

A search of the literature therefore fails to produce data showing major discord between spouses over family planning. Nevertheless, persistent evidence that a significant share of women appear to use oral pills or the IUD surreptitiously does not permit this psychic cost to be wholly dismissed.

TABLE 5   Husband-Wife Agreement over Contraception:
Illustrative Data from Egypt, 1980

| | Attitude of Respondent | | |
|---|---|---|---|
| Attitude of Spouse | Total | Approves | Neutral | Dis-approves |
| Approve | 86.2 | 84.4 | 0.4 | 1.4 |
| Neutral | 2.9 | 1.7 | 0.9 | 0.3 |
| Disapprove | 6.4 | 4.2 | 0.5 | 1.7 |
| Don't know | 4.6 | 3.3 | 0.4 | 0.9 |
| Total | 100.1 | 93.6 | 2.2 | 4.3 |

Note:  Figures do not add up to 100 because of rounding.

Source:  State Information Service (Population I-E-C Unit), Arab
Republic of Egypt, and the Social Development Center, Chicago.

## Contraception as Undermining Family Security and Status

Where the family is the principal unit of social organization, its continuity and strength may be believed to
depend on the number of children born.  For a couple that
has achieved its desired family size, but which lacks a
son, the practice of contraception could generate considerable psychic and normative costs.  Where status in
the clan and the community is enhanced by having many
grandchildren of both sexes, curtailment of childbirth
represents an opportunity cost.  In these ways, contraception can create fears about the weakening or extinc-
tion of the lineage (see Fawcett, in these volumes).  It
is plausible to expect that these feelings of insecurity
about family status will tend to diminish as family
organization changes from the extended to the nuclear
form.

## Contraception as Foregoing Perceived
## Benefits of Childbearing

An obvious major psychic and normative cost of contraception is the foregoing of benefits believed to derive
from having children.  Even where the net balance of
beliefs and attitudes strongly favors a decision to

practice family planning (to satisfy economic or other needs), there may be sadness or regret at having to make this choice.

### Contraception as a Threat to Self-Fulfillment and Security in the Family Role

In marriage, each partner achieves a sense of self-worth and self-fulfillment by playing a social role perceived as satisfying, socially acceptable, and reflective of his or her self.  For most adults (in all cultures), child-bearing and childrearing are integral aspects of this role (see Fawcett, in these volumes).

In high-fertility societies, the cost for a woman of practicing contraception may be fear that her entire role or status will be undermined, and that her husband will abandon her or take another wife.  At a deeper level, Lidz (1969) believes that many women undergo psychological and normative suffering when they use modern contraceptives precisely because the risks of childbirth have been removed.  They may suffer feelings of frustration or guilt over having sexual intercourse "for no purpose" other than its enjoyment.

A man, on the other hand, may fear that if he fails to continue fathering children, his friends will perceive him as being an inadequate male and family head.  The wife's management of fertility (by oral pills, IUD, or sterilization) may also be seen as undermining the husband's authority and possibly leading her to unfaithful or promiscuous behavior (Hollerbach, 1980).  Her seeking to enter the labor force may in addition be ego-deflating to the male and a further threat to sexual exclusivity. Thus, contraceptive use can generate psychic tensions within individuals and between couples by affecting their sexual adjustment.  Not practicing contraception, using unreliable methods, or "taking chances" with reliable methods may be ways to release or express these tensions.

### Contraception as a Loss of Enjoyment of Children

Children can be a great source of joy and satisfaction; contraception, whether for economic or other reasons, may therefore thwart or frustrate these pleasures of parent-hood, requiring psychic sacrifices of considerable magnitude (Fawcett, in these volumes).  Although the

deep-seated need to bear children and the demand to enjoy
parenthood are universal, they appear to be largely
satisfied by the first two or three children who survive
to age 2 (Bulatao, 1981). Beyond that point, the decision
to begin contraception or to bear additional children
appears to be determined by factors other than child
enjoyment. Consequently, adoption of contraception at
higher parities should have only small normative and
psychic costs of this sort.

### Contraception as Making the Family
### Vulnerable to Infant Mortality

Infant mortality is so common in many developing societies
that some observers cite it as a major reason for non-
adoption of contraception. In these circumstances,
practicing family planning could cause a couple to be
anxious that they might end up with fewer children than
desired. Infant death rates have been falling in Third
World countries for the past two decades (Chen, in these
volumes); this is the major factor in the increased life
expectancies in these countries. As the public becomes
aware of this trend, there should be less resistance to
family planning because of the fear of infant mortality.
The limited research that has been done shows that, to
date, large segments of the public tend to be only partially informed of these trends or are skeptical of the
claims. Fear of infant death as a reason for desiring
many children is often cited in fertility surveys.
Bulatao (1975), for example, found this to be a leading
reason for wanting more children. CELADE/CFSC found
moderate support for this factor, although they found
other social-psychological variables more powerful.

It may also be noted that contraception is correctly
perceived in many Third World countries as promoting
infant survival because it permits longer intervals
between births. This is used as a major argument for
family planning in sub-Saharan Africa.

Table 6 presents data from Egypt on the fear of infant
mortality and awareness of changing mortality trends.
Only about one-fifth of the respondents had a correct
estimate of the level of infant mortality; more than 40
percent had an exaggerated estimate; and more than one-
third did not know. There was widespread awareness of
the fact that infant mortality is declining; however,
about one-fifth of respondents perceived it as remaining

TABLE 6    Fear of Infant Death as a Normative or Psychic
Cost of Contraception: Illustrative Data from Egypt, 1980

| Question | Prevalence (Percent distribution) | Impact (Percent using contraception) |
|---|---|---|
| Out of every 10 babies born in this (village/neighborhood), how many of them do you think will die before they are 5 years old? | 100 | 56 |
| Zero or one (correct) | 22 | 65 |
| Two (incorrect) | 19 | 53 |
| Three (very wrong) | 13 | 48 |
| Four or more (very wrong) | 10 | 42 |
| Don't know | 36 | 58 |
| (Chi square = 25.8 with 4 d.f., sig. at .0001) | | |
| Do you believe that babies die more often or less often than they did 10 years ago? | 100 | 56 |
| The same or more often today | 21 | 44 |
| Less often today | 69 | 60 |
| Don't know | 10 | 50 |
| (Chi square = 21.0 with 2 d.f., sig. at .0001) | | |

Note:  See note to Table 1.

Source:  State Information Service (Population I-E-C Unit), Arab
Republic of Egypt, and the Social Development Center, Chicago.

unchanged or even rising in comparison with a decade
ago.  The potency of such misunderstanding is indisput-
able:  the practice of family planning is much lower
among those with exaggerated estimates of infant mortality
or those who are unaware that it is declining.

## CONTRACEPTION AS BEHAVIOR INCONSISTENT WITH PERSONAL VALUES AND NORMS

Even in the absence of any of the psychic and normative
constraints discussed above, there may be some conflict
between the overt contraceptive behavior required and an
individual's long-term commitment to certain values and
norms.

Contraception as Implying "Inner Control" or "Efficacy"

Noncontraceptors often tend to believe that family size
is determined by God, fate, or chance--and is hence
outside their sphere of responsibility. Adoption of
contraception requires abandoning this philosophy of
"external control" and assuming personal responsibility
for family size. This has wide ramifications: once this
inner control is assumed, cognitive consistency requires
equal self-reliance in other spheres.

Rotter (1960) has explored the ways in which this
conflict affects innovation and acceptance of new ideas.
Because traditional village people are thought to be
highly fatalistic, it was hypothesized early in family
planning efforts that overcoming this fatalism would be
an important psychic cost for potential users of contraception. A number of research studies in fact show that
a fatalistic outlook toward childbearing and family size
is a prevalent and powerful impediment to contraception.
As early as 1967, Groat and Neal (1967:958) stated, "For
those high in powerlessness, fertility seems likely to
constitute an occurrent, a chance happening, an unmanaged
event." Clifford and Ford (1974) found that fatalism was
associated with nonuse of contraception, and with lowered
effectiveness of fertility control among those who were
contracepting. Sinquefield (1974:31) applied the Rotter
scale of internal-external control to a sample of low-
income black women in rural Alabama and found "the lower
a woman's degree of internal control, the higher the
probability is that she will resist family planning."
Niehoff and Anderson (1966) saw peasant fatalism as a
serious but not insurmountable barrier to adoption of new
behaviors, pointing out that much fatalism is based on
religious philosophy, which is revered but not practiced
for pragmatic reasons. Much of it is based on situational factors; if these change, fatalism diminishes.
Bulatao's (1975) Value of Children study in the Philippines suggested that the effect of personal efficacy on
family planning may be mediated by its effect on values
and costs: the more efficacious respondents gave more
weight to the costs of children and were more likely to
disregard social pressures to have children.

Table 7 reports data from Egypt that support the
"efficacy" hypothesis: only about two-thirds of the
Egyptians of reproductive age surveyed have a feeling of
control over family size; among the one-third who are
fatalistic or not sure, the rate of contraceptive use is
comparatively low.

TABLE 7   Inner Versus External Control as a Normative or
Psychic Cost of Contraception:   Illustrative Data from
Egypt, 1980

| Question | Prevalence (Percent distribution) | Impact (Percent using contraception) |
|---|---|---|
| Do you really believe that a person can limit his family size to any number he chooses or do you think this is something you don't really have any control over? | 100 | 56 |
|   A person can control family size | 66 | 65 |
|   It is something a person cannot control | 38 | 35 |
|   Not sure, don't know | 6 | 0 |
|     (Chi square = 89.9 with 1 d.f., sig. at .001) | | |

Note:  See note to Table 1.

Source:   State Information Service (Population I-E-C Unit), Arab
Republic of Egypt, and the Social Development Center, Chicago.

## Contraception as a Threat to Sex Roles and Sexual Adjustment

Couples often perceive the practice of contraception as a
threat to the enjoyment of sex.  Contraceptive appliances
may be perceived as nuisances that interfere with or
reduce pleasure; the pill and sterilization are sometimes
mistakenly believed to weaken libido.  In such cases,
these psychic costs may be a very strong and direct
impediment to contraceptive use.  In other cases, elimination of the pregnancy risk may remove sexual inhibi-
tions, an observation made about the pill, the IUD, and
male and female sterilization.

The little empirical evidence available indicates that
good sexual adjustment and the practice of contraception
are positively correlated.  Sinquefield (1974) found
strong support for this hypothesis:  women who wished
they were married to someone else or did not enjoy sex
tended to be nonusers.  Keller (1970) found that
"defensive masculinity" (covert anxiety over sexual
adequacy) was linked to nonuse of contraception.

The Egyptian survey investigated this issue with
respect to condoms by asking the question reported in
Table 8.  A majority of Egyptians said they believe that

TABLE 8   Interference of Contraception With Sex Life as a
Normative or Psychic Cost of Contraception:   Illustrative
Data from Egypt, 1980

| Question | Prevalence (Percent distribution) | Impact (Percent using contraception) |
|---|---|---|
| Some people think that using condoms will interfere with the pleasure and naturalness of sex. Other people say that modern condoms are so good that people are not aware of any difference. What do you think? Do you think that condoms: | 100 | 77 |
| Greatly interfere with sex life | 20 | 78 |
| Interfere to some degree | 35 | 81 |
| Do not interfere with sexual pleasure | 10 | 77 |
| Don't know, no opinion | 35 | 72 |
| (Chi square = 4.5 with 3 d.f., not sig.) | | |

Note:   See note to Table 1.

Source:   State Information Service (Population I-E-C Unit), Arab
Republic of Egypt, and the Social Development Center, Chicago.

condoms do interfere with sex, and only 10 percent were
willing to declare unilaterally that they do not.
Because this belief is so widespread and the use rate of
condoms is extremely low, there is no correlation between
this attitude and the general practice of contraception.

## Contraception as Violating Modesty and Privacy in Sexual Matters

The practice of contraception may require a certain
amount of manipulation of the sexual organs and sub-
mission to medical examination.   For women who are very
shy about sex, this may create distress.   In many clinics
providing contraceptive services, a woman must have a
pelvic examination; because of a shortage of female
physicians, these examinations are often performed by a
male physician.   To the extent that women dread this
examination, it is a psychic cost of contraception,
although this distress has seldom been measured.

In Egypt, women were asked a question about examination by a female and a male physician (Table 9).   There

TABLE 9  Embarrassment at Pelvic Examination as a
Normative or Psychic Cost of Contraception:  Illustrative
Data from Egypt, 1980 (female respondents only)

| Question | Prevalence (Percent distribution) | Impact (Percent using contraception) |
|---|---|---|
| How would you feel about getting a physical examination from a female doctor? | 100 | 54 |
| Too embarrassed to permit it | 3 | 43 |
| Very embarrassed but would permit it | 17 | 47 |
| A little embarrassed | 8 | 59 |
| Not embarrassed | 72 | 55 |
| (Chi square = 3.7 with 3 d.f., not sig.) | | |
| How would you feel about getting a physical examination from a male doctor? | 100 | 54 |
| Too embarrassed to permit it | 20 | 49 |
| Very embarrassed but would permit it | 49 | 53 |
| A little embarrassed | 8 | 68 |
| Not embarrassed | 23 | 54 |
| (Chi square = 5.8 with 3 d.f., not sig.) | | |

Note:  See note to Table 1.

Source:  State Information Service (Population I-E-C Unit), Arab
Republic of Egypt, and the Social Development Center, Chicago.

was a comparatively low level of embarrassment with
female physicians, but a very high level with male
physicians.  One-fifth declared they could not undergo
such an examination, and an additional one-half said they
would permit it, but would feel very embarrassed; only
about one-fourth of the women would feel it to be an
unembarrassing, normal medical procedure.  However, the
impact of this psychic cost upon the practice of contraception appears to be small.  As shown in the right-hand
column of Table 9, the practice of family planning among
those who would feel embarrassment is somewhat lower than
among those who would not feel embarrassment, but these
differences are too small to be statistically significant, either for male or female physicians.

ANXIETY COSTS OF PRACTICING CONTRACEPTION

Another category of constraints on the adoption of contraception is anxieties and fears about effects upon the user.

## Anxiety about Temporary Side Effects

Every method of contraception thus far invented has caused at least some temporary physical discomfort or side effect among a significant minority of users (see Schearer, in these volumes). These side effects are perceived as mild and temporary by most users in Europe and North America, who receive medical counsel on their transitory and harmless nature. In sharp contrast, in Third World countries, side effects are often greatly exaggerated and feared: symptoms cited are frequently not verified by clinical trials, and their effects are perceived as debilitating and harmful; moreover, many do not believe that they are temporary. The pill, the IUD, and sterilization (the most effective of the modern methods) tend to have especially strong fears attached to them. These fears are clearly based on misinformation and rumor. Whether they arise from inadequate counseling, medical neglect of unusual cases of strong reaction, sensationalism in newscasts, or deliberate diffusion by opponents of family planning, they should not simply be dismissed as irrational fears; they exact a high toll in psychic costs and in refusal to adopt modern contraception.

Bogue (1962:533) early advised as a basic premise that "in order to avoid backfires, the limitations, weaknesses and disadvantages of using family planning must be admitted and discussed openly." Holmes (1973:24) reported the following for Thailand:

By far the most important health-related factor causing people to avoid birth control measures was the fear of possible side effects from using various methods. . . . There is considerable evidence that beliefs about negative side effects make up a large proportion of villages' "total knowledge" about family planning. . . . These are circulated in one form or another as rumors. . . . Peer communication or gossip works very rapidly.

Shevasunt and Hogan (1979:105) found in northern Thailand
that "medical reasons" (side effects) were given by
nearly one-half of all women who had discontinued use of
the pill, IUD, or injection.  Keller (1973:37) reports
that follow-up interviews with dropouts from family
planning clinics found "side effects were almost exclusively mentioned as the first reason, and often other
reasons followed."  The potential psychic cost of these
exaggerated fears is great--both to the public and to
population programs.

    That exaggerated fears of side effects continued to be
a major psychic cost is illustrated in Table 10 by data
from Egypt.  Most respondents had heard of the side
effects of oral pills; however, more than 70 percent were
either incorrectly or insufficiently informed about these
effects.  Those who incorrectly believed that these side
effects are not temporary were much less inclined to
practice family planning than those who were correctly
informed.


### Fears of Permanent Damage to Health

Despite massive research evidence that permanent damage
to health is very rare when contraceptives are provided
with appropriate medical supervision (see Schearer, in
these volumes), there is widespread belief in developing
countries that permanent damage to health will almost
inevitably result from long-term use.  This belief is
particularly prevalent for the most effective methods--
the pill, the IUD, and sterilization.

    Intense fears about the long-term effects of contra-
ception on health, based on rumor and half-truths, are
reported from many parts of the world.  Keller (1973)
found that dropouts from family planning programs in the
U.S. were likely to have accepted negative rumors about
such harmful effects.  Stycos and Marden (1973) found
that two-thirds of the women who had heard of oral
contraceptives before coming to clinics (in Honduras) had
heard that the method was harmful; an even higher percentage had negative views about the IUD.  They concluded
that "the source of such beliefs is primarily gossip" (p.
81).  Mundigo (1973) confirmed that this was a major
factor in discontinuation, and blamed clinics for inadequate counseling.  In rural Guatemala, Bertrand et al.
(1978:55) found that "the greater one's exposure to
negative rumors about the pill, the less likely one is to

TABLE 10   Threats to Physical Well-Being as Normative or
Psychic Costs of Contraception:   Illustrative Data from
Egypt, 1980

| Question | Prevalence (Percent distribution) | Impact (Percent using contraception) |
|---|---|---|
| A few women feel a little sick when they first start to take the pill. Have you ever heard about this?   IF YES: How long do these symptoms last? | 100 | 59 |
|   Two months or less | 29 | 67 |
|   More than two months | 58 | 58 |
|   Don't know | 13 | 36 |
|     (Chi square = 35.8 with 2 d.f., sig. at .001) | | |
| Can using birth prevention pills cause any disease if a woman is in good health when she starts using the pills? | 100 | 57 |
|   Yes | 32 | 52 |
|   Maybe, don't know | 18 | 52 |
|   No | 50 | 62 |
|     (Chi square = 11.0 with 2 d.f., sig. at .004) | | |
| Index of misinformation about safety of methods | -- | 56 |
|   Low misinformation | -- | 74 |
|   Moderate misinformation | -- | 59 |
|   High misinformation | -- | 26 |
|     (Chi square = 112.0 with 2 d.f., sig. at .0001) | | |

Note:   See note to Table 1.

Source:   State Information Service (Population I-E-C Unit), Arab
Republic of Egypt, and the Social Development Center, Chicago.

approve of family planning."   Numerous studies of reasons
for discontinuation of contraception have found large
proportions of such responses as "medical reasons--
other," which imply that the client (rather than the
doctor) prescribed the discontinuation.   How to maintain
continuation of contraception in the face of these
powerful rumors has been a major problem for family
planning programs in Third World countries.

Table 10 provides data from Egypt on fear of the
long-term health risks of contraception.   Women who had

TABLE 11  Percentage of Respondents Considering Each
Contraceptive Method Safe or Unsafe:  Illustrative Data
from Egypt, 1980

| Method | Safe | Unsafe | Method | Safe | Unsafe |
|---|---|---|---|---|---|
| Oral pill | 25 | 75 | Creams and jellies | 72 | 28 |
| IUD | 40 | 60 | Male sterilization | 75 | 25 |
| Diaphragms | 62 | 38 | Female sterilization | 78 | 22 |
| Vaginal Tablets | 63 | 37 | Rhythm | 95 | 5 |
| Injections | 71 | 29 | | | |

such fears had an adoption rate 10 percentage points
below that of women who did not.  In addition, respondents were asked, "How safe for a person's health is
the _____ method?"  Results for people who knew the
method and had an opinion are in Table 11.  The correct
answer, in every case, is very nearly 100 percent safe.
That fears of the oral pill and the IUD (the two leading
methods available) are pandemic is clearly evident.
These responses to detailed questions about the effects
of oral pills, the IUD, and sterilization on health were
combined to form an "index of misinformation" about
health safety (Table 10).  Those with high scores on
misinformation were only about one-third as likely to be
practicing family planning as those with low scores.
This wide disparity, combined with the high prevalence of
misinformation, leads the Egypt report to conclude, "This
combination of responses lays bare what appears to be the
single greatest obstacle to the progress of family
planning in Egypt" (SIS/SDC, Report 2).

## Anxiety about Contraceptive Failure

The decision to practice contraception generates a new
desire--the desire not to have an unwanted accidental
pregnancy.  Because of misinformation and rumors, many
people greatly underestimate the reliability of modern
methods of contraception; those who only a few months
before may have been unconcerned about pregnancy may
experience considerable anxiety that the method they have
chosen will fail.  This may be particularly true for
couples who greatly increase their sexual activity as a
consequence of adopting a modern method.  The other
psychic and normative costs may not seem to be worth
enduring if the probability of success is low.

TABLE 12   Perceptions of Contraceptive Unreliability as
Normative or Psychic Costs of Contraception:   Illustrative
Data from Egypt, 1980

| Method | Prevalence (Percent distribution) | | |
|---|---|---|---|
| | Reliable | Unreliable | Don't know |
| How reliable (effective in preventing pregnancy) do you think the _____ method is? | | | |
| Oral pill | 77 | 13 | 10 |
| IUD | 52 | 27 | 21 |
| Injections | 40 | 10 | 50 |
| Diaphragm | 31 | 22 | 47 |
| Foaming tablet | 23 | 23 | 54 |
| Vaginal creams and jellies | 24 | 23 | 53 |
| Condom | 38 | 37 | 25 |
| Female sterilization | 70 | 5 | 25 |
| Male sterilization | 44 | 5 | 51 |
| Rhythm method | 32 | 48 | 20 |

| Index of misinformation about reliability | Prevalence (Percent distribution) | Impact (Percent using contraception) |
|---|---|---|
| Total | 100 | 56 |
| Low misinformation | 12 | 74 |
| Moderate misinformation | 55 | 65 |
| High misinformation | 33 | 36 |
| (Chi square = 114.0 with 2 d.f., sig. at .0001) | | |

Note:   See note to Table 1.

Source:   State Information Service (Population I-E-C Unit), Arab
Republic of Egypt, and the Social Development Center, Chicago.

Data for Egypt illustrate the underestimation of the
reliability of modern contraceptive methods (and
overestimation of the reliability of traditional or folk
methods) in many--if not most--Third World countries.
Table 12 reports the perceptions of an Egyptian sample
about the reliability of the various methods.   The
correct answer for all methods is "reliable," which
includes all responses from "very reliable" to "moderately reliable."   Obviously, there is massive under-
appreciation of the efficacy of modern contraceptives in

avoiding pregnancy.  Those who use these methods can only
suffer needless anxiety and worry; this anxiety is part
of the price faced by potential users who hold these
popular views.

An "index of misinformation about reliability," compiled by combining all items of understatement of efficacy
(and overstatement of efficacy of spermicides, condoms,
and rhythm), is reported in the bottom panel of Table
12.   One-third of the population is highly misinformed
on this index, and an additional 55 percent moderately
so; only one adult in eight can be said to be adequately
informed.  The impact of this misinformation on the use
of contraception is clear:  the rate of contraceptive use
is only one-half as high among those who are poorly
informed as among the very few who are not misinformed.

### PSYCHOLOGISTICS:  PERCEIVED ACCESSIBILITY OF CONTRACEPTIVE SERIVCES

Some form of family planning service is "available" (at a
cost) to a very high percentage of fertile couples in
developing countries.  Even where there are no organized
family planning programs, contraceptives can be obtained
in pharmacies and/or from private physicians in nearby
cities.  Instead of being objective statements of reality,
discussions of availability tend to become subjective
studies of potential user's knowledge and perceptions; if
services are perceived as being nonexistent or too incon-
venient and costly, it is as if they did not in fact
exist.

Tsui et al. (1981) found that perceived availability
was significantly linked to contraceptive use in three
developing countries (Bangladesh, Korea, and Mexico).
Lightbourne et al. (1982) report World Fertility Survey
data indicating that, in most Asian and Latin American
countries surveyed, high proportions of the respondents
(49 to 92 percent) knew of an outlet where family planning services could be obtained.  Brackett and Ravenholt
(1980) found that this knowledge is related to travel
time to the nearest sources:  perceived availability
declines with greater distance, and is also linked with
actual use.  (Lightbourne et al. [1982] confirm this.)

Perceived availability of contraception can involve a
number of dimensions.  Monetary cost is obviously important:  if people believe they cannot afford contraception
at current prices, it is inaccessible to them.  Family

planning programs around the world are subsidizing
supplies and services in order to overcome this psychic
cost. Another dimension is follow-up medical care.
Where clinics have a reputation for not answering questions or not showing concern for women with symptoms of
side effects of contraception, it is logical to expect
reluctance to adopt. Also significant is the general
treatment clients receive when they attend clinics--
waiting time, cordiality of staff, willingness to answer
questions, privacy, and confidentiality. Finally, some
clinics, biased in favor of or against particular methods,
may recommend and provide only one kind of contraceptive,
giving the client no choice.

Research on these dimensions is extremely limited,
despite awareness of their importance on the part of
experts in the management of contraceptive services.
Some programs have sought to provide the ultimate in
accessibility--delivery of the service to individual
homes, free of charge. Such "saturation" experiments
have usually resulted in increased acceptance and use, at
least temporarily.

A special dimension of accessibility is whether to
integrate family planning with other health or social
development programs, thereby providing wider coverage
and greater acceptability, or to maintain specialized
family planning programs. Experience in some countries
has shown that busy and overworked public health clinics
tend to give contraception a lower priority and to show
less initiative and consistency in offering it than
specialized family planning agencies.

All of the international agencies dealing with contraception are dedicated to the principle that perceived
accessibility--in its physical, financial, and human
relations dimensions--must be improved. Thus, they are
seeking to promote accessibility as part of their technical assistance, training, and advisory services.


                    SYNTHESIS AND CONCLUSIONS

The normative and psychic costs of contraception reviewed
above can be categorized according to level of prevalence
and impact:

    Level 1:  Minor normative and psychic costs
    Level 2:  Moderate normative and psychic costs
    Level 3:  Major normative and psychic costs

It should be noted that there is great country-to-country variability, and that only crude data exist for some areas.  Because so little is known of the situation in sub-Saharan Africa, it is prudent to limit the classification to the Third World nations in Asia, Latin America, and Northern Africa and the Middle East.

Level 1:  Minor Normative and Psychic Costs   The empirical evidence indicates that the following four sources of psychic and normative costs are not highly prevalent and do not have a strong impact on contraceptive practice:

    Disharmony with the extended family system
    Loss of enjoyment of children
    Threat to sex roles and sexual adjustment
    Violation of modesty and privacy in sexual matters

The wide dissemination of information about population and contraception over the past decade, combined with the increasing availability of a wide variety of reliable modern contraceptives and rising material expectations, appear to have negated the impact of these factors.

Level 2:  Moderate Normative and Psychic Costs   These normative and psychic costs appear to be moderately prevalent in Third World societies; in most nations, only a minority of the population is affected by each.  Within that minority, these factors usually have a moderate or weak impact, so that, overall, they have a strong impact on only a small fraction of the total.

    Nonconformity with religious and moral beliefs
    Provoking discord between spouses
    Undermining family security and status
    Making the family vulnerable to infant mortality
    Perceived accessibility of contraceptive services

Level 3:  Major Normative and Psychic Costs   The following costs appear to have a major effect on a very large share of those couples in Third World countries who are not now contracepting.  Thus they may be identified as the major barriers to greater adoption of family planning, in the following order of importance:

Fears of permanent damage to health
Anxiety about temporary side effects
Requiring communication about sex between spouses
Implying "inner control" or "efficacy"
Socially illegitimate behavior
A threat to self-fulfillment and security in the
family role

Because of the fragmentary and varied nature of the
empirical data, this synthesis is necessarily highly
informal and approximate.  However, it should provide
hypotheses for further research efforts; these efforts
need to be multivariate, with all of the normative and
psychic costs considered simultaneously to measure the
independent impact of each.

A few other concluding points might be made.  First,
in Third World nations, certain fundamental, noneconomic
social changes associated with modernization appear to be
taking place that have only a low correlation with changes
in the per-capita gross national product (the usual
indicator of economic development).  All have the effect
of reducing the psychic and normative costs of contraception.  These changes may be identified as follows:

a.  Progressive nuclearization of the family, with
    diminishing power of the extended family
b.  Urbanization of the population, with increasing
    secularization and individualization
c.  Decreasing infant mortality rates
d.  Increasing democracy in the status of women
e.  Extensive mass media exposure to modern ("Western")
    models of husband-wife interaction and decision
    making
f.  Increasing internal control and decreasing external
    control in a wide sphere of activity, including
    health
g.  Rapid accumulation of knowledge, accompanied by
    increased pressures for long-range planning and
    decision making

With these changes, decreasing prevalence and impact of
the contraceptive costs discussed in this paper can be
anticipated, even where economic development stagnates.

Second, most of the "major" and "moderate" costs
(including family vulnerability to infant mortality,
socially illegitimate behavior, anxiety about temporary
side effects, fears of permanent damage to health,

anxiety about contraceptive failure, perceived physical accessibility, and perceived organizational availability) can be affected by well-planned programs of public information based on scientific fact, without "propaganda" either for or against any particular population policy.

Finally, this discussion has treated each of the psychic and normative costs as if its relationship to contraception were inherently negative. To the extent that these costs are based on norms, once the pronatalist position of a society becomes a minority point of view, the direction of influence of all of the culture-based costs is reversed. For example, the social legitimacy factor can (and does) turn into social disapproval and gossip about people who bear excessive numbers of children. Such a reversal may be expected for disharmony with the extended family system, loss of enjoyment of children, nonconformity in religious and moral beliefs, threat to self-fulfillment and security in the family role, socially illegitimate behavior, requiring communication about sex between spouses, and implying "inner control" or "efficacy." Survey evidence is showing that already, pronatalist values are a minority view in many Third World countries. Thus, as worldwide discussion of the topic continues, one can expect many costs of contraception to turn into costs of noncontraception.

## BIBLIOGRAPHY

Ager, J. W. (1976) Multiple regression and facet techniques in psychological research on population. Pp. 87-103 in S. H. Newman and V. D. Thompson, eds., Population Psychology: Research and Educational Issues. Washington, D.C.: U.S. Department of Health, Education, and Welfare.

American Psychological Association (1972) Task force on psychology, family planning, and population policy report. American Psychologist 27:1000-1005.

Arnold, F., and J. T. Fawcett (1976) The Value of Children: Hawaii, Vol. 3. Honolulu: East-West Population Institute.

Back, K. W., and P. H. Hass (1973) Family structure and fertility control. In J. T. Fawcett, ed., Psychological Perspectives on Population. New York: Basic Books.

Bagozzi, R. P., and F. Van Loo (1978)  Toward a general theory of fertility:  A causal modeling approach. Demography 15:301-319.

Bakare, C. G. (1974)  An appraisal of psychology research in family planning. Professional Psychology 5:346-351.

Bakker, C. B., and C. R. Dightman (1964)  Psychological factors in fertility control. Fertility and Sterility 15:559-567.

Beckman, L. J. (1981)  The relationship between sex roles, fertility, and family size preferences. Psychological Abstracts 65:18-49.

Bertrand, J. T., M. A. Pineda, and E. Soto (1978) Communicating Family Planning to Rural Guatemala. Chicago:  Community and Family Study Center, University of Chicago.

Bogue, D. J. (1962)  Some tentative recommendations for a "sociologically correct" family planning communication and motivation program in India.  Pp. 503-538 in C. V. Kiser, ed., Research in Family Planning.  Princeton, N.J.:  Princeton University Press.

Bogue, D. J. (1967)  Sociological Contributions to Family Planning Research.  Chicago:  Community and Family Study Center, University of Chicago.

Bogue, D. J., ed. (1970)  Further Sociological Contributions to Family Planning Research.  Chicago: Community and Family Study Center, University of Chicago.

Boldt, E., and A. H. Latif (1977)  Contraceptive careers:  Towards a subjective approach to fertility regulating behavior. Journal of Comparative Family Studies 8:357-367.

Brackett, J. W., and R. T. Ravenholt (1980)  The potential demand for voluntary sterilization:  Some findings from the World Fertility Survey.  In M. E. Schima and I. Lubell, eds., Voluntary Sterilization: A Decade of Achievement.  New York:  Association for Voluntary Sterilization.

Brody, E. B. (1974)  Psychocultural aspects of contraceptive behavior in Jamaica:  Individual fertility control in a developing country. Journal of Nervous and Mental Disease 159:108-109.

Brody, E. B., F. Ottey, and J. LaGranada (1974)  Couple communication in the contraceptive decision making of Jamaican women. The Journal of Nervous and Mental Disease 159:407-412.

Bulatao, R. A. (1975)  The Value of Children: Philippines, Vol. 2.  Honolulu:  East-West Population Institute.

Bulatao, R. A. (1981) Values and disvalues of children in successive childbearing decisions. Demography 18:1-25.

Buripakdi, C. (1977) The Value of Children: Thailand, Vol. 4. Honolulu: East-West Population Institute.

Caldwell, J. C. (1976) Toward a restatement of demographic transition theory. Population Development Review 2:321-366. (Reprinted in J. C. Caldwell, The Persistance of High Fertility, 1977.)

Cawte, J. (1975) Psychosexual and cultural determinants of fertility choice behavior. American Journal of Psychology 132:750-753.

CELADE and CFSC (1972) Fertility and Family Planning in Metropolitan Latin America. Chicago: Community and Family Study Center, University of Chicago.

Chung, B. M., J. A. Palmore, S. J. Lee, and S. L. Lee (1972) Psychological Perspectives: Family Planning in Korea. Seoul: Korean Institute for Research in the Social Sciences.

Cicourel, A. V. (1967) Fertility, family planning, and social organization: Some methodological issues. Journal of Social Issues 23.

Clifford, W. B., and T. R. Ford (1974) Variations in value orientations and fertility behavior. Social Biology 21:185-195.

Cochrane, S. H., and F. D. Bean (1976) Husband-wife differences in the demand for children. Journal of Marriage and the Family 38:297-307.

Cogswell, B. E., and M. B. Sussman (1974) Changing roles of women, family dynamics, and fertility. Pp. 11-26 in H. Y. Tien and F. D. Bean, eds., Comparative Family and Fertility Research. Leiden: Brill.

Coombs, L., and D. Fernandez (1978) Husband-wife agreement about reproductive goals. Demography 15:57-73.

Crawford, T. J., R. Heredia, and E. Stocker (1970) Family planning attitudes and behavior as a function of the perceived consequences of family planning. In D. J. Bogue, ed., Further Sociological Contributions to Family Planning Research. Chicago: Community and Family Study Center, University of Chicago.

Davidson, A. R., and J. J. Jaccard (1975) Population psychology: A new look at an old problem. Journal of Personality and Social Psychology 31:1073-1082.

Davidson, A. R., and J. J. Jaccard (1976) Social psychological determinants of fertility intentions. In S. H. Newman and V. D. Thompson, eds., Population

Psychology:  Research and Educational Issues.
Washington, D.C.:  U.S. Department of Health,
Education, and Welfare.
DuBois, C. A. (1963)  Socio-cultural aspects of
population growth.  Pp. 251-265 in R. O. Greep, ed.,
Human Fertility and Population Problems.  Cambridge,
Mass.:  Shenkman.
Elliott, R. (1973)  Advertising family planning.  In
Readings on Population Information and Education.  New
York:  Ford Foundation.
Fawcett, J. T. (1970)  Psychology and Population.  New
York:  Population Council.
Fawcett, J. T., ed. (1973)  Psychological Perspectives on
Population.  New York:  Basic Books.
Fawcett, J. T. (1974)  Psychological research on family
size and family planning in the United States.
Professional Psychology 5:334-344.
Figa-Talamanca, I., L. W. Green, and A. Fisher (1974)
Social and Psychological Aspects of Family Planning
Communication and Attitude Change Strategies.  Paper
presented at Expert Group Meeting on Social and
Psychological Aspects of Fertility Behavior, ESCAP,
Bangkok.
Fishbein, M., and J. Jaccard (1973)  Theoretical and
methodological considerations in the prediction of
family planning intentions and behavior.
Representative Research in Social Psychology 4:37-51.
Freedman, D. S., R. Freedman, and P. K. Whelpton
(1960-61)  Size of family and preference for children
of each sex.  American Journal of Sociology 66:141-159.
Freedman, R. (1962)  American studies of family planning
and fertility:  A review of major trends and issues.
Pp. 211-227 in C. V. Kiser, ed., Research in Family
Planning.  Princeton, N.J.:  Princeton University
Press.
Freedman, R., and J. Y. Takeshita (1969)  The program
setting, results, and implications.  Pp. 171-200 in
Family Planning in Taiwan.  Princeton, N.J.:
Princeton University Press.
Freedman, R., and P. K. Whelpton (1952)  Fertility
planning and fertility rates by adherence to
traditions.  In P. K. Whelpton and C. V. Kiser, eds.,
Social and Psychological Factors Affecting Fertility,
Vol. 3.  New York:  Milbank Memorial Fund.
Freedman, R., and P. K. Whelpton (1952)  The relationship
of general planning to fertility planning and
fertility rates.  Pp. 549-574 in P. K. Whelpton and C.

V. Kiser, eds., Social and Psychological Factors
Affecting Fertility, Vol. 3. New York: Milbank
Memorial Fund.

Friedman, H. L., R. L. Johnson, and H. P. David (1976)
Dynamics of fertility choice behavior: A pattern for
research. In S. H. Newman and V. D. Thompson, eds.,
Population Psychology: Research and Educational
Issues. Washington, D.C.: U.S. Department of Health,
Education, and Welfare.

Groat, N. T., and A. G. Neal (1967) Social psychological
correlates of urban fertility. American Sociological
Review 32:945-959.

Hass, P. H. (1974) Wanted and unwanted pregnancies: A
fertility decision-making model. Journal of Social
Issues 30:125-165.

Hill, R., J. M. Stycos, and K. Black (1959) The Family
and Population Control. Chapel Hill, N.C.:
University of North Carolina Press.

Hoffman, L. W., and F. Wyatt (1960) Social change and
motivations forhaving larger families: Some
theoretical considerations. Merrill-Palmer Quarterly
6:235-244.

Hollerbach, P. E. (1980) Power in Families:
Communication and Fertility in Decision-Making.
Center for Policy Studies Working Papers No. 53. New
York: Population Council.

Holmes, H. (1973) Human Factors which Influence
Responses to Family Planning among Northeastern Thai
Villagers. UNDP/UNICEF Development Support
Communication Service.

Insko, C. A., R. R. Blake, R. B. Cialdini, and S. A.
Mulaik (1970) Attitude toward birth control and
cognitive consistency: Theoretical and practical
implications of survey data. Journal of Personality
and Social Psychology 16:228-237.

Iritani, T. (1979) The Value of Children: Japan, Vol.
6. Honolulu: East-West Population Institute.

Keller, A. B. (1970) Psychological sources of resistance
to family planning. In D. J. Bogue, ed., Further
Sociological Contributions to Family Planning
Research. Chicago: Community and Family Study
Center, University of Chicago.

Keller, A. B. (1973) Patient attrition in five Mexico
City family planning clinics. In J. M. Stycos, ed.,
Clinics, Contraception and Communication: Evaluation
Studies of Family Planning Programs in Four Latin
American Countries. New York: Appleton-Century-
Crofts.

Laing, J. E. (1970)  The relationship between attitudes and behavior:  The case of family planning.  In D. J. Bogue, ed., Further Sociological Contribution to Family Planning Research.  Chicago:  Community and Family Study Center, University of Chicago.

Lee, R. P. L. (1974)  Social Change and Changes in Fertility Motivation.  Paper presented at Expert Group Meeting on Social and Psychological Aspects of Fertility Behavior, ESCAP, Bangkok.

Lee, S. J., and J. Kim (1979)  The Value of Children: Korea, Vol. 7.  Honolulu:  East-West Population Institute.

Lehfeldt, H. (1971)  Psychology of contraceptive failure.  Medical Aspects of Human Sexuality 5:68–77.

Leibenstein, H. (1974)  An interpretation of the economic theory of fertility:  Promising path or blind alley? The Journal of Economic Literature 12:456–487.

Lidz, R. (1969)  Emotional factors in the success of contraception.  Fertility and Sterility 20:761–771.

Lightbourne, R., S. Singh, and C. Green (1982)  The World Fertility Survey:  Charting global childbearing. Population Bulletin 37(1).  Washington, D.C.: Population Reference Bureau.

MacDonald, A. P., Jr. (1970)  Internal–external locus of control and the practice of birth control.  Psychology Reports 27:206.

Miller, W. B. (1973)  Personality and Ego Factors Relative to Family Planning and Population Control. Unpublished report.  Department of Psychiatry, Stanford University, Stanford, Calif.

Miller, W. B., and R. K. Godwin (1977)  Psyche and Demos:  Individual Psychology and the Issues of Population.  New York:  Oxford University Press.

Morgan, R. W., J. Kocher, and M. Carvajal (1976)  New Perspectives in the Demographic Transition. Occasional Monograph Series No. 4.  Washington, D.C.: Interdisciplinary Communications Program, Smithsonian Institution.

Mundigo, A. I. (1973)  Honduras revisited:  The clinic and its clientele.  In J. M. Stycos, ed., Clinics, Contraception, and Communication:  Evaluation Studies of Family Planning Programs in Four Latin American Countries.  New York:  Appleton-Century-Crofts.

Newman, S. H., and V. D. Thompson, eds. (1976) Population Psychology:  Research and Educational Issues.  Washington, D.C.:  U.S. Department of Health, Education, and Welfare.

Niehoff, A. H., and J. C. Anderson (1966)  Peasant fatalism and socioeconomic innovation. <u>Human Organization</u> 25:273-282.

Olson-Prather, E. (1976)  Family planning and husband-wife relationships in Turkey. <u>Journal of Marriage and the Family</u> 38:379-385.

Palmore, J. A. (1976)  Demographic evaluation systems and psychological research designs.  In S. H. Newman and V. D. Thompson, eds., <u>Population Psychology:  Research and Educational Issues</u>. Washington, D.C.:  U.S. Department of Health, Education, and Welfare.

Palmore, J. A., P. M. Hirsch, and A. B. Marzuki (1971) Interpersonal communication and the diffusion of family planning in West Malaysia. <u>Demography</u> 8:411-425.

Piotrow, P. T. (1973)  <u>World Population Crisis:  The United States Reponse</u>. New York:  Praeger.

Poffenberger, T. (1969)  <u>Husband-Wife Communication and Motivational Aspects of Population Control in an Indian Village</u>. New Delhi:  Central Institute of Family Planning.

Pohlman, E. (1969)  <u>The Psychology of Birth Planning</u>. Cambridge, Mass.:  Schenkman Publishing Company, Inc.

Polgar, S. (1966)  Some socio-cultural aspects of family planning in the United States today. <u>Human Organization</u> 25:321.

Polgar, S. (1975)  Cultural development, population, and the family.  Pp. 239-251 in Department of Economic and Social Affairs, <u>The Population Debate:  Dimensions and Perspectives</u>.  Papers of the World Population Conference, Bucharest, 1974.  New York:  United Nations.

Pratt, L., and P. K. Whelpton (1953)  Extra-familial participation of wives in relation to interest in and liking children, fertility planning, and actual and desired family size.  In P. K. Whelpton and C. V. Kiser, eds., <u>Social and Psychological Factors Affecting Fertility</u>. New York:  Milbank Memorial Fund.

Presser, H. B. (1977)  Early motherhood:  Ignorance or bliss? <u>Family Planning Perspectives</u> 9.

Presser, H. B. (1977)  Guessing and misinformation about pregnancy risks among urban mothers. <u>Family Planning Perspectives</u> 9.

Rainwater, L. (1965)  <u>Family Design:  Marital Sexuality, Family Size, and Contraception</u>. Chicago:  Aldine.

Rogers, E. M. (1971)  Incentives in the diffusion of family planning innovations. <u>Studies in Family Planning</u> 2:241-248.

Rogers, E. M. (1973)  Communication Strategies for Family Planning. New York:  The Free Press.

Rosario, F. Z. (1971)  A Survey of Social Psychological Variables Used in Studies of Family Planning. Paper No. 11.  Honolulu:  East-West Communications Institute.

Ross, J. A., and R. G. Potter (1980)  Changes in acceptors' and users' ages:  A test of an explanatory mechanism. Population Studies 34:367-380.

Rotter, J. B. (1960)  Generalized expectancies for internal versus external control reinforement. Psychological Monographs 80:1-28.

Sandberg, E. C., and R. I. Jacobs (1971)  Psychology of the misuse and rejection of contraception. American Journal of Obstetrics and Gynecology 110:227-242.

Shedlin, M. G., and P. E. Hollerbach (1981)  Modern and traditional fertility regulation in a Mexican community:  The process of decision making. Studies in Family Planning 12:278-296.

Shevasunt, S., and D. P. Hogan (1979)  Fertility and Family Planning in Rural Northern Thailand. Chicago:  Community and Family Study Center, University of Chicago.

Sinquefield, J. C. (1974)  A Social-Psychological Study of Resistance to Family Planning in Rural Alabama. Chicago:  Community and Family Study Center, University of Chicago.

Smith, M. B. (1965)  Motivation, communications research, and family planning. Pp. 70-92 in M. Sheps and J. C. Ridley, eds., Public Health and Population Change. Pittsburgh, Pa.:  University of Pittsburgh Press.

Steinlauf, B. (1979)  Problem-solving skills, locus of control, and the contraceptive effectiveness of young women. Child Development 50:268-271.

Stoeckel, J. E. (1970)  A socio-demographic analysis of family planning in a rural area of East Pakistan. In D. J. Bogue, ed., Further Sociological Contributions to Family Planning Research. Chicago:  Community and Family Study Center, University of Chicago.

Stycos, J. M. (1962)  A critique of the traditional Planned Parenthood approach in underdeveloped areas. Pp. 477-501 in C. V. Kiser, ed., Research in Family Planning. Princeton, N.J.:  Princeton University Press.

Stycos, J. M. (1968)  Contraception and Catholicism in Latin America. In J. M. Stycos, ed., Human Fertility in Latin America. Ithaca, N.Y.:  Cornell University Press.

Stycos, J. M. (1971)  Opinion, ideology, and population problems:  Some sources of domestic and foreign opposition to birth control.  Pp. 533-566 in National Academy of Sciences, Rapid Population Growth, Consequences and Implications.  Baltimore, Md.:  The Johns Hopkins Press.

Stycos, J. M., ed. (1973)  Clinics, Contraception, and Communication:  Evaluation Studies of Family Planning Programs in Four Latin American Countries.  New York:  Appleton-Century-Crofts.

Stycos, J. M. (1977)  Indexing birth control.  Family Planning Perspectives 9:286-292.

Stycos, J. M., and K. W. Back (1964)  The Control of Human Fertility in Jamaica.  Ithaca, N.Y.:  Cornell University Press.

Stycos, J. M., and P. G. Marden (1973)  Health and family planning in a Honduran barrio.  In J. M. Stycos, ed., Clinics, Contraception, and Communication:  Evaluation Studies of Family Planning Programs in Four Latin American Countries.  New York:  Appleton-Century-Crofts.

Sujono, H. (1974)  The Adoption of an Innovation in a Developing Country:  The Case of Family Planning in Indonesia.  Chicago:  Community and Family Study Center, University of Chicago.

Thompson, L., and G. B. Spanier (1978)  Influence of parents, peers, and partners on the contraceptive use of college men and women.  Journal of Marriage and the Family 40:481-491.

Thompson, V. D., and H. P. David (1977)  Population psychology in perspective.  International Journal of Psychology 12:135-146.

Tien, H. Y., and F. D. Bean, eds. (1974)  Comparative Family and Fertility Research.  Leiden:  Brill.

Tobin, P. L. (1976)  Conjugal role definition, value of children, and contraceptive practice.  Social Quarterly 17:314-322.

Townes, B., F. L. Campbell, L. R. Beach, and D. C. Martin (1976)  Birth planning values and decisions:  Preliminary findings.  In S. H. Newman and V. D. Thompson, eds., Population Psychology:  Research and Educational Issues.  Washington, D.C.:  U.S. Department of Health, Education, and Welfare.

Tsui, A. O., D. P. Hogan, J. D. Teachman, and C. Welti-Chanes (1981)  Community availability of contraceptives and family limitation.  Demography 18:615-625.

Wanty-Pancot, M. C., and G. Rucquoy (1975) Psychological resistance of women to the principal feminine contraceptive methods: Toward a clinical classification. Acta Psychiatrica Belgica 75:49-73.

Westoff, C. F., R. G. Potter, P. C. Sagi, and E. G. Mishler (1961) Family Growth in Metropolitan America. Princeton, N.J.: Princeton University Press.

Westoff, C. F., R. G. Potter, and P. C. Sagi (1963) The Third Child. Princeton, N.J.: Princeton University Press.

Whelpton, P. K., and C. V. Kiser, eds. (1946, 1950, 1954, 1958) Social and Psychological Factors Affecting Fertility. New York: Milbank Memorial Fund.

Williams, P. (1970) Traditionalism and change receptivity: A study of reactions to a fertility reduction campaign. In D. J. Bogue, ed., Further Sociological Contributions to Family Planning Research. Chicago: Community and Family Study Center, University of Chicago.

Wood, R. J., F. L. Campbell, B. D. Townes, and L. R. Beach (1977) Birth Planning Decisions. American Journal of Public Health 67:563-565.

World Health Organization Task Force on Psychosocial Research in Family Planning and Task Force on Service Research in Family Planning (1980) User preferences for contraceptive methods in India, Korea, the Philippines, and Turkey. Studies in Family Planning 11:267-273.

World Health Organization Task Force on Psychosocial Research in Family Planning, Special Programme of Research, Development, and Research Training in Human Reproduction (1981) A cross-cultural study of menstruation: Implications for contraceptive development and use. Studies in Family Planning 12:3-16.

World Health Organization Task Force on Psychosocial Research in Family Planning, Special Programme of Research, Development, and Research Training in Human Reproduction (1981) Women's bleeding patterns: Ability to recall and predict menstrual events. Studies in Family Planning 12:17-27.

Wu, T.-S. (1977) The Value of Children: Taiwan, Vol. 5. Honolulu: East-West Population Institute.

Wyatt, F. (1967) Clinical notes on the motives of reproduction. Journal of Social Issues 23:29-56.

Yaukey, D., W. Griffiths, and B. J. Roberts (1967) Couple concurrence and empathy on birth control motivation in Dacca, East Pakistan. American Sociological Review 32:716-726.

Chapter 5

# Abortion: Its Prevalence, Correlates, and Costs

HENRY P. DAVID*

## INTRODUCTION

Induced abortion is one of the oldest forms of fertility regulation;[1] it is also one of the most controversial.[2] No other elective surgical procedure has evoked as much worldwide debate, generated such emotional and moral controversy, or received greater sustained attention from members of the public concerned with women's rights and well-being. Although some developing countries have achieved significant fertility declines in recent years, actual family size continues to exceed total desired family size in most (Harrison, 1980; Westoff, 1981; World Fertility Survey, 1980). In many countries, abortion is a traditional method of fertility regulation, especially where modern contraceptives are only gradually becoming accessible. The World Fertility Survey (WFS) obtained little information on abortion, in part because the host governments decided against using the WFS abortion module; however, evidence strongly suggests that nearly everywhere, women of all backgrounds resort to abortion to some extent, regardless of legal codes, religious sanctions, or personal dangers.[3]

*It gives me much pleasure to acknowledge the support and encouragement extended over many years by Christopher Tietze (Population Council). Considerable assistance in preparing this paper was generously provided by Sev Fluss (Health Legislation Subunit, Office of Publications, World Health Organization, Geneva), the Population Reference Bureau (Washington), and the Population Information Program of Johns Hopkins University (Baltimore). The opinions expressed and remaining errors are solely the author's responsibility.

193

Because of the illegality, social ambivalence, and political sensitivity associated with abortion, empirical data about its role within the total context of fertility regulation still pose numerous questions. It is the purpose of this paper to summarize what is known about prevalence, costs, and correlates of abortion in developing countries. An overview of abortion procedures is followed by a discussion of research data sources and constraints. The legal status and actual practice of abortion in 144 countries are then summarized. This is followed by a discussion of the worldwide incidence of abortion and perceptions of its prevalence, as well as its effects on fertility rates, the abortion-contraception relationship, and the role of repeat abortions. Characteristics of clients and service providers are also noted. Next, available data on mortality and morbidity are reviewed within the context of the legal status of abortion. This is followed by a discussion of economic, social, and psychological costs for the woman, her family, and society; the costs of denied abortion are also considered. The paper concludes with a list of propositions summarizing the major points presented and suggesting areas for further research.

## Abortion Procedures

As used by the medical profession, the term "abortion" denotes the termination of a pregnancy "after the implantation of the blastocyst in the endometrium but before the fetus has attained viability, that is, before it has become capable of surviving, with appropriate life support, the neonatal period and eventually maintaining an independent extrauterine life" (Tietze, 1981). The two major categories of abortions are the induced and the spontaneous. The former are initiated voluntarily to terminate a pregnancy that is known or believed to exist; all other abortions are deemed spontaneous, even if an external cause is involved, such as an injury or high fever. This paper addresses only induced abortion, whether legal or illegal according to the prevailing legislation in each country.

Three primary abortion methods are currently used by physicians: (1) instrumental evacuation by the vaginal route, (2) uterine surgery, and (3) medical induction of labor. In the first category, surgical curettage has been progressively replaced in recent years by suction

curettage, also known as vacuum aspiration, which has
been shown to be simpler, quicker, and less traumatic
(Tietze, 1981). The average time required for instrumental evacuation is less than five minutes. "Menstrual
regulation" is a variant of suction curettage that is
generally limited to the first two weeks after a missed
menstrual period when pregnancy cannot yet be reliably
diagnosed. It has become popular in many developing
countries with restrictive abortion legislation whose
statutes make proof of pregnancy an essential element of
the so-called crime of abortion (Dunshee de Abranches,
1976; Paxman and Barberis, 1980). "Dilatation and
evacuation" is the use of instrumental evacuation
procedures early in the second trimester, usually at 13
to 15 weeks of gestation. In the second category, the
two major uterine surgical procedures for the termination
of pregnancy are hysterotomy and hysterectomy. Finally,
medical induction of labor is generally used to terminate
second-trimester pregnancies, beginning in the 16th week
of gestation. Methods range from replacement of amniotic
fluid by a hypertonic solution of sodium chloride to
intraamniotic injections of prostaglandins. (For a
detailed description of these procedures and their
relative advantages and disadvantages, see Tietze, 1981).

Of course, persons without medical training also have
methods for inducing abortion. These include spells and
incantations, a variety of traditional medications that
tend to be either ineffective or toxic, and various
procedures designed to damage or destroy the conceptus,
leaving its expulsion to natural forces. The most widely
used method is probably the insertion of a foreign body
into the uterus. Twigs, roots, clothes hangers, rubber
tubes (catheters), and other objects have been used for
this purpose (e.g., Figa-Talamanca, 1977, 1980; Tietze,
1981). In Southeast Asia, abdominal massage is practiced
by indigenous midwives to induce bleeding (Narkavonnakit,
1979b; Narkavonnakit and Bennett, 1981; Gallen, 1982;
Gallen et al., 1981). Elsewhere, injections of soapy
water or readily available household disinfectants may be
used (Tietze, 1981).

The differential diagnosis between spontaneous and
illegal or self-induced abortion is sometimes impossible:
the latter cannot be identified without either evidence
of manipulation, such as injury to the cervix or perforation of the uterus, or information from the woman,
members of her family, or the person performing the
abortion. Most septic abortions are believed to be

induced; however, many illegally induced abortions show
no signs or symptoms, whereas some spontaneous abortions
do (Tietze, 1981).  Incomplete abortion is the most
common diagnosis when women are admitted to hospitals for
aftercare, usually for postabortal bleeding caused by
retention of placental tissue.


## Data Sources and Constraints

Although abortion is common, it is extremely difficult to
assess empirically.  Legal, religious, and cultural constraints vary widely, giving the term different meanings
from country to country and over time within the same
country.  Only recently and in a few countries has it
been possible to distinguish the costs of abortion (both
granted and denied) from other consequences of unwanted
pregnancy (Illsley and Hall, 1976; Moore, 1974, 1976;
David et al., 1978).

Research is most representative, valid, and reliable
in countries where abortion is legal, and where efficient
population registration systems include information on
fertility and related health services, for example in
Cuba, Czechoslovakia, Hungary, Denmark, and the United
Kingdom (e.g., Tietze, 1981).  However, few developing
countries have statistical systems that integrate abortion
and other health services data.  In countries where
abortion is illegal, most information on the health,
socioeconomic, and psychological costs of abortion is
derived from four sources:  hospital records, death
certificates, retrospective surveys of women, and
interviews with abortion service providers.  Terms and
measurements used in abortion research are defined in
Figure 1.

Hospital records generally report the number of women
admitted for treatment of abortion complications and the
number of subsequent deaths in a given period of time.
Such records can suggest a minimum incidence of mortality,
and reflect the public costs of illegal abortion (Figa-
Talamanca, 1979).  Among the major disadvantages of this
information source are frequent failure to differentiate
between spontaneous and induced abortion (WHO, 1979a),
inaccuracy of official records (Lopez-Escobar et al.,
1978), and the selectivity of women admitted to hospitals,
who represent an unknown proportion of the total number
of women obtaining abortions.  Thus, although hospital
records document the considerable expenses involved in

caring for women admitted for abortion-associated complications, conclusions based on these data are tenuous because they seldom consider the much larger proportion of women whose abortions do not necessitate hospitalization. With the growing availability of simpler methods for terminating early pregnancies, medical, paramedical, and nonmedical abortionists can be expected to improve their skills. Complications may be further reduced if present clinical trials with prostaglandin analogues lead to a low-cost vaginal suppository for safe, self-administered, first-trimester abortion (e.g., Foster, 1980).

Although death certificates can provide a minimum figure for abortion mortality, their completeness and validity varies greatly among developing countries. For example, deaths may be ascribed to other causes or simply not be registered.

Retrospective surveys of abortion incidence permit selection of representative samples and, if repeated, extrapolation to population subgroups over time. However, even in countries where abortion is legal, such as Hungary, Japan, and Yugoslavia, it has been noted that women either selectively "forget" to mention abortions in their pregnancy histories (e.g., Hungary, 1969b; Hogue, 1975, 1978), or do not include medication taken to bring on a late period (e.g., Newman, 1980). Another difficulty is the lack of comparability due to differences in design, as well as in age and marital status of respondents, and a lack of specificity in questions asked (e.g., Gaslonde, 1976). Prospective surveys are more valid, but are also much more costly (e.g., Santee, 1975). Another approach is the "randomized response technique," which permits respondents to give information on highly sensitive topics without revealing the actual facts to the interviewer (Warner, 1965). However, although numerous modifications have been explored, results have been mixed. In general, there are no reliable broad-based statistical data on illegal abortion (Tietze, 1981).

Recently published surveys of abortion service providers in Korea (Hong and Tietze, 1979), Thailand (Narkavonnakit, 1979a, 1979b), the Philippines (Gallen, 1982), and Mexico (Tomaro, 1981; Gallen et al., 1981) are more promising sources of abortion data. By developing rapport and guaranteeing anonymity, researchers have obtained reliable data about the abortion experience of selected married and unmarried women, confirmed by local interviews with women seeking abortions.

FIGURE 1   Terms and Measurements Used in Abortion Research

---

Terms

ABORTION:  The termination of a pregnancy before the fetus is capable
of extrauterine life (medical definition).

INDUCED ABORTION:  Deliberate interference with a pregnancy, with the
intention of terminating it, by the pregnant woman herself or by
another person.

SPONTANEOUS ABORTION:  All abortions not induced are spontaneous even
if an external cause such as trauma or disease is involved; also
called miscarriage.

SEPTIC ABORTION:  Abortion that is followed by infection.  The
majority of septic abortions are thought to be induced, but infection
can occur after spontaneous abortion.

INCOMPLETE ABORTION:  The presence of retained products of conception
in the uterus after a spontaneous or induced abortion.  Incomplete
abortion is the most common diagnosis when women are hospitalized for
abortion complications.

ABORTIFACIENT: A drug or other substance used to cause a pregnant
woman to abort.

Measurements

Abortion is usually measured by RATES, which relate numbers of
abortions to population, or by RATIOS, which relate numbers of
abortions to numbers of events such as livebirths, deliveries, or
pregnancies.

PREVALENCE RATE:  The proportion of women who have had one or more
abortions in their lifetimes, usually expressed as a percentage.  This
is the most common measurement reported by surveys.

ABORTION RATE (INCIDENCE RATE):  The number of abortions in a given
period, usually a year relative to a whole population or to a
population of women.  This measurement of incidence is usually
expressed as a number of abortions per 1,000 women of reproductive
age, 15-44 or 15-49.  Incidence rates can also be age- or
parity-specific.

HOSPITALIZED ABORTION RATE:  The number of women hospitalized in a
given period, usually one year, for abortion complications relative to
the population of all women or of women of fertile age.

ABORTION RATIO:  The number of abortions relative to the number of
live births, pregnancies, or deliveries in a given period (usually one
year), expressed as the number of abortions per 1,000 events.
Sometimes ratios are reported as the number of abortions in women's
lifetimes per 1,000 lifetime live births.

FIGURE 1 (continued)

---

ABORTION-MORTALITY RATIO:  The number of deaths associated with or
attributed to abortion per 100,000 abortions (also known as a
death-to-case rate).  When complete data are not available, the ratio
is often expressed as the number of in-hospital deaths attributed to
abortion per 1,000 cases of abortion complications.

ABORTION-MORTALITY RATE:  The number of deaths associated with or
attributed to abortion per 100,000 women of fertile age.

---

Sources:  Liskin (1980); Tietze (1981).

   Finally, abortion-related psychosocial research is
constrained by sociocultural ambiguities and political
sensitivities.  In the United States, for example, more
statistics are available on legal abortion than on any
other surgical procedure.  However, problems in interpretation persist, due partly to the difficulty of
obtaining representative population samples from the
range of public and private service providers.  These
problems are compounded by the lack of comparability
between local and regional studies, the complexities of
obtaining adequate follow-up access to the woman and her
partner, and the absence of standardized instruments for
assessing psychosocial and economic determinants and
costs (David, 1978a).  Reported sociodemographic information is usually very limited in the national surveys
conducted by the Centers for Disease Control (1980) or
the Alan Guttmacher Institute (Forrest et al., 1979;
Henshaw et al., 1981, 1982).  Similar limitations have
been noted in other developed countries where abortion is
legal (IUSSP, 1977).


## ABORTION POLICIES, LAWS, AND PRACTICES

As of April 1982, the worldwide legal status of abortion
ranges from complete prohibition to elective abortion at
the request of the woman during the first trimester of
pregnancy, usually defined as the first twelve weeks of
gestation beginning with the first day of the last menstrual period.  Figure 2 summarizes the current legislative situation in 144 countries, both developed and
developing, according to four major categories of abortion
availability and grounds.  In the 25 nations where
abortion is entirely illegal, no grounds for pregnancy
termination are cited in the legislation.  In 39

FIGURE 2   Legal Status of Abortion by Grounds April 1982:   144 Countries

| ILLEGAL | Belgium | Gabon | Monaco | Somalia |
|---|---|---|---|---|
| | Burundi | Haiti | Mongolia | Spain |
| Not allowed | Central | Indonesia | Niger | Tonga |
| regardless of | African Rep. | Iran | Panama | Upper Volta |
| indications | Colombia | Mali | Philippines | Western Samoa |
| | Dominican | Malta | Portugal | Zaire |
| N = 25 | Republic | Mauritania | Rwanda | |

| RESTRICTIVE | Afghanistan | Ireland | Mozambique | Sudan |
|---|---|---|---|---|
| | Bahrein | Ivory Coast | Nauru | Syria |
| Allowed under | Bangladesh | Kenya | Nicaragua | Togo |
| narrow life- | Benin | Laos | Nigeria | United Arab |
| threatening | Botswana | Lebanon | Pakistan | Emirate |
| conditions | Burma | Lesotho | Paraguay | Uruguay |
| only | Chad | Libya | Saudi Arabia | Vanuatu |
| | Chile | Madagascar | Senegal | Venezuela |
| N = 39 | Guatemala | Malawi | Sierra Leone | Yemen, North |
| | Iraq | Mauritius | Sri Lanka | Yemen, South |

| CONDITIONAL | Albania | Egypt | Jamaica | Peru |
|---|---|---|---|---|
| | Algeria | El Salvador | Jordan | Seychelles |
| Allowed under | Argentina | Ethiopia | Korea, Rep. of | South Africa |
| broad health, | Australia | Fiji | Kuwait | Swaziland |
| eugenic, and | Bahamas | Gambia | Liberia | Tanzania |
| juridical | Barbados | Ghana | Malaysia | Thailand |
| indications | Bolivia | Greece | Mexico | Trinidad and |
| | Brazil | Grenada | Morocco | Tobago |
| N = 48 | Cameroon | Guinea | Namibia | Turkey |
| | Canada | Guyana | Nepal | Uganda |
| | Congo | Honduras | New Zealand | Zimbabwe |
| | Costa Rica | Hong Kong | Papau-New | |
| | Ecuador | Israel | Guinea | |

| ELECTIVE | Austria | German Dem. | Korea, Dem. | Switzerland |
|---|---|---|---|---|
| | Bulgaria | Rep. | People's Rep. | Tunisia |
| Allowed on | China | German Fed. | Luxembourg | USSR |
| request or for | Cuba | Rep. | Netherlands | United Kingdom |
| social indica- | Cyprus | Hungary | Norway | USA |
| tions in first | Czechoslovakia | Iceland | Poland | Viet Nam |
| trimester | Denmark | India | Romania | Yugoslavia |
| | Finland | Italy | Singapore | Zambia |
| N = 32 | France | Japan | Sweden | |

Sources:   Official Gazettes:   International Digest of Health Legislation; Law
Files of the International Planned Parenthood Federation; Transnational Family
Research Institute; Cook and Dickens (1979); Stepan (1979); Paxman (1980a); and
David (1981).

countries, the availability of legal abortion is specifically restricted to situations threatening the woman's
life.  Conditional reasons for abortion are stated in the
laws of 48 lands; these conditions include risk to the
woman's mental or physical health beyond that normally
associated with pregnancy, some degree of likely impairment of the fetus or the child, and pregnancy resulting
from incest or rape.  In 32 lands, abortion is available
on request in the first 10 or 12 weeks of gestation, for
specific social or socioeconomic indications, or for
reasons of failure of a routinely used contraceptive
method.

Seen in historical perspective, a social revolution
has occurred in abortion legislation in recent decades.
In 1954, abortion was illegal in all countries except
Iceland, Denmark, Sweden, and Japan.[4]  In the subsequent
27 years, more than 30 countries, including such major
developing nations as China, India, Singapore, and
Tunisia, changed their formerly restrictive laws or
policies to permit abortion on a woman's request or for a
broad range of social indications.  These changes can be
traced, in part, to increased recognition of the health
dangers of illegal abortion, and to growing support for a
woman's right to terminate an unwanted pregnancy early in
gestation under safe conditions.  During the same period,
four Eastern European countries (Bulgaria, Czechoslovakia,
Hungary, and Romania) rerestricted their liberal legislation somewhat as part of a well organized pronatalist
effort (David and McIntyre, 1981; David, 1982a), while
New Zealand and Israel succumbed to conservative pressures
in making abortion for social reasons less accessible.
In Iran, the Revolutionary Government revoked implementation of the liberal legislation.  Only China, Singapore,
and Tunisia openly acknowledged legalizing abortion for
the purpose of limiting population growth and enhancing
social and economic development.  Presently, about two-
thirds of the world's population live under conditions of
liberal legislation, mostly in Europe, North America, and
parts of Asia.

In actual practice, abortion remains illegal, restrictive, or difficult to obtain in many of the larger and
more populous developing countries of Asia; all of Latin
America, except Cuba; all of sub-Saharan Africa; and all
the Moslem countries of the Middle East and North Africa,
except Tunisia and Kuwait.  In a number of countries
where abortion is legal, it is also extremely difficult
to obtain.  Legalization does not require health author-

ities to meet existing demand or ensure service availability at the earliest stage of pregnancy.[5] The
American and European experience of administrators
unwilling to comply with existing legislation, or health
personnel asking to be excused from providing abortion
services, can be duplicated in many developing countries.
Abortions continue to be enmeshed in more regulatory
requirements than most other medical procedures (Paxman,
1980a). In Brazil, Mexico, and Peru, where the legislation is conditional (covering only rape, incest, or
broadly defined health reasons), the process of obtaining
a legal abortion is so cumbersome that "conditional"
really is equivalent to illegal. Abortion is legally
available on request in India; however, it is in fact
largely unavailable in most rural areas where the majority of the population lives. In Zambia, bureaucratic
requirements and limited available resources complicate
legal abortion availability. The Kuwait legislation is
too recent to permit a judgment.

Conversely, in some countries, strict anti-abortion
laws are unenforced. In Chile, Korea, and Taiwan,
abortions are performed by physicians with little legal
risk. In Thailand, most identified rural abortionists
were wives of government civil servants (Narkavonnakit,
1979a). In Panama, law enforcement officials are known
to look the other way when physicians terminate early
pregnancies under the name "menstrual regulation."[6]
Elsewhere, definitions of legal grounds for abortion may
be so clouded and confusing as to preclude legal action
against physicians. Abortion to save a woman's life can
be authorized under the general principles of criminal
law applicable to a given state of necessity (Stepan,
1979); this probably explains why some abortions on
medical grounds are tolerated even in those few countries
where prohibitions against illegal abortions are said to
be strictly enforced.

In sum, evolving societal trends, coupled with the
increasingly well-organized women's movement and its male
supporters, gradually moved many legislators toward
abortion liberalization. However, because significant
segments of the population still oppose both abortion and
freer access to contraception, which could reduce the
need for abortion, termination of unwanted pregnancies
continues to be restricted for many women in developed
and developing countries, particularly the young and the
economically disadvantaged (Jaffe et al., 1981; David,
1981a).

INCIDENCE AND FERTILITY EFFECTS OF ABORTION

Worldwide Incidence and Perceived Prevalance

The total number of abortions performed each year
throughout the world is not known and perhaps never will
be.  Estimates range from 13.7 million (Rochat et al.,
1980) to 55 million (International Planned Parenthood
Federation, 1974, 1978), suggesting abortion ratios
ranging from 207 to 450 per 1,000 live births.  Moreover,
these estimates combine information from countries where
abortion is legal and reliably reported and those where
it is illegal or in which nationwide abortion data are
not reported.[7]

No reliable method has yet been devised to estimate
the incidence of illegal abortions (Tietze, 1981).[8]
However, on the basis of data cited by Tietze (1981),
International Planned Parenthood Federation (1974, 1978),
and Liskin (1980), as well as information gathered for
Abortion Research Notes (1972), it is possible to suggest
some broad patterns and trends in developing countries
where access to abortion is illegal or legally restricted.
Induced abortion is probably more frequent in Asia and
Latin America than in Africa and the Middle East.  It is
also perhaps more common in those countries of Southeast
Asia where it is legally restricted but widely available
in practice (e.g., South Korea, Thailand) than in those
countries where it is legal but actual access is very
limited (e.g., India).  Rates of illegal abortion are
probably increasing in most developing countries as a
larger proportion of women decide to terminate unwanted
pregnancies regardless of legal technicalities.  For
example, it has been suggested that every year in rural
Thailand, one in seven women of fertile age has an illegal
abortion, typically by means of abdominal massage provided
by a traditional practitioner residing in the woman's
village (Narkavonnakit, 1979a, 1979b, 1980; Narkavonnakit
and Bennett, 1981).

The situation in India is particularly noteworthy
because of the comparatively low incidence of legal
abortion since the Medical Termination of Pregnancy Act
made legal abortion available on request in 1972:  the
reported number of legal terminations increased from
24,000 in 1972 to 278,100 in 1977, while the number of
illegal abortions was estimated at between four and six
million (Goyal, 1978).  Indian researchers suggest that
women continue to resort to illegal abortion because of

insufficient information about legal termination services
(Chandrasekhar, 1978; Krishna Menon, 1979); limited
publicity about the law and the widely held misperception
that abortion is illegal (Goyal, 1978); lack of adequate
facilities, particularly in rural areas (Padubidri and
Kotwani, 1979); impersonal and unattractive abortion
services at approved centers, with long waiting periods
(P.S. David, 1978; Krishna Menon, 1979); and reluctance
of unmarried women to register for abortions at hospitals
and clinics (Bhatt, 1980). Since access to legal abortion
is limited, illegal abortion remains a major health
problem. This is in sharp contrast with South Korea,
where abortion is often perceived to be available on
request although its legal availability is conditional
(Hong and Watson, 1976): a 1975 national abortion survey
yielded an abortion ratio of 667 abortions per 1,000 live
births (Park et al., 1979); a 1977-78 survey of abortion
providers in Seoul suggested an abortion ratio of 2,750
per 1,000 live births in the capital city (Hong and
Tietze, 1979).

Most information on the extent of illegal abortion in
the Middle East from the 1960s and early 1970s is of
limited quality. More recent information from Tunisia
(where elective abortion is legal) and from Turkey (where
abortion is widely available) indicates that increasing
numbers of women have resorted to abortion to terminate
unwanted births (Nazer, 1980; Tecsan et al., 1980).

In sub-Saharan Africa, Zambia's legislation is similar
to that of Britain. The requirement that requests must
be approved by three physicians and that procedures must
be performed in hospitals, except under certain specified
circumstances, has kept the number of legal abortions
low--173 in 1976 (Mhango and Grech, 1979). Surveys have
not been particularly successful in eliciting information
on illegal abortion, in part because few women are willing
to admit flaunting strong tribal sanctions and legal
restrictions. Still, in many parts of Africa, abortion
is said to be a traditional form of birth control (Ndeti,
1973; Waife, 1978).


### Characteristics of Clients and Service Providers

### Clients

Major demographic characteristics reported from some of
the countries where abortion is legal include the woman's

age, number of prior births, and marital status. Among the women seeking abortions, the proportion of those under 20 years of age ranges between 25 and 30 percent in the United States, Canada, England and Wales, and Norway; in recent years, the United States has reported the highest proportion of teenagers and unmarried women among all women obtaining pregnancy terminations (CDC, 1979; Tietze, 1981). Conversely, the proportion of older, parous, and married women is high in Tunisia, India, Japan, Czechoslovakia, and Hungary. Intermediate positions are represented by Denmark, Finland, the German Federal Republic, and Singapore.

These patterns tend to reflect differences in adolescent sexual activity, societal disapproval of premarital pregnancies and births, and the customary age at first marriage, together with differences in the availability and accessibility of contraceptive and abortion services (Tietze, 1979b, 1981). Determinants of choice behavior in resolving an unwanted pregnancy--whether to terminate or not--also vary widely across and within cultures, influenced in part by considerations related to the present partner situation, postponement of initial childbearing, desire to extend childspacing, or the wish not to exceed the "completed" number of children (e.g., David, 1980; Miller, 1981).

As with all other data on illegal abortion, information on the social and demographic characteristics of women resorting to illegal abortions is fragmentary. Some data are available for Latin America (IFRP, 1980a). These data show that 18 percent of users were single and that 47 percent wanted no additional children. It might also be noted that the women in this study were markedly younger and of lower parity than those reported in Latin American studies published in the 1960s. Data for Asia (Liskin, 1980) showed that the number of abortions tended to increase with the wife's education and the husband's occupational status; 20 percent of users were single. A carefully designed study in a rural province in Thailand (Narkavonnakit, 1980) showed that nearly one-third of the married users had not completed their families and sought abortions for childspacing purposes; more than 50 percent had completed their families; and the remaining 10 percent cited marital or economic problems as their motive in seeking abortion. Finally, some data are available for Africa. Most African women using abortion tend to come from selected population subgroups and to practice abortion early in their reproductive careers (Liskin,

1980). The majority of those hospitalized for abortion complications are less than 25 years old, usually unmarried, and of low parity. Many young African women resort to abortion because pregnancy constitutes grounds for expulsion from most African schools (Siwale, 1977).


Service Providers

Surveys of illegal abortion practitioners have recently been reported from Thailand (Narkavonnakit, 1979a, 1979b; Narkavonnakit and Bennett, 1981) and from the Philippines (Gallen, 1982). These surveys show that most practitioners are women, generally without medical training. Most do not state their primary motive as making money, but regard or claim to regard what they are doing as a community service.[9] Moreover, most are seldom harrassed by local authorities. Sometimes, the performance of illegal abortions is seen by practitioners as a way to reduce health risks associated with many conditions under which such abortions are sought and as an opportunity to encourage the use of contraception (see Faundes and Hardy, 1978).

On the other hand, the reverse can also be true. In countries where abortion is legal, a woman's request to terminate an unwanted pregnancy presents an ethical and moral dilemma for many physicians and nurses, posing conflicts between the woman's decision and a personal commitment to saving life (e.g., Nathanson and Becker, 1977, 1980). In some respects, the process of obtaining an abortion differs markedly from traditional medical practice. Women wishing to terminate an unwanted pregnancy are usually "healthy"; some physicians are prepared to perform abortions to save a woman's physical health, but not to preserve the economic well-being of her family (Potts, 1979). These conflicts play a significant part in the abortion debate. Moreover, conditions of practice, perceptions of professional roles, and the woman's economic status are often interrelated. Historically, women with greater economic resources have had far fewer difficulties in obtaining abortions from qualified physicians than have economically disadvantaged women, whether the abortion sought was legal or illegal. Inequity is increased when private prejudice is permitted to become public policy because physicians and hospital administrators refuse to perform or permit legal abortions.

Effects on Fertility Rates

It has been suggested that no developed country has
achieved a decline in its birth rate without considerable
recourse to abortion, whether legal or illegal, and that
a similar situation prevails in developing countries
(Potts, 1972). This statement is supported by an extensive review of the available research literature (van der
Tak, 1974). In examining fertility trends, consideration
was given to availability of abortion in practice as well
as in law, to the extent of concurrent contraceptive
practice, and to the degree to which legal abortions
displaced previously illegal abortions. Note was also
taken of other factors bearing upon observed fertility
trends, such as changes in age at marriage and in sexual
behavior; age/sex and rural/urban population structure;
and concurrent socioeconomic and infant mortality levels.
The most dramatic recorded declines in fertility over
relatively short time periods occurred when elective
abortion was made available to a population already
strongly motivated to control family size, and practicing
only traditional or no contraception at the time of
abortion legalization.

Extensive surveys conducted over several years in
Korea demonstrate that abortion played an important role
in that country's national fertility decline and served
as a major stimulant for more effective contraceptive
practice (Hong and Watson, 1976). Presently, legal
abortion is widely used to supplement contraception,
especially by older women at higher parities and by urban
women with higher education (KIFP, 1979). In Latin
America, Cuba has achieved the lowest birth rate, 14.7
per 1,000 population in 1979. Recent fertility declines
have been associated with improved access to legal abortion and contraceptive services within the socialized
system of public health care. While the number of
induced abortions peaked in 1975, the abortion ratio
continued to rise, reaching 745 abortions per 1,000 live
births in 1978 (Hollerbach, 1980). Similarly, in the
People's Republic of China, abortion ratios in major
cities are increasing with declining birth rates (Tien
and Shao, 1980; Chen, 1981; Chen and Kols, 1982).


Abortion/Contraception Interrelationships

Studies of abortion are incomplete unless they consider
the complementary relationship between abortion and

contraception as methods of fertility regulation.
Successful contraception requires the coordination of
three distinct human forces:  the drive to have sexual
intercourse, the wish to have or not to have a child, and
the will to regulate the consequences of sexual behavior
(David et al., 1978). Although these forces may be
logically linked, they are not psychologically related.
Contraception requires a considerable and ever-vigilant
effort, typically with a longer-term reward that appears
only as the absence of an event. Although improvements
have been and continue to be made in fertility-regulating
methods and delivery systems, universal availability and
acceptability remain elusive goals.

All known societies use a mixture of contraception and
abortion to control their fertility (Potts, 1970).  Historically, the notion of preventing conception is relatively recent, requiring adherence to a new level of
shared responsibility in sexual behavior, exposure to and
acceptance of contraceptive information and education,
and conscious precoital planning.  In contrast, abortion
requires little prior educational effort; moreover, a
missed period and anxiety about an unwanted pregnancy
usually provide sufficient motivation.  Unlike most
contraceptives, abortion is a 100 percent effective,
one-time, coitus-independent operation, based on certainty rather than probability (Moore, 1971).  Abortion
also avoids interference with sexual activity and spares
the woman the health dangers believed by some to be
associated with modern contraceptives.  Furthermore,
where guilt is associated with abortion, at least some
guilt may also be associated with contraceptives, which
often require a continual rather than a single violation
of a value system.

The relative roles of contraception and abortion vary
within and between countries.  In some countries, abortion
is the primary means of fertility control; in others,
increased use of contraception lowers the incidence of
abortion; in still others, abortion and contraception
increase together.  These patterns suggest a possible
transitional path from high to lower abortion rates:
with the passage of time, contraceptive practice improves,
and resort to abortion declines, although it is never
eliminated.  Such has been the experience reported for
some countries of Western, Northern, and Eastern Europe,
Latin America, and Japan (e.g., Requena, 1970; van der
Tak, 1974; Potts et al., 1977; David and McIntyre, 1981).
Many developing countries are at an earlier phase in the

evolution of abortion practice, but may be moving more
rapidly to more effective contraceptive practice (David,
1982b).

In those countries where abortion and modern contraceptives are equally available, it is important to learn why
some women continue to rely on abortion rather than on
contraception.  Findings from Yugoslavia indicate a
greater degree of personal efficacy or control, future
planning, and husband-wife consensus in the group of
successful contraceptors.  A low sense of efficacy
threatens the effective use of contraceptive methods,
which require a woman's initiative and consistent discipline (Kapor-Stanulovic and Friedman, 1978; Bogue, in
these volumes).

Numerous studies have shown that women who are highly
motivated to control family size will use both abortion
and contraception (e.g., David et al., 1978; Potts et
al., 1977).  Women who have practiced contraception are
more likely to resort to abortion than those who have
not, and vice versa.  These relationships have been
documented in surveys of women in developed and developing countries where abortion is legal, for example,
Hungary (e.g., Klinger and Szabady, 1978; Klinger, 1979),
Japan (e.g., Muramatsu and van der Tak, 1978), Singapore
(e.g., Tan, 1978), Tunisia (e.g., Nazer, 1980), the
United States (Zelnik and Kantner, 1978), and Yugoslavia
(e.g., Kapor-Stanulovic and Friedman, 1978).  Similar
findings have been reported from countries where abortion
is technically illegal but easily available, for example,
South Korea (e.g., Hong and Watson, 1976), the Philippines
(e.g., Flavier and Chen, 1980), and Turkey (e.g., Tecsan
et al., 1980).  Other studies document the shift to more
vigilant contraceptive practice following hospitalization
for abortion or abortion complications (e.g., Miller et
al., 1976; Liskin, 1980).

Chile provides a particularly instructive example of
what can be accomplished when an intensive family planning
program is initiated at a time when contraceptive practice
is low and resort to illegal abortion high (Onetto, 1980).
Between 1964 and 1978, the percentage of women using
contraceptives increased seven-fold from 3.2 to 23
percent.  During the same period, the number of women
admitted to Chilean hospitals for abortion complications
declined from over 56,000 to 37,900, and abortion-related
maternal mortality decreased from 11.8 to 4.2 per 10,000
live births.  These observations, plus steady declines in
the total maternal mortality rate, the neonatal and infant

death rate, and the birth rate, suggest a gradual increase
in the number of women relying on contraception rather
than illegal abortion to control their fertility (Liskin,
1980).

Experience in different countries with varied abortion
legislation and access to modern contraceptives indicates
that the use of abortion or contraception is greatly
influenced by the availability of various methods and by
such personal characteristics as the woman's age and
parity (David et al., 1978). In general, if modern
contraceptives are readily obtainable, more women who
previously relied on ineffective methods, backed by legal
or illegal abortion, will shift to more efficient contraceptive practice (Liskin, 1980; David and McIntyre, 1981).
Part of the problem is that in numerous countries where
abortion is highly restrictive, hospitals and service
providers are, for diverse reasons, reluctant to offer
contraceptives to women hospitalized with complications
of illegal abortions (e.g., IFRP, 1980a; Gallen, 1982).
Under such circumstances, resort to repeat abortion is
almost inevitable.

Although the number of unmarried women included in
abortion studies in developing countries is generally
small, when meaningful comparison is possible, married
women are usually more likely to accept contraception
(e.g., Hardy and Herud, 1975; Miller et al., 1976,
1977). This may reflect women's differing perceptions of
their immediate need for contraception, as well as cultural attitudes about sexual activity and the acceptability of contraceptive use among unmarried women. However,
in a study of women under age 20 discharged from 39
hospitals in nine Latin American countries, the same
percentage of married as unmarried women were practicing
contraception when interviewed several weeks after treatment for abortion complications (IFRP, 1980a). The data
show that, in general, women over age 20 at higher parity
accept contraceptives after abortion more frequently than
women under age 20 at lower parity (e.g., Hardy and Herud,
1975; IFRP, 1980a; Miller et al., 1976, 1977).[10]

Women interviewed in hospitals after admission for
abortion complications at times represent a perplexing
group for advocates of family planning. For example, in
the Dominican Republic, such women were highly motivated
to prevent births of unwanted children and were generally
aware of the availability of modern contraceptives, but
gave little indication of adopting such methods. Illogi-
cal as it seems, women hospitalized with abortion

complications were fearful of health hazards believed to be associated with the longer-term use of contraceptives and preferred the risks of illegal abortion (Ramirez et al., 1978). This may be partly explained by the taboo nature of abortion, which impedes the dissemination of information through the media or by word of mouth; as one result, the same misinformation keeps recirculating. The true relationship between the risks of illegal abortion and contraception needs to be more fully communicated.

Abortion-related medical and behavioral research has focused almost entirely on women; men are often the forgotten sexual partner. Very few studies have reported on the couple decision-making process in developed or developing countries, and even fewer on male perceptions of and experiences with abortion (Miller and Godwin, 1977; David, 1980; Shostak, 1979). In numerous developing countries, many men continue to insist on having the sole right to decide whether or when to have a child, deny their wives access to contraception, and oppose changes in women's traditional roles (Stokes, 1980). For example, in the Dominican Republic, a sizable proportion of husbands either did not know or did not want to know their wives' abortion histories, preferring to let them take responsibility for such decisions (Friedman et al., 1975). Secretive abortion where male disapproval of contraception is perceived has also been reported from Jamaica (Brody et al., 1976; Brody, 1981) and Colombia (Browner, 1976).

Given reasonable availability of contraceptives, there is no evidence of competition between abortion and contraceptive practice. Women experiencing contraceptive failure followed by unintended conception and unwanted pregnancy are often prepared to go to any length to seek an abortion, whether legal or not. Observations from many countries suggest that "abortion is the horse that pulls contraceptive practice into the community" (Potts et al., 1977).

## Repeat Abortions

Five factors combine to make women with previous abortion experience more likely candidates for future abortions than other women (Tietze, 1978a; Tietze and Jain, 1978). First is the age factor: among women who have had at least one abortion, as compared to those who have not, more are in the sexually most active prime reproductive

age group (20-29 years), and fewer are teenagers and
older women. Second, it can be assumed that nearly all
women who have had abortions were sexually active and
probably resume sexual activity after their abortions.
Third, all women with abortion experience have been able
to conceive; this compares to the 40 percent of all women
aged 15 to 44 without abortion experience who are unable
to conceive, have undergone surgical sterilization, are
married to vasectomized men, or are not sexually active.
Fourth, women who have had one abortion are likely to
resort to another to avoid a future birth, whereas women
at risk of having a first abortion probably include a
substantial number who would not choose to terminate an
unintended conception. Finally, there is a very small
group of women who consciously prefer to rely on abortion
rather than on contraception, plus a larger number who
find it difficult to practice contraceptive vigilance
consistently and effectively. These women are at high
risk for both first and repeated abortions.

The proportion of repeat abortions among all abortions
has increased most rapidly in those countries, such as
the United States, where restrictive abortion laws and
practices have only recently been replaced by relatively
easier access to pregnancy termination. For example, in
the United States, the proportion of repeat abortions
rose from about 15.2 percent of all reported abortions in
1976 to 29.5 percent in 1978 (Tietze, 1981).[11] This
phenomenon should not be interpreted as a decrease in the
practice of contraception or motivational deficiencies.
Indeed, Tietze (1978a) concludes that, after experiencing
their first abortion, "a substantial majority" of women
"did in fact practice contraception with a high degree of
consistency and success." This finding has been substantiated by more recent U.S. studies (e.g., Howe et al.,
1979; Shepard and Bracken, 1979).

## MORTALITY AND MORBIDITY

### Mortality from Illegal Abortion

Illegal abortions are associated with greater mortality,
morbidity, and other long-term complications when performed by inexperienced practitioners or under unhygienic
conditions than when induced by skilled operators using
modern methods. Although, as previously noted, sources
of data are inaccurate and unreliable, review of avail-

able studies shows that abortion is a major cause of
maternal mortality in developing countries (Liskin,
1980). Mortality associated with illegal abortions is
probably about 50 to 100 deaths per 100,000 abortions.
Even at the lowest estimate, the death-to-case rate is
almost 50 times higher than that associated with legal
curettage procedures in the United States.

Since recorded hospital admissions often include women
with spontaneous abortions, which are less likely to be
life-threatening than illegal abortions, and generally
exclude women who do not come to the hospital after an
illegal abortion, the reported ratios may overestimate
mortality from illegally induced pregnancy terminations.
This observation is confirmed by studies from hospitals
in India and Thailand reporting mortality only among
women with admitted or presumed illegal abortions.  These
ratios range from 8 to 307 deaths per 1,000 admissions
for complications of illegal abortion (e.g., Bhatt and
Soni, 1973; Chatterjee, 1977; Malhotra and Devi, 1979;
Philips and Ghouse, 1976; Koetsawang, 1975, 1976).
Registered deaths attributed to complications of induced
and spontaneous abortion as a proportion of all registered
maternal deaths for the years 1970-78 show an annual
average of 20 percent or higher for several developing
countries.  However, such data are of questionable value
because many deaths are not registered; moreover, in some
countries, where overall maternal mortality is low, a few
deaths attributed to abortion may constitute a large proportion of all maternal deaths (Tietze, 1981).

Finally, it should be noted that medically safe abortions are available in nearly every country, dependent on
the ability to pay.  It is the large group of economically
disadvantaged women most in social need who, unable to
pay the price of safety, may pay with their health and
sometimes with their lives.


## Mortality from Legal Abortion

Data from countries where abortion is legal are usually
fairly complete, although they may underestimate the
number of abortions performed and associated deaths
(Moore, 1974; Potts et al., 1977).  In the United States,
more epidemiological data have become available for the
mortality and morbidity of legal abortion than for any
other surgical procedure. The mortality ratio from legal
abortion was shown to be lowest of all (Cates and Tietze,

1978; Grimes and Cates, 1979),[12] with the rate increasing as the abortions were performed later in the gestation period (Centers for Disease Control, 1980). When performed under ideal conditions, first-trimester abortion has a mortality as low as one per 100,000 (IFRP, 1980b). In Cuba, where access to legal abortion was gradually liberalized in the 1960s and there is a good registration system, the mortality ratio was 1.2 deaths per 100,000 legal abortions during 1971-1974. Total abortion deaths per 100,000 women age 15 to 44 years declined from 3.6 in 1968 to 1.6 in 1974, falling further to 0.2 in 1978 as illegal abortions were sharply reduced (David, 1979; Hollerbach, 1980).[13]

The risk-benefit considerations of abortion depend not only on the relative advantages or disadvantages of illegal and legal abortion, but also on the disadvantages of being pregnant, especially in the developing countries. In many of these countries, particularly in rural areas, maternal mortality remains high because of a lack of medical resources (including personnel), the unwillingness or inability of women to seek prenatal care, and the large number of high-parity older women having further pregnancies (IFRP, 1980b). For those countries for which reliable data are available, United Nations estimates indicate that maternal death rates during pregnancy (including abortion), childbirth, and the puerperium are up to ten times higher in developing than in developed countries (United Nations, 1976, 1977). This discrepancy in the risks of pregnancy makes the legality or illegality of abortion a variable of particular importance (IFRP, 1980b).

## Morbidity from Illegal Abortion

Complications of abortion are more difficult to measure than mortality; however, the incidence of serious complications appears to be higher with illegal abortions performed by untrained practitioners using unsafe methods, especially in advanced stages of pregnancy. The most frequent major complications of illegal abortion are pelvic infection, hemorrhage, and shock, requiring postoperative care (WHO, 1978). Another frequently reported complication is trauma to the pelvic organs, including cervical lacerations, uterine perforation, and damage to the bladder and intestines. Moreover, although there are no systematic studies of longer-term complications of

illegal abortion, published reports often cite adverse
effects on subsequent pregnancies (e.g., Liskin, 1980).

Particular complications are frequently associated
with the method used to induce abortion. For example,
chemical substances inserted into the cervical os can
cause burns and bleeding and may lead to the formation of
bladder or rectal fistulas (Potts et al., 1977; Schwarz,
1968); abdominal massage, frequently practiced in Southeast Asia and Africa, can cause internal bleeding and
organ damage (Gallen, 1979; Mwambia, 1973; Sambhi, 1977);
mechanical methods, such as the insertion of a twig or
other object into the cervix, may lead to uterine and
intestinal perforation and subsequent peritonitis (Lwanga,
1977; Philips and Ghouse, 1976). Other nonmedical methods
include eating or drinking quinine, laundry whiteners, or
any one or a combination of potions or chemicals that can
lead to poisoning, renal failure, or intense vomiting
requiring immediate medical attention. These should not
be confused with folk medicines that may bring on a late
menstrual period early during gestation when women are
less certain about their pregnancy (Browner, 1980). The
far less dangerous methods of suction curettage are
generally practiced by physicians or by experienced
midwives and nurses. However, in developing countries
where abortion is illegal, the choice of method is frequently limited by a woman's knowledge of and access to
service providers, the means at the provider's disposal,
and financial costs. Thus safety considerations may
become secondary to the urgent need to terminate an
unwanted pregnancy.

Women admitted to hospitals for complications are not
typical of all those receiving illegal abortions; they
are representative only of those whose complications are
sufficient to require medical treatment and who choose to
request such care. Moreover, less skilled practitioners
are becoming increasingly experienced in the use of modern
abortion methods, offer to perform earlier abortions at
lower cost, and more often give their clients antibiotics
after the procedure to reduce the likelihood of sepsis
and associated complications (Potts, 1980).

In view of the paucity of data on rural illegal abortions, the data from Thailand are of particular importance
(Narkavonnakit, 1980; Narkavonnakit and Bennett, 1981).
First, the total number of indigenous procedures performed during the year (17,228) was estimated. This
figure was then compared with the total number of hospital
admissions for incomplete abortions during the same period

(415) plus the total number of abortion clients who were
not hospitalized but were incapacitated for a while
(3,970). The total complication rate thus derived was
25.4 percent; only 2.4 percent experienced complications
serious enough to require hospitalization. Most dangerous
were self-administered traditional medications (orally
ingested abortifacients), followed by intramuscular
injections. Abdominal massage, the most frequently used
method, was also the least debilitating, followed by
uterine injections (Narkavonnakit and Bennett, 1981).

Although complication rates for illegal abortions
cannot be readily determined because of a lack of reliable
data, it is instructive to note changes in hospital admissions for septic or incomplete abortions in areas where
legal restrictions have been eased. For example, data
from New York City municipal hospitals show that some
6,500 women were admitted in 1969 for treatment of incomplete spontaneous or illegally induced abortions. In
1971, the year following abortion legalization, the
figure was 3,600, and by 1975 (the most recent year for
which data are available), the number of women admitted
had fallen to 2,700, mostly for miscarriages (Alan
Guttmacher Institute, 1980). Similar findings have been
reported from other U.S. cities (Liskin, 1980), from
England (Soskice and Trussell, 1973), and from Yugoslavia
(Stampar, 1973-74).


## Morbidity from Legal Abortion

In countries where abortion is legal, the use of more
reliable abortion methods helps account for generally
much lower complication rates. In the United States, for
example, curettage during the first trimester appears to
be safest, with suction (vacuum aspiration) curettage
causing fewer major complications than sharp (D&C)
curettage (Grimes and Cates, 1979). Other techniques
used later in pregnancy have higher complication rates.

Longer-term complications of legal abortion have been
studied extensively in diverse countries, often with
conflicting results (Belsey, 1979; Edstrom, 1975; WHO,
1978, 1979b; Cates, 1982). One reason is the multiple
variables involved, including different abortion methods
(suction versus sharp curettage), different stages of
gestational development in women of diverse age and
parity, different levels of skill and experience among
medical service providers, the possible influence of

smoking during pregnancy, and selective "forgetting" among women questioned about prior abortions (Hogue, 1975, 1978; Grimes and Cates, 1979). Moreover, the absence of international standards for recording and evaluating the severity of symptoms makes comparisons between studies difficult (Cates, 1979; Tietze, 1981). Some comparative data are provided by Tietze (1981), who summarized findings of nine major studies on the outcome of the first pregnancy following one or more abortions performed in medical settings. These studies were conducted in 16 locations and involved a total of about 12,000 women with abortion experience and 90,000 women in comparison groups. In general, the data do not show a significantly higher risk of an adverse outcome of pregnancy for those having prior abortion experience. Risks for women with one prior abortion are generally higher than those for women having experienced a previous live birth; however, this can be explained by a shift of the dangers of first pregnancy to the second pregnancy when abortion takes place.

Abortion in the second trimester of gestation requires more skill and is associated with higher mortality, complication rates, and costs (e.g., Tietze, 1978b, 1979a; Cates et al., 1979; Cates and Tietze, 1978; Berger et al., 1981). In recent years, "dilatation and evacuation" procedures have become an increasingly acceptable option for such abortions; these procedures can be done at 13–15 weeks of gestation, whereas medical induction cannot be safely performed until 16 weeks. The advantages and disadvantages of using these procedures in developing countries have been reviewed by Cates et al. (1980). Although perceived as emotionally stressful by operating room staff, they offer many psychological advantages for the patient, who does not experience labor (Rooks and Cates, 1977; Hern and Corrigan, 1978).[14]

Observations in developed countries where second-trimester abortions are legal suggest that the highest proportion of delayed abortion occurs among women under age 20. Partially as a function of age, these women tend to be single, pregnant for the first time, and low in education and socioeconomic status (David, 1981d; Berger et al., 1981). External conflicts likely to delay the abortion decision include lack of information on the availability or location of services, financial difficulties, bureaucratic and service provider bias, parental/guardian consent requirements, and inaccurate medical diagnosis. Psychological conflicts include

ambivalence about the abortion decision, hesitation or
fear to confide in partner or parents, a history of
irregular menstrual periods, and late recognition or
denial of pregnancy (David, 1981d). Fortunately, the
proportion of second trimester abortions in the United
States declined steadily from 17.9 percent of all
abortions in 1972 to 8.6 percent in 1978 (CDC, 1980).
The trend observed in all countries for which data are
available shows a decline in legally induced second-
trimester abortions.[15]

In conclusion, review of available findings from
countries where abortion is legal shows that, when performed by competent providers in aseptic conditions,
abortion is a comparatively safe procedure involving less
risk of mortality and morbidity than carrying a pregnancy
to term. However, additional research is needed to
identify more precisely the longer-term complications, if
any, that may be associated with different abortion
techniques and with particular groups of women at risk.

OTHER COSTS:  ECONOMIC, SOCIAL, AND PSYCHOLOGICAL

Economic and Social Costs

In developing countries where legal abortions are easily
and safely available on request during the first trimester
of pregnancy, financial costs to the woman are quite low.
For example, no charges are made in Cuba (David, 1979),
for married women in China (Wolfson, 1976), or in public
hospitals in Tunisia (Nazer, 1980). In India, costs vary
with the type of facility and service provider sought
(David, 1975). Costs of government-provided legal abortion services are deemed far lower than those of medical
services made necessary by illegal abortion complications.[16]

In developing countries with restrictive legislation,
the price of an illegal abortion varies widely from no
fee to whatever the traffic will bear (Liskin, 1980).
Traditional birth attendants and less-skilled practitioners generally charge lower fees and at times accept
goods in payment (Flavier and Chen, 1980; Gallen, 1982;
Gallen et al., 1981; Sampoerno and Sadli, 1975); gestational age is the determining factor for most practitioners who charge on a per-month-of-pregnancy basis
(e.g., Narkavonnakit, 1979a). The highest charges are
usually requested by physicians, who use more modern and

safer methods. Thus economically disadvantaged women often have no choice but to seek the services of less-skilled practitioners relying on more dangerous procedures (e.g., Viel, 1979).

The financial costs of an illegal abortion can include far more than the service provider's fee. For example, there may be charges for drugs used to alleviate subsequent complications or for transportation to a hospital. When hospitalization is involved, there may be concomitant loss of pay from missed work and additional costs of services rendered while the woman is incapacitated (e.g., Ramirez et al., 1978; Narkavonnakit and Bennett, 1981). Complications of illegal abortion also burden both governmental and nongovernmental medical facilities. Since it is often impossible to distinguish between spontaneous and illegally induced abortions, costs of treatment can seldom be determined exactly; however, available evidence suggests that most abortions resulting in complications are illegally induced and that complicated cases are more costly than uncomplicated ones (Liskin, 1980). In the Dominican Republic, for example, the cost of treating complications was deemed to be nearly 50 percent of the maternal hospital budget; moreover, hospital treatment of an abortion complication cost more than 12 times as much as a normal hospital delivery (Ramirez and Garcia, 1975). In many developing countries, hospitals are hard-pressed to provide quality care to meet the needs created by the dual impact of high birth rates and high rates of admission for abortion complications. As one consequence, women are often discharged too soon, resuming household and other responsibilities before they have fully recuperated, and placing themselves at greater risk for subsequent problems (e.g., Viel, 1976).

## Psychological Costs

Of all the complications of abortion, psychological costs are the most difficult to assess (Potts et al., 1977). Early research on abortion of necessity focused on small groups of women who had been granted therapeutic abortions under restrictive conditions or who had procured illegal abortions (Osofsky et al., 1975). Studies conducted prior to liberalization in the United States yielded inconsistent findings, ranging from frequent or severe psychological sequelae, to occasional direct or indirect problems, to no noticeable difficulties (David,

1978a). There was little research evidence to support
the warnings of psychiatrists regarding the alleged
frequency of serious depression following illegally
induced abortions (Osofsky et al., 1973). Studies
conducted following liberalization have been summarized
from time to time (e.g., Institute of Medicine, 1975;
Illsley and Hall, 1976; David, 1978a). However, many of
these studies consist of impressionistic case reports,
often without addressing rudimentary methodological
concerns. Inconsistencies of interpretation stem from a
lack of consensus regarding symptoms, severity, and
duration of mental disorder; opinions based on clinical
case studies without regard to the vast number of women
who do not come to therapeutic attention after abortion;
and a lack of adequate follow-up studies (Adler, 1976).
Indeed, health professionals' perceptions of the psychological consequences of abortions, what they expect women
to experience, are not always matched by the experiences
reported by the women themselves (Baluk and O'Neill,
1980). Review of the diverse literature from countries
where abortion is legal suggests that, for the vast
majority of women, feelings of guilt, regret, and
sadness, when noted, are mild and transitory, usually
followed by a sense of relief associated with successful
crisis resolution (David, 1981b).

One reason for the sometimes conflicting opinions on
the psychological costs of abortion is a lack of epidemiological data in the international research literature on
the incidence of either postabortion or postpartum psychotic reactions. By means of computer linkage, it
recently became possible to screen all women in Denmark
under age 50 terminating a pregnancy or carrying to term
in 1975 for admission to psychiatric hospital within
three months after abortion or delivery. Data were also
obtained on admissions to psychiatric hospital for all
Danish women aged 15 to 49 over a similar time period.
Admission to psychiatric hospital was deemed a measurable
event, reflective of severe stress associated in time
with delivery and abortion, and less subject to diverse
interpretations than visits to clinical practitioners
(David et al., 1981). For never married and currently
married women, the postpregnancy-related risk of admission to psychiatric hospital was around 12 per 10,000
abortions or deliveries, compared with an overall admission rate of 7.5 per 10,000 Danish women of similar age.
The postabortion rate of admission to psychiatric hospital
adds only slightly to the risk for major medical abortion

complications (estimated in the United States at 50 per
10,000 abortions) when the procedure is performed by
skilled practitioners using modern methods during the
first trimester (Tietze, 1981).

In sum, it may well be a truism that there is no
psychologically painless way to cope with unintended
conceptions and unwanted pregnancies (David, 1972a,
1972b). For some women, abortion elicits doubts and
feelings of guilt and remorse that must be considered
psychological costs, regardless of their duration or
whether they come to the attention of mental health
specialists (Lamanna, 1980). The decision to terminate
an unwanted pregnancy is seldom easy (David, 1980);
however, alternatives such as forced marriage, bearing an
out-of-wedlock child, giving a child up for adoption, or
adding an unwanted child to an already strained marital
relationship are also likely to create psychological
problems for the woman, the child, the family, and society
(David, 1973, 1981c). In general, more research needs to
focus on the conditions that may influence the intensity
and duration of postpregnancy-related depression, including desire for pregnancy; stress before or during pregnancy; first- or second-trimester abortion; social support
for the abortion decision or coercion by family, friends,
or the medical community; religious or moral opposition;
previous emotional health, etc. (Hollerbach, 1979).

The scant evidence available from developing countries
suggests that religious attitudes, beliefs, or practices
do not prevent motivated women from seeking abortions,
regardless of legal status. Abortion is an often dramatic, comparatively expensive, and sometimes dangerous
event of considerable personal significance, but is
largely invisible to society. At a time of need, a woman
makes decisions in her private world, sharing sometimes
with her male partner, but expecting little help from the
community. When deemed necessary, the physical and mental
health risks of a more dangerous illegal procedure are
preferred to the alternative of carrying an unwanted
pregnancy to term.

## Costs of Denied Abortion

Although the dynamics of intended and unintended conceptions and wanted and unwanted pregnancies and childbearing
have long been debated (e.g., Pohlman, 1969; Hass, 1974;
Miller, 1978), it has seldom been possible to systemati-

cally follow women denied abortion or the children they
were compelled to bear. The only longitudinal study with
matched controls ever reported is still in progress in
Prague, Czechoslovakia (Dytrych et al., 1975, 1978;
David, 1981c; David and Matejcek, 1981). Unique circumstances combined to make available for detailed medical,
psychological, and social assessment 110 boys and 110
girls born in 1961-63 to Prague women twice denied
abortion for the same pregnancy, and a matched control
group of children whose mothers had not applied for
pregnancy termination. The control group was formed on
the basis of pair-matching according to age, sex, number
of siblings, birth order, and school class; the mothers
were matched for age, marital status, and socioeconomic
status as determined by the husband's occupation and his
presence in the family. The research staff was not
involved in the matching process and did not know which
child belonged to what subgroup.

The children were about 9 years old at the time of
original psychological, educational, and medical assessment, and were subsequently followed up at varied time
intervals (Matejcek et al., 1978, 1979, 1980). Initially,
aggregate differences between the study and control children were not statistically significant. However, differences observed in school, family, and social life were
highly consistent and cumulatively in disfavor of the
study children. Group differences have persisted through
16 to 18 years of family life; they have actually widened
and become more significant statistically. A review of
all the data from this unique and continuing longitudinal
study suggests that "unwantedness" during early pregnancy
constitutes a not-negligible factor for the subsequent
development of the child (David, 1981c).


PROPOSITIONS

The following propositions are based on the previous
sections, where references to the literature will be
found.

1. In many developing countries, abortion is a
traditional method of fertility regulation, especially
where modern contraceptives are only gradually becoming
available and more widely accessible. Women resort to
abortion to terminate unwanted pregnancies regardless of
socioeconomic or cultural background, legal codes,
religious sanctions, or risks to physical or mental
well-being.

2. Influenced by different legal, social, and political ambiguities, abortion has different meanings from country to country and over time within the same country. Findings should therefore be judged in terms of the constraints under which they were obtained. In countries where abortion is illegal, the advantages and disadvantages of available data sources should be considered, as should the observation that most women obtaining illegal abortions may never come to the attention of the hospital system, or may "forget" their experiences in retrospective interviews. Locally initiated surveys of known service providers offer the best hope for reliable information on illegal abortion.

3. The worldwide legal status of abortion ranges from complete prohibition to elective abortion at the request of the woman during the first trimester of pregnancy. However, restrictive abortion legislation has rarely, if ever, been effective in preventing abortion. In certain countries, strict abortion laws are not enforced; some abortions on medical grounds are tolerated even in those few countries which adhere to strict legal prohibitions. Conversely, liberalization of abortion legislation does not ensure ready access to services or abandonment of humiliating restrictions, especially for economically disadvantaged women.

4. No reliable method has yet been demonstrated for estimating at reasonable cost the incidence of illegal abortion and associated health risks. However, the frequent statement that abortion is the world's leading method of fertility regulation has no basis in verifiable fact and is almost certainly wrong. No developed country has achieved a significant decline in birth rates without considerable recourse to abortion, whether legal or not, and it is likely that the experience of developing countries will be similar.

5. Given reasonable availability of contraceptives, the relationship between abortion and contraception is complementary rather than competitive; therefore, the most efficient approach to achieving voluntary reduction in birth rates is a national program providing ready access to modern contraceptives, backed by widely available legal or quietly condoned abortion. Abortion is rarely preferred to contraception; it is usually sought as the only possible way of avoiding a birth at that time. There is strong evidence that a substantial majority of women are more efficient contraceptors after abortion. However, in countries where abortion is highly

restrictive, service providers are often reluctant to offer contraceptives to women hospitalized with complications of illegal abortion, thus setting the stage for continued resort to illegal abortion; moreover, women hospitalized with complications stemming from illegal abortions are also fearful of the alleged health hazards of modern contraceptives.

6.   An increasing proportion of repeat abortions among all legal abortions and a repeat rate higher than the first-abortion rate can be expected for several years after abortion has been legalized, as the pool of women at risk for repeat abortion continues to rise to an eventual plateau.  Age, sexual activity, ability to conceive, decision to terminate a previous pregnancy, and a conscious preference for abortion as the chosen method of fertility regulation are the major factors influencing the incidence of repeat abortion.

7.   Sociodemographic characteristics of abortion-seeking women differ greatly among countries reporting such data.  These diverse findings reflect differences in adolescent sexual activity, societal disapproval of premarital pregnancies and births, and the customary age at first marriage, plus differences in the availability and accessibility of modern contraceptives and abortion services.  Determinants of choice behavior resolving an unwanted pregnancy, whether to terminate or carry to term, vary widely within and across cultures.

8.   Attitudes of medical and allied health personnel are central to the equitable provision of legal abortion services and to resolution of special problems faced in countries where abortion is illegal.  The process of obtaining an abortion differs markedly from traditional medical practice.  Women asking to terminate an unwanted pregnancy are usually "healthy," seeking technical assistance to implement their own decision rather than seeking a medical diagnosis or medical treatment for a medically identifiable disease.  The resultant role conflict with the more traditional orientations of medical decision makers is a major divisive influence.

9.   When performed by untrained practitioners or under unhygienic conditions, illegal abortions are associated with greater mortality and morbidity and longer-term complications than when induced by skilled operators using modern methods.  Illegal abortion is a major cause of maternal mortality in many developing countries. Although medically safe abortions are available nearly everywhere, they are not easily accessible to poor women,

who, unable to pay the price of safety, may pay with their health and sometimes with their lives.

10.  Data from developed and developing countries where abortion is legal indicate that the mortality ratio associated with first-trimester abortion is far lower than that associated with carrying a pregnancy to term; in the United States, for example, abortion is safer than a tonsillectomy.  However, the risks of pregnancy vary greatly among developed and developing countries, making the legality or illegality of abortion a variable of particular importance, in relative health risks.  In countries where abortion is legal, the methods used by competent service providers also influence the much lower complication rates.  Suction curettage appears to be safest in the first trimester; additional research is needed to identify more precisely the longer-term complications, if any, that may be associated with different abortion techniques and with particular groups of women at risk.  Abortion in the second trimester of gestation requires more skill and is associated with higher mortality, complication rates, and costs.

11.  In developing countries, a woman's choice is frequently limited by her knowledge of and access to service providers, the means at the provider's disposal, and financial costs.  Within that context, considerations of safety (and subsequent morbidity) may become secondary to the urgent need to terminate an unwanted pregnancy.  However, as illegal service providers become increasingly skilled in the use of modern methods, women admitted to hospital for abortion-associated complications may no longer be typical.

12.  In developing countries with restrictive legislation, the financial cost of an illegal abortion varies widely.  Ability to pay and gain access to medical care are closely associated with reduced risks or complications; economically disadvantaged women often have no choice but to seek the services of lesser skilled practitioners relying on more dangerous procedures.  If complications occur, additional personal costs are incurred, including the loss of pay for missed work and the expense of providing services to the family.  Complications of illegal abortions also burden medical facilities, requiring longer and more expensive care than other obstetrical and gynecological events.  As one consequence, women may be discharged too soon, assuming household and other responsibilities before they have fully recuperated, and placing themselves at greater risk for subsequent health problems.

13.  There is no psychologically painless way to cope with an unwanted pregnancy. Of all the costs of abortion, legal or illegal, obtained or denied, the psychological ones are the most difficult to assess. For the vast majority of women, feelings of guilt, regret, or sadness, when noted, are mild and transitory, usually followed by a sense of relief associated with successful crisis resolution; few women come to the attention of mental health services and fewer still experience a psychotic reaction. When abortion is deemed personally necessary, the physical and mental health risks of more dangerous illegal procedures are preferred to the alternative of carrying an unwanted pregnancy to term.

14.  Denial of an abortion request constitutes a not-negligible risk factor for the subsequent life of a child born to a woman compelled by society to deliver an unwanted pregnancy.

15.  Overall, findings suggest that a liberal abortion policy is likely to reduce problems of fertility control confronting women, families, and society, especially the young and the poor. In the final analysis, the legality of induced abortion is a political issue. Although universally practiced, tolerated, or approved by large population groups, and most effective in meeting individual fertility objectives, abortion is often the least politically acceptable means of fertility regulation.

## NOTES

1.  Perhaps the first published reference to pregnancy termination as a means of fertility regulation appeared in Aristotle's (384-322 BC) Politics. Abortion was recommended as a means of maintaining the ideal size of the city state wherever couples already had sufficient children (Aristotle, 1932; Farr, 1980).

2.  No major religion has a unified or unbroken history of support or opposition to induced abortion. It was not until 1869 that Pope Pius IX "made a sharp change in church law by eliminating any distinction between a formed and unformed fetus in meting out the penalty of excommunication for abortion," even to save the life of the woman (Callahan, 1970). A variety of opinions can be found in each of the major Western and nonWestern religions, most of which altered their views over time (e.g., Moore, 1974; David, 1980, 1981a).

3.  Motivation to control fertility is at times so strong
    that women who are otherwise law-abiding, have little
    or no money to spare, and are concerned about their
    health are willing to break the law, borrow money,
    and risk their physical and psychological well-being
    to avoid unwanted births (e.g., David et al., 1978;
    David, 1981b; Liskin, 1980; Gallen et al., 1981).
4.  The USSR pioneered in the liberalization of abortion
    legislation in 1920, restricted abortion again in
    1936, and then reliberalized it in 1955, an action
    eventually followed by all the socialist countries of
    Central and Eastern Europe except Albania.  Despite
    evidence that the USSR abortion rate may be the
    highest in the world--well above the birth rate in
    most cities at least--the liberal law of 1955 has
    remained in force.
5.  None of the countries which liberalized its laws
    since 1967 authorized trained nonphysicians to
    perform pregnancy termination (Paxman, 1980b).  In
    China, early abortions are often performed by nurses,
    "barefoot doctors," or midwives.  In Bangladesh,
    despite the absence of authorizing legislation, "lady
    health visitors" have received training and are
    performing menstrual regulation procedures during
    early gestation when determination of pregnancy is
    less certain.
6.  In some Middle Eastern countries, physicians and
    midwives benefiting financially from performing
    illegal abortions are said to be reluctant to support
    proposals for legislative changes (Nazer, 1970).
7.  The numbers of legal abortions, abortion rates per
    1,000 women 15 to 44 years of age, and abortion
    ratios per 1,000 live births six months later are
    regularly compiled by Tietze (e.g., 1981) for all
    countries reporting such information.  Among
    developing lands, only Cuba, India, Singapore, and
    Tunisia provide national data on an annual basis,
    with Cuba having perhaps the most complete
    information.  Fragmentary data are also coming from
    China, where abortion is available on request.
8.  Although there is little doubt that desperate women
    will resort to abortion no matter what the legal
    circumstances or risks to well-being, the frequent
    statement that induced abortion is the world's
    leading method of fertility regulation has no basis
    in verifiable fact and is almost surely wrong
    (Berelson et al., 1979).

9. Motivations for providing illegal abortion range from "making money" to "helping poor women." Although the former attitude may prevail in major cities and in much of Latin America, the latter seems more prevalent in rural sectors of those Asian countries where abortion is technically illegal and service providers are seldom disturbed by the authorities.

10. The importance of educational level to postabortion contraceptive practice in developing countries appears to vary, with no clear trends emerging from the limited research literature (Liskin, 1980).

11. All such reports must be considered cautiously since women's responses to questions about repeat abortion are notoriously subject to error, selective "forgetting," and deliberate denial, regardless of the legal status of abortion (Hogue, 1975, 1978).

12. The mortality ratio was 1.4 deaths per 100,000 abortions in 1977 (CDC, 1979), compared with 12 maternal deaths from all causes per 100,000 live births in 1972 to 1975 (Cates and Tietze, 1978), and 16 deaths per 100,000 tonsillectomies in 1977 (National Center for Health Statistics, 1979). More recent data have been reviewed by Tietze (1981) and by Cates (1982).

13. Similar patterns have been observed elsewhere. Despite large increases in the annual number of abortions in Singapore after legislative reforms in 1970 and 1974, the total number of abortion deaths decreased from 51 in 1968-70 to 26 in 1974-76 as the incidence of illegal abortions dropped (Lim et al., 1979). By contrast, rerestriction of a very liberal abortion policy in Romania in late 1966 resulted in an increase in the number of deaths attributed to abortion from 64 in 1965 to 170 in 1967 and 432 in 1976 (Tietze, 1979a; WHO, 1965, 1967, 1980). A dramatic contrast is reported from India, giving a mortality rate of 660 per 100,000 for medically induced abortions and 780 per 100,000 among women admitted to the same hospital for incomplete abortions during the same time period (IFRP, 1980b). Overall, illegal abortion mortality probably varies from 100 per 100,000 when performed by qualified medical practitioners to over 1,000 per 100,000 when induced by unskilled persons.

14. The use of prostaglandin analogues in 12,500 late terminations without fatality in London has been reported by Atherton (1980).

15. Although there are no systematic studies from developing countries where abortion is illegal, there is no reason to doubt that mortality and morbidity increases with abortion delay into the second trimester.
16. The cost-effectiveness of alternative service-delivery models by skilled and experienced paramedical personnel is being explored in several countries, including the rural areas of China (PIACT, 1980).

## BIBLIOGRAPHY

Abortion Research Notes (1972)  Bethesda, Md.:  Transnational Family Research Institute.

Adler, N. E. (1976)  Sample attrition in studies of psychosocial sequelae of abortion:  How great a problem?  Journal of Applied Social Psychology 6:240-259.

Adler, N. E. (1979a)  Abortion:  A social-psychological perspective.  Journal of Social Issues 35:100-119.

Adler, N. E. (1979b)  Psychosocial issues of therapeutic abortion.  Pp. 159-177 in D. Youngs and A. Ehrhardt, eds., Psychosomatic Obstetrics and Gynecology.  New York:  Appleton-Century-Crofts.

Akingba, J. B. (1977)  Abortion, maternity and other health problems in Nigeria.  Nigerian Medical Journal 7:465-471.

Alan Guttmacher Institute (1980)  Safe and Legal:  10 Years' Experience with Legal Abortion in New York State.  New York:  Alan Guttmacher Institute.

Ampofo, P. A. (1973)  Epidemiology of Abortion in Selected African Countries.  Paper presented at the IPPF Conference on the Medical and Social Aspects of Abortion in Africa, Accra, Ghana.

Aristotle (1932)  Politics.  Cambridge, Mass.:  Harvard University Press.

Attherton, R. D. (1980)  12,500 late terminations.  Abortion Research Notes 9:8.

Baluk, U., and P. O'Neill (1980)  Health professionals' perceptions of the psychological consequences of abortion.  American Journal of Community Psychology 8:67-75.

Begum, F., A. R. Khan, and S. Jahan (1978)  Experience with Abortion Related Admissions in Dacca Medical College Hospital.  Technical Report No. 8.  Dacca:  Bangladesh Fertility Research Programme.

Belsey, M. A. (1979)  Long term sequelae of induced
    abortion:  Considerations in interpretations of
    research.  Pp. 156-162 in G. I. Zatuchni, J. J.
    Sciarra, and J. J. Speidel, eds., Pregnancy
    Termination.  Hagerstown, Md.:  Harper and Row.
Berelson, B., W. P. Mauldin, and S. J. Segal (1979)
    Population:  Current Status and Policy Options.
    Center for Policy Studies Working Papers No. 44.  New
    York:  Population Council.
Berger, G. S., W. E. Brenner, and L. Keith, eds. (1981)
    Second Trimester Abortion:  Perceptions After a Decade
    of Experience.  Boston:  Wright/PSG.
Bhatt, R. V. (1980)  Personal communication to L. Liskin,
    15 March.
Bhatt, R. V., and J. M. Soni (1973)  Criminal abortion in
    Western India.  Journal of Obstetrics and Gynecology
    of India 23:243-246.
Bhuiyan, N., R. Begum, and S. Begum (1979)  Character-
    istics of Abortion Cases Admitted in Chittagong
    Medical College in 1978.  Technical Report No. 33.
    Dacca:  Bangladesh Fertility Research Programme.
Brody, E. B. (1981)  Sex, Contraception, and Motherhood
    in Jamaica.  Cambridge, Mass.:  Harvard University
    Press.
Brody, E. B., F. Ottey, and J. LaGrande (1976)  Fertility
    related behavior in Jamaica.  ICP Occasional
    Monographs, No. 6.
Browner, C. (1976)  Poor Women's Fertility Decisions:
    Illegal Abortion in Cali, Colombia.  Unpublished Ph.D.
    dissertation.  University of California, Berkeley.
Browner, C. (1980)  The management of early pregnancy:
    Colombian folk concepts of fertility control.  Social
    Science and Medicine 14B:25-32.
Callahan, D. (1970)  Abortion:  Law, Choice, and
    Morality.  New York:  Macmillan.
Cates, W., Jr. (1979)  Late effects of induced abortion:
    Hypothesis or knowledge?  Journal of Reproductive
    Medicine 22:207-212.
Cates, W., Jr. (1982)  Legal abortion:  The public health
    record.  Science 215:1586-1590.
Cates, W., Jr., and C. Tietze (1978)  Standardized
    mortality rates associated with legal abortion:
    United States, 1972-1975.  Family Planning
    Perspectives 10:109-112.
Cates, W., Jr., K. F. Schulz, D. A. Grimes, and C. W.
    Tyler, Jr.  (1979)  The effect of delay and method
    choice on the risk of abortion morbidity.  Family
    Planning Perspectives 9:266-272.

Cates, W., Jr., K. F. Schulz, and D. A. Grimes (1980)
Dilatation and evacuation for induced abortion in
developing countries: Advantages and disadvantages.
Studies in Family Planning 11:128-133.
Centers for Disease Control (1979) Abortion
Surveillance, 1977. Atlanta, Ga.: Centers for
Disease Control.
Centers for Disease Control (1980) Abortion
Surveillance, 1978. Atlanta, Ga.: Centers for
Disease Control.
Chandrasekhar, S. (1978) Population and Law in India,
2nd ed. Dehli: Macmillan.
Chatterjee, P. (1977) Induced abortion and its hazards.
Journal of the Indian Medical Association 69:173-175.
Chen, P. C. (1981) Rural Health and Birth Planning in
China. Research Triangle Park, N.C.: International
Fertility Research Program.
Chen, P. C., and A. Kols (1982) Population and birth
planning in the People's Republic of China.
Population Reports, Series J, No. 25.
Cook, R. J., and B. M. Dickens (1979) Abortion laws in
commonwealth countries. International Digest of
Health Legislation 30:395-502.
David, H. P. (1972a) Unwanted pregnancies: Costs and
alternatives. Pp. 439-466 in C. F. Westoff and R.
Parke, Jr., eds., Demographic and Social Aspects of
Population Growth. Vol. 1 of the Commission on
Population Growth and the American Future Research
Reports. Washington, D.C.: U.S. Government Printing
Office.
David, H. P. (1972b) Abortion in psychological
perspective. American Journal of Orthopsychiatry
42:61-68.
David, H. P. (1973) Psychological studies in abortion.
Pp. 241-273 in J. T. Fawcett, ed., Psychological
Perspectives on Population. New York: Basic Books.
David, H. P. (1978a) Psychosocial studies of abortion in
the United States. Pp. 77-115 in H. P. David, H. L.
Friedman, J. van der Tak, and M. Sevilla, eds.,
Abortion in Psychosocial Perspective: Trends in
Transnational Research. New York: Springer.
David, H. P. (1978b) Healthy family functioning: A
cross-cultural overview. Bulletin of the World Health
Organization 55:327-342.
David, H. P. (1979) Notes from Cuba. Abortion Research
Notes 8(1-2).

David, H. P. (1980) The abortion decision: National and international perspectives. Pp. 57-98 in J. T. Burtchaell, ed., Abortion Parley. Kansas City, Mo.: Andrews and McMeel.

David, H. P. (1981a) Abortion policies. Pp. 1-40 in J. E. Hodgson, ed., Abortion and Sterilization: Medical and Social Aspects. London: Academic Press.

David, H. P. (1981b) Worldwide abortion trends. Pp. 75-192 in P. Sachdev, ed., Abortion: Readings and Research. Toronto: Butterworths.

David, H. P. (1981c) Unwantedness: Longitudinal studies of Prague children born to women twice denied abortion for the same pregnancy and matched controls. Pp. 81-102 in P. Ahmed, ed., Coping with Medical Issues: Pregnancy, Childbirth and Parenthood. New York: Elsevier.

David, H. P. (1981d) Second trimester: Social issues. Pp. 221-237 in G. S. Berger, W. E. Brenner, and L. Keith, eds., Second Trimester Abortion Perspective After a Decade of Experience. Boston: Wright/PSG Publishing Co.

David, H. P. (1982a) Eastern Europe: Pronatalist policies and private behavior. Population Bulletin 36.

David, H. P. (1982b) Incentives, reproductive behavior, and integrated community development in Asia. Studies in Family Planning 13:159-173.

David, H. P., and Z. Matejcek (1981) Children born to women denied abortion: An update. Family Planning Perspectives 13:32-34.

David, H. P., and R. J. McIntyre (1981) Reproductive Behavior: Central and Eastern European Experience. New York: Springer.

David, H. P., H. L. Friedman, J. van der Tak, and M. J. Sevilla, eds. (1978) Abortion in Psychosocial Perspective: Trends in Transnational Research. New York: Springer.

David, H. P., N. K. Rasmussen, and E. Holst (1981) Postpartum and postabortion psychotic reactions. Family Planning Perspectives 13:88-92.

David, P. S. (1975) India. Pp. 8-20 in H. P. David and B. Shashi, orgs., Psychosocial Aspects of Abortion in Asia. Washington, D.C.: Transnational Family Research Institute.

David, P. S. (1978) Abortion: The Indian experience. People 5:16-17.

Denmark, National Board of Health (1978) Statistics on Legal Abortion, 1977 (and earlier years). Copenhagen: National Board of Health.

Dunshee de Abranches, C. A. (1976)  Menstrual regulation
    in Latin America:  The language of the law.  Pp. 89-91
    in H. H. Holtrop, R. S. Waife, W. Bustamante, and A.
    Rizo, eds., New Developments in Fertility
    Regulation.  Chestnut Hill, Mass.:  Pathfinder Fund.
Dytrych, Z., Z. Matejcek, V. Schuller, H. P. David, and
    H. L. Friedman (1975)  Children born to women denied
    abortion.  Family Planning Perspectives 7:165-171.
Dytrych, Z., Z. Matejcek, and V. Schuller (1978)
    Children born to women denied abortion in
    Czechoslovakia.  Pp 201-224 in H. P. David, H. L.
    Friedman, J. van der Tak., M. Sevilla, eds., Abortion
    in Psychosocial Perspective:  Trends in Transnational
    Research.  New York:  Springer.
Edstrom, K. G. B. (1975)  Early complications and late
    sequelae of abortion:  A review of the literature.
    Bulletin of the World Health Organization 52:123-139.
Farr, A. D. (1980)  The Marquis de Sade and induced
    abortion.  Journal of Medical Ethics 6:7-10.
Faundes, A., and E. Hardy (1978)  Contraception and
    abortion services at Barros Luco Hospital, Santiago,
    Chile.  Pp. 284-297 in H. P. David, H. L. Friedman, J.
    van der Tak, and M. Sevilla, eds., Abortion in
    Psychosocial Perspective:  Trends in Transnational
    Research.  New York:  Springer.
Figa-Talamanca, I. (1977)  Social and psychological
    factors in the practice of induced abortion as a means
    of fertility control in an Italian population.  Genus
    27:99-266.
Figa-Talamanca, I. (1979)  Health and economic effects of
    illegal abortion:  Preliminary findings from an
    international study.  Pp. 361-369 in G. I. Zatuchni,
    J. J. Sciarra, and J. J. Speidel, eds., Pregnancy
    Termination.  Hagerstown, Md.:  Harper and Row.
Figa-Talamanca, I. (1980)  Personal communication, March.
Flavier, J. M., and C. H. C. Chen (1980)  Induced
    abortion in rural villages of Cavite, the
    Philippines:  Knowledge, attitudes, and practice.
    Studies in Family Planning 11:65-71.
Forrest, J. D., E. Sullivan, and C. Tietze (1979)
    Abortion in the United States, 1977-1978.  Family
    Planning Perspectives 11:329-341.
Foster, H. W. (1980)  Suppository to induce abortion in
    1-7 hours undergoing trials.  Ob/Gyn News, 15 November.
Friedman, H. L., and R. L. Johnson (1978)  Methodological
    issues in psychosocial abortion research.  Pp. 301-305
    in H. P. David, H. L. Friedman, J. van der Tak, and M.

Sevilla, eds., <u>Abortion in Psychosocial Perspective:</u>
<u>Trends in Transnational Research</u>. New York: Springer.

Friedman, H. L., A. Ramirez-Medina, and E. Garcia-Tatis
(1975) Attitudes of a sample of male heads of
household in the Central, Oriental, Sur, and Cibao
regions, Dominican Republic. Pp. 89-99 in
<u>Epidemiology of Abortion and Practices of Fertility</u>
<u>Regulation in Latin America: Selected Papers</u>.
Scientific Publication No. 306. Washington, D.C.:
Pan American Health Organization.

Friedman, H. L., R. L. Johnson, and H. P. David (1976)
Dynamics of fertility choice behavior: A pattern for
research. Pp. 171-198 in S. H. Newman and V. D.
Thompson, eds., <u>Population Psychology: Research and</u>
<u>Educational Issues</u>. DHEW Publication No. (NIH)
76-574. Washington, D.C.: Center for Population
Research.

Gallen, M. (1979) Massage abortion. <u>People</u> 6:2.

Gallen, M. (1982) Abortion in the Philippines: A study
of clients and practitioners. <u>Studies in Family</u>
<u>Planning</u> 13:35-44.

Gallen, M., T. Narkavonnakit, J. B. Tomaro, and M. Potts
(1981) <u>Traditional Abortion Practices: Three Studies</u>
<u>of Illegal Abortion in the Developing World</u>. Research
Triangle Park, N.C.: International Fertility Research
Program.

Gaslonde, S. (1976) Abortion research in Latin America.
<u>Studies in Family Planning</u> 7:211-217.

Goyal, R. S. (1978) Legalization of abortion: A social
perception. <u>Health and Population: Perspectives and</u>
<u>Issues</u> 1:302-308.

Grimes, D. A., and W. Cates, Jr. (1979) Complications
from legally induced abortions: A review.
<u>Obstetrical and Gynecological Survey</u> 34:177-191.

Hall, M., ed. (1977) Abortion Systems and Patient
Needs: A Cross-National Research Design. Paper
presented at the World Health Organization Scientific
Group on Abortion, Geneva.

Hardy, E., and K. Herud (1975) Effectiveness of a
contraceptive education program for postabortion
patients in Chile. <u>Studies in Family Planning</u>
6:188-191.

Harrison, P. (1980) Unwanted births: A new perspective.
<u>People</u> 7:15-16.

Hass, P. H. (1974) Wanted and unwanted pregnancies: A
fertility decision-making model. <u>Journal of Social</u>
<u>Issues</u> 30:125-165.

Henshaw, S., J. D. Forrest, E. Sullivan, and C. Tietze (1981)  Abortion in the United States, 1978-1979. Family Planning Perspectives 13:6-18.

Henshaw, S. K., J. D. Forrest, E. Sullivan, and C. Tietze (1982)  Abortion services in the United States, 1979 and 1980. Family Planning Perspectives 14:5-15.

Hern, W. M., and B. Corrigan (1978)  What About Us? Staff Reactions to the D&E Procedure.  Paper presented at the 16th Annual Meeting of the Association of Planned Parenthood Physicians, San Diego, Calif.

Hogue, C. J. R. (1975)  Low birth weight subsequent to induced abortion: A historical prospective study of 948 women in Skopje, Yugoslavia. American Journal of Obstetrics and Gynecology 123:675-681.

Hogue, C. J. R. (1978)  Review of postulated fertility complications subsequent to pregnancy termination. Pp. 356-367 in J. J. Sciarra, G. I. Zatuchni, and J. J. Speidel, eds, Risks, Benefits, and Controversies in Fertility Control.  Hagerstown, Md.: Harper and Row.

Hollerbach, P. E. (1977)  Parental choice and family planning: The acceptability, use, and sequelae of four methods.  Pp. 189-222 in Y. E. Hsia, K. Hirschhorn, R. L. Silverberg, and L. Godmilow, eds., Counseling in Genetics.  New York: Liss.

Hollerbach, P. E. (1979)  Parental choice and family planning: The acceptability, use, and sequelae of four methods.  Pp. 189-222 in Y. E. Hsia, K. Hirschhorn, R. L. Silverberg, and L. Goldman, eds., Counseling in Genetics.  New York: Liss.

Hollerbach, P. E. (1980)  Recent trends in fertility, abortion, and contraception in Cuba. International Family Planning Perspectives  6:97-106.

Hong, S. B., and C. Tietze (1979)  Survey of abortion providers in Seoul, Korea. Studies in Family Planning 10:161-163.

Hong, S. B., and W. B. Watson (1976)  The Increasing Utilization of Induced Abortion in Korea.  Seoul: Korea University Press.

Howe, B., H. R. Kaplan, and C. English (1979)  Repeat abortions: Blaming the victims. American Journal of Public Health 69:1242-1246.

Hungary, Central Statistical Office (1969a)  Survey Techniques in Fertility and Family Research: Experience in Hungary.  Budapest: Central Statistical Office.

Hungary, Central Statistical Office (1969b)  The concealment of induced abortions: An estimate of

induced abortions. Pp. 110-118 in Survey Techniques
in Fertility and Family Research. Budapest: Central
Statistical Office.

Illsley, R., and M. H. Hall (1976) Psychosocial aspects
of abortion: A review of issues and needed research.
Bulletin of the World Health Organization 53:83-106.

Institute of Medicine (1975) Legalized Abortion and the
Public Health. Washington, D.C.: National Academy of
Sciences.

International Fertility Research Program (1980a)
Abortion in Latin America. Research Report No. DDX
005. Research Triangle Park, N.C.: International
Fertility Research Program.

International Fertility Research Program (1980b) Ramos.
Research Triangle Park, N.C.: International Fertility
Research Program.

International Planned Parenthood Federation (1974)
Survey of World Needs in Population. London:
International Planned Parenthood Federation.

International Planned Parenthood Federation (1978) Unmet
needs. People 5:25-32.

International Union for the Scientific Study of
Population (1977) Recommendations for Comparative
Abortion Statistics in Countries Where Induced
Abortion is Legalized. IUSSP Papers No. 7. Liege:
International Union for the Scientific Study of
Population.

Jaffe, F. S., B. L. Lindheim, and P. R. Lee (1981)
Abortion Politics: Private Morality and Public
Policy. New York: McGraw-Hill.

Kapor-Stanulovic, N., and H. L. Friedman (1978) Studies
in choice behavior in Yugoslavia. Pp. 119-144 in H.
P. David, H. L. Friedman, J. van der Tak, and M.
Sevilla, eds., Abortion in Psychosocial Perspective:
Trends in Transnational Research. New York: Springer.

Klinger, A. (1979) Birth control and family planning in
Hungary in the last two decades. World Health
Statistics 32:257-268.

Klinger, A., and E. Szabady (1978) Patterns of abortion
and contraceptive practice in Hungary. Pp. 168-200 in
H. P. David, H. L. Friedman, J. van der Tak, and M.
Sevilla, eds., Abortion in Psychosocial Perspective:
Trends in Transnational Research. New York: Springer.

Koetsawang, S. (1975) Annual Statistics 2511-2518/
1968-1975: Illegal Abortion. Bangkok: Siriraj
Family Planning Research Unit, Mahidol University.

Koetsawang, S. (1976)  Annual Statistics 2519/1976: Abortion. Bangkok:  Siriraj Family Planning Research Unit, Mahidol University.

Korean Institute for Family Planning (1979)  The Korean National Fertility Survey, 1974.  First country report, Seoul, 1977.  Summarized in International Family Planning Perspectives 5:35-36.

Krishna Menon, M. K. (1979)  A recent program of legal abortion in India.  Pp. 395-398 in G. I. Zatuchni, J. J. Sciarra, and J. J. Speidel, eds., Pregnancy Termination. Hagerstown, Md.:  Harper and Row.

Lamanna, M. A. (1980)  Science and its uses:  The abortion debate and social science research.  Pp. 101-158 in J. T. Burtchaell, ed., Abortion Parley. Kansas City, Mo.:  Andrews and MeMeel.

Lim, L. S., M. C. E. Cheng, M. Rauff, and S. S. Ratnam (1979)  Abortion deaths in Singapore (1968-1976). Singapore Medical Journal 20: 391-394.

Liskin, L. S. (1980)  Complications of abortions in developing countries. Population Reports, Series F., No. 7.

Lopez-Escobar, G., C. Riano-Gamboa, and N. Lenis-Nicholls (1978)  Abortion: Questions, Commentaries, and Partial Results of Some Colombian Research (in Spanish).  Monograph No. 8.  Bogota:  Corporacion Centro Regional de Poblacion.

Lozano, C. A., A. M. T. Peralta, M. F. Reyes, P. R. Alvarado, and J. Saravia (1979)  Morbidity-Mortality: Classification and Treatment of Septic Abortion (in Spanish).  Bogota:  Facultad de Medicina, Universidad Nacional de Colombia.

Lwanga, C. (1977)  Abortion in Mulago Hospital, Kampala. East African Medical Journal 54:142-148.

Malhotra, S., and P. K. Devi (1979)  A comparative study of induced abortions before and after legalization of abortions. Journal of Obstetrics and Gynecology of India 29:598-601.

Matejcek, Z., Z. Dytrych, and V. Schuller (1978) Children from unwanted pregnancies. Acta Psychiatrica Scandinavica 57:67-90.

Matejcek, Z., Z. Dytrych, and V. Schuller (1979)  The Prague study of children born from unwanted pregnancies. International Journal of Mental Health 7:63-77.

Matejcek, Z., Z. Dytrych, and V. Schuller (1980) Follow-up study of children born from unwanted pregnancies. International Journal of Behavioral Development 3:243-251.

Mhango, C. G., and E. S. Grech (1979)  Family planning
    programme and abortion laws in Zambia.  In N. Mwaniki,
    M. Marasha, J. K. G. Mati, and M. K. Mwaniki, eds.,
    Surgical Contraception in Sub-Sahara Africa.  Chestnut
    Hill, Mass.:  Pathfinder Fund.
Miller, E. R., S. Pachauri, and A. Saha (1976)  Patterns
    of Contraceptive Acceptance after Abortion:  A Study
    in Four Asian Hospitals.  Chapel Hill, N.C.:
    International Fertility Research Program.
Miller, E. R., V. McFarland, M. S. Burnhill, and I. W.
    Armstead (1977)  Impact of abortion experience on
    contraceptive practice.  Advances in Planned
    Parenthood 12:15-28.
Miller, W. B. (1978)  The intendedness and wantedness of
    the first child.  Pp. 209-243 in W. B. Miller and L.
    F. Newman, eds., The First Child and Family
    Formation.  Chapel Hill, N.C.:  Carolina Population
    Center.
Miller W. B. (1981)  The Psychology of Reproduction.
    Springfield, Va.:  National Technical Information
    Service.
Miller W. B., and R. K. Godwin (1977)  Psyche and Demos.
    New York:  Oxford University Press.
MINSAP (Ministry of Public Health) (1980)  Annual reports
    and personal communications from Havana, Cuba.
Mohlake, S. (1980)  Personal communication, May.
Moore, E. C. (1971)  Induced abortion and contraception:
    Sociological aspects.  Pp. 131-155 in S. H. Newman, M.
    B. Beck, and S. Lewit, eds., Abortion Obtained and
    Denied:  Research Approaches.  New York:  Population
    Council.
Moore, E. C. (1974)  International Inventory of
    Information on Induced Abortion.  New York:  Columbia
    University International Institute for the Study of
    Human Reproduction.
Moore, E. C. (1976)  Abortion, Including Review of
    Current Status.  New Delhi:  World Health
    Organization, Regional Office for South-East Asia.
Muramatsu, M., and J. van der Tak (1978)  From abortion
    to contraception:  The Japanese experience.  Pp.
    145-167 in H. P. David, H. L. Friedman, J. van der
    Tak, and M. Sevilla, eds., Abortion in Psychosocial
    Perspective:  Trends in Transnational Research.  New
    York:  Springer.
Mwambia, S. P. K. (1973)  The Meru of Central Kenya.  In
    A. Molnos, ed., Cultural Source Materials for
    Population Planning in East Africa, Vol. 3.  Nairobi:
    East African Publishing House.

Narkavonnakit, T. (1979a) <u>Rural Abortion in Thailand: A</u>
<u>National Survey of Practitioners</u>. Bangkok: Research
and Evaluation Unit, National Family Planning Program.

Narkavonnakit, T. (1979b) Abortion in rural Thailand: A
survey of practitioners. <u>Studies in Family Planning</u>
10:223-229.

Narkavonnakit, T. (1980) A Study of 110 Women who
Experienced an Abortion Performed by a Traditional
Practitioner in the Province of Chayapoon, Thailand,
1980. Unpublished manuscript. Research and
Evaluation Unit, National Family Planning Program,
Bangkok.

Narkavonnakit, T., and T. Bennett (1981) Health
consequences of induced abortion in rural Northeast
Thailand. <u>Studies in Family Planning</u> 12:58-65.

Nathanson, C. A., and M. H. Becker (1977) The influence
of physicians' attitudes on abortion performance,
patient management and professional fees. <u>Family</u>
<u>Planning Perspectives</u> 9:158-163.

Nathanson, C. A., and M. H. Becker (1980) Obstetricians'
attitudes and hospital abortion services. <u>Family</u>
<u>Planning Perspectives</u> 12:26-32.

National Center for Health Statistics (1979) <u>Detailed</u>
<u>Diagnoses and Surgical Procedures for Patients</u>
<u>Discharged from Short-Stay Hospitals: United States,</u>
<u>1977.</u> Hyattsville, Md.: U.S. Department of Health,
Education, and Welfare.

Nazer, I. R. (1970) Abortion in the Near East. Pp.
267-273 in R. E. Hall, ed., <u>Abortion In A Changing</u>
<u>World</u>, Vol. 1. New York: Columbia University Press.

Nazer, I. R. (1980) The Tunisian experience in legal
abortion. <u>International Journal of Gynecology and</u>
<u>Obstetrics</u> 17:488-492.

Ndeti, K. (1973) Abortion in Traditional Societies: A
Sociological Review of Abortion in Six East African
Societies. Paper presented at the International
Planned Parenthood Federation Conference on the
Medical and Social Aspects of Abortion in Africa,
Accra, Ghana.

Newman, L. F. (1980) Widespread use of emmenagogues.
Cited in <u>Population Reports</u>, Series F., No. 7.

Ng, K. H., and T. A. Sinnathuray (1975) Maternal
mortality from septic abortions in University
Hospital, Kuala Lumpur from March 1968 to February
1974. <u>Medical Journal of Malaysia</u> 30:52-54.

Ojo, O. A., and V. Y. Savage (1974) A ten year review of
maternal mortality rates in the University College

Hospital, Ibadan, Nigeria. American Journal of Obstetrics and Gynecology 118:517-522.

Onetto, E. (1980) Abortion in Chile, 1964-1979. Unpublished paper in the files of the Population Information Program.

Osofsky, J. D., J. H. Osofsky, and R. Rajan (1973) Psychological effects of abortion: With emphasis upon immediate reactions and follow up. Pp. 188-205 in H. J. Osofsky and J. D. Osofsky, eds., The Abortion Experience. Hagerstown, Md.: Harper and Row.

Osofsky, J. D., H. J. Osofsky, R. Rajan, and D. Spitz (1975) Psychosocial aspects of abortion in the United States. Mount Sinai Journal of Medicine 42:456-468.

Padubidri, V., and B. G. Kotwani (1979) Septic abortions: 5 years' review. Journal of Obstetrics and Gynecology of India 29:593-597.

Palmer, S. J. (1978) Abortion in Africa: An expert group report. Pp. 23-27 in F. T. Sai, ed., A Strategy for Abortion Management: Report of an IPPF Africa Regional Meeting. London: International Planned Parenthood Federation.

Pan American Health Organization and Transnational Family Research Institute (1975) Epidemiology of Abortion and Practices of Fertility Regulation in Latin America: Selected Reports. Scientific Publication No. 306. Washington, D.C.: Pan American Health Organization.

Park, B. T., B. M. Choi, and H. Y. Kwon (1979) The 1976 National Fertility and Family Planning Evaluation Survey. Seoul: Korean Institute for Family Planning.

Pauls, F. (1973) Abortion Profile in Kinshasa, Zaire. Paper presented at the International Planned Parenthood Conference on Medical and Social Aspects of Abortion in Africa, Accra, Ghana.

Paxman, J. M. (1980a) Law and Planned Parenthood. London: International Planned Parenthood Federation.

Paxman, J. M. (1980b) Roles for non-physicians in fertility regulation: An international overview of legal obstacles and solutions. American Journal of Public Health 70:31-39.

Paxman, J. M., and M. Barberis (1980) Menstrual regulation and the law. International Journal of Gynecology and Obstetrics 17:493-503.

Philips, F. S., and N. Ghouse (1976) Septic abortion: Three year study 1971-1973. Journal of Obstetrics and Gynecology of India 26:652-656.

Pohlman, E. W. (1969)  The Psychology of Birth Planning.
   Cambridge, Mass.:  Schenkman.
Potts, M. (1970)  Postconceptive control of fertility.
   International Journal of Gynecology and Obstetrics
   8:957.
Potts, M. (1972)  Introduction:  Problems and strategy.
   Pp. 1-16 in M. Potts and C. Woods, eds., New Concepts
   in Contraception. Baltimore, Md.:  University Park
   Press.
Potts, M. (1979)  Perspectives on fertility control.
   International Journal of Gynecology and Obstetrics
   16:449-455.
Potts, M. (1980)  Personal communication, November.
Potts, M., P. Diggory, and J. Peel (1977)  Abortion.
   Cambridge, Mass.:  Cambridge University Press.
Program for the Introduction and Adapatation of
   Contraceptive Technology (PIACT) (1980)  Contraceptive
   use in China.  PIACT Product News 2(1):6.
Ramirez, A., and E. Garcia (1975)  Study of Abortion in
   200 Women in the Dominican Republic.  Santo Domingo:
   Universidad Nacional Pedro Henriquez Urena.
Ramirez, C. E., A. Russin, and R. L. Johnson, with A.
   Ramirez, E. Garcia, A. E. Noboa Mejia (1978)  The
   preferred risk of illegal abortion in the Dominican
   Republic. Pp. 225-240 in H. P. David, H. L. Friedman,
   J. van der Tak, and M. Sevilla, eds., Abortion in
   Psychosocial Perspective:  Trends in Transnational
   Research. New York:  Springer.
Requena, M. (1970)  Abortion in Latin America.  Pp.
   338-352 in R. E. Hall, ed., Abortion in a Changing
   World, Vol. 1.  New York:  Columbia University Press.
Riano-Gamboa, G., J. G. Ferguson, and A. Goldsmith
   (1975)  Clinical Management of Incomplete Abortion in
   the University Hospitals of Colombia (in Spanish).
   Conference Paper Series No. 79.  Chapel Hill, N.C.:
   International Fertility Research Program.
Rochat, R. W., D. Kramer, P. Senanayake, and C. Howell
   (1980)  Induced abortion and health problems in
   developing countries.  Lancet 2:484.
Rooks, J. B., and W. Cates, Jr. (1977)  Emotional impact
   of D&E vs. instillation.  Family Planning Perspectives
   9:276-277.
Rushwan, H. M. E., J. G. Ferguson, Jr., Z. M. El Nayal,
   E. H. E. El Nahas, and R. P. Bernard (1975)  Three
   Center Study on Incomplete Abortion in Khartoum,
   Sudan.  Unpublished manuscript.  International
   Fertility Research Program, Chapel Hill, N.C..

Sai, F. T. (1974)  Sub-Saharan black Africa.  Pp. 243-249
    in H. P. David, ed., Abortion Research:  International
    Experience. Lexington, Mass.:  Heath.
Sambhi, J. S. (1977)  Abortion by massage:  "Bomoh."
    IPPF Medical Bulletin 11(1).
Sampoerno, D., and S. Sadli (1975)  Indonesia.  Pp. 21-28
    in H. P. David and B. Shashi, orgs., Psychosocial
    Aspects of Abortion in Asia. Washington, D.C.:
    Transnational Family Research Institute.
Santee, B. (1975)  A prospective abortion study in
    Santiago, Chile.  Pp. 30-38 in Epidemiology of
    Abortion and Practices of Fertility Regulation in
    Latin America:  Selected Reports.  Scientific
    Publication No. 306.  Washington, D.C.:  Pan American
    Health Organization.
Sauvy, A. (1969)  General Theory of Population.  London:
    Weidenfeld and Nicolson.
Schwarz, R. H. (1968)  Septic Abortion.  Philadelphia:
    Lippincott.
Shepard, M. J., and M. B. Bracken (1979)  Contraceptive
    practice and repeat induced abortion:  An
    epidemiological investigation.  Journal of Biosocial
    Science 11:289-302.
Shostak, A. B. (1979)  Abortion as fatherhood lost:
    Problems and reforms.  The Family Coordinator
    28:569-574.
Siwale, S. H. (1977)  View from Africa:  Zambia.  In D.
    J. Bogue, K. Oettinger, M. Thompson, and P. Moore,
    eds., Adolescent Fertility.  Chicago:  University of
    Chicago Commmunity and Family Study Center.
Soskice, D. W., and J. J. Trussell (1973)  Effects of the
    abortion act.  British Journal of Hospital Medicine
    299-302.
Stampar, D. (1973-74)  An investigation concerning the
    reliability of data on the frequency of induced
    abortion (in Serbo-Croation).  Stanovnistno
    3-4:273-277.
Stepan, J., ed. (1979)  Survey of Laws on Fertility
    Control.  New York:  United Nations Fund for
    Population Activities.
Stokes, B. (1980)  Men and Family Planning.  Paper No.
    41.  Washington, D.C.:  World Watch Institute.
Tan, S. B. (1978)  The Psychosocial Aspects of Abortion
    in Singapore.  Ottawa:  International Development
    Research Centre.
Tecsan, S., C. E. Carpenter-Yaman, and N. H. Fisek
    (1980)  Abortion in Turkey.  Ankara:  Institute of
    Community Medicine, Haceteppe University.

Tien, H. Y., and X. W. Shao (1980)  How China meets its population problem. *International Family Planning Perspectives* 6:65-73.

Tietze, C. (1978a)  Repeat abortions--why more?  *Family Planning Perspectives* 10:286-288.

Tietze, C. (1978b)  Safety and health hazards of abortion. *Journal of Obstetrics and Gynecology* (Singapore) 9:49-56.

Tietze, C. (1979a)  *Induced Abortion: 1979*, 3rd ed.  New York: Population Council.

Tietze, C. (1979b)  Legal abortion in the world today. Pp. 406-415 in G. I. Zatuchni, J. J. Sciarra, and J. J. Speidel, eds., *Pregnancy Termination: Procedures, Safety, and New Developments*. Hagerstown, Md.: Harper and Row.

Tietze, C. (1981)  *Induced Abortion: A World Review*, 4th ed. New York: Population Council.

Tietze, C., and A. K. Jain (1978)  The mathematics of repeat abortion: Explaining the increase. *Studies in Family Planning* 9:294-299.

Tomaro, J. B. (1981)  Mexico. In M. Gallen, T. Narkavonnakit, J. B. Tomaro, and M. Potts, *Traditional Abortion Practices: Three Studies of Illegal Abortion in the Developing World*. Research Triangle Park, N. C.: International Fertility Research Program.

United Nations (1976)  *Demographic Yearbook, 1975*, Table 28. New York: United Nations.

United Nations (1977)  *Demographic Yearbook, 1976*, Table 16. New York: United Nations.

van der Tak, J. (1974)  *Abortion, Fertility, and Changing Legislation: An International Review*. Lexington, Mass.: Lexington Books.

Viel, B. (1976)  *The Demographic Explosion: The Latin American Experience*. New York: Irvington.

Viel, B. (1979)  The health consequences of illegal abortion in Latin America. Pp. 353-360 in G. I. Zatuchni, J. J. Sciarra, and J. J. Speidel, eds., *Pregnancy Termination: Procedures, Safety, and New Developments*. Hagerstown, Md.: Harper and Row.

Waife, R. S. (1978)  *Traditional Methods of Birth Control in Zaire*. Chestnut Hill, Mass.: Pathfinder Fund.

Warner, S. L. (1965)  Randomized response: A survey technique for eliminating evasive answer bias. *Journal of the American Statistical Association* 60:63-69.

Westoff, C. (1981)  Unwanted fertility in six developing countries. *International Family Planning Perspectives* 7:43-52.

Wolfson, M. (1976) Planning for people. People 3:18-21.

World Fertility Survey (1980) Summary of major findings presented at the World Fertility Conference, London, July. International Family Planning Perspectives 6:114-116.

World Health Organization (1965) World Health Statistics Annual, Vol. 1. Vital Statistics and Causes of Death. Geneva: World Health Organization.

World Health Organization (1967) World Health Statistics Annual, Vol. 1. Vital Statistics and Causes of Death. Geneva: World Health Organization.

World Health Organization (1978) Induced Abortion. Technical Report Series No. 623. Geneva: World Health Organization.

World Health Organization (1979a) World Health Statistics Annual, Vol. 3. Vital Statistics and Causes of Death. Geneva: World Health Organization.

World Health Organization (1979b) Special Programme of Research, Development, and Research Training in Human Reproduction: Eighth Annual Report. Geneva: World Health Organization.

World Health Organization (1980) Statistics on file in data bank. World Health Organization, Geneva.

Zelnik, M., and J. F. Kantner (1978) Contraceptive patterns and premarital pregnancy among women aged 15-19 in 1976. Family Planning Perspectives 10:135-144.

Zipper, J. (1915) Chilean experience with IUDs: Updating the programme. Pp. 217-324 in F. Hefnawi and J. J. Segal, eds., Analysis of Intrauterine Contraception. Amsterdam: North Holland.

Chapter 6

# Infanticide as Deliberate Fertility Regulation

SUSAN C. M. SCRIMSHAW*

Infanticide has been practiced by human populations at least since the upper Paleolithic era (Carr-Saunders, 1922). It is recorded in ancient literature, from the Bible (Moses) to the plays of Sophocles (Oedipus); in archeological records (Carr-Saunders, 1922; Valois, 1961); in past and contemporary anthropological accounts (Ellis, 1827; Balikci, 1967; Wagley, 1969); and in historical anthropological and demographic literature (Langer, 1974; Trexler, 1973a; Shorter, 1977). In fact, the practice has been so common that one anthropologist has called infanticide "the most widely used method of population control during much of human history" (Harris, 1977:5).

Despite the many past and present accounts of infanticide, the practice has seldom been quantified. It is difficult enough to obtain accurate fertility data in much of the world; it is more difficult still to get accurate infant mortality data, and nearly impossible to obtain accurate data on the deliberate killing of infants and children. Moreover, the discussion of infanticide in relation to fertility is constrained by the fact that there are many stated reasons for infanticide, ranging from characteristics of the infant at birth (twins, deformities, wrong sex) to explicit familial or societal concerns about overpopulation, large families, or close spacing. Although only these latter concerns are overtly linked to fertility, many of the other reasons may be "excuses" for eliminating an unwanted child or maintaining population growth at specific levels.

*I wish to thank Mildred Dickeman and the reviewers and the editors for their helpful comments on this paper.

With these constraints in mind, this paper will
discuss the available evidence on the use of infanticide
as a fertility control measure. First, definitions and
forms of infanticide will be presented, followed by an
examination of its incidence. The discussion will then
focus on infanticide in relation to fertility. Under
this heading, the relationships between fertility and
infant mortality will be explored, particularly as regards
behavioral interventions affecting mortality. Infanticide
as a form of fertility control at both the societal and
individual or familial levels will also be discussed
under the same heading. Finally, conclusions and
suggestions for needed research will be presented.

## DEFINITIONS AND FORMS OF INFANTICIDE

Definitions of infanticide in the literature range from
"the willful destruction of newborn babies through
exposure, starvation, strangulation, smothering or . . .
lethal weapon" (Langer, 1974:353) to killing of "a child
within the first year of life" (Kluge, 1978:33) to "child-
killing" without reference to age (Trexler, 1973a:98).
Although strictly speaking, infanticide should mean the
willful destruction of <u>infants</u>, it has come to refer to
both infants and children. Nevertheless, in most
societies where overt infanticide is practiced, it occurs
very early in the child's life, before it has the status
of a real person in the society. Thus the problem of
defining infanticide is similar to that of defining the
beginning of life in induced abortion. Once a society
has the technology to intervene in utero to save a life,
the failure to do so could be labeled infanticide, as has
induced abortion. As Williamson points out, "the line
between abortion and infanticide is not always clear."
She mentions that both the Kamchadal of Siberia and the
Yanomamo of Venezuela kill the fetus through the wall of
the abdomen at some point during the last few months of
pregnancy (1978:62). In fact, the definition of when
life is taken usually depends on a cultural definition of
when life begins. In modern U.S. society, this is often
the age at which a fetus can survive outside the mother's
uterus, although technological developments are constantly
lowering that age. Among the Machigenga, a newborn is
not accepted until its mother has nursed it, often a day
after birth (Johnson, 1981:63). Among Andean Indian
groups, a child may not be acknowledged until it has

survived its first year (Whitehead, 1968). In the past in Japan, a child was not named until the seventh day after birth (Bacon, 1891:63). Williamson (1978) says the Peruvian Amhuaca do not consider children fully human until they are three years old. In other societies, the acknowledgement of a newborn as a member of the society with a right to life may take days or even weeks (Ford, 1964:74).

The definition of infanticide is also complicated by the fact that it does not necessarily involve the deliberate or violent killing of a child. In the past, it has also been taken to include both abandonment and "negligence in the care of children" (Carr-Saunders, 1922). One could argue that abandonment does not constitute infanticide. However, while it is certainly not overt killing, it is the discarding of the child under circumstances which may mean its death. The demographic and historical literature contains many examples of infant and child abandonment in Europe during the 17th, 18th, and 19th centuries, with mortality rates as high as 90 percent (Trexler, 1973a; Kellum, 1974; Shorter, 1977; Langer, 1974). Current definitions can also include "passive infanticide" in the form of what has been called benign neglect (Cassidy, 1980) or underinvestment (Scrimshaw, 1978; Ware, 1977, 1981), which leads to child mortality that might otherwise have been avoided. This concept of negligence or underinvestment is itself complicated by the fact that in some situations, it is not the result of a conscious decision. Parents may simply favor some children over others, and because resources are scarce, the results are sometimes fatal for the neglected child (see Neel, 1970; Chandrasekar, 1959: 124-125; Harris, 1977:16; Ware, 1977, 1981; Scrimshaw, 1978). In other instances, parents may decide a child is "not for this world" and refuse to seek medical treatment for or invest resources in that child (Gutierrez de Pineda, 1955:19). In today's world, both developed and developing, such unconscious underinvestment is more prevalent than the deliberate killing of a child (Dickeman, 1975:133).

This unconscious underinvestment or passive infanticide can be more precisely defined as any combination of medical, nutritional, physical, or emotional neglect of an infant or young child in comparison to other children in the family or to children of families in similar socioeconomic and educational circumstances. In many instances, this neglect will lead to death, but

there will also be many survivors, who may be physically
and/or emotionally compromised because of the neglect
they experienced.  It is important to note that underinvestment is defined in <u>relative</u> terms:  the best an
impoverished family can provide would frequently be
considered inadequate by modern medical and nutritional
standards; neglect in fact occurs only when an infant or
child receives <u>less</u> than the family might be able to
provide, and less than family members know should be
provided.

Infanticide, then, can comprise a number of behaviors.
These include the following, which are not necessarily
mutually exclusive:

    Deliberate killing
    Placing the child in a dangerous situation
    Abandonment where the child might survive
    "Accidents"
    Excessive physical punishment
    Lowered biological support
    Lowered emotional support

In all but perhaps the first of these situations, failure
is possible; thus infanticide may be attempted, but
unsuccessful.  Such attempted infanticide must be discussed along with actual deaths, just as a discussion of
contraceptive use would normally include contraceptive
failure rates.


## INCIDENCE OF INFANTICIDE

The scarcity of accurate data on actual frequencies of
infanticide has already been mentioned.  There are no
such data in the demographic literature reviewed for this
paper.  The anthropological literature includes analyses
of a data set called the Human Relations Area Files
(HRAF), which contains data on over 300 societies organized by topic.  Because of the nature of anthropological
research, these societies tend to be small, although they
often include representatives of fairly large populations,
such as the Ibo of Nigeria, the Eskimo of Alaska and
Canada, and the Aymara of Bolivia and Peru.  The data
were collected from the 18th century on, but come
primarily from the 20th century.

Divale and Harris (1976) analyzed this data set for
populations for which there was information on age-sex

structure and presence (or recent presence) of warfare.
Their analysis of 112 societies (561 populations) meeting
these criteria also included a discussion of infanticide.
Although their sample is not random, they feel it is generally representative of preindustrial societies because
it is so large, and because the set of HRAF societies is
reasonably representative of the world's major geographic
regions.  Table 1 is based on their listing of societies.
Unfortunately, they do not specify what they mean by words
such as "common" and "occasional;" however, they still
give a rough idea of the incidence of infanticide.  All
of the Asian societies they list practiced infanticide
"commonly," as did 58 percent of the African societies.
Oceania had the lowest proportion of societies "commonly"
practicing infanticide, although there are no data on
infanticide for 58 percent of those societies, and the
actual figure may therefore be higher.  On a global
basis, 36 percent of the preindustrial cultures in the
sample practiced infanticide commonly, and 15 percent
practiced it occasionally or rarely.  It was clearly
identified as <u>not</u> practiced in only 9 percent of the 112
cultures.  This supports what the historical and archeological literature cited at the beginning of this chapter
suggests--that human societies have practiced infanticide
for a long time.  It does not, however, tell us whether
the practice was intended to curb population growth or
limit family size, rather than to destroy malformed
infants or accomplish other similar purposes.  The societies where the former reasons have been documented will
be listed later in this discussion.

Table 1 relates to overt or admitted infanticide for
which, as noted, the data are scarce.  Evidence of differential care or passive infanticide is even more difficult to come by.  The best evidence emerges from the
examination of sex differentials in mortality and morbidity.  On a strictly biological basis, slightly more
males than females are born.  Thus, if there were any sex
differential in mortality, males should have the higher
rates (Stolnitz, 1956).  India provides an example of the
opposite.  Findings from the Khanna study indicate that
boys receive more food and medical care than girls (Singh
et al., 1965).  Also, in the first five years of life,
the female death rate was 74 per 1000 per year while the
male death rate was 50 (Wyon and Gordon, 1971).  Welch
(1974) reports similar data from Bangladesh, where a girl
is more likely to survive in a family with more boys than
girls than one with the opposite balance.  Also reporting

TABLE 1   Frequency of Infanticide in 112 Societies, by
World Area

| World Area | Common | Occasion-al or not common | Not practiced | No infor-mation | Total |
|---|---|---|---|---|---|
| Asia | 6 | 0 | 0 | 0 | 6 |
| Africa | 7 | 0 | 0 | 5 | 12 |
| North America | 11 | 4 | 3 | 5 | 23 |
| Oceania | 12 | 5 | 6 | 32 | 55 |
| South America | 4 | 7 | 1 | 4 | 16 |
| Total | 40 | 16 | 10 | 46 | 112 |
| Percent | 36 | 15 | 9 | 40 | 100 |

Source:   Based on data in Divale and Harris (1976:533-535) from the
Human Relations Area Files.   Societies with no information on
infanticide are included because of the possibility that the absence
of information is related to the absence of infanticide.

on Bangladesh, D'Souza and Chen found "pronounced excess
female mortality over male mortality" (1980:258).   For
example, in 1975 the postneonatal mortality rate for
males was 98.4 per 1000 live births, while the female
rate was 126.3.   Overall, the mortality rates for females
were "significantly higher" through age 4, and then were
normal through age 14.   Ware (1981) adds that in Asia,
Jordan, Pakistan, and Sabah, infant mortality is higher
for female babies; female mortality is also higher for
ages 1 through 4 in nine populations--Bangladesh, Burma,
India, Jordan, Pakistan, Sabah, Sarawak, Sri Lanka, and
Thailand.   Kaku (1975) suggests that, as recently as
1966, there is evidence for "passive" female infanticide
in Japan based on a significant rise in the rate of
female infant mortality, partly due to accidents.   It is
noteworthy that this was a temporary, one-year rise; the
rates for males remained unchanged for the period from
1961 through 1967 examined by Kaku.   Kaku speculates that
the rise in female mortality was due to differential care
based on the belief that girls born in that year, the
year of the Firehorse, were ill-fated and supposedly
destined to murder their husbands.   A recent report on
China (Wren, 1982) states that female babies are still
sometimes drowned, and that mothers of daughters (first-
born) are sometimes beaten and ill-treated.   For Arab
areas, data for Jordan, Lebanon, Syria, and the

Palestinian Arabs document poorer nutritional status and higher mortality rates for girls than for boys from ages 1 to 5 (Cook, 1964; Kimmance, 1972). For Africa and Latin America, there is less evidence for higher female infant and young child mortality with the exception of some Latin American Indian groups (Scrimshaw, 1978:389).

In sum, the data on differential infant and young child mortality by sex strongly indicate behavioral differences in the care of male and female children in some cultures under some circumstances. The extent to which this differential care reflects either societal or individual "population policies" will be discussed in the following section.

INFANTICIDE AND FERTILITY

Relationships Between Fertility and Infant Mortality

The current literature on the relationship between fertility and infant mortality includes theories about both behavioral and biological factors. First, the theory of demographic transition states that mortality declines are eventually followed by fertility declines (Notestein, 1945; Davis, 1945). The child replacement hypothesis states that children who die will be replaced as quickly as possible (Omran, 1971), while the child survival hypothesis states that couples must produce enough children to ensure the survival of a given number to adulthood (Taylor et al., 1976). The health approach indicates that couples will not reduce their fertility until they are convinced that infant mortality levels have indeed dropped (Preston, 1978); it also posits that family-size limitation and greater birth spacing will contribute to improvements in the nutritional and health status of mothers and children (Berg, 1970; Zeitlin et al., 1982). However, another potential factor in the fertility-infant mortality equation is seldom mentioned: that in some societies, infant mortality may be an overt or even a completely unconscious way of attaining a given family size (Ware, 1977; Scrimshaw, 1978).

Figure 1 illustrates the relationships between infant mortality and fertility. The solid lines represent relationships that are acknowledged and frequently discussed. Thus, high fertility affects infant mortality through biological mechanisms (maternal depletion, early weaning) and is in turn affected by those same mechanisms

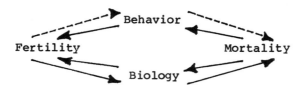

FIGURE 1  Behavioral and Biological Relationships Between
Fertility and Infant Mortality

Note:  Solid lines indicate relationships often discussed, broken lines behavioral relationships seldom
discussed.

(when an infant dies during the lactation period, the
mother resumes ovulation and can become pregnant sooner
than if she continued nursing).  Mortality is assumed to
influence fertility behavior through the child survival
and replacement effects discussed above.  Behavioral
links from high fertility to infant mortality (represented in the figure by dotted lines) have been largely
omitted from previous discussions.  Even though overt
infanticide has been in the literature for a long time,
differential care and child neglect have rarely been
discussed in relation to fertility.  As Ware (1977:3)
states, "if parents kill or neglect their children as a
means of limiting family size, then any relationship
between fertility control and involuntary child loss will
be totally obscured in all available statistics."  An
important concept behind Ware's statement is that of
family size.  To a demographer, the number of pregnancies
and live births is an important variable; to an individual
or family, the bottom line is the number of living
children--the current, and eventually the completed
family size.
     The influence of family size on infant mortality and
fertility can be seen in a closer examination of the
hypotheses on relationships between infant mortality and
fertility.  Both the child replacement and the child
survival hypotheses are useful for explaining fertility
behavior in some societies; however, neither hypothesis
alone nor the two taken together are sufficient to
describe fertility-mortality relationships in many
societies.

Taylor et al. (1976) maintain that there is little direct evidence for the child survival hypothesis, and question a direct causal link between the decline of child mortality and a decline in fertility. They point out that reduced child mortality has not been a precondition for lower fertility in some situations; moreover, it is difficult to prove that parents replace each child. They sugggest that "no single factor can be expected to explain the totality of complex motivations which lead to or inhibit fertility reduction" (p. 263), and that the balance of factors varies with the society and its stage in the process of demographic transition. Thus the child survival hypothesis tends to have some validity at the point in the transition where there has been a drop in mortality. This article is one of the few that acknowledges the possibility of mortality as a family-size control strategy. The authors suggest that the relative degree of unwantedness of children is a factor in infant mortality and fertility. The spectrum of infant mortality may range from lower-parity children who die but were wanted, to children at higher parities whose births exceed family-size desires.

The child replacement hypothesis is closely linked to the child survival hypothesis, and there is frequently little distinction made between them. However, the child survival hypothesis relates to the need to believe that children will survive to adulthood before fertility regulation is accepted, whereas the child replacement hypothesis addresses the more immediate, micro-level attempt of a couple to replace as quickly as possible a child who dies. Preston (1978) defines replacement rates as the average ratio of additional births to additional deaths. He points out that in no population are as many as 50 percent of child deaths replaced by additional births, and suggests a variety of reasons for this: there may not be a target number of surviving children; the targets may be so high that fertility couldn't possibly be any higher; the targets may be for one sex only; the couple may have fecundity problems; the child's death may result in a downward modification of ideal family size; and the child's death may have been anticipated and protected by insurance strategies of "overproduction" (pp. 12-14). Of these explanations, only the one related to targets for one sex allows for the possibility that every effort may not be made to prevent some child deaths. Other studies provide examples of the failure to replace dead children. In

Guatemala, Teller et al. (1975:338-343) conclude that
"women do not seem to be overcompensating for an intra-
interval death by hastening the coming of the next conception." In Colombia and Mexico, it has been suggested
that parity levels may in fact decrease with increased
child deaths (Rutstein and Medica, 1978).

One of the most interesting analyses of child survival
and replacement is provided by Chowdhury et al. (1976)
for Pakistan and Bangladesh. They address complications
in assessing the impact of child mortality on fertility
arising from the fact that high fertility can contribute
to high mortality. Although their data show that women
with fewer living children experience shorter birth intervals, it is difficult to sort out whether those shorter
intervals are due to conscious efforts to replace dead
children, result from shorter lactation amenorrhea following an infant death, or contribute to the deaths
through shortening lactation and maternal depletion (see
also Heer, in these volumes; Chen, in these volumes). In
an attempt to eliminate some of these biases, they
analyzed birth intervals according to previous child
deaths, excluding those deaths that had occurred just
prior to the birth interval examined. They found no
statistically significant difference in birth intervals
between women who had experienced at least one child
death and those who had not. They concluded that "in the
context of these two South Asian societies with moderately
high levels of fertility and mortality, there is no evidence that child deaths generate a desire to replace
children" (Chowdhury:255-258).

The inadequacy of the theory of demographic transition
for characterizing a number of populations has been suggested (Preston, 1978; Ware, 1977), and is evident from
the preceding discussion. This may be because there is a
certain amount of infant mortality in many societies which
cannot be assumed to result solely from factors beyond
the control of individuals.


## Infanticide as Fertility Control

### At the Societal Level

Historically, infanticide has been directly linked to
fertility regulation. One of the most common reasons
given for overt infanticide in the literature is regulation of either societal or familial fertility (Abernethy,

1979:52; Dickeman, 1975; Carr-Saunders, 1922). Specifically, this often involves limiting population to avoid food shortages. For example, Firth (1961:202) writes that the Tikopia practiced infanticide in proportion to the available food; this was done unwillingly, "with limited resources in mind," and only after the family already had at least one child of each sex. Some societies limit population according to the scarcity of other goods that have become associated with prestige: "Competition for essential resources is replaced by competition for socially valued goods" (Wilkenson, 1973:48). Thus, for example, the money that must be set aside for a dowry can make a female child less attractive to her parents.

A number of societies acknowledge explicitly that they practice infanticide to limit population. These include ancient cultures such as the Greeks (Langer, 1974), large societies of the recent past such as Japan and China (Lorimer, 1954; Langer, 1974), and recent and current preindustrial cultures such as the Eskimo (Freeman, 1971), the McKenzie Dene (Helm, 1980), the Australian aborigines (Howitt, 1904; Goodale, 1971), and the Jakun and Sakai of Malaya (Skeet and Blagden, 1906). Others, such as the Yaudapu Enga of New Guinea (Gray, 1981) and the Kung Bushmen (Howell, 1979; Lorimer, 1954), practice infanticide to increase spacing, which has the effect of reducing completed fertility rates.

When infanticide is consciously related to the need to regulate population size in relation to scarce resources, it is easy to see the link between the behavior and biological adaptation to a specific environment (Dickeman, 1975:120-129). Anthropological ecologists theorize that "beliefs and behaviors that affect fertility, death and disease rates are major factors in the adaptations of human societies. Over time, every society develops behavioral strategies which maximize gains and minimize losses in its population size relative to particular environments" (Alland, 1970:203). For any given biocultural adaptation, there is a maximum population level beyond which food energy extraction may damage the environment enough to threaten the survival of the group. When a population approaches this level, called carrying capacity, Malthusian checks on size may begin to operate, and the group may or may not evolve successful stategies for averting environmental degradation (Alland, 1970). Most human groups do not wait until the Malthusian checks begin to operate, but reduce fertility or increase

mortality through behaviors designed to improve the quality of life of the existing population. These theories
help explain why behavior that is detrimental to individual survival (such as infanticide) may be practiced:
the possibility of survival or the quality of life of the
entire group may be enhanced if fewer individuals are
present (Scrimshaw, 1978:399).

In a discussion of individual and group fertility
stategies, Wrigley (1978:135) labels as "unconscious
rationality" those "patterns of behavior in animals which
bring an apparent benefit to the species of which individual members of the population are unaware. What is true
of societies of animals may be true equally of societies
of men." He (along with others such as Alland) suggests
that particular behaviors may develop as a result of a
trial and error process comparable to the economic concept
of the "invisible hand of the marketplace." In an example
of this sort of reasoning, Freeman (1971:1016) writes of
Eskimo infanticide that the practice has ecological advantages, but that it is "doubtful" whether Eskimos are
"aware of such ecologic/biologic implications. . . .
However, because the implications are adaptive, the trait
itself (infanticide) is all the more likely to persist."

Female infanticide, the most common, can be seen either
as an intermediate mechanism for population control or as
an end to itself. If infant mortality is a means of
population control, it is, of course, more efficient to
eliminate females given the existence of polygamy, since
a few males could keep a population of females reproducing. In discussing the relationships between social
structure, fertility, female infanticide, and warfare,
Divale and Harris (1976) suggest that both warfare and
female infanticide operate as population-regulating
mechanisms, but that warfare and male-dominated social
structures provide the <u>motive</u> for female infanticide,
which is the <u>real</u> population regulation mechanism. Their
analysis can be challenged. Hirshfeld et al. (1978) and
Lancaster and Lancaster (1978) have questioned the
precision of Divale and Harris' data and their interpretation of the value of women. Divale and Harris (1976)
admit that the link with warfare appears weak, and that
female infanticide can occur in the absence of warfare.
Moreover, it is not clear that either sex ratios or rates
of infanticide are precisely reported for many of the 393
societies they examined. Nevertheless, it is unarguable
that female infanticide will have a greater impact on
population growth than will male infanticide, as long as
polygamy is practiced.

It is also clear that in ord
infanticide to exist, the sociel
value on male than on female infa
for example, in harsh environmenta
strength is important.  In a detail
Eskimo tribes, Riches (1974) showed
the harshness of the environment and
where tribes under the greatest press
highest sex ratio.  In a very few cult
are turned, and women are perceived as
their gathering or farming skills.  This
Tiwi of Australia (Goodale, 1971) and the
ela (Wilbert, 1982), both of which practic
commonly than female infanticide.

Other discussions of female infanticide i    ~ledge
that its ultimate function may be the reduction of rates
of population growth, but that its proximate utility may
be maintenance of the social structure.  The most detailed
discussion of this is provided by Dickeman (1975, 1979).
In some cases, female infanticide served to offset heavy
male mortality rates from hunting and warfare; in other
instances, however, it could be attributed to "asymetrical
marriage alliances."  In societies such as India, China,
and Europe, the preferential marriage form was hypergamy,
with women marrying men of higher castes or classes.  To
do this, women needed large doweries.  This created an
excess of women at the top, and encouraged the practice
of preferential female infanticide.

Whether infanticide is practiced for population control
or for other reasons, it must be recognized that it is a
more adaptive mechanism for fertility and population
control than induced abortion.  Induced abortion often
carries with it higher risks of maternal mortality and
subsequent infertility due to infections.  Although this
is not true under modern medical conditions, such conditions did not exist in the past and are not legally
available in many societies today.  Although infanticide
carries a higher risk for the mother than if she had not
undergone the risks of pregnancy and birth in the first
place, it is still safer than inducing an abortion under
poor conditions (Tietze et al., 1976).

The theories discussed in this section are rather
easily applied to small, isolated populations whose
relationship to the environment is direct and relatively
unchanging, although a precise measure of carrying
capacity has proved extremely elusive.  Given the current
interdependence of human societies as well as rapidly

...nologies for extracting food and energy ...ironment, direct relationships between adap-...d environment are much more difficult to observe. ...elationships may persist in some peasant communi-...s, and behaviors that evolved in the past may also persist in the present; however, in the current world, behaviors such as overt or passive infanticide may be better understood at the micro level of individuals or families.

## At the Individual or Familial Level

When infanticide is mandated or clearly encouraged at the societal level for purposes of population control, birth spacing, or family-size limitation, individuals will be pressured by other members of the society to follow those norms. When such mandates are not present or explicit, individuals may still choose overtly, covertly, or unconsciously to reduce their family size or influence spacing through behaviorally induced infant mortality.

Infanticide, either active or passive, is extremely difficult to document at the individual level, particularly when the practice is not officially sanctioned or is forbidden. Nevertheless, there is evidence that in addition to occasional cases of overt infanticide, individuals in many societies practice abandonment, neglect, and differential care (Dickeman, 1975; Neel, 1970). There are reports of widespread abandonment in Latin American countries, for instance, though estimates of the number of abandoned children are difficult to credit (Hollsteiner and Tacon, 1982).

In addition to actual abandonment, a major means of passive infanticide is differential care. For example, in a Guatemalan community, a woman who felt she already had too many children tried unsuccessfully to abort a pregnancy. When a perfectly healthy baby was born, she declared that it was weak and sickly and would die soon. It did, probably due to a lack of feeding and nurturing (M. Scrimshaw, 1977). As defined earlier, differential care involves the withholding of scarce resources from the less valued children. These may be children of a less-preferred sex, as discussed above. They may also include children of a higher birth order who are not as well integrated into the family, or members of a closely spaced pair.

Parity above five is associated with higher infant mortality in many studies (Wyon and Gordon, 1971; Radovic, 1966; Roberts and Tanner, 1963), as is being the second in a closely spaced pair of children (Wolfers and Scrimshaw, 1975). In both cases, however, there are many other behavioral and biological factors involved, so that the impact of differential care cannot be established on the basis of current evidence.

Nevertheless, cases of differential care are reported in the literature. Aguirre (1966) cites incidents of infants and young children being "allowed to die" when attacked by disease, calling this "masked infanticide." Chagnon (1968) mentions a Yanomamo mother who did not feed her baby, saying it had stopped eating because of a bad case of diarrhea. He found that the baby would eat, but the mother was starving it. In discussing differences between the mothers of normal and malnourished children in India, Graves (1977) notes that mothers of malnourished children felt significantly more negative about their pregnancies.

In a discussion of differential mortality in India, Simmons et al. (1980:14) state that "other things being equal, a child's survival will be determined by how much it is wanted," in relation to the number of children the parents have and the child's sex. In an analysis of sex differentials for infectious causes of death in Bangladesh, D'Souza and Chen (1980) state that the reason for these differentials is probably neglect, especially in feeding, which then renders an infant more susceptible to infection. In Korea, one study showed that for 100 male children under the age of 5, there were 85 visits to the health center in a year, but only 50 visits a year for 100 female children (Ware, 1981:57).

In sum, methods of passive infanticide include outright abandonment, as well as neglect in the areas of feeding (including breastfeeding and supplementation), sanitation, medical care, supervision, and attention. The undesirability of a particular child may be explicitly voiced by parents as they discuss their ill or deceased children; more often, however, the occurrence of passive infanticide must be estimated by the researcher, either through direct observation or by inference.

## CONCLUSIONS AND RECOMMENDED RESEARCH

It is clear that the data on infanticide are scattered and incomplete. Anthropologists have documented its occurrence in many pre-industrial societies, but have not provided quantitative information. Demographers and historians have provided some quantitative information for societies in the past, but little for the present. In fact, the existence of infanticide in the present has been largely ignored or denied. This is regrettable because unless it is acknowledged that some infant mortality is behaviorally induced or influenced, many theories, such as the child replacement hypothesis, fail to offer adequate explanations of fertility and mortality patterns in some societies. Passive infanticide has further implications related to child health since the many survivors of such attempts are often physically, mentally, and emotionally compromised.

Several areas of needed research on the subject of infanticide may be identified.

1. <u>Improved Quantification</u> Anthropologists and others observing or being told of infanticide should strive for both precision and quantification. How frequently does it occur per 1000 live births and per family? Why is it done? How is it done? Who decides it must be done? How do people feel about it? In the case of passive infanticide, the researcher should try to document differential care and attitudes toward specific infants and children as precisely as possible.

2. <u>Better Analysis of Existing and New Quantitative Data</u> Some of the questions raised in this chapter on such problems as the relationship between maternal age, maternal health, and higher infant mortality can be addressed through multivariate analysis. Studies that include objective data on the mother's health status are rare, but they exist and should be exploited. Even in the absence of such information, more can be done with questions of correlation and causality in the relationship between fertility and infant mortality.

3. <u>Further Examination of the Current Hypotheses on Relationships Between Fertility and Infant Mortality</u> Omran (1971) mentions the scarcity of studies specifically designed to investigate either direct or indirect effects of child survival on fertility. Similarly, Schultz (1976:280) states: "No one, to my knowledge, has yet estimated . . . the separate fertility effects of a child's death attributable to behavioral and biological factors while holding constant the more important socio-

economic determinants of reproductive demands." In sum,
questions such as the impact of maternal age, weight,
health status, and nutritional status on perinatal,
infant, and child mortality must be addressed. Differential mortality must be assessed while controlling for
birth order, number of living children in the family,
contraception, lactation, and other related variables.
On the behavioral side, particular attention needs to be
paid to the impact on children of the family's economic
situation and the resultant choices that must be made
related to food, medical care, and attention or care
while the mother works.

4. Quantification and Better Understanding of Infant
and Child Abandonment How extensive is it? Under what
circumstances do parents abandon children? How does child
abandonment relate to birth spacing, parity, attempts at
contraception or abortion, and family economic status?
Are some children retained while others are abandoned?
How do parents perceive the fate of abandoned children?

5. Further Investigation of Passive Infanticide The
family context of infants and children who show signs of
malnutrition, untreated disease, abuse, and neglect needs
to be examined. Attention should be paid to factors such
as sex, birth order, number of surviving siblings, parental family-size desires, and spacing when such children
appear in health centers or as research subjects. Parents
should be observed and interviewed to elicit their attitudes and behaviors towards these children, with every
effort made to quantify and analyze the resulting data.

To summarize, some of the data needed to better understand both overt and passive infanticide as they relate
to the relationships between fertility and infant mortality already exist, but have not been properly exploited.
Other types of information need to be collected. Most
important, if this is to be done, researchers and health
care providers must change their view of parent/child
relationships to admit the possibility that both overt
and passive infanticide still exist.

BIBLIOGRAPHY

Abernethy, V. (1979) Population Pressure and Cultural
    Adjustment. New York: Human Sciences Press.

Aguirre, A. (1966) Colombia: The family in Candelaria. Studies in Family Planning 1(11).

Alland, A. (1970) Adaptation in Cultural Evolution: An Approach to Medical Anthropology. New York: Columbia University Press.

Bacon, A. M. (1891) Japanese Girls and Women. New York: Gordon Press.

Balikci, A. (1967) Female infanticide on the Arctic coast. Man 2:615-625.

Berg, A. (1970) Toward survival: Nutrition and the population dilemma. Interplay 24-27.

Carr-Saunders, A. M. (1922) The Population Problem. A Study in Human Evolution. London: Clarendon Press.

Cassidy, C. M. (1980) Benign neglect and toddler malnutrition. In L. Greene and F. Johnson, eds., Social and Biological Predictors of Nutritional Status, Physical Growth, and Development. New York: Academic Press.

Chagnon, N. (1968) Yanomamo: The Fierce People. New York: Holt, Rinehart, and Winston.

Chandrasekhar, S. (1959) Infant Mortality in India 1901-1955. London: George Allen and Unwin, Ltd.

Chowdhury, A. K. M. A. et al. (1976) The effect of child mortality experience on subsequent fertility: Pakistan and Bangladesh. Population Studies 30:249-261.

Cook, R. (1964) Nutrition and mortality of females under 5 years of age compared with males in the greater Syria region. Journal of Tropical Pediatrics 10:76-81.

Davis, K. (1945) The world demographic transition. Annals of the American Academy of Political and Social Science 237:1-11.

Dickeman, M. (1975) Demographic consequences of infanticide in Man. Annual Review of Ecology and Systematics 6:100-132.

Dickeman, M. (1979) Female infanticide, reproductive strategies and social stratification: A preliminary model. In N. A. Chagnon and W. Irons, eds., Evolutionary Biology and Human Social Behavior: An Anthropological Perspective. North Scituate, Mass.: Duxbury Press.

Divale, W. T., and M. Harris (1976) Population, warfare and the male supremicist complex. American Anthropologist 78:521-538.

D'Souza, S., and L. C. Chen (1980) Sex differentials and mortality in rural Bangladesh. Population and Development Review 6:257-270.

Ellis, W. (1827) Narrative of a Tour Through Hawaii. London.

Firth, R. (1957) We, the Tikopia. London: Allen and Unwin.

Firth, R. (1961) Elements of Social Organization. Boston: Beacon Press.

Ford, C. S. (1945) A Comparative Study of Human Reproduction. Yale University Publications in Anthropology No. 3. New Haven, Conn.: Yale University Press.

Ford, C. S. (1964) A Comparative Study of Human Reproduction. Human Relations Area Files Press No. 32. New Haven, Conn.: Yale University Press.

Freeman, M. (1971) A social and economic analysis of systemic female infanticide. American Anthropologist 73:1011-1018.

Goodale, J. (1971) Tiwi Wives. Seattle, Wash.: University of Washington Press.

Graves, P. L. (1977) Nutrition, infant behavior and maternal characteristics: A pilot study in West Bengal, India. American Journal of Clinical Nutrition 30:242.

Gray, B. (1981) Personal communication.

Gulick, J., and M. E. Gulick (1975) Kinship, contraception and family planning in the Iranian city of Isfahan. Pp. 241-293 in M. Nag, ed., Poulation and Social Organization. The Hague: Mouton.

Gutierrez de Pineda, V. (1955) Causas culturales de la mortalidad infantil. Revista Colombiana de Antropologia 4:11-86.

Harris, M. (1977) Cannibals and Kings: The Origins of Cultures. New York: Random House.

Helm, J. (1980) Female infanticide, European diseases, and population levels among the McKenzie Dene. American Ethnologist 7:259-285.

Hirschfeld, L. A., J. Howe, and B. Levin (1978) Warfare, infanticide and statistical interference: A comment on Divale and Harris. American Anthropologist 80:110-115.

Hollsteiner, M. R., and P. Tacon (1982) Urban Migration in Developing Countries: Consequences for Families and Their Children. New York: United Nations.

Howell, N. (1979) Demography of the Dobe/King. New York: Academic Press.

Howitt, A. W. (1904) The Native Tribes of South-East Australia. London.

Johnson, O. (1981) The socioeconomic context of child abuse and neglect in native South America. Pp. 55-70 in J. E. Korbin, ed., Child Abuse and Neglect:

_Cross-Cultural Perspectives_. Berkeley, Calif.: University of California Press.

Kaku, K. (1975) Were girl babies sacrificed to a folk superstition in 1966 in Japan? _Annals of Human Biology_ 2:391-393.

Kellum, B. (1974) Infanticide in England in the later Middle Ages. _History of Infanticide Quarterly_ 1:367-388.

Kimmance, K. J. (1972) Failure to thrive and lactation failure in Jordanian villages in 1970. _Environmental Child Health_ 18:313-316.

Kluge, E.-H. (1978) Infanticide as the murder of persons. In M. Kohl, ed., _Infanticide and the Value of Life_. Buffalo, N.Y.: Prometheus Books.

Lancaster, C., and J. Lancaster (1978) On the male supremicist complex: A reply to Divale and Harris. _American Anthropologist_ 80:115-117.

Langer, W. (1974) Infanticide: A historical survey. _History of Childhood Quarterly_ 1:353-365.

Lorimer, F. (1954) _Culture and Human Fertility_. Zurich: UNESCO.

Neel, J. V. (1970) Lessons from a "primitive" people. _Science_ 170:815-822.

Newcombe, H. (1965) Environmental versus genetic interpretations of birth order effects. _Eugenics Quarterly_ 12:90-101.

Notestein, F. W. (1945) Population--The Long View. In T. W. Schultz, ed., _Food for the World_. Chicago: University of Chicago Press.

Omran, A. R. (1971) _The Health Theme in Family Planning_. Carolina Population Center Monograph No. 16. Chapel Hill, N.C.: University of North Carolina.

Oxhorn, H. (1955) Hazards of grand multiparity. _Obstetrics and Gynecology_ 5:150-156.

Preston, S. H. (1972) Interrelations between death rates and birth rates. _Theoretical Population Biology_ 3:162-185.

Preston, S. H. (1978) _The Effects of Infant and Child Mortality on Fertility_. New York: Academic Press.

Radovic, P. (1966) Frequent and high parity as a medical and social problem. _American Journal of Obstetrics and Gynecology_ 94:583-585.

Riches, D. (1974) The Netsilik Eskimo: A special case of selective female infanticide. _Ethnology_ 13:351-362.

Roberts, D. F., and R. E. S. Tanner (1963) Effects of parity on birth weight and other variables in a Tanganyika Bantu Sample. _British Journal of Preventive and Social Medicine_ 17:209-215.

Rutstein, S., and V. Medica (1978)  The Latin American experience.  In S. Preston, ed., The Effects of Infant and Child Mortality on Fertility.  New York:  Academic Press.

Schultz, T. P. (1976)  Interrelationships between mortality and fertility.  In R. G. Ricker, ed., Population and Development:  The Search for Selective Interventions.  Baltimore, Md.:  The Johns Hopkins University Press.

Scrimshaw, M. (1977)  Personal communication.

Scrimshaw, S. C. M. (1978)  Infant mortality and behavior in the regulation of family size.  Population and Development Review 4:383-403.

Shorter, E. (1977)  The Making of the Modern Family.  New York:  Basic Books.

Simmons, G. B., C. Smucker, S. Bernstein, and E. Jenson (1980)  Post-Neonatal Mortality in Rural India: Implications of an Economic Model.  Paper presented to the annual meeting of the American Public Health Association, Detroit.

Singh, F., J. E. Gordon, and J. B. Wyon (1965)  Cause of death at different ages by sex and by season in a rural population of the Punjab 1957-1959:  A field study.  Indian Journal of Medical Research 53:906-917.

Skeet, W. W., and C. O. Blagden (1906)  Pagan Races of the Malay Peninsula, Vol. 2.  London.

Stolnitz, G. (1956)  A century of international mortality trends:  II.  Population Studies 10:1742.

Taylor, C. E., J. S. Newman, and N. U. Kelley (1976)  The child survival hypothesis.  Population Studies 30:263-278.

Teller, C., W. Butts, C. Yarborough, A. Lechtig, J.-P. Habicht, H. Delgado, and R. Martorell (1975)  Effects of declines in infant and child mortality on fertility and birthspacing:  Preliminary results from retrospective data in four villages.  Pp. 338-343 in Seminar on Infant Mortality in Relation to the Level of Fertility. Committee for International Coordination of National Research in Demography.  Bangkok:  CICRED.

Tietze, C., J. Bongaarts, and S. B. Schearer (1976)  Mortality associated with a control of fertility.  Family Planning Perspectives 8:6-14.

Trexler, R. (1973a)  Infanticide in Florence:  New sources and first results.  History of Childhood Quarterly 1:98-116.

Trexler, R. (1973b)  The foundlings of Florence 1395-1455.  History of Childhood Quarterly 1:259-284.

Valois, H. V. (1961)  The social life of early Man:  The
    evidence of skeletons.  In S. L. Washburn, ed., The
    Social Life of Early Man.  Chicago:  Aldine.
Wagley, C. (1969)  Cultural influences on population:  A
    comparison of two Tupi tribes.  Pp. 268-280 in A. P.
    Vayda, ed., Environment and Cultural Behavior.  New
    York:  The Natural History Press.
Wagley, C. (1977)  Welcome of Tears.  New York:  Oxford
    University Press.
Ware, H. (1977)  The relationship between infant
    mortality and fertility:  Replacement and insurance
    effects.  Proceedings of the International Population
    Conference, Liege, 1977, Vol. 1.  Liege:
    International Union for the Scientific Study of
    Population.
Ware, H. (1981)  Women, Demography and Development.
    Development Studies Center Demography Teaching Notes.
    Canberra:  Australian National University.
Welch, F. (1974)  Sex of Children, Prior Uncertainty, and
    Subsequent Fertility Behavior.  R-1510-RF.  Santa
    Monica, Calif.:  Rand Corporation.
Whitehead, L. (1968)  Altitude, fertility and mortality
    in Andean countries.  Population Studies 22:335-346.
Wilbert, J. (1982)  Personal communications.
Wilkenson, R. G. (1973)  Poverty and Progress.  London:
    Methuen.
Williamson, L. (1978)  Infanticide:  An anthropological
    analysis.  Pp. 61-75 in M. Cohl, ed., Infanticide and
    the Value of Life.  Buffalo, N.Y.:  Prometheus Books.
Wolfers, D., and S. C. M. Scrimshaw (1975)  Child
    survival and intervals between pregnancies in
    Guayaquil, Ecuador.  Population Studies 29:479-496.
Wren, C. S. (1982)  Old nemesis haunts China on birth
    plan.  New York Times, July 29.
Wrigley, E. A. (1978)  Fertility strategy for the
    individual and the group.  Pp. 135-154 in C. Tilley,
    ed., Historical Studies of Changing Fertility.
    Princeton, N.J.:  Princeton University Press.
Wyon, J., and J. Gordon (1971)  The Khanna Study:
    Population Problems in Rural Punjab.  Cambridge,
    Mass.:  Harvard University Press.
Yeats, W. B. (1928)  King Oedipus.  New York:  MacMillan.
Zeitlin, M. F., J. D. Wray, J. B. Stanbury, N. P.
    Schlossman, M. H. Meurer, and P. J. Weinthal (1982)
    Nutrition and Population Growth:  The Delicate
    Balance.  Cambridge, Mass.:  Oelgeshlager, Gunn and
    Hain, Inc.

# Chapter 7

# Population Programs and Fertility Regulation

W. PARKER MAULDIN

MEASURING THE IMPACT OF FAMILY PLANNING PROGRAMS

Over the past two decades, there has been a tremendous
increase in official attention to population issues.
This is reflected in awareness and concern, in policies
and programs, in training of personnel and development of
institutions, and in growing research efforts. Antigrowth
and profamily planning policies have been established in
35 countries (with nearly 80 percent of the population of
the developing world), usually accompanied by some form
of program, though these are still weak in many.[1]
Training and research programs in demography/social
science and biomedicine/contraceptive development have
been undertaken in Asia and Latin America, and to a
lesser extent in Africa.

A population assistance community has emerged, with
the objectives of promoting and supporting population
activities. Net funding is now over $500 million per
year from international, national, and private sources
(see Table 1). Funds are devoted to

a wide range of population activities, including
national censuses, demographic surveys and research;
information and education programs; delivery of family
planning services; construction of training centers,
and maternal and child health and family planning
clinics; training of doctors; paramedical personnel
and village health workers; supply of contraceptives,
equipment and vehicles; programs for marketing non-
clinical contraceptives; and staff and institutional
development (Kanagaratnam, 1978:11).

TABLE 1    Assistance for Population Activities by Major
Donors, 1971 and 1980 (in thousand U.S. dollars)

| Donor | 1971 | 1980 |
|---|---|---|
| Total Governmental | $133,744 | $413,070 |
| United States | 109,567 | 195,000 |
| Norway | 3,870 | 47,260 |
| Sweden | 7,446 | 40,080 |
| Germany | 1,657 | 35,000 |
| Japan | 2,090 | 30,700 |
| Netherlands | 1,106 | 15,109 |
| Canada | 2,496 | 13,521 |
| United Kingdom | 2,311 | 13,000 |
| Denmark | 1,918 | 12,490 |
| Others | 1,283 | 10,910 |
| Total Multilateral | $23,547 | $338,029 |
| UNFPA | 8,937 | 157,518 |
| World Bank | 1,600 | 77,800 |
| WHO | 2,823 | 41,878 |
| United Nations | 6,995 | 37,892 |
| UNICEF | 2,382 | 9,331 |
| UNESCO | 38 | 6,652 |
| ILO | 165 | 6,001 |
| FAO | 607 | 3,957 |
| Others | | 7,000 |
| Total Private Agencies | $60,798 | $117,432 |
| IPPF | 15,202 | 50,956 |
| Family Planning International Assistance | 276 | 18,800 |
| Population Council | 16,347 | 14,436 |
| Ford Foundation | 21,261 | 5,400 |
| Rockefeller Foundation | 5,981 | 4,534 |
| Mellon Foundation | | 3,500 |
| Hewlett Foundation | | 1,465 |
| Other | 1,731 | 18,341 |
| Aggregate Total | $218,089 | $868,531 |
| Net Total (eliminating double counting) | $168,553 | $519,895 |

Source:  Adapted from tables compiled by UNFPA.

A large proportion of such funding, roughly three-quarters, goes to family planning activities.

This increased attention to population issues has in turn generated an interest in evaluating the impact of family planning programs on contraceptive use and on fertility levels (Marshall, 1977).

There is an extensive literature on measuring the impact of family planning programs on fertility using both micro and macro analytical approaches (United Nations, 1978, 1979; Forrest and Ross, 1978; Ross and Forrest, 1978; Chandrasekaran and Hermalin, 1975; Gorosh and Wolfers, 1979; Potter, 1969, 1977). Despite this large literature, however, there are substantial problems in performing such measurements. Perhaps the most serious problem is that on a national scale, one cannot know what would have happened without the family planning program. In experimental programs and matching studies, this problem can be largely overcome by comparison of the experimental and control or matched groups. On a national scale, one can construct models taking into account changes in socioeconomic factors, but different models give different results. It is generally acknowledged that institutional, including cultural, factors are important determinants of fertility; however, we do not yet know how to quantify the effects of institutional factors, and in particular we do not know how to identify those factors that "trigger" a fertility decline.

Because of these methodological problems, both the International Union for the Scientific Study of Population and the Population Division of the United Nations are actively seeking to improve techniques for measuring program impact. To this end, Forrest and Ross classify methods of analyzing the impact of family planning programs under seven categories: decomposition, correspondence of timing of program activity and fertility change, matching studies, experimental and control areas, multiple regression and areal units, births averted among acceptors, and simulation methods. The Chandrasekaran and Hermalin volume and the United Nations Manual IX use slightly different but highly similar categories.

The problems addressed and raised by these methodologies are illustrated in the case of decomposition techniques. Basically, changes in age structure affect crude birth rates, but not total fertility rates; changes in marital patterns affect both. One of the first steps in analyzing the determinants of changes in fertility is therefore to standardize rates, or decompose changes in

fertility that are attributable to changes in age structure, in marital patterns, and in marital fertility (see
Shryock and Siegel, 1971; United Nations, 1979; Kitagawa,
1955; Cho and Retherford, 1973). Because family planning
programs are often thought to affect marital fertility,
but not age structure or marital patterns, such decomposition is useful to separate out that part of fertility
change that is presumed not to be affected by population
programs.

There are a number of limitations to this methodology,
however. First, although family planning programs do not
affect age structure significantly in the short run, if a
program has helped reduce fertility over a period of 10
to 15 years, the changing age composition, with fewer
people in the younger age groups, is a factor in the
increasing proportion of women of reproductive age.
Analysts have generally ignored this possible effect of
population programs. Similarly, most analysts assume
that population programs should not be credited with
affecting changes in marital patterns. Increasingly,
however, population programs seek to influence attitudes
about the appropriate age of first marriage (notably in
China), and the age of marriage itself. There have not
been attempts to quantify this relationship.

Finally, most developing countries have rather poor
statistical systems, and data are often unavailable that
are required for decomposing changes in crude birth rates
during recent periods.[2] With these limitations in
mind, the present paper reviews the available literature,
focusing first on the general relationship between family
planning programs and prevalence of contraceptive use,
and then on empirical studies both across and within
countries of the relationship between family planning
programs and fertility decline.

## FAMILY PLANNING PROGRAMS AND
## PREVALENCE OF CONTRACEPTIVE USE

The annual number of family planning acceptors in
large-scale programs has increased from a few tens of
thousands around 1960 to about 2.5 million in 1965 and
approximately 25 million in 1980. Estimates of prevalence
of use are now available from the World Fertility Survey,
contraceptive prevalence surveys by Westinghouse Health
Systems (Lewis and Novak, 1982) and the Centers for
Disease Control (Morris and Anderson, 1982), and national

surveys in a number of countries.  These data demonstrate
very rapid increases in contraceptive prevalence rates in
some countries with national family planning programs
(Table 2 and Figure 1).  In some countries, however--
Ghana, Kenya, Morocco, Bangladesh, Nepal, and Pakistan,
for example--contraceptive prevalence rates remain low
after many years of a national family planning program.[3]

Global, regional, and country estimates of prevalence
rates have been made using regression equations based on
the relationship between crude birth rates and prevalence
rates, as reported in surveys; this relationship is
strong, as indicated by an $R^2$ of 0.91 (Nortman and
Hofstatter, 1980).  However, this approach overestimates
prevalence of use in countries with high proportions of
sterility caused by venereal disease and in countries
with a high incidence of induced abortion.  Moreover,
prevalence estimates derived from surveys or regression
equations include both program and nonprogram sources,
and thus do not give direct evidence on the impact of
family planning programs.

Although continuation rates vary with the particular
method used and characteristics of the user, in practice
the average period of use in most developing countries is
two years.  Accordingly, the estimated number of current
users of fertility control methods directly attributable
to a national program may be estimated as double the
number of reported annual acceptors.  This estimation
procedure gives a figure of about 50 million couples in
developing countries (excluding China) using contraception from program sources in 1978-79; an estimate based
on a regression equation gives a figure of more than 80
million (Larson, 1981; Diaz-Briquets, 1980).  These
figures suggest that (1) about 60 percent of contraceptive use in developing countries (excluding China) is
from program sources; and (2) about 20 percent of couples
in the reproductive ages are using a contraceptive method
(34 percent including China, where the prevalence rate is
thought to be about 68 percent).

The major issue remains, however, of whether and to
what extent government programs lead to an increase in
prevalence of use.  Government programs typically make
contraceptives available at a subsidized price or at no
monetary cost to the user.  One would expect, therefore,
that some users who previously purchased supplies in the
commercial sector would shift to the public sector when
available.[4]  Many former users of privately supplied
fertility control methods switch to program sources of

TABLE 2   Percent of Current Contraceptive Users Among
Married Couples, Wife Aged 15-44, by Specified Year

| Country and Year | Percent | Country and Year | Percent | Country and Year | Percent |
|---|---|---|---|---|---|
| Colombia | | Mexico | | South | |
| 1969 | 21 | 1973 | 13 | Korea | |
| 1976 | 45 | 1976-77 | 32 | 1964 | 9 |
| 1978 | 49 | 1978 | 41 | 1968 | 19 |
| | | | | 1976 | 44 |
| Taiwan | | Thailand | | 1979 | 54 |
| 1965 | 13 | 1969-70 | 14 | | |
| 1970 | 26 | 1975 | 37 | | |
| 1976 | 46 | 1979 | 48 | | |
| 1980 | 70 | | | | |

Sources:
Colombia--Bureau of the Census (1979); Colombia, Departamento
   Administrativo Nacional de Estadistica (1977); Larson (1981).
Mexico--Nortman and Hofstatter (1980); Population Information Program
   (1981).
South Korea--Ross and Smith (1970:225-230); Keeny (1972:102); Cho and
   Retherford (1982).
Taiwan--Freedman et al. (1982); Taiwan Provincial Institute of Family
   Planning (1980).
Thailand--Knodel et al. (1982).

supply initially; this is sometimes called the substitution effect.  Although most evaluation studies collect
information on what methods an acceptor used prior to
enrollment in the family planning program, providing a
correction factor, there may be either under- or over-
reporting of former use.  Also, many program administrators and evaluators believe, with some evidence, that a
larger proportion of those switching from nonprogram to
program supplies also switch from an inefficient to a
modern and more efficient method of fertility control.
Another aspect of the substitution effect is that some
former nonusers who first turn to a program source would
have gone to a private or commercial source if the
program were unavailable.[5]

A related question is how effective commercial avenues
of distributing contraceptives would have been without
the program.  Most private donors and many governments
have recognized the potential importance of the commercial
sector, encouraging it to expand its activities; in some
instances they have subsidized commercial contraceptives
to reduce their costs.  Although there is no satisfactory

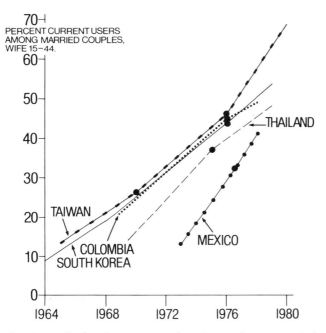

FIGURE 1   Growth in Contraceptive Prevalence:   Selected
Countries, 1964-1980

empirical evidence relating to this question, most
informed observers conclude that government programs have
led to availability of supplies much more rapidly and at
much lower cost than would otherwise have been the case.

The precise extent of the substitution effect, and of
the general effect of family planning programs on levels
of contraceptive use, is therefore a complex and difficult
question.  However, though these effects are difficult to
measure with any exactitude, evidence presented in Figure
2 indicates that "the gross contribution of the government to the prevalence rate is substantial at all levels
of the rate" (Nortman, 1982:31).

Some empirical studies have been done to explore the
relationship between contraceptive availability and
levels of use.  Of course, this issue is clouded by the
factor of motivation.  One extreme position is that,
without strong motivation to limit family size, availability of methods will have no effect; conversely, with
sufficient motivation, couples will control their fertil-

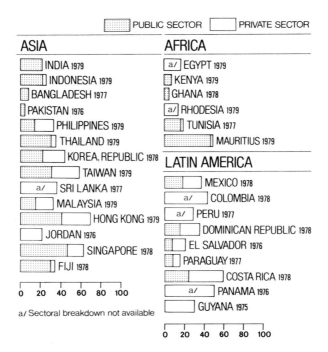

FIGURE 2    Percent of Married Women of Reproductive Age
Using Contraception in Specified Year (countries listed
in order of population size)

Source:    Nortman (1982:29).

ity whether or not methods are readily available.  For
example, much of the fertility decline in the Western
world was accomplished by the use of coitus interruptus,
the condom, and possibly abortion.  Another view is that
there is a considerable demand, largely unexpressed, for
fertility control methods.  The availability of supplies
and services, accompanied by an informational program,
can therefore appreciably accelerate the adoption of
fertility control.  This view is disputed by authors such
as Davis (1967), Driver (1972), and Petersen (1981).
Assessment of the relationship between availability and
use is further complicated by the argument that data will
not answer the question because program administrators
would not go to the expense of establishing facilities if

there were no demand; thus a high correlation between
availability and use does not indicate that use results
from availability.

The data that do exist on trends in availability and
their relationship to use are limited.  Macro data sets
show that the number of service points in national family
planning programs was about 110,000 in 29 countries in
the late 1970s (Nortman and Hofstatter, 1980); although a
comparable figure is not available for the early 1960s,
far fewer service points and fewer national family planning programs existed at that time.  As was noted above,
there was a very large increase in the number of users of
contraceptive methods in developing countries during this
period.  This lends some support to the view that increased availability often leads to increased use.  It
should also be noted that information programs typically
accompany an increase in service outlets, and such programs are thought to legitimize and popularize contraceptive use.

Another approach was to ask knowledgeable persons to
estimate the extent to which various types of contraceptive services were available within 33 developing countries, and then to relate availability to fertility
decline from 1960 to 1973.  The responses indicated a
moderately strong relationship between these two factors.
However, there were deficiencies in the data used, and it
was concluded that "many programs might be much more
effective if the entire range of fertility regulation
methods were generally available in rural, as well as
urban areas, and many service points, at convenient
hours, and at low or no cost" (Mauldin, 1975:33).

Along related lines, a study carried out by the World
Fertility Survey reported average "time of travel to
perceived nearest outlet" for methods of fertility
control as shown in Table 3.  The data are taken from
in-depth pilot studies designed to determine the feasibility of obtaining information on household and community availability of fertility control methods, and
should therefore be regarded as illustrative (Rodriguez,
1977).  Data on perceived time to the nearest outlet for
contraceptive supplies have been collected in a number of
World Fertility Surveys and in prevalence surveys carried
out under the auspices of the Centers for Disease Control
(Morris and Anderson, 1982) and Westinghouse Health
Systems (Lewis and Novak, 1982).  The analysis of those
data reported in Rodriguez (1977) is largely limited to
the relationship between knowledge of the location of a

TABLE 3   Average Travel Time (in minutes) to Nearest
Known Family Planning Outlet by Country and Urban-Rural
Residence

| Country | Median | | Mean | |
|---|---|---|---|---|
| | Urban | Rural | Urban | Rural |
| India | 15 | 30 | 26 | 51 |
| Panama | 15 | 30 | 19 | 31 |
| Turkey | 10 | 30 | 13 | 57 |

Source:   Rodriguez (1977:52, Table 3.9.1).

source of supply for oral contraceptives and their use or
nonuse.  Within urban areas, location of residence does
not affect the perception of time required to travel to a
source of oral contraceptives; within rural areas, perceived travel times do vary, and where they are relatively
high, use is generally low.  Thus, although these data
only weakly support the hypothesis that use increases
with availability in urban areas, there is some support
for the hypothesis in rural areas.

## EMPIRICAL STUDIES OF THE RELATIONSHIP BETWEEN
## FAMILY PLANNING PROGRAMS AND FERTILITY DECLINE

A number of empirical studies have attempted to assess
the relationship between family planning programs and
fertility decline, especially relative to the effects of
socioeconomic variables (see Retherford and Palmore, in
these volumes, for a detailed discussion of this issue).
Of these studies, evaluations of experimental programs
are most important, and will be discussed first.  Other
single-country studies will be considered next, followed
by studies across countries.

### Experimental Programs

There have been many experimental and demonstration programs relating to various aspects of family planning; 96

of these are reviewed by Cuca and Pierce (1977), who classified them as follows:

- 46 were concerned with the type and characteristics of personnel suited for certain functions or the type of remuneration that would elicit the most favorable performance.
- 19 were concerned with the contribution of mass media campaigns to the effectiveness of programs.
- 16 related to the effectiveness of integration of health programs and family planning services.
- 10 were attempts to determine whether intensive campaigns increase the acceptance and practice of family planning.
- 14 sought to measure the impact of various schemes for increasing the availability of contraceptives, mostly community-based distribution (CBD) programs.
- 6 tested the impact of incentives.

Most of these experimental and demonstration programs measured changes in the number of acceptors rather than changes in fertility. A substantial number of these programs were successful in increasing acceptance of family planning, and elements of them were incorporated into national programs. There also have been a sizable number of experimental programs in which the results were inconclusive, and of course, some notable failures.

Among the programs that were successful in reducing fertility are the following:

- The Comilla Organizer Study, in which the total fertility rate was reduced from 8.5 to 6.2 or by 27 percent from 1958-59 to 1966-67.
- The San Gregorio experiment, in which fertility was reduced by 20 percent from 1962 to 1966.
- The Greenland experiment, in which the birth rate decreased from about 45 to 20 between 1967 and 1969, a reduction of 50 percent.
- The Koyang/Kimpo experiment, in which the general fertility rate fell by 38 percent in Koyang and 13 percent in Kimpo over a period of about two and a half years from 1962 to 1964.
- The Cerro de Pasco experiment in which the total fertility rate decreased 18 percent from 8.06 to 6.58 from 1966 to 1970.

Experiments designed to reduce fertility but which failed to do so include the well-known Khanna experiment in India, the Lulliani experiment in Pakistan, and probably the Sweden-Ceylon experiment in what is now Sri Lanka. (In the last case, Cuca and Pierce say that, despite some decrease in the birth rate, there was no evidence that this decline was related to the experimental treatment.) The Gandhigram experiment in India is often cited as a successful intervention program, and it is reported that the crude birth rate declined from 43 in 1959 to 31 in 1971. However, the reports containing those figures are so skimpy that one is not comfortable in accepting the results. Jain obtained and analyzed some additional data, but these were not adequate to resolve the questions nor to warrant publication. Therefore, the results of the Gandhigram Experiment are classified here as indeterminate.

In recent years, there has been much interest in community-based distribution programs. One such program in Bangladesh, its eventual successor, and another program in South Korea are discussed below. The Bangladesh studies were conducted among a very poor and uneducated rural population in Matlab Thana from 1975 to 1981 to test the hypothesis that contraceptive services can reduce fertility (Phillips et al., 1982; Chen et al., 1981). The initial study, known as the Contraceptive Distribution Project (CDP), tested a pill and condom household contraceptive distribution approach; the second study, known as the Family Planning Health Services Project (FPHSP), augmented that strategy with better training of workers, a wider selection of methods, more intensive follow-up and referral services, and ancillary health care.

In the CDP project, nonclinical methods of contraception (oral pills and condoms) were distributed in 153 villages with a population of 135,000, while 80 villages were serviced by the regular government programs and designated as the comparison area. Since village-based government services have not yet been fully implemented, the studies represent a de facto test of the effects of services vis-a-vis no services at all. In all, 154 lady village workers (LVWs), mostly illiterate, elderly, and widowed women, were recruited and instructed in the distribution of oral contraceptives. Each worker was responsible for maintaining lists of women eligible for contraception and for conducting household visits to all of these women to offer six months of pill supplies and

replenish stocks when needed. The project was launched
in October 1975 with minimum worker training in motivation and follow-up, in accordance with the hypothesis
that distribution alone would increase contraceptive use
and reduce fertility.

A baseline survey of eligible women showed that about
33 percent of the respondents were either current users
of contraception or expressed a desire to cease childbearing and an interest in using contraception in the
future. In a survey conducted three months after contraceptive distribution was started, however, only 17
percent of the respondents were using oral pills. Moreover, prevalence of pill use had declined to 9 percent by
the end of the first 18 months of the study. Overall
prevalence was correspondingly low: 18 percent at 3
months and 13 percent at 18 months. Overall prevalence
in comparison area villages remained at 4 percent throughout the study. It is likely that the overall impact of
CDP during its first year ranged between 5 and 17 percent.
CDP had an effect, though modest, on fertility in Matlab
in its first impact year; in the second CDP project year,
the program had no effect (Stinson et al., 1982).

The limitations of CDP led to a reformulation of
contraceptive research in Matlab and the FPHSP. The
overall goal of the FPHSP service system was to shift
from the CDP emphasis on contraceptive technology to an
emphasis on comprehensive contraceptive care, including
frequent and regular visits to all women, whether contracepting or not, providing a wide choice of methods, and
ancillary health services. The initial emphasis was on
comprehensive family planning services rather than
maternal and child health. The most important change was
the addition of the injectable depo-provera to the bat-
tery of methods available in the village. The principal
link established between health and family planning services was a three-tiered referral system for the detection
and treatment of side effects, with FVWs treating minor
side effects and referring more serious problems to sub-
centers for treatment or further referral to a physician.[6]

Introduction of this new system was followed by a
sharp rise in contraceptive prevalence from 10 percent in
October 1977 to 34 percent by the end of 1978, where use
prevalence remains to date. The general fertility rates
in the treatment and control areas were almost identical
at the beginning of these experiments, but differed by 25
percent in 1978. The crude birth rates were 34.7 and
46.9, respectively. This is an impressive result from a

relatively simple, apparently easily replicable program
that was carried out in a high-fertility, low-income,
poorly educated population.  However, because high-quality
management may have played more of a role in the experiment than is apparent, the replicability of this program
cannot be assessed until larger programs similar or
identical in design are carried out.

The Korean Population Policy and Program Evaluation
Study used local canvassers to register "at risk" women
and keep those lists up to date.  These women were visited
at home and offered either a free three-month supply of
oral pills or condoms or a coupon for a free IUD insertion
or tubal ligation.  The canvasser who made the initial
contacts continued to provide information to couples and
operated a resupply depot out of her home.  This service
only provided contraceptives; no integration with other
health or social services was sought.

A baseline survey was taken about a year before the
program began; the program lasted forty months, and a
year after it ended another survey was taken.  Thus there
were two surveys five years apart.  The study was carried
out in the province of Cheju.  Its population of 420,000
had appreciably lower rates of contraceptive use than did
all of Korea at the beginning of the study--21 percent as
compared with 36 percent among women 15 to 44 years of
age--and higher fertility--a total fertility rate of 4.6
as compared with 3.9 for all of Korea.  Five years later,
contraceptive use had more than doubled from 21 to 45
percent, as compared with a substantial but smaller
increase from 36 to 54.5 percent for all of Korea.
Fertility fell slightly more rapidly in Cheju than in all
of Korea--30 percent as compared with 28 percent.  The
changes in fertility were more rapid in the experimental
area than in rural Korea:  there was a decrease of 32
percent in the total fertility rate in South County, of
40 percent in North County, and 29 percent in rural Korea
as a whole (Park et al., 1982).


## Single-Country Studies

Although there are many nonexperimental studies of fertility decline in individual countries, for the most part
these analyses do not attempt to quantify how much of the
decline is attributable to specific independent variables.
Chen and Fawcett (1979), for example, attribute fertility
decline in Singapore to employment opportunities for women

and constraints on the availability of housing, on the one hand, and family planning and governmental disincentives for childbearing on the other. Their analysis, though convincing, is qualitative rather than quantitative.

Similar conclusions were drawn for Malaysia, where Jones (1982) found that, although family planning played a lesser role than socioeconomic factors in the fertility decline, it was nevertheless an important force. Again, however, its effect cannot be quantified. Parallel findings were made for the Philippines (Concepcion, 1982), and for Thailand, where Knodel et al. (1982:30-31) made the following observation:

> The development of an active program corresponds closely with the timing of the fertility decline in rural areas; the vast majority of Thai women report receiving their contraceptive supplies or services through the program; analysis of services statistics indicates that the number of estimated births averted through the program can account for most of the observed decline in fertility, and the presence of a program outlet in a village, and to a lesser extent, in a subdistrict, is generally associated with higher contraceptive use and lower fertility, after controlling for other factors than is the absence of an outlet.

The authors also note that socioeconomic development, at least as conventionally defined, does not seem to account for much of the decline; rather, they emphasize the rapid expansion of mass communication and transportation systems that has considerably reduced the isolation of village life.[7] Similar studies in Taiwan by Freedman et al. (1982) and in the Republic of Korea by Cho and Retherford (1982) assign more importance to socioeconomic factors than do the Philippine and Thai analyses, but also credit the family planning programs with having important effects. One analysis in the Republic of Korea indicated that the national family planning program accounted for about 37 percent of the decline in the birth rate per thousand women aged 15-44 between 1963 and 1973.

Another illustrative example is provided by contrasting fertility decline in Brazil and China. In the former there has been no national population program, only a private family planning program that was restricted to a few states. Carvalho et al. (1982:24) note that "the

occurrence of fertility reduction practically without
family planning programs makes Brazil an important case
for the discussion of the effects of institutional efforts
on fertility." Their analysis is interesting and
provocative:

> Beginning in the second half of the 1960s, there
> appears to have been a very sharp acceleration in the
> falling trend in fertility levels of the Brazilian
> population. . . . This acceleration occurred mainly
> due to increased use of contraception. From an
> economic point of view, there seem to have been two
> principal causes for the acceleration in the decline
> in fertility: one structural--the intensification in
> the process of proletarianization; and the other
> cyclical--the fall in the standard of living among
> large segments of the population.
>     . . . the process of proletarianization increased
> the cost of subsistence for the labor force through
> the substitution of foodstuffs purchased in the market
> for domestically produced foodstuffs, even though this
> did not involve a change in the composition of the
> consumer basket. In addition, other items placed new
> burdens on the family, such as housing and transporta-
> tion. These transformations had the effect of dis-
> couraging large families (Carvalho et al., 1982:48-50).

In China, just the opposite seems to have occurred. Yuan
Fang et al. (1982:50) conclude an analysis of fertility
decline in China by saying they had analyzed the demographic and socioeconomic factors affecting the birth
rate: "None of these factors is conducive to declines in
the birth rate. . . . The determinative factor fostering
a decline in the birth rate in new China has been the
party and government birth planning policy." According
to reports, there has been a decrease in the crude birth
rate of China from about 37 to about 18, which suggests
that, based on today's population, there are 19 million
fewer births per year than there would have been without
the fertility decline. Most of this change can probably
be attributed to China's determined efforts to decrease
rates of growth, including the structure of incentives
and disincentives designed to limit the size of its
population in the twenty-first century.

Finally, a good illustrative case is provided by
Zachariah (1981) in a study of Kerala. Between 1966 and
1978, the crude birth rate in rural Kerala declined from

37 to 26, and in the three districts of Palghat, Ernakulam, and Alleppey, which were studied intensively, from 42 in 1965 to just under 20 in 1979. The most significant decline for the three districts began after 1976, coinciding with the intensified family planning program. A regression analysis that included socioeconomic variables of caste, household expenditures, land owned, years of schooling, roofing material, source of water, toilet facilities, and family planning explained just over one-half of the variance in fertility measured as parity or children ever born. The main conclusion from this analysis was that the principal variables responsible for the decline were education, caste, and family planning.

Zachariah uses three approaches in his effort to determine the relative influence of Kerala's planning program: comparison of Kerala with Sri Lanka, analysis of the characteristics of family planning users and those among whom fertility has declined, and analysis of the relationship between the official family planning output and fertility decline by district and period. Kerala and Sri Lanka are similar in socioeconomic development, and both had relatively weak family planning programs until the mid 1960s. The two areas have very similar prevalence rates for use of conventional contraceptive methods, but differ sharply in their sterilization rates. From 1975 to 1980, Kerala's total marital fertility rate declined by 1.77, and just over half (52 percent) of this decline is attributed to higher sterilization rates. Support for this conclusion is found in the prevalence rates of sterilization in different socioeconomic groups: prevalence rates were higher among those with 1-4 years of schooling; among Ezawa and scheduled caste communities, not among the Naira; and among women from households with lower monthly per capita expenditures. "We attribute this higher sterilization rate among the lower strata of society to the official Family Planning program, especially with its economic incentives" (Zachariah, 1981:59). A third piece of empirical evidence supporting a substantial contribution by the official family planning program to Kerala's fertility decline is the high correlation in particular districts and periods between official family planning output and fertility levels. Zachariah concludes that "the official family planning program has played a significant role in the fertility reduction in Kerala. About 40 percent of the fertility decline can be attributed directly to the official family planning program" (1981:70).

## Intercountry Studies

One of the earliest intercountry studies aimed at
determining the relative impact of socioeconomic and
family planning variables on fertility decline was done
by the World Bank (King, 1974). This study of 19 countries, which also contains a separate analysis of 16
states of India, examines the association between the
output of family planning programs, on the one side, and
socioeconomic and program input variables, on the other.
Socioeconomic variables included were per capita GNP,
female secondary school enrollment, death rate, proportion of population in urban areas, newspaper circulation,
and density of population; program input variables included the number of service points, personnel, physicians, and funds expended or allocated for the family
planning program.

The study found that socioeconomic variables appeared
to have slightly greater explanatory power than program
input variables in accounting for variations in total
user rates. However, service points alone accounted for
62 percent of the total variance. Although the number of
service points was associated with socioeconomic variables, the degree of dependence was not very high. Interaction effects accounted for about a third, or a little
more, of the total variation. The study concludes that
both social change and family planning programs have a
positive role in promoting increased contraceptive
practice and a decline in fertility.

Srikantan (1977) analyzed fertility decline in 20
countries, and also in the states of India. He used a
variety of socioeconomic indicators; two program input
variables--medical personnel per 10,000 population, and
family planning program expenditure per acceptor; and
five program output variables--percent of married women
in the reproductive ages who are acceptors of family
planning, who use program contraceptives, and who use any
contraceptive, acceptors of contraception and sterilization, and cumulative number of acceptors of contraception and sterilization. He concluded that demographic
and socioeconomic variables in the 20-country study were
directly responsible for 32 percent of the fertility
decline, and with indirect effects counted, were responsible for 52 percent. Program input had a small effect
of 9 percent, while the program output effect was 39
percent. He notes that the small program input effect
partly reflects the lack of suitable program input indi-

cators on a comparable basis for the different countries, and suggests that the results may be interpreted to mean that the program had an impact on fertility that was at least as large as the direct effect of the socioeconomic indicators. There was also positive interaction between these two sets of factors in their fertility impact: on the one hand, socioeconomic change facilitated program implementation; on the other, program inputs had a net spillover effect beyond the program that more than offset program substitution.

Mauldin and Berelson (1978) carried out an analysis of fertility decline from 1965 to 1975 in a large number of developing countries. Their analysis focuses on how much of the fertility decline is associated with "modernization," including such socioeconomic variables as health, education, economic status, and urbanization, and how much with population policies and programs (primarily family planning programs) designed to reduce rates of growth. The study found that, although modernization has a substantial, and usually a more important effect on fertility decline, "on balance family planning programs have a significant, independent effect over and above the effect of socioeconomic factors" (Mauldin and Berelson, 1978:124; see Table 4).[8] The authors go on to draw the following conclusions:

> The key finding probably is that the two--social setting and program effort--go together most effectively. The joint analysis appears to "explain" or predict about 83 percent of the total variance in fertility decline. Countries that rank well on socioeconomic variables and also make substantial program effort have on average much more fertility decline than do countries that have one or the other, and far more than those with neither. The policy implications are that, if a country wants to reduce its fertility, it should seek a high degree of modernization (which of course all do, and find costly and difficult) and it should adopt a substantial family planning program; for countries at or near the bottom of the socioeconomic scale, however, the results would probably be slight and the administrative implementation very difficult. In such settings it requires a special kind of determination--as found in India, Indonesia, and China in the early to mid-1970s-- to implement a strong program effort in a deprived setting.

TABLE 4  Crude Birth Rate Declines (in percents), by Social Setting and Program Effort:  94 Developing Countries, 1965-75

| Social Setting | Program Effort | | | | | | | | Total |
|---|---|---|---|---|---|---|---|---|---|
| | Strong (20+) | | Moderate (10-19) | | Weak (0-9) | | No Program | | |
| | Country | Decline | Country | Decline | Country | Decline | Country | Decline | |
| High | Singapore | 40 | Cuba | 40 | Venezuela | 11 | Korea, North | 5 | |
| | Hong Kong | 36 | Chile | 29 | Brazil | 10 | Kuwait | 5 | |
| | Korea, South | 32 | Trinidad and Tobago | 29 | Mexico | 9 | Peru | 2 | |
| | Barbados | 31 | Colombia | 25 | Paraguay | 6 | Lebanon | 2 | |
| | Taiwan | 30 | Panama | 22 | | | Jordan | 1 | |
| | Mauritius | 29 | | | | | Libya | -1 | |
| | Costa Rica | 29 | | | | | | | |
| | Fiji | 22 | | | | | | | |
| | Jamaica | 21 | | | | | | | |
| | Mean | 30 | Mean | 29 | Mean | 9 | Mean | 3 | 19 |
| | Median | 30 | Median | 29 | Median | 9.5 | Median | 2 | 22 |
| Upper Middle | China | 24 | Malaysia | 26 | Egypt | 17 | Mongolia | 9 | |
| | | | Tunisia | 24 | Turkey | 16 | Syria | 4 | |
| | | | Thailand | 23 | Honduras | 7 | Zambia | -2 | |
| | | | Dominican Republic | 21 | Nicaragua | 7 | Congo | -2 | |
| | | | Philippines | 19 | Zaire | 6 | | | |
| | | | Sri Lanka | 18 | Algeria | 4 | | | |
| | | | El Salvador | 13 | Guatemala | 4 | | | |
| | | | Iran | 2 | Morocco | 2 | | | |
| | | | | | Ghana | 2 | | | |
| | | | | | Ecuador | 0 | | | |
| | | | | | Iraq | 0 | | | |
| | Mean | 24 | Mean | 18 | Mean | 6 | Mean | 2 | 10 |
| | Median | 24 | Median | 20 | Median | 4 | Median | 1 | 7 |

Lower
Middle

| | Vietnam, North | 23 | India | 16 | Papua–New Guinea | 5 | Angola | 4 |
|---|---|---|---|---|---|---|---|---|
| | | | Indonesia | 13 | Pakistan | 1 | Cameroon | 3 |
| | | | | | Bolivia | 1 | Burma | 3 |
| | | | | | Nigeria | 1 | Yemen, P.D.R. | 3 |
| | | | | | Kenya | 0 | Mozambique | 2 |
| | | | | | Liberia | 0 | Kampuchea | 2 |
| | | | | | Haiti | 0 | Ivory Coast | 1 |
| | | | | | Uganda | −4 | Senegal | 0 |
| | | | | | | | Saudi Arabia | 0 |
| | | | | | | | Vietnam, South | 0 |
| | | | | | | | Madagascar | 0 |
| | | | | | | | Lesotho | −4 |
| | Mean | 23 | Mean | 14 | Mean | 1 | Mean | 1 |
| | Median | 23 | Median | 14.5 | Median | 0.5 | Median | 1.5 |

Low

| | Tanzania | 5 | Laos | 5 |
|---|---|---|---|---|
| | Dahomey | 3 | Central African Rep. | 5 |
| | Bangladesh | 2 | Malawi | 5 |
| | Sudan | 0 | Bhutan | 3 |
| | Nepal | −1 | Ethiopia | 2 |
| | Mali | −1 | Guinea | 2 |
| | Afghanistan | −2 | Chad | 2 |
| | | | Togo | 2 |
| | | | Upper Volta | 1 |
| | | | Yemen | 1 |
| | | | Niger | 1 |
| | | | Burundi | 1 |
| | | | Sierra Leone | 0 |
| | | | Mauritania | 0 |
| | | | Rwanda | 0 |
| | | | Somalia | 0 |
| | Mean | 1 | Mean | 2 |
| | Median | 0 | Median | 1.5 |

| | | | | |
|---|---|---|---|---|
| Mean | 29 | 21 | 4 | 2 |
| Median | 29 | 22 | 2 | 3 |

Source:  Mauldin and Berelson (1978:110).  Program effort scores run from 0 to 30 on their scale.

Another intercountry study (Faruqee, 1979) uses factor
analysis as the principal analytical tool, concentrating
on fertility decline from 1970 to 1975 in 62 developing
countries. This study uses 12 socioeconomic and 3 family
planning variables (number of years a government family
planning program has been in operation, family planning
personnel per million females aged 15-44, and number of
family planning facilities per million females 15-44).
The factors in this type of analysis represent different
variables: factor 1 represents the level of development,
including such variables as percent of population living
in urban areas, per capita GNP, percentage of gross
national product from the primary sector, population per
doctor, life expectancy, and the crude death rate; factor
2 is an index of government expenditures (total, for
health, education, and government consumption); factor 3
is called the family planning input dimension, and
includes the three variables listed above; and factor 4
represents the actual and potential rate of growth of an
economy. In the results of this analysis, factor 1 is
associated with 30 percent of the variance in the crude
birth rate decline, factor 2 with an additional 17
percent, factor 3 with an additional 17 percent, and
factor 4 with an additional 11 percent. The four factors
together are associated with or "explain" 75 percent of
fertility decline.

"Factor analysis does not treat any variable as a
dependent variable. Thus, the relationship of a particular variable with the emerging factors is somewhat
affected by inclusion of that variable in the same rotated
matrices," Faruqee (1979:30) argues. Therefore, he also
used multiple regression in his analysis, with the four
factors being treated as independent variables. A much
smaller proportion of the variance in the crude birth
rate decline is explained in this manner--an $R^2$ of only
.28 using all four factors plus the crude birth rate in
1970. The $R^2$ with factor 1 only is .14, and with factor
3 (family planning input) .21. Thus, economic development "explains" more of the variance in crude birth rate
decline than does any other factor, and family planning
inputs explain about half as much. The author concludes
that his analysis "confirms the significant role of
family planning, but development clearly emerges as the
more important of the two in influencing fertility
decline" (Faruqee, 1979:38). It should also be noted
that, if socioeconomic variables such as literacy, school
enrollment, infant mortality, and composition of the

labor force (e.g., percent in agriculture or nonagricul-
ture) had been included in Faruqee's analysis, the variance in crude birth rate decline that is associated with
socioeconomic variables probably would have been increased
significantly.

## CONCLUSION

Family planning programs vary in coverage, intensity, and
quality, and there have been few systematic efforts to
measure program inputs.  This is an area of research
offering significant potential rewards.  Many of the
problems and issues raised in this paper are not likely
to be resolved to the satisfaction of all analysts;
however, efforts of the United Nations, of the International Union for the Scientific Study of Population,
and of individual scholars are promising.  The consensus
of most analysts appears to be that, though precise
quantitative credit cannot be allocated among socioeconomic factors, institutional factors, and policies and
programs, there is considerable empirical evidence that
large-scale family planning programs, when well managed,
have a substantial effect on fertility independent of the
influence of socioeconomic factors.

## NOTES

1. At the same time, an upsurge of serious pronatalist
   policies in Eastern Europe and continued pronatalist
   policies of lesser intensity characterize some
   developed countries.
2. Data are available for 13 countries (Mauldin, 1981);
   although there is considerable variation among these
   countries, changes in marriage patterns account for
   one-third or more of changes in crude birth rates for
   7 of the 13, and for 20 percent or more in 4 other
   countries.
3. Although trend data are not available for most
   countries with national programs, prevalence rates are
   available for a relatively recent year, e.g., 1975 or
   later (Larson, 1981).
4. Two general patterns have been observed.  In such
   countries as Korea, Taiwan, Hong Kong, Costa Rica, and
   Mexico, the public sector grew quickly in relation to
   the private sector at first, and then more slowly once

prevalence rates became relatively high. In India, Indonesia, Thailand, Fiji, and Mauritius, the public sector has remained predominant even with increased prevalence rates.

5. The reverse also happens, namely, a program user decides to use a private or commercial source because of convenience or anonymity, to avoid travel or waiting time, etc.

6. In mid-1979, development of maternal and child health services lapsed because of the departure of the principal investigator, a physician, from the project. For this reason, the FPHSP is now more a family planning project than an integrated health services scheme.

7. They also believe the pace of fertility decline has been facilitated by certain aspects of the Thai cultural context, in particular the Buddhist outlook on life and the position of women in Thai society.

8. Hernandez (1981) argues that the effect of family planning programs is considerably less than Mauldin and Berelson estimate, based on his regression analyses. His analysis was restricted, however, to multiple regression, and did not deal with exploratory data analysis, cross classification analysis, etc., as did that of Mauldin and Berelson.

## BIBLIOGRAPHY

Bureau of the Census (1979) Colombia. Country Demographic Profiles. ISP-DP-20. Washington, D.C.: U.S. Department of Commerce.

Carvalho, J. A. M., P. T. A. Paiva, and D. Sawyer (1982) The recent sharp drop in fertility in Brazil: Economic boom, social inequality and baby bust. In W. P. Mauldin, ed., Fertility Decline in Developing Countries: Case Studies, forthcoming.

Chandrasekaran, C., and A. I. Hermalin (1975) Measuring the Effect of Family Planning Programs on Fertility. Liege: Ordina Editions.

Chen, L. C., J. Chakraborty, A. M. Sardar, and M. D. Yunus (1981) Estimating and partitioning the mortality impact of several modern medical technologies in basic health services. Pp. 113-140 in International Population Conference, Manila, 1981, Vol. 2. Leige: International Union for the Scientific Study of Population.

Chen, P. S. J., and J. T. Fawcett (1979)  Public Policy
    and Population Change in Singapore.  New York:
    Population Council.
Cho, L. J., and R. D. Retherford (1973)  Comparative
    analysis of recent fertility trends in East Asia.
    International Population Conference, Liege, Vol. 2.
    Liege:  International Union for the Scientific Study
    of Population.
Cho, L. J., and R. D. Retherford (1982)  Fertility
    transition in the Republic of Korea.  In W. P.
    Mauldin, ed., Fertility Decline in Developing
    Countries: Case Studies, forthcoming.
Colombia, Departamento Administrativo Nacional de
    Estadistica (1977)  Encuesta Nacional de Fecundidad,
    Colombia, 1976, Resultados Generales.  Bogota.
Concepcion, M. B. (1982)  Changing fertility in the
    Philippines:  When, how, why.  In W. P. Mauldin, ed.,
    Fertility Decline in Developing Countries: Case
    Studies, forthcoming.
Cuca, R., and C. S. Pierce (1977)  Experiments in Family
    Planning:  Lessons from the Developing World.
    Baltimore, Md.:  The Johns Hopkins University Press.
Davis, K. (1967)  Population policy:  Will current
    programs succeed?  Science 158.
Diaz-Briquets, S. (1980)  Memo of 19 November, 1980 from
    Diaz-Briquets of Population Reference Bureau,
    Washington, D.C. to John Chao of USAID.
Driver, E. (1972)  Social ideology, social organization,
    and family planning:  A world view.  In E. Driver,
    ed., Essays on Population Policy.  Lexington, Mass.:
    Heath.
Fang, Y., C. Fenghuan, and Z. Lizhong (1982)  A
    preliminary analysis of birth planning and birth rate
    reduction in new China.  In W. P. Mauldin, ed.,
    Fertility Decline in Developing Countries:  Case
    Studies, forthcoming.
Faruqee, R. (1979)  Sources of Fertility Decline:  Factor
    Analysis of Inter-Country Data.  World Bank Staff
    Working Paper No. 318.  Washington, D.C.:  World Bank.
Forrest, J. D., and J. A. Ross (1978)  Fertility effects
    of family planning programs:  A methodological
    review.  Social Biology 25:145-163.
Freedman, R., A. Hermalin, K. K. C. Liu, and T. H. Sun
    (1982)  The role of socioeconomic development and the
    family planning program in Taiwan's fertility
    decline.  In W. P. Mauldin, ed., Fertility Decline in
    Developing Countries: Case Studies, forthcoming.

Gorosh, M. and D. Wolfers (1979)  Standard couple-years
    of protection.  Pp. 34-47 in The Methodology of
    Measuring the Impact of Family Planning Programmes on
    Fertility, Manual IX.  ST/ESA/SER. A/66.  New York:
    United Nations.
Hernandez, D. J.  (1981)  A note on measuring the
    independent impact of family planning programs on
    fertility declines.  Demography 18:627-634.
Jones, G. W.  (1982)  Fertility decline in peninsula
    Malaysia.  In W. P. Mauldin, ed., Fertility Decline in
    Developing Countries: Case Studies, forthcoming.
Kanagaratnam, D.  (1978)  Approaches to the Population
    Problem and Accomplishments of Population Activity:
    An Overview.  Presentation to the Population and
    Development Course of the Economic Development
    Institute, World Bank, Washington, D.C.
Keeny, S. M.  (1972)  East Asia review, 1971.  Studies in
    Family Planning 3:102.
King, T., coordinating author (1974)  Population Policies
    and Economic Development.  Baltimore, Md.:  The Johns
    Hopkins University Press.
Kitagawa, E. M.  (1955)  Components of a difference
    between two rates.  Journal of the American
    Statistical Association 50:1168-1194.
Knodel, J.  (1979)  From natural fertility to family
    limitation:  The onset of fertility transition in a
    sample of German villages.  Demography 6:493-521.
Knodel, J., N. Debavalya, and K. Peerasit (1982)
    Thailand's continuing fertility decline.  In W. P.
    Mauldin, ed., Fertility Decline in Developing
    Countries: Case Studies, forthcoming.
Larson, A.  (1981)  Patterns of Contraceptive Use Around
    the World.  Washington, D.C.:  Population Reference
    Bureau.
Lewis, G. L., and J. A. Novak (1982)  An approach to the
    measurement of availability of family planning
    services.  Pp. 241-278 in A. I. Hermalin and B.
    Entwisle eds., The Role of Surveys in the Analysis of
    Family Planning Programs.  Liege:  Ordina Editions.
Marshall, J. F.  (1977)  Acceptability of fertility
    regulating methods:  Designing technology to fit
    people.  Preventive Medicine 6:65.
Mauldin, W. P.  (1975)  Assessment of national family
    planning programs in developing countries.  Studies in
    Family Planning 6:30-36.
Mauldin, W. P.  (1981)  The determinants of fertility
    decline in LDCs:  An overview of the available

empirical evidence. In <u>International Population Conference, Manila, 1981</u>. Liege: International Union for the Scientific Study of Population.

Mauldin, W. P., and B. Berelson (1978)  Conditions of fertility decline in developing countries, 1965-75. <u>Studies in Family Planning</u> 89-148.

Morris, L., and J. E. Anderson (1982)  The use of contraceptive prevalence survey data to evaluate family planning program service statistics.  Pp. 149-170 in A. I. Hermalin and B. Entwisle, eds., <u>The Role of Surveys in the Analysis of Family Planning Programs</u>. Liege:  Ordina Editions.

Nortman, D. L. (1982)  Empirical patterns of contraceptive use:  A review of the nature and sources of data and recent findings.  Pp. 25-49 in A. I. Hermalin and B. Entwisle, eds., <u>The Role of Surveys in the Analysis of Family Planning Programs</u>. Liege: Ordina Editions.

Nortman, D. L., and E. Hofstatter (1980)  <u>Population and Family Planning Programs:  A Compendium of Data through 1978</u>, 10th ed.  New York: Population Council.

Park, C. B., J. A. Palmore, L.-J. Cho, and J.-Y. Park (1982)  The Korean Experience.  Paper prepared for the annual meeting of the Population Association of America, San Diego, Calif.

Petersen, W. (1981)  American efforts to reduce the fertility of less developed countries.  In N. Eberstadt, ed., <u>Fertility Decline in the Less Developed Countries</u>. New York:  Praeger Publishers.

Phillips, J. F., W. S. Stinson, S. Bhatia, M. Rahman, and J. Chakraborty (1982)  The demographic impact of the family planning-health services project in Matlab, Bangladesh.  <u>Studies in Family Planning</u> 13:131-140.

Population Information Program (1981)  Contraceptive prevalence surveys:  A new source of family planning data.  <u>Population Reports</u>, Series M, Number 5. Baltimore, Md.:  The Johns Hopkins University.

Potter, R. G. (1969)  Estimating births averted in a family planning program.  Pp. 413-434 in S. J. Behrman et al., eds., <u>Fertility and Family Planning:  A World View</u>.  Ann Arbor, Mich.:  University of Michigan.

Potter, R. G. (1977)  Use of models in evaluating changing effects of contraceptive behavior.  Pp. 273-284 in <u>International Population Conference, Mexico City</u>, Vol. 1.  Liege:  International Union for the Scientific Study of Population.

Potter, R. G. (1979) Analysis of reproductive process. Pp. 76-96 in The Methodology of Measuring the Impact of Family Planning Programmes on Fertility, Manual IX. ST/ESA/SER/. A/66. New York: United Nations.

Rodriguez, G. (1977) Assessing the Availability of Fertility Regulation Methods: Report on a Methodological Study. WFS Scientific Reports No. 1. London: World Fertility Survey.

Ross, J. A., and J. D. Forrest (1978) The demographic assessment of family planning programs: A bibliographic essay. Population Index 44(1).

Ross, J. A., and D. Smith (1970) Korea: Trends in Four National KAP Surveys, 1964-1967. Population and Family Planning in the Republic of Korea 1:225-230. Seoul: Ministry of Health and Social Affairs, Republic of Korea.

Shryock, H. S., and J. S. Siegel (1971) The Methods and Materials of Demography, Vol. 2. Bureau of the Census. Washington, D.C.: U.S. Department of Commerce.

Srikantan, K. S. (1977) The Family Planning Program in the Socio-Economic Context. New York: Population Council.

Stinson, W. S., J. F. Phillips, M. Rahman, and J. Chakraborty (1982) The demographic impact of the contraceptive distribution project in Matlab, Bangladesh. Studies in Family Planning 13:141-158.

Taiwan Provincial Institute of Family Planning (1980) Annual Report, July 1979-June 1980. Taipei.

United Nations (1978) The Methodology of Measuring the Impact of Family Planning Programmes on Fertility: Problems and Issues. ST/ESA/Ser.A/61. New York: United Nations.

United Nations (1979) The Methodology of Measuring the Impact of Family Planning Programmes on Fertility, Manual IX. ST/ESA/Ser.A/66. New York: United Nations.

Zachariah, K. C. (1981) Anomaly of the Fertility Decline in Kerala: Social Change, Agrarian Reform, or the Family Planning Programs? Population and Human Resources Division, Discussion Paper No. 81-17. Washington, D.C: World Bank.

Chapter 8

# Diffusion Processes Affecting Fertility Regulation

ROBERT D. RETHERFORD and JAMES A. PALMORE*

The timing and speed of fertility transition depend
primarily on two factors:  economic and social development (including mortality decline), which, through a
variety of mechanisms, reduces the number of births that
couples want; and diffusion of birth control, which to
some extent proceeds independently of development.
Development is more fundamental than diffusion in
explaining fertility transition, in the following sense:
an advanced state of development is a sufficient condition for fertility decline, whereas the spread of birth
control knowledge and services is not (as, for example,
when desired fertility exceeds natural fertility).  Nevertheless, evidence presented in this paper suggests that
the independent effects of diffusion can be significant.
Assessing the magnitude of these effects is of considerable policy interest, since programs aimed at diffusion
of birth control have been and continue to be the principal instrument of population policy in countries
wishing to limit population growth.
  This paper first explores the general concept of diffusion.  It then suggests how models of diffusion and
fertility transition can be integrated to provide a
theoretical framework for discussions of the diffusion
process.  Next, it examines the relationship between
diffusion and social integration, as well as the various
networks of communication through which diffusion takes
place.  This is followed by a discussion of the magnitude
and significance of the effects of diffusion on fertility

*We are grateful to John Knodel, Peter Smith, George
Beal, and the reviewers for helpful comments and
suggestions.

295

transition. Finally, some research issues are raised,
along with some policy implications of the discussion.


THE CONCEPT OF DIFFUSION

Diffusion models have been used to analyze the spread of
a wide range of innovations, from new farming methods to
new consumer products to family planning programs. The
principal features of such models have been reviewed by
Rogers (1962, 1973), Rogers and Shoemaker (1971), and
Brown (1981). The following discussion draws especially
on Brown's review.

Diffusion is the process by which innovations spread
from one locale, social group, or individual to another.
In diffusion models, the term innovation is used broadly
to refer to a product, technique, practice, or idea that
is intrinsically new (an invention), or new only to a
particular setting, as is the case with some forms of
birth control whose practice dates back to ancient times
(Himes, 1936). Innovations may be classified as discontinuous, involving the introduction of something dramatically new, or continuous, involving modification of
something that already exists. At the start of marital
fertility transition, birth control is best viewed as a
discontinuous innovation for the vast majority of the
population; subsequently, as contraceptive methods and
services improve, it may be viewed as a continuous innovation. As a further distinction, consumer innovations
are those adopted by individuals or households; technological or producer innovations are those adopted by
entrepreneurs or firms; and institutional innovations are
those adopted by governments or other nonprofit organizations or agencies. Although birth control innovations
encompass all three types, in recent decades some of the
most important have been institutional innovations related
to the establishment of family planning programs.

Many diffusion studies distinguish factors related to
the effective flow of information, employing such concepts
as interpersonal networks, two-step flows (opinion leaders
and followers), and multi-step flows. In the case of
birth control diffusion, it is helpful to conceptualize
such flows hierarchically: one level, for example, consists of local interpersonal networks; a second level is
the network of family planning and related services within
each country; a third level consists of international
agencies, private organizations operating at the inter-

national level, and counterpart agencies and officials in national governments. Not only information, but also influence and resources flow through these networks.

Also relevant to information flow is resistance or barriers to diffusion. Analysis of these barriers addresses variations in individual propensity to adopt innovations (or innovativeness) and congruence between a particular innovation and the social, economic, and psychological characteristics of the potential adopter. Also emphasized in this connection have been population factors (e.g., density of emitters and potential receptors), distance factors (both geographic and social),[1] and the role of social norms.[2] The demographic literature, discussed in more detail below, has emphasized barriers associated with such cultural factors as language, ethnicity, and religion.

Diffusion is sometimes studied according to certain key attributes of the innovation itself that influence its rate of adoption. In Rogers and Shoemaker's (1971: 138ff.) paradigm, the first of these is relative advantage, the degree to which the innovation is perceived to be better, or perhaps less costly, than its alternatives or predecessors, if any. This factor helps explain why, in contemporary less developed countries, modern contraceptive methods such as the pill have been adopted much more quickly than coitus interruptus, which historically was very important in Europe, but has the considerable relative disadvantage of high psychic costs. A second attribute is compatibility with existing values, norms, technology, and practices, mentioned above for values and norms in connection with barriers to diffusion. A third is complexity. Some complex birth control methods, such as sophisticated forms of the rhythm method requiring careful date keeping, temperature recording, and observation of cervical mucous, have been slow to spread. A fourth attribute is trialability, the degree to which an innovation may be tried on a limited basis. This factor helps explain why sterilization, for example, usually does not become popular until after simple reversible methods such as the pill have become widely accepted. A fifth attribute is the observability of the innovation and its results. One of the major effects of contemporary family planning programs is to increase greatly the observability of birth control innovations, thereby speeding up the diffusion process. Without such programs, birth control has very low observability, partly because it is practiced in the privacy of the home, and partly

because it is usually a somewhat taboo subject of conversation, especially when normative barriers to adoption
are present.

Characteristics specifically affecting the diffusion
of contraceptive innovations have been listed by Freedman
and Berelson (1976:14). These include medical safety,
clinical effectiveness, reversibility, simplicity and ease
of use, absence of side effects, one-time administration
for long-lasting effect, protection of privacy, no effect
on libido and sexual pleasure, cultural (especially religious) acceptability, simplicity of supply lines, ease of
access to supplies, and low cost. Freedman (1979:74) has
argued further that attractive methods help legitimize
the idea of family limitation.

Analyses of lags in adoption usually distinguish several major stages of diffusion. These vary in number,
depending on the particular study, but they usually
include an awareness stage; a knowledge-gathering and
evaluation stage, leading to a decision whether to try
the innovation; a trial stage, involving experimentation
with the innovation to determine its utility; and a
confirmation stage, involving either continuation or
discontinuation, depending on whether the utility of the
innovation is confirmed (see, e.g., Rogers, 1962, 1973;
Rogers and Shoemaker, 1971). Some innovations, such as
sterilization, have zero trialability, in which case the
last two stages are combined.

The rate of adoption is usually conceptualized and
measured as the number or percentage who adopt within a
given time span. Measures of adoption are usually based
on either new adopters or contraceptive prevalence (see,
for example, Mauldin, 1975); a less frequently used
alternative when more direct data are not available is
Coale and Trussell's (1974, 1978) demographic index of
marital fertility control (used, for example, by van de
Walle and Knodel, 1980). Any of several measures of
marital fertility, or, more properly, departures of
marital fertility from the natural level, may also be
used. These are indirect indicators of contraception; on
the other hand, fertility is the ultimate variable of
interest. In the case of adoption stages, one may also
examine changes in the percentage who know about, or have
ever used, a particular method within a given time span.

Adoption (or awareness, or trial) curves, with the
percentage who have adopted (or know about, or have ever
tried) graphed against time, usually resemble a logistic,
or an elongated S-shaped curve. Initially, only a small

proportion use the innovation. The rate of use gradually
accelerates, then slows down again as saturation is
approached. Many individuals are cautious and wait for
the innovation to be perfected or demonstrated as effective before trying it, preferring to let others take the
initial risks. As van de Walle and Knodel (1980:29) have
noted, once some couples in a community adopt family
limitation, it is increasingly easy for other couples to
follow suit.

Diffusion situations may also be classified according
to whether propagators with an interest in diffusion are
present or absent. Today's propagators of birth control,
as mentioned earlier, include a broad mix of international
agencies, government family planning programs, private
foundations, private family planning associations, and
commercial enterprises that market birth control products.
Evidence presented below suggests that diffusion of birth
control information and services usually begins sooner
and proceeds more rapidly when propagators are present
than when they are not. Purposive, organized programs
for diffusing birth control include not only family planning programs but also legislation (e.g., China's one-
child family law) and incentive programs for limiting
family size.

Purposive diffusion has been conceptualized as
involving two essential steps: first, the establishment
of diffusion agencies (e.g., family planning clinics),
the location of which influences the spatial pattern of
adoption; and second, the formulation and implementation
of a strategy to induce adoption in the service area.
Diffusion strategies include such aspects as infrastructure, price, promotional communications, and market
selection and segmentation (see, e.g., Roberto, 1975).
Diffusion agencies can change norms as well as work
around them, or, in some cases, use them as positive
incentives or reinforcements. This is especially true
for government family planning programs: government
endorsement of family planning can have a legitimizing
effect that often seems to substantially reduce normative
barriers against birth control, resulting in an earlier
onset and a faster rate of adoption.

Analysis of lags between invention and adoption has
emphasized not only stages of adoption, but also the
notion of complementarities, the idea that an innovation
may not be practical until complementary products, technologies, practices, or ideas appear or are perfected.
If the innovation in question is a marketable product or

service, then analysis of profitability, which is closely
related to the Rogers and Shoemaker concept of relative
advantage, mentioned above, is important because it provides a summary indicator of whether an innovation will
be adopted. However, profitability is not so relevant in
the case of family planning (except in private-sector
marketing of contraceptives) because such programs are
not interested in commercial profit, though they are
usually established and located with some concern for the
balance of costs and potential benefits.[3]

Implicit in the notions of complementarities, profitability, and cost-benefit analysis is the idea that certain preconditions related to level of economic and social
development must exist if there is to be a demand for the
innovation. Thus, although level of development alone
does not determine the timing and rate of diffusion (this
would be an unwarranted reductionist view that simply does
not fit the facts), it does place important constraints
on that process.

## THE INTEGRATION OF DIFFUSION
## AND FERTILITY TRANSITION MODELS

Given the substantial literature on diffusion, including
numerous applications to the spread of birth control,[4]
it is astonishing that fertility transition models have
slighted the role of diffusion processes. Developments
in the two areas have proceeded rather independently, perhaps because of disciplinary isolation: diffusion models
have been the province mainly of geographers, communication specialists, and rural sociologists, whereas fertility transition models have been the province mainly of
demographers, nonrural sociologists, and economists.
There is therefore a clear need to integrate these two
traditions.

The time seems ripe for such an integration. As
economists have become more interested in fertility
transition models, these models have relied increasingly
on demand concepts involving the utilities and costs of
alternative family sizes. This emphasis is reflected in
the framework for these volumes (see Easterlin, 1975).
Diffusion models have similarly relied increasingly on
profitability, cost-benefit, and utility-cost concepts to
explain rates of adoption. Another pertinent development
is that economic models increasingly consider information
costs, a factor that is, of course, essential to any
realistic modeling of diffusion processes.

It would seem, then, that transition and diffusion models can be integrated through the basic utility-cost concepts common to both. A start in this direction is provided by a highly simplified model of sudden and rapid fertility decline that emphasizes both developmental and diffusion processes, proposed recently by Retherford (1979, 1980). The basic idea, following Easterlin (1975, 1978), is that demanded family size is a function of the costs and utilities of achieving each alternative size.[5] These are specified by family-size utility and cost functions, with demanded family size being the number of children that maximizes net utility, computed as the difference between these two functions. The cost of achieving a given family size includes the cost of birth control, which is itself a significant determinant of demand and acts to increase it, especially in pretransition situations where birth control costs are high. Retherford's model defines demanded family size in conformance with general economics usage to include consideration of birth control costs; therefore, demanded family size is not the same as desired or wanted family size.

For simplicity and convenience, the model conceptualizes all utilities and costs in psychic equivalents so that all costs of birth control, whether monetary or psychic, can be considered together as a single variable. Economists usually restrict the concept of cost to what is objectively measurable, such as money and time costs, and denote psychic costs as disutility; however, psychic costs are central to birth control diffusion processes, and a more flexible concept of costs is therefore useful in studying this area of human behavior. Moreover, whether psychic costs are conceptualized as costs or disutility is irrelevant to the problem of how to measure them.

In the model, two fundamental changes cause populations to approach the threshold of marital fertility control. One of these is mortality decline, which increases the number of surviving children (the number that would occur in the absence of deliberate birth control).[6] The other is decline in the production utility of children (Leibenstein, 1957), which reduces desired family size; this decline is in turn tied to a number of facets of economic and social development, especially the rise of mass education (see Caldwell, in these volumes).[7]

For a period of time, as the threshold of marital fertility control is approached, desired family size (which does not take birth control costs fully into account and hence is less than demanded family size) is lower than natural family size, yet no birth control is practiced. This condition of latent receptivity to birth control seems to be observed in many contemporary developing countries just before fertility transition begins, when desired family size is commonly about four and natural family size between five and six. In this situation, which may persist for some time, the high cost of birth control raises effective demand to the natural family size.

Under the most common circumstances, the model's threshold condition for adoption of birth control is that the birth control cost of preventing the last naturally occurring child must fall below the net cost (without birth control costs taken into account) of acquiring that child. If the cost of prevention exceeds the net cost of acquisition, birth control is not practiced. In the model, as development proceeds, the cost of prevention falls and the net cost of acquisition rises.

The costs of birth control for the typical individual or couple are conceptualized as having a fixed and a variable component. The former consists mainly of normative costs (the psychic costs of violating social norms against the use of birth control) and initial resistance costs (psychic costs associated with ignorance and fear of birth control). The variable component consists mainly of the money, time, inconvenience, and health risk costs of birth control that accumulate the more one restricts family size. If withdrawal or abstinence is used, both the fixed and variable components consist mainly of psychic costs, which are by no means inconsequential if these methods are to be used effectively. Thus the graph of birth control costs by family size declines comparatively gradually between zero and the natural family size; it then drops suddenly and steeply to zero at the natural family size by an amount equal to the fixed cost of birth control, since no birth control at all is necessary to achieve the natural family size. Before marital fertility transition begins, the fixed cost of birth control is very high. (The variable cost of birth control can also be quite high, as discussed in Schearer's article in these volumes.)

A shift is precipitated when the higher social strata of the population attain the threshold condition and adopt birth control. If a high degree of social integration prevails, the model posits that the pace-setting behavior of the higher social strata quickly stimulates collapse of the normative and initial resistance costs of birth control throughout the population.[8] The more socially integrated the population is, the more quickly this process occurs. By social integration is meant good communication and shared values, norms, and institutions, usually associated with such characteristics as geographic compactness; common political authority; and cultural homogeneity in such areas as language, ethnicity, and religion (Retherford, 1979, 1980; see also Rogers and Shoemaker, 1971, who distinguish between homophilous and heterophilous populations).

When the normative and initial resistance costs of birth control collapse, the fixed cost of birth control, which is initially very high, falls suddenly and dramatically. As a result, a large proportion of the remaining population attains the threshold condition shortly after the dominant stratum does, despite considerable variability in couple perceptions of the various costs and utilities of children. Thus the stage is set for rapid diffusion of birth control innovation, and all the diffusion mechanisms mentioned above come into play. In a well-integrated society, the result is sudden and rapid fertility decline; in less-integrated populations, fertility decline may be more gradual.

The speed of birth control diffusion is also generally faster the later in history that fertility transition begins (Kirk, 1971). There are several reasons for this. First, the later the start, the earlier mortality falls relative to the general level of development, due largely to the importation of advanced health technology, itself a diffusion process of great demographic significance (Davis, 1956; Preston, 1975). Hence increases in natural family size play an increasingly important role, compared with other aspects of economic and social development, in attainment of the threshold condition for adoption of birth control. Natural family size at the start of transition tends to be higher the later in history transition begins, thus raising the potential distance that family size can fall in a short time.

A second reason why diffusion is faster the later in history it begins is that some aspects of economic and social development appear to proceed faster the later they get underway, again because of the increased potential for rapid importation of technology and know-how from more industrialized nations. This works in two ways. First, and rather obviously, all the development-related determinants of fertility decline evolve more

rapidly. Second, and less obviously, the normative and
initial resistance costs of birth control have less time
to attenuate as the threshold of fertility transition is
approached ever more rapidly; the less attenuated the
fixed cost of birth control is when the threshold is
reached, the larger it is, and the farther it can potentially fall when it finally collapses.

The attenuation of normative birth control costs is an
important aspect of cultural lag. Although norms tend to
be rooted in the conditions of everyday life, to some
extent they have a life of their own, especially if they
become institutionalized in, for example, church doctrine
or civil law. Pronatalist and anti-birth control norms
are rooted in such conditions as high mortality and the
high production and security utility of children. When
these underlying conditions change, it takes time for the
norms to adjust (Roman Catholic doctrine on birth control
and the family is a case in point). Knowledge, too, tends
to be rooted in the conditions of everyday life. When
birth control is not needed, knowledge of methods is not
widespread, and erroneous ideas abound. Again, when
underlying conditions change, it takes time for knowledge
and ideas to catch up. Thus attenuation of initial
resistance costs associated with ignorance of birth
control is also an aspect of cultural lag. Generally
speaking, the later in history transition begins, the
faster underlying conditions change, the greater cultural
lag becomes, and the larger and more rapid the "catch-up"
is once diffusion of knowledge and practice of birth
control finally start.

A third reason why diffusion proceeds more rapidly the
later in history fertility transition begins relates to
the appearance of cheaper and more effective contraceptives and medically safe sterilization and abortion,
increasingly propagated through government family planning
programs. The later transition begins, the more likely a
government is to quickly implement or greatly expand a
family planning program to meet the surge in demand for
cheap and effective birth control services; thus the
money, time, inconvenience, and health risk costs of
birth control are driven down at the same time that the
normative and initial resistance costs fall. (The discussion below of international population assistance is
relevant in this connection.) The overall drop in birth
control costs is then especially great, and diffusion
especially rapid. Moreover, if government and private
agencies inaugurate family planning programs before fer-

tility transition begins in the mass of the population,
the consequent reduction in birth control costs (particularly in normative and initial resistance costs because
of government endorsement and legitimation) may precipi-
tate adoption of birth control and fertility decline much
sooner than would otherwise be the case.  Thus diffusion
processes may advance the timing of fertility transition
as well as speed it up once it starts.

Finally, the later in history that transition begins,
the more advanced the means of communication, implying
that a high degree of social integration characterizes
larger population aggregates than before.  Therefore,
rapid diffusion of birth control innovation and the
related phenomenon of sudden and rapid fertility decline
can be expected in these larger aggregates.

Once transition begins and birth control starts to
spread rapidly, norms favoring large families weaken;
couples are more likely than before to perceive advantages
of fewer children (another aspect of cultural lag), and
thus to reduce family-size desires.  Thus, rapid diffusion
of birth control and rapid fertility decline often precede
rather than follow declines in desired family size (as,
for example, in Taiwan and Thailand; see Freedman and
Berelson, 1976; Sun et al., 1978; Knodel and Debavalya,
1978; and Freedman, 1978:381).  Actual and wanted family
size fall almost concurrently, so that the proportion of
fertility reported as unwanted does not necessarily
change much, at least for a while (Westoff, 1978).

The starting or threshold date of marital fertility
transition is usually fairly well defined.  However, it
is clear from the model just described (which should be
viewed as a set of plausible hypotheses, not a proven set
of propositions) that the threshold of marital fertility
decline may not be so easily defined according to associated levels of economic and social indicators.  The model
suggests that the threshold date of marital fertility
decline is a complex function of such variables as mortality level; economic and social development factors
relating to utility of children to parents; and economic,
social, cultural, geographic, and political factors
influencing the rate of diffusion of birth control.
Nothing in the model suggests that there is a unique
combination of these factors that determines the onset of
marital fertility transition; thus the onset of transition
is compatible with a wide range of levels of development,
which is in fact what is observed, as discussed later in
this paper.

Given this theoretical model, the discussion below examines several aspects of the diffusion process:   how it is facilitated by social integration; the networks through which it operates at the local or personal, national or family planning, and international levels; and the extent of its effects on both the timing and pace of the fertility transition.

## THE IMPORTANCE OF SOCIAL INTEGRATION
## AS A FACILITATOR OF DIFFUSION

As mentioned earlier, a high degree of social integration, associated with geographic compactness, common political authority, and cultural homogeneity in such areas as language, ethnicity, and religion, speeds the diffusion process.  The province-level Princeton study of historical demographic transition in Europe found sudden onset of rapid fertility decline most noticeable in populations with precisely these features (see, e.g., Coale, 1973; Lesthaeghe, 1977; Livi-Bacci, 1971, 1977; Coale et al., 1979).[9]  From the point of view of resistance to adoption, the Princeton study also shows that linguistic, ethnic, and religious boundaries often pose formidable barriers to diffusion:   maps of these boundaries coincide remarkably well with ones that distinguish provinces according to date of onset of rapid marital decline (Lesthaeghe's study of Beligum, cited above, provides an especially dramatic example).

In contemporary less developed countries, the most spectacular instances of rapid diffusion of birth control and sudden and rapid fertility decline have also occurred in comparatively small geographic areas,[10] in populations with a high degree of cultural homogeneity.  Well-known examples are Taiwan, South Korea, Hong Kong, Singapore, Thailand, and a number of Caribbean islands, such as Barbados, Jamaica, and Trinidad and Tobago (Mauldin, 1978); Japan, at the time its fertility fell decisively, is a less recent but still notable example.  A common political authority, especially as manifested in an aggressive national family planning program, is also evident in most of these examples.  As in Europe historically, rapid diffusion of birth control and sudden and rapid fertility decline are even more pronounced in subgroups within countries, where social integration is greater than at the national level.  In Northern Thailand, for example, the total fertility rate in Chiang Mai province fell from approximately 5.2 in 1960 to 2.7 in 1975, much more rapidly than the rate for Thailand as a whole (Pardthaisong, 1978); in Singapore, the crude birth rate for Malays fell from 45 per thousand in 1964 to 17 in 1975, again much more rapidly than for Singapore as a whole (Chang, 1978).

A salient aspect of highly integrated populations is the absence of organized institutional resistance representing minority interests. Such resistance, even by a small minority, can be very effective in slowing diffusion of birth control. The role of the Catholic Church in many Western countries is an example. In developing countries, this influence has been weaker than it was historically in Europe, but it can still be observed; for example, during the 1970s an elaborate social marketing scheme for condoms in the Philippines was halted by the Catholic Women's League before it even got off the ground (Repetto, 1977). The inclusion of sympathetic religious leaders on national family planning coordinating boards has helped to counter such opposition; this was done, for example, in Korea (Keeney, 1975). International agencies have frequently pursued a similar approach. For example, in some South Pacific countries, such as Tonga, the United Nations Fund for Population Activities (UNFPA) has provided financial aid to the Catholic Church for promoting the rhythm method; this has had the effect, intended or not, of promoting Church tolerance of other approaches also supported by UNFPA.

The importance of social integration to diffusion is also illustrated by the tendency, seldom studied but well-known among family planning programs, for villages not only to adopt contraception as units, but also to discontinue as units. This may occur, for example, because of rapidly spreading rumors about side effects. Although marital fertility decline at the national level appears to be irreversible once it begins (Knodel and van de Walle, 1979), small localities may sometimes be integrated enough to show reversibility, just as individuals do.

Another relevant dimension of social integration is political integration and power, particularly the degree to which government is centralized. Highly centralized systems, such as those found in China and Indonesia, are conducive to rapid diffusion of family planning through government-sponsored programs. Central government authority reaches down to the production brigade level in China and to the village headman in Indonesia, both of which

have been utilized with great effectiveness by their
respective central governments to promote family planning
(Freedman, 1978; Keeney, 1975:12, 105).  Such political
influences can sometimes overcome lack of integration in
other areas, such as ethnicity, language, and religion.


## DIFFUSION NETWORKS

As noted above, diffusion operates through a hierarchy of
networks at several levels:  the local or personal, the
national or family planning, and the international.  These
networks are examined in the subsections below.


### Local or Personal Networks

Small, local populations, such as villages, are generally
characterized by a high degree of social integration.  As
noted earlier, when normative birth control costs collapse
in a highly integrated population, the threshold condition
for adoption of birth control is achieved almost simultaneously by a large proportion of the population despite
wide variation in couples' perceptions of the utilities
and costs of children, and thus in socioeconomic status.
In this situation, couple differences in fertility
behavior depend a great deal on their location in social
networks, and network variables such as information
access and relationship to opinion leaders may account
for a great deal of the variance in fertility behavior.
Later in transition, when the birth control diffusion
process is essentially complete, network variables may be
less important.
     Although the study of local network diffusion relates
to several areas of fertility research, both economic
(e.g., Easterlin, 1975, 1978; Retherford, 1979, 1980) and
psychosocial (e.g., Miller and Godwin, 1977; Miller and
Hollerbach, 1979; Burch, 1980), its principal distinctive
emphasis is on social influences.  In this connection,
three topics should be discussed:  opinion leadership,
social networks, and social press or climate.
     Communications researchers have long been concerned
with the first two of these topics, studying extensively
the relationships between message sources and message
receivers (e.g., Shannon and Weaver, 1949).  In the early
1960s, when many national family planning program were
beginning, communication efforts were modeled after the

findings from studies of other innovations.  Only in the middle and late 1960s did research focus specifically on opinion leadership and social networks in the area of family planning (e.g., Palmore 1967).  Even now, studies in this area are scarce and involve few researchers (e.g., Palmore, 1967; Palmore et al., 1971; Palmore et al., 1977; Fisher, 1978; Placek, 1974-75).  Recent family planning program emphasis on "accessibility" and "community-based distribution systems" (Foreit et al., 1978) is consistent with the findings of the opinion leadership and network research that has been done.  This research has shown that, although the mass media facilitate awareness and basic information about contraception, adoption itself is more likely to be encouraged or discouraged by opinion leaders "closer to home" who share many of the same characteristics as the couples who have not yet adopted a method.

Several generalizations summarize the currently prevalent views on family planning opinion leadership. First, opinion leadership in family planning is a multistep flow, with opinion leaders likely to appear at any step.  Second, there is a range of opinion leadership from those who merely inform others about fertility regulation, to legitimizers who not only inform but also recommend, to implementers who are active in promoting use (Palmore, 1967; Palmore et al., 1976).  Third, opinion leaders tend to have several characteristics as communicators:  they generally participate in social situations, are sensitive to various information sources, are well informed about family planning, are innovators in family planning, and give advice.  In particular, they have generally tried and discussed methods themselves, and are well informed about side effects, so that they may discourage use of a particular method or advocate an alternative method.

Analysis of local social networks involves construction of measures from sociometric data, usually obtained from sample surveys with the proviso that whole villages (or other small areas) are included in the sample (for a recent review of network research, see Rogers and Kincaid, 1981).  The question on which the sociometry is based varies widely from study to study.  In some studies, respondents are asked with whom they have discussed family planning; in others, more general sociometric questions are asked, such as who are the five persons with whom the respondent has closest contact.  Of these, the latter approach is probably preferable (Kim and Palmore, 1978).

Using answers to these questions, the analyst proceeds to establish the patterns of links among individuals in the area under study. Typically, respondents are represented as circles on a sociometric map of the study area, with lines joining those who say they have close contact with each other. One-headed arrows represent nonreciprocal links, and two-headed arrows represent reciprocal links (i.e., each of the respondents named the other as a close contact). An example of a sociometric map from a study in Korea is shown in Figure 1.

Many types of measures are possible based on such data. For example, the data may be used to define groups that can be used instead of individuals as the focus of analysis. Although such defining of groups can be done in several ways, some standard definitions seem to be emerging in the literature. Richards (1975), principal originator of the popular NEGOPY computer package for network analysis, defines a group as a set of individuals that satisfies five criteria: (1) there must be three or more members; (2) each member must have more than 50 percent of his or her links with other members of the group; (3) there must be at least one way to reach each member from each other member by tracing links between the members; (4) there can be no single person who, when removed from the group, causes the rest of the group to fail to meet any of the first three criteria; and (5) there must be no single link which, if omitted, causes the group to fail to meet any of the above criteria. (Figure 1 shows five groups so defined.)

Many measures can be devised at the group level, such as connectiveness (the number of directed links in a group divided by the maximum possible number of directed links for a group of that size), openness (the number of links group members have with persons outside that group divided by the number of people in the group), and one-step zone size (the number of other groups directly linked to the group of reference). More complex measures, such as zone integration and zone connectiveness, can also be constructed (see, for example, Richards, 1975; Rogers et al., 1976; Rogers and Kincaid, 1981; Danowski, 1976; Kim and Palmore, 1978). It is also possible to construct measures solely from the links themselves. For each respondent, one can count the number of incoming links (those with many are operationally defined as opinion leaders), the number of outgoing links, links to persons who use contraception, links to highly educated persons, and so on. Both the group and individual link measures

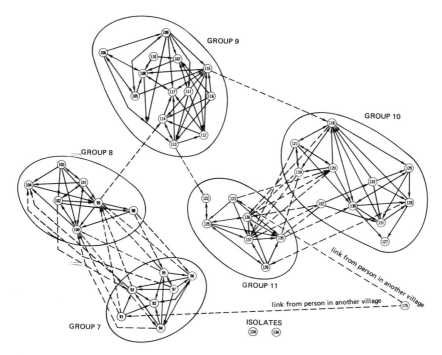

FIGURE 1   An Illustration of Personal Networks:   Sangchon
Village, Kyeongsangnam Province, Korea, 1975

can then be related to suitable dependent variables, such
as knowledge or use of contraception.

Using measures of the type just discussed, Lee (1977),
Kim and Palmore (1978), Rogers and Kincaid (1981), and
others have found strong relationships between these
measures and contraceptive use.   Kim and Palmore, for
example, included thirteen network measures in an analysis
that also included blocks of indicators of sociodemographic status, family planning program measures, and
indices of social climate.   They found that network
variables explained 38 to 100 percent as much variance as
did sociodemographic variables; relative to program
variables, the comparable range was 29 percent to 80
percent, while relative to social climate variables, the
range was 54 percent to 114 percent.

Closely related to the social network perspective are
the notions of social climate and social press, based on
the idea that the relevant part of a person's social

environment is not only the objective reality, but also
the perception of that reality. Social climate or
"press" refers to the individual's perception of social
pressure to use contraception. Measures of this perception generally rely on a series of questions of the form,
"How many of your friends, relatives, and neighbors favor
family planning?" Although the idea of climate or press
dates back at least to W. I. Thomas and his "definition
of the situation" (Thomas and Thomas, 1928), its application to population research is more recent. Palmore and
Freedman (1969) and Kinderman (1969) found perceptions of
others' contraceptive use levels important in determining
individual adoption in Taiwan. Chung et al. (1972), using
a scale of ten items, found that birth control press was
among the two best psychological variables correlating
with family planning use.

The three research topics of opinion leadership, social
networks, and social climate are complementary rather than
distinct. Social climate measures are related to the
social network approach since they simply reflect individual perceptions of what those in the network think. As
noted above, there are also social network measures for
opinion leadership, so that studies showing the importance
of opinion leadership variables to family planning behavior are also related to the social network approach. To
date, however, few studies have integrated these
approaches.

## National or Family Planning Networks

Beyond the local or interpersonal level, national-level
diffusion, particularly in the form of family planning
programs, is central to the spread of birth control
information and adoption. The effectiveness of such
programs in promoting the use of birth control varies
widely, as do their modes of operation. Although no one
type of program or organization is uniformly superior,
given the divergence in institutional settings involved,[11]
some generalizations about more effective approaches can
be made.

First, integration of services is often helpful in
overcoming normative and modesty barriers at the start of
a program. Such integration may be with health services
(e.g., block extension educators in India), or community
development services (e.g., the semaul, or community
development, movement in Korea), or even broader. A good

example of how integration can help is in most South Pacific countries, where there is a highly developed public health nurse network well suited to assuming family planning functions. Women can get contraceptives through the nurse without their neighbors' knowledge, which would be difficult if contraceptives were distributed by a separate group of family planning workers. This advantage is especially great for injectables, which make family planning even less observable (there is no evidence of use in the home after the nurse leaves), and which are very popular in Tonga and Western Samoa, for example. There are also obvious cost advantages to integrated programs, as long as medical control is not too tight. (For example, if medical prescriptions for drug store purchases are rigidly required, and if nurses and paramedical personnel are prohibited from dispensing most kinds of contraceptives, diffusion of family planning may be greatly impeded.) The degree of integration with health services that is desirable depends a great deal on the local situation.

There is abundant evidence that reliance on a variety of methods and delivery systems has also contributed to higher family planning performance rates in many countries (for a review of evidence relating mainly to community-based distribution, see Gardner et al., 1976, and Foreit et al., 1978). For example, numerous studies of barriers to adoption posed by time and distance have confirmed the importance of outreach workers and community-based distribution (see, e.g., Fawcett et al., 1966; Fawcett et al., 1967; Fuller 1972; Laing, 1979). Tables 1 and 2 summarize the prevailing wisdom regarding the proper mix of methods and delivery systems and the relation of method mix to life-cycle stage of clients.[12]

In contrast, little is known about the most effective ways to use the mass media to promote family planning. Programs have employed such varied approaches as spot announcements on radio or television; short dramas and discussions on radio and, less often, television; slides and short film strips shown in public movie theaters; slides, film strips, and movies shown by mobil vans; stories and advertisments in newspapers and magazines, especially women's magazines; comic books; match book covers; family planning fans; billboards and posters; flip charts; pamphlets; books; drug store displays; and introduction of family planning messages into the acts of touring magicians, play companies, and the like. Media use has varied widely from country to country. In some

TABLE 1   Appropriateness of Contraceptive Methods by
Delivery System

| Contraceptive Method | Delivery System | | | | |
| --- | --- | --- | --- | --- | --- |
| | Private Family Planning Clinic | Private Physician | Health System | Subsidized Commercial Distribution | Community-Based Distribution |
| Condom | * | | * | *** | *** |
| Vaginal Methods | * | | * | *** | *** |
| Oral Contraceptive | ** | ** | * | *** | *** |
| IUD | *** | *** | *** | | |
| Injectable | *** | ** | *** | ** | ** |
| Sterilization | *** | *** | *** | | |
| Abortion or Menstrual Regulation | *** | *** | ** | | |

*Less appropriate
**Appropriate
***Most appropriate

Source:   Perkin and Saunders (1979:1).

countries, media have been used sparingly to keep a low
profile for the program and avoid attracting opposition;
in others, virtually all of the approaches have been
used.  Unfortunately, the effectiveness of these various
approaches and campaign intensities has not been well
researched.  This is partly because such research is
difficult to carry out when extensive interpersonal communication is likely to contaminate the assessment of
media impact.
     Because of this lack of research, only a few general-
izations can be advanced on the role of the media in the
diffusion process.  One such generalization is that information, education, and communication (IEC) campaigns can
be effective in the early stages of a family planning
program:  they can increase awareness and knowledge of
methods and services, and reduce resistance to birth
control by helping to legitimize the idea of family-size
limitation (Schramm, 1971).[13]  Once knowledge is widespread and birth control begins to be accepted, the impact
of such campaigns diminishes, since they do not seem to
be very effective in motivating couples to reduce preferred family size.[14]

TABLE 2   Appropriateness of Contraceptive Methods by Stage
in Life Cycle

| Contraceptive Method | Reproductive Life Stage | | | |
| | Post Menarche | Pre First Birth (delay) | Post First Birth (spacing) | Termination |
|---|---|---|---|---|
| Condom | ** | * | | |
| Vaginal Methods | * | * | | |
| Oral Contraceptive | * | ** | * | |
| IUD | | * | ** | |
| Injectable | | | ** | * |
| Sterilization | | | | ** |
| Abortion or Menstrual Regulation | - - - - - - - Back-up Throughout - - - - - - | | | |

*Appropriate
**Most appropriate

Source:  Perkin and Saunders (1979:9).

IEC campaigns can also help to combat rumors.  A number of rumors about birth control are common (see Rogers
[1973:303ff.] for a partial list):  that the IUD moves
inside the body; that the IUD or pill or injection causes
cancer; that any given method decreases sexual satisfaction or leads to a loss of sexual desire; that the pill
leads to weight gain, discoloration of the skin, or
nausea; that any chemical method may have long-range
genetic effects; that vasectomy leads to impotence; that
a method which, in reality, is reversible is not; that
all government methods are designed to eliminate certain
minority groups or that foreign-supplied drugs are
designed to have a negative effect on Third World users;
and that government-supplied contraceptives are inferior
to those available in the private sector.  Some of these
fears have some basis in fact, but are frequently exag-

gerated through rumors (see Schearer, in these volumes; Bogue, in these volumes).

Semantics has also played an important role in IEC campaigns. What used to be called birth control came to be called family planning in the 1950s. Contraceptives were portrayed as medical instrumentalities, reflecting a conscious attempt to associate birth control with family welfare and health, which are virtually universally valued (Davis, 1971). More recently, one notes the choice of the term "menstrual regulation" in place of "early abortion."

## International Networks

At the international level, the catalytic role of international population assistance, which grew from about U.S. $2 million in 1960 to more than U.S. $644 million in 1978 (UNFPA, 1979:17, 20; see also Mauldin, in these volumes), has assumed major significance. Such assistance currently covers about half of the actual costs of population activities in developing countries (see Schearer, in these volumes). It often has provided the critical spark to get things moving and helped overcome bottlenecks to keep things moving (Gille, 1977:88). Its effect on the starting times of fertility transition has already been discussed.

Despite this significance, international population assistance has received remarkably little attention from academic researchers, perhaps because analysis in this area requires an institutional approach that emphasizes case studies of particular donor agencies. Such a particularistic approach is somewhat alien to demography, sociology, and economics, the disciplines that have dominated population research. Practitioners in these fields are trained to base explanation on more generalized variables, such as education, per capita income, family planning inputs, and the like, and to emphasize statistical evidence and statistical models. This mode of analysis has been extremely fruitful in analyzing individual and areal data, but it becomes less fruitful as one progresses to more complex units of analysis such as family planning programs and international donor agencies. The analysis of the latter is in many ways not amenable to quantitative methods (although these are still useful), but requires instead a more qualitative approach. For the most part, research of this nature has been carried out not by academics, but by persons associated with donor agencies or action programs themselves.

One excellent study of this kind chronicles the first 25 years of Population Council activities, between 1952 and 1977 (Population Council, 1978). During this period, the Council devoted considerable resources to building indigenous leadership in the population field, promoting demographic data collection and analysis in developing countries, conducting a large biomedical research program, providing technical and organizational assistance to emerging national family planning programs, and promoting the international exchange of information through a major publications program. Although there is little doubt that the Population Council has been very effective as a family planning diffusion agency, its overall impact on fertility is difficult to assess quantitatively because most of its activities have long-term multiplier effects and are several steps removed from individual decisions to limit family size.

Under the aegis of the Population Council, Kim et al. (1972) have provided a valuable history of the early stages of the Korean family planning program, in which Population Council support played an important role. Particularly interesting is the discussion of how private groups, including the International Planned Parenthood Federation and the Planned Parenthood Federation of Korea, laid the foundation for the national program, and then how they worked closely with the government in addressing those aspects of the program that were either politically sensitive (such as the early IEC campaigns) or required a degree of flexibility difficult to attain in large government bureaucracies (e.g., pilot projects, evaluation activities, and channeling of external assistance funds). More case studies of this kind are needed, since strategies have varied from country to country.

A few other studies are available. A history of the UNFPA has been prepared (Salas, 1979). The World Bank (1972) has described the major thrusts of its program in what was originally prepared as an in-house working paper. Only scant information is available on the evolution of the United States Agency for International Development's (USAID) international population assistance program; this is unfortunate since AID provides close to one-third of all international population assistance (Gille, 1977:81). Historical information on the population programs of the many private foundations involved in the population field, such as the Ford Foundation, is similarly fragmentary. A comprehensive history of the entire international population assistance effort, emphasizing an analysis of its impact, would certainly be extremely useful.

Several aspects of international population assistance worthy of further investigation emerge from the literature that is available. One is international demonstration effects, which practitioners in the field seem to agree are quite important. For example, both Korea and Taiwan have international training programs in family planning (headquartered at the Korean Institute for Family Planning in Seoul--recently reorganized and renamed the Korean Institute of Population and Health--and at the Chinese Center for International Training in Family Planning in Taichung). A great number of government officials from other countries have attended these programs, which have apparently been effective in stimulating the founding and improvement of family planning programs in other countries. In addition to supporting these formalized international training programs, donor agencies have also funded many individual tours enabling high government officials to observe successful programs in other countries. These training programs and tours have been important not only in providing technical and organizational information, but also in generating enthusiasm and making the idea of a family planning program more tangible to those who have never observed one. International conferences have played a complementary role by keeping family planning officials up to date with new developments in other countries, and by encouraging a sense of professionalism and commitment. Again, little research has been done on such demonstration effects; both the case study approach and quantitative analysis would be appropriate.

Similarly, little attention has been paid to the mechanisms by which donor agencies cooperate with one another to minimize duplication and maximize effectiveness of aid funds. One mechanism of cooperation has been international conferences designed explicitly for this purpose, most notably the Bellagio conferences sponsored by the Rockefeller Foundation (see, e.g., Rockefeller Foundation, 1977). Another mechanism has been needs-assessment missions, which have been pioneered mainly by UNFPA and the World Bank. Because of their broad membership, which typically includes members from a cross-section of public and private agencies and a variety of professional backgrounds, these missions have provided a way to coordinate and integrate population planning with other agencies and other aspects of development planning (UNFPA, 1979:21); these missions also perform important evaluative functions. World Bank missions, reflecting World Bank management views, have sometimes generated pressure by requiring

sound family planning programs as a condition of development loans (Keeney, 1975:24), and it seems likely that
this has contributed to speeding the diffusion of family
planning through government programs. The needs-
assessment strategy itself should be more systematically
evaluated as a mechanism for family planning diffusion.

The role of international agencies in the development
of particular aspects of national programs is also worth
investigating. For example, the close relationship of
the Population Council to the programs in South Korea and
Taiwan helps explain the early reliance of those programs
on the IUD, which the Council was instrumental in developing. Similarly, the emphasis on oral contraceptives in
the early stages of the Malaysian program can be traced
to the population assistance of the Swedish International
Development Agency (SIDA), which provided the contraceptives.

Research and evaluation activities have been very
important in accelerating and maintaining the momentum of
international population assistance. Such work done in
the early stages of the Taiwan program has served to a
considerable extent as a model; results from the Taiwan
studies were extremely important in persuading donor
agencies that family planning programs were effective and
worth supporting (Cernada, 1970; Cernada and Sun, 1974).
Agencies such as the Population Council, UNFPA, and USAID
have contributed heavily to basic demographic data collection and demographic research around the world (Gille,
1977) for precisely this reason. Thus research and evaluation have played a very important role in the diffusion
of family planning at the international level (and, to a
lesser extent, within countries), although again the
impact is difficult to assess quantitatively.

Ultimately, diffusion of family planning at the international level reduces the cost of birth control and feeds
into the simplified individual-level utility-cost models
mentioned earlier. However, the process by which this
occurs is complex and frequently indirect. The institutional mechanisms involved, though important, are several
steps removed from individual birth control decisions and
difficult to capture by quantitative statistical methods.


EFFECTS OF DIFFUSION ON THE TIMING AND PACE
OF FERTILITY TRANSITION

The process of diffusion occurs through the hierarchy of
networks described above. Its speed and extent will vary

according to the degree of social integration in a given
culture, the effectiveness of the various networks, and
the presence or absence of barriers to the process, many
of which are related to levels of social and economic
development.  Given these variations, a central question
becomes the relative significance of the effects of diffusion and development on fertility decline.  The subsections below address this question first for the timing
or onset of fertility decline, and then for its pace.

## Effects on Timing

A good deal of debate continues to focus on the relative
effects of diffusion and development on the timing of
fertility transition, and the evidence is not conclusive.
Some dismiss diffusion, and family planning programs in
particular, as having rather insignificant effects (e.g.,
Davis, 1963, 1967; Demeny, 1975, 1979a, 1979b), while
others assign them major importance (e.g., Freedman,
1978; Mauldin and Berelson, 1978; Bogue and Tsui, 1979a,
1979b).

In an early article bearing directly on this question,
Carlsson (1966) argued that fertility decline is basically
a process of adjustment to economic and social change,
rather than a process of innovation and diffusion of
radically new birth control behavior.  Carlsson interpreted the existence of substantial urban-rural and
regional variations in pretransition marital fertility in
Sweden as evidence that birth control was practiced widely
before marital fertility transition began.

Knodel (1977) subsequently disputed this conclusion and
presented evidence that innovation-diffusion processes, as
well as adjustment processes, are important in explaining
the timing of marital fertility decline.  In making his
argument, he distinguished between parity-independent
birth control, which affects only birth spacing and is
consistent with a natural-fertility regime, and parity-
dependent birth control, or family limitation, which
involves conscious stopping behavior and departures from
natural fertility.  According to Knodel's interpretation,
urban-rural and regional differences in pretransition
marital fertility stemmed mainly from regional variations
in parity-independent birth control, mostly through mechanisms involving no conscious effort to reduce fertility.
Among these mechanisms, regional variations in the customary length of breastfeeding, which affects birth inter-

vals through its inhibitory effects on ovulation, appear
to have been especially important. The association of
pretransition marital fertility fluctuations with economic fluctuations (e.g., in the harvest) stemmed mainly
from temporary abstinence aimed at postponing births
during hard times, and from reduced libido, fecundity,
and coital frequency associated with famine, malnutrition, and epidemic diseases. All these parity-independent
mechanisms involve spacing but not stopping behavior, and
have little or no effect on the age pattern of natural
fertility. Some parity-dependent control may have been
practiced by small elites or subgroups prior to marital
fertility transition, but not by the mass of the
population.

Knodel's evidence in support of this interpretation
hinges mainly on use of Coale and Trussell's (1974)
demographic index of marital fertility control, m,
mentioned earlier. This index measures departures from
the typical age pattern of natural fertility, and requires
as input only a set of age-specific marital birth rates.
Thus m is an indirect measure of parity-dependent birth
control that is unaffected by parity-independent birth
control. In Sweden, m was constant, with minor fluctuations, for 150 years prior to 1880, when marital fertility began its secular decline. In 1880, m began to
increase and continued to do so steadily until a much
lower level of marital fertility was attained. If parity-
dependent birth control were purely an adjustment process,
then m should have gradually increased over the entire
period for which data are available, since Sweden was
developing economically and socially over this entire
period. Instead, m followed an elongated S-shaped trajec-
tory over time, which is typical of an innovation-
diffusion process.

Carlsson's interpretation has also been questioned by
Mosk (1978), who examined Swedish urban-rural fertility
differences with a more extensive data set, by province.
Mosk found that, in 1880, the earliest date for which he
had data, the rural index of marital fertility was lower
than the urban index in about half the cases. The index
of overall fertility was lower in urban than in rural
areas, but mainly because of later age at marriage. Thus
the urban-rural and regional variations in marital fertility in 1880 were not closely associated with level of
development, and offer no support for a purely adjustment
hypothesis.

Other evidence cited by Knodel in support of his interpretation comes from individual-level data from historical
family reconstitution studies; these data show that, prior
to marital fertility transition, mother's age at the birth
of her last child is unaffected by the survivorship of
previous children. If parity-dependent birth control were
widespread, as Carlsson concludes, then one should observe
some stopping behavior at earlier ages among those whose
previous births all survived. Knodel also cites the fact
that in European countries for which data are available,
legitimate and illegitimate fertility started to decline
at the same time. Since illegitimate births are unwanted
regardless of level of economic development, adjustment
processes cannot explain either the decline in illegitimate fertility or its coincidence with the decline in
legitimate fertility. Innovation and diffusion of birth
control knowledge, skills, and means, however, do provide
a plausible explanation. Knodel also observes that in
contemporary developing countries, desired family size
often does not decline rapidly until after marital fertility begins to fall. This phenomenon is difficult to
reconcile with a purely adjustment perspective, but it
does make sense if one views parity-dependent birth
control as an innovation. In the innovation-diffusion
perspective, when parity-dependent control, or family
limitation, becomes viewed as acceptable behavior and
marital fertility starts to fall, people are more likely
to perceive the advantages of smaller families; thus the
innovation of family limitation triggers a decline in
desired family size. Finally, Knodel notes that the
incredible rapidity of marital fertility decline in many
contemporary developing countries cannot be explained
purely by adjustment processes, because the pace of
development does not at all match the pace of marital
fertility decline. In sum, the evidence cited by Knodel
suggests that both innovation and adjustment processes
are involved in marital fertility transition. Pretransition fluctuations and differentials in marital fertility
appear to stem from fluctuations and differentials in
natural fertility, relating to the potential supply of
children.

Findings from the Princeton study of European fertility transition, mentioned earlier and covering many more
countries than those mentioned by Knodel (1977), also
suggest that diffusion can have a great effect on advancing the timing of transition. As noted, this study
revealed that some two-thirds of European province-sized

administrative areas started marital fertility transition within a 30-year period between 1880 and 1910, despite widely different levels of mortality and development (Knodel and van de Walle, 1979). Judging from the results of the Princeton study, diffusion processes may have advanced the timing of fertility transition in the less developed areas of Europe by as much as 50 years, and perhaps more in some cases. Systematic examination of the Princeton data is needed to evaluate more precisely the magnitude of these effects.

Knodel's (1979) study of German villages also sheds light on the possible effect of diffusion on the timing of transition. Although most of his villages were rather similar in economic and social characteristics, fertility transition began almost 100 years sooner in some villages than in others. Barriers to diffusion may well account for much of this difference in timing.

Further evidence is available from contemporary less developed countries, where there seems to be a good deal of diffusion of birth control knowledge and methods from urban to rural areas, especially since organized family planning programs almost invariably begin in urban areas. In Thailand, for example, McCormick Hospital established a high-quality private family planning program in the Chiang Mai area of Northern Thailand; apparently as a result, fertility fell in this area about ten years sooner than in the rest of Thailand (Pardthaisong, 1978). The time gap probably would have been even longer had not the government established a national family planning program about ten years after the McCormick program began. Given Thailand's high rate of population growth, this ten-year difference is not inconsequential, even though it may seem rather insignificant from a long-term historical perspective. The South Korean family planning program, which started out stronger in rural than in urban areas, is a notable exception that actually proves the point, because South Korea is one of the few countries where rural fertility decline has not lagged behind urban decline (Keeney, 1975:35).

A striking characteristic of the contemporary situation in developing countries, compared with the historical situation in Europe, is the presence of an enormous international family planning diffusion effort, discussed earlier, financed in large part by the developed countries (for monetary figures, see Mauldin, in this volume). Partly as a consequence of this effort, there is today in the developing countries a striking parallel to what

Knodel and van de Walle observed in Europe historically, but on a world-wide scale. In slightly less than 30 years, between 1950 and 1979, the proportion of the developing world's population covered by family planning programs has increased from zero to over 90 percent (Nortman and Hofstatter, 1980:17). During the 1960s and 1970s, many of these countries began marital fertility transition, and it appears very likely that, for the 30-year period between 1960 and 1990, at least three-quarters of the developing world's population will have begun the transition. In both cases, historical and contemporary, there is tremendous variability in culture and level of development at the start of transition; in both cases, diffusion offers a plausible explanation of the compression in time of starting dates for the diffusion of birth control and marital fertility transition.

From the point of view of causality, it is important to note that the international population assistance effort is itself basically a consequence of rapid mortality decline after World War II, which, as noted above, occurred largely because of the diffusion of inexpensive but very effective modern public health technology from developed countries (Davis, 1956; Preston, 1975). This astonishing mortality decline caused rapid increases in population that impeded development efforts, causing alarm at both national and international levels. Thus, at the global level, the diffusion effort itself is largely a consequence of mortality decline and population pressure on economic and organizational resources, stemming ultimately from historical economic and social development in the developed countries. Thus we return to the point made at the beginning of this paper, that development is more fundamental than diffusion in explaining fertility transition. Nevertheless, it is still true that the international family planning diffusion effort has gained considerable momentum of its own, and that it has had major effects in particular settings that have been quite independent of local levels of economic and social development.

The above discussion suggests that many of the disagreements about the relative importance of development and diffusion may be more apparent than real. Proponents on both sides of this argument can probably agree that diffusion processes can advance the timing of fertility transition by at least 10 to 20 years and perhaps as much as 50 or more years in some circumstances. The disagreement seems to be not so much about these magnitudes as

about their significance. Certainly over the long sweep
of history, development is the basic explanation of fertility transition, and a 10- to 20-year advance in the
timing of transition is perhaps not very significant. In
the short run, however, especially if population is
pressing against resources and growing at close to 3
percent a year (implying a doubling time of 23 years),
advancing the timing of transition by 10 to 20 years or
more by means of an organized diffusion program is of
major significance.

As noted above, diffusion processes help explain why
threshold levels of mortality and socioeconomic indices
at the beginning of fertility transition vary so much
from one country to the next. Besides the Knodel and van
de Walle (1979) study of such variations in historic
Europe, there are several similar studies in contemporary
developing countries. Studies prior to 1978 have been
reviewed by Mauldin and Berelson (1978:92). More
recently, it has become apparent that Thailand and
especially Indonesia have begun marital fertility
transition at levels of development (except for mortality) substantially lower than those observed in earlier
studies of other less developed countries. Freedman has
noted that objective development changes much smaller than
those that characterized the West can provide motivation
for lower fertility today.[15]


Effects on Pace

How much can diffusion compress the transitional section
of the S-shaped adoption curve in time? The answer is
complicated by the fact that the rate of diffusion depends
also on the speed of decline of desired family size, which
is strongly influenced by the speed of economic and social
development. Kirk (1971) has shown that fertility declines in contemporary developing countries, where they
have begun, are proceeding much more rapidly than they
did historically in the developed countries (about three
times faster, if one compares transitions starting in
1875-99 with those starting after 1950); however, whether
diffusion of birth control has contributed substantially
to this acceleration is not evident from his results.
Subsequent studies have more clearly demonstrated that
family planning programs can greatly accelerate fertility
decline. Mauldin and Berelson (1978), for example,
regressed fertility change between 1965 and 1975 in a

number of developing countries (anywhere between 38 and 94 countries, depending on which of several statistical models was used) against a number of economic and social indicators. They consistently found that family planning input and effort variables greatly increased the proportion of variance explained (usually by at least 15 percentage points), over and above the usual economic and social variables. In the basic regression, seven socioeconomic factors (including mortality level) explained 66 percent of the variance, rising to 83 percent when family planning program effort variables were added.

One can find many instances where program implementation or program improvements have clearly speeded up fertility decline, although it is usually difficult to ascertain by precisely how much because of a lack of control groups. In Korea, for example, the percentage of eligible women (married women of reproductive age) who knew of some contraceptive method increased from 51 percent in 1964, just as the national family planning program was getting into full swing, to 87 percent in 1968; knowledge of the IUD rose from 11 to 84 percent during the same period (Mauldin, 1975:31). Between 1965 and 1973, the percentage who had ever practiced contraception among eligible women with no education increased from 16 to 53 percent and among rural residents from 19 to 58 percent (Freedman and Berelson, 1976:22). As noted above, Korea is one of the few countries where rural fertility decline has not lagged behind urban fertility decline, evidently because in its initial stages, the national family planning program effort was stronger in rural than in urban areas (Keeney, 1975:35; Chung et al., 1972); this pattern also suggests that the program had substantial effects. Between 1965 and 1973, the proportion practicing contraception among those wanting no more children increased from 31 to 54 percent. Between 1972 and 1977, female sterilizations increased from near zero to 22 percent of all new acceptors, due to the introduction of laparoscopy (a simplified outpatient procedure) and a tripling of government subsidies that had the effect of making sterilization virtually free (Westoff et al., 1980:130-137; Korean Institute for Family Planning, 1978:291; Cho and Retherford, 1982). Many other examples could be cited, but are more properly covered in other papers in these volumes having to do with the assessment of family planning program impact (Mauldin, in these volumes).

RESEARCH ISSUES

This paper has raised a number of questions about the diffusion of birth control--the channels through which it occurs, the magnitude and significance of its effects-- that cannot be adequately answered without further research. This section addresses several issues related to that needed research.

First, the study of diffusion of birth control in contemporary less developed countries would benefit from more longitudinal and time series data with small areas as the units of analysis. Presently, fertility studies in less developed countries are overwhelmingly based on cross-sectional analyses of single surveys, an approach not suited to the study of diffusion, which is preeminently a time-dependent process. Greater use of comparable cross-sectional surveys large enough to have areal detail would be much more useful. The Princeton study of historical fertility transition in Europe, based on time series of areal data, has proven extremely valuable for the study of diffusion processes even though the data were only of the most elementary kind (Coale, 1973). Today's time series data are, potentially at least, immensely richer.

A related problem concerns the interpretation of statistical findings relating to the effects of development variables and family planning programs on fertility. Statistical findings based on cross-sectional data depend a great deal on the stage of transition from which the data come. Because of diffusion, fertility differentials by, say, education can change dramatically within just a few years. This implies that the coefficient of the educational variable in a cross-sectional multiple regression analysis of fertility can change just as dramatically and quickly. However, this does not mean that the causal relation of education to fertility has changed in any fundamental way during the interim. A similar point can be made regarding apparent changes in the effects of other socioeconomic and family planning program variables. Time-series data and related analysis techniques, because of the insight they provide into diffusion processes, can aid in the interpretation of such findings.

Better measures of the potential for birth control diffusion also need to be developed. One measure frequently used is the difference between the natural and the desired number of surviving children (see for example, Easterlin, 1975). However, this is not a very good measure because

the relative intensity of preference for the desired
number over the natural number is highly variable:  in
today's developing countries that have not yet begun
fertility transition, it is common, as mentioned above,
for the desired number of children to be about four and
the natural number between five and six; Pakistan and
Thailand, for example, were both in this situation in the
late 1960s (Shah and Palmore, 1979; Knodel and Debavalya,
1978).  It is plausible in retrospect, however, that the
relative intensity of preference for four over six was
much stronger in Thailand than in Pakistan, since rapid
adoption of birth control and rapid fertility decline
began shortly afterward in Thailand but not in Pakistan,
despite a massive contraceptive campaign in the latter.
Better measurement of the potential for birth control
diffusion might be accomplished by supplementing survey
questions on desired family size with at least one additional question designed to assess intensity of preference
for the desired number over either the natural number, or
one or two more than the desired number (Retherford,
1980).  If N is the desired number, the basic question
might be of the form:  "How much do you prefer N children
over N+1 children?  Just barely, a little, some, very
much, or extremely much?"  If responses were scored from
1 to 5, an average score near 5 would indicate that diffusion of birth control and fertility decline were immi-
nent, whereas an average score near 1 would indicate that
even very low birth control costs would probably be enough
to discourage use.  Although this approach has the virtue
of being very simple to apply and easy to interpret, it
is as yet untested.  Other, more established approaches
to psychometric measurement of preference intensities,
though considerably more complex and difficult to interpret, might also be useful for better measurement of the
potential for diffusion of birth control (see, for
example, Coombs et al., 1975; Terhune and Kaufman, 1973;
Myers and Roberts, 1968; Bulatao, 1981).

In some circumstances, family planning programs initially emphasize contraception as a means of improving
maternal and child health through longer birth intervals.
To date, research has paid little attention to diffusion
of birth control for such purposes.  Such research is less
important than that on diffusion for family limitation,
but it deserves more attention than it has so far
received.

## POLICY IMPLICATIONS

A high level of development appears to be a sufficient but not a necessary condition of fertility transition. Diffusion processes that reduce the costs and facilitate the use of fertility regulation also can have a significant impact on the timing and pace of fertility transition. This is even more true in today's less developed countries than in the industrial countries historically because of the innovation in recent decades of organized family planning programs as purposive diffusion agencies. The policy relevance of diffusion research is obvious since purposive diffusion, mainly through family planning programs, is the principal avenue by which governments and other agencies attempt to reduce fertility. Considerable debate continues to focus on the relative significance of the effects of diffusion and economic and social development. The evidence is not conclusive, and more research is needed in this area.

## NOTES

1. Physical distance is less important now than it was historically because of improvements in transportation and communication; moreover, existing health networks are sometimes used to provide large areas, if not the entire country, with new birth control information and services within a relatively short period. Nevertheless, birth control costs associated with distance factors have by no means become insignificant (Schearer, in these volumes).
2. Of course, some norms facilitate, rather than impede, diffusion.
3. The weighing of costs and benefits can be a very complex process, especially in government-sponsored programs where service location decisions must take into account such factors as regional political interests and the organization and location of pre-existing health facilities. Such cost-benefit considerations replace profitability considerations in the public and private nonprofit sectors (see Schearer, in these volumes).
4. See, e.g., Rogers, 1973, for an extensive review of the family planning communication and diffusion literature prior to the early 1970s.

5. Family size is defined as the number of children surviving to some criterion age.

6. Note, however, that insofar as infant neglect is a response to unwanted children, infant mortality rates may remain high until contraception becomes acceptable (see Scrimshaw, 1978; in these volumes; van de Walle and Knodel, 1980).

7. The old age security utility of children also falls as a consequence of development (see Potter, in these volumes; Lee and Bulatao, in these volumes), but usually not significantly until well after marital fertility transition first gets underway. Another factor of interest is diffusion of the Western nuclear family ideal, which Caldwell (1976, 1978) has argued plays an important role in stimulating marital fertility control. However, Caldwell's hypothesis, while perhaps valid in some African countries, is highly controversial if held valid for all developing countries. For example, Freedman (1979:69) has noted in rebuttal that, in Taiwan, major fertility decline has occurred in the presence of traditional family values that are changing slowly but are still very different from Western family values.

8. Van de Walle and Knodel (1980) refer to this process somewhat more generally as "diffusion of the idea of family limitation."

9. To some extent, Europe itself constitutes a common cultural area. Indeed, a precipitous and rapidly diffusing decline in the normative and initial resistance costs of birth control, associated mainly with the adoption of coitus interruptus, offers a plausible explanation of why fully two-thirds of European province-sized administrative areas experienced a sudden onset of rapid marital fertility decline within a 30-year period beginning around 1880, despite a tremendous variety of fertility levels (due to variations in spacing behavior, not stopping behavior), mortality levels, and economic and social conditions just prior to the decline (Knodel and van de Walle, 1979; van de Walle and Knodel, 1980).

10. This is not to say that rapid fertility decline cannot occur also in large populations (e.g., China).

11. Perkin and Saunders (1979:7) observe that the evolution of family planning delivery systems has been from single-purpose to multi-purpose outlets, from private to government to both private and

government operations, and from health agencies to commercial and community organizations. The self-contained, single-purpose clinic of the 1960s, often operated by a private family planning association, was supplemented first by the addition of "change agents," usually known as family planning workers; later in the late 1960s and early 1970s by integrated health, postpartum, maternity-centered, and high-risk clinical approaches; and more recently by subsidized marketing and community-based and household distribution. In some countries, additional delivery channels operate through government social security facilities, labor unions and factories, local organizations such as mothers' clubs, and religious communities.

12. The literature on organizational aspects of family planning programs is large, and more extensive treatment of it is beyond the scope of this paper. For further discussion, see United Nations, 1972, 1976, 1977; Inter Governmental Coordinating Committee, 1974.

13. Radio is a useful and inexpensive medium for IEC, since cheap transistor radios are now common throughout most of the developing world and can reach illiterate as well as literate persons (Keeney, 1975).

14. Somewhat on the margin of the IEC effort has been population education in the schools. The impact of such programs on the diffusion of family planning is long-term and therefore difficult to measure (see Kee, 1981, for a recent review of the population socialization literature, including population education).

15. One important reason for exceptions such as Pakistan, Bangladesh, or Afghanistan is that the governments have been unable to set up administrative, communication, and transportation systems capable of reaching the village masses, either with the ideas of the outside world that would revolutionize expectations, or with the minimal services and goods that make the new ideas and aspirations credible (Freedman, 1978:380). Another reason is that these are Muslim countries where the extremely subordinate position of women is a barrier to the adoption of family limitation; because of the seclusion of women, family planners often find themselves in the position of offering their messages and methods, which are usually female methods, to a largely inaccessible and unreceptive audience (van de Walle and Knodel, 1980:39-40).

BIBLIOGRAPHY

Bogue, D. J., and A. O. Tsui (1979a)  A reply to Paul
    Demeny's "On the end of the population explosion."
    Population and Development Review 5:479-494.
Bogue, D. J., and A. O. Tsui (1979b)  Zero world
    population growth?  The Public Interest 55:99-113.
Brown, L. A. (1981)  Innovation Diffusion:  A New
    Perspective. New York:  Methuen, Inc.
Bulatao, R. A. (1981)  Values and disvalues of children
    in successive childbearing decisions.  Demography
    18:1-26.
Burch, T. K., ed. (1980)  Demographic Behavior:
    Interdisciplinary Perspectives on Decision-Making.
    Boulder, Colo.:  Westview Press.
Caldwell, J. C. (1976)  Toward a restatement of
    demographic transition theory.  Population and
    Development Review 2:321-366.
Caldwell, J. C. (1978)  A theory of fertility:  From high
    plateau to destablization.  Population and
    Development Review 4:553-578.
Carlsson, G. (1966)  The decline of fertility:
    Innovation or adjustment process.  Population Studies
    20:149-174.
Cernada, G. P., ed. (1970)  Taiwan Family Planning
    Reader:  How a Program Works.  Taichung, Taiwan:
    Chinese Center for International Training in Family
    Planning.
Cernada, G. P., and T. H. Sun (1974)  Knowledge into
    Action:  The Use of Research in Taiwan's Family
    Planning Program.  Paper No. 10.  Honolulu:
    East-West Communication Institute.
Chang, C. T. (1978)  Fertility Transition, Nuptiality
    Changes, and Family Planning in Singapore.  Paper
    presented at the Conference on Comparative Fertility
    Transition in Asia, Nihon University, Tokyo.
Cho, L.-J., and R. D. Retherford (1982)  Fertility
    transition in the Republic of Korea.  In W. P.
    Mauldin, ed., Fertility Decline in Developing
    Countries:  Case Studies.  Forthcoming.
Chung, B. M., J. A. Palmore, S. J. Lee, and S. J. Lee
    (1972)  Psychological Perspectives:  Family Planning
    in Korea.  Seoul:  Hollym Publishers.
Coale, A. J. (1973)  The demographic transition.  Pp.
    53-72 in International Population Conference, Liege
    1973, Vol. 1.  Liege, Belgium:  International Union
    for the Scientific Study of Population.

Coale, A. J., and T. J. Trussell (1974)  Model fertility
    schedules:  Variations in the age structure of
    childbearing in human populations.  Population Index
    41:185-258.  (See also Erratum, Population Index
    41:572.)
Coale, A. J., and T. J. Trussell (1978)  A new procedure
    for fitting optimal values of the parameters of a
    model schedule of marital fertility rates.
    Population Index 44:203-211.
Coale, A. J., B. A. Anderson, and E. Harm (1979)  Human
    Fertility in Russia since the Nineteenth Century.
    Princeton, N.J.:  Princeton University Press.
Coombs, C. H., L. C. Coombs, and G. H. McClelland (1975)
    Preference scales for number and sex of children.
    Population Studies 29:  273-298.
Danowski, J. A. (1976)  Communication network analysis
    and social change.  Pp. 277-306 in G. C. Chu, S. A.
    Rahim, and D. L. Kincaid, eds., Communication for
    Group Transformation in Development.  Honolulu:
    East-West Communication Institute.
Davis, K. (1956)  The amazing decline of mortality in
    underdeveloped areas.  Journal of the American
    Economic Association 46:305-318.
Davis, K. (1963)  The theory of change and response in
    modern demographic history.  Population Index
    29:345-366.
Davis, K. (1967)  Population policy:  Will current
    programs succeed?  Science 158:730-739.
Davis, K. (1971)  The nature and purpose of population
    policy.  Pp. 3-29 in K. Davis and F. G. Styles, eds.,
    California's Twenty Million:  Research Contributions
    to Population Policy.  Berkeley:  Institute of
    International Studies, University of California.
Demeny, P. (1975)  Observation on population policy and
    population program in Bangladesh.  Population and
    Development Review 1:307-321.
Demeny, P. (1979a)  On the end of the population
    explosion.  Population and Development Review
    5:141-162.
Demeny, P. (1979b)  On the end of the population
    explosion.  A rejoinder.  Population and Development
    Review 5:495-504.
Easterlin, R. A. (1975)  An economic framework for
    fertility analysis.  Studies in Family Planning
    6:54-63.
Easterlin, R. A. (1978)  The economics and sociology of
    fertility:  A synthesis.  In C. Tilly, ed.,

Historical Studies of Changing Fertility. Princeton,
N.J.: Princeton University Press.

Fawcett, J. T., A. Somboonsuk, and S. Khaisang (1966)
Diffusion of Family Planning Information by Word of
Mouth Communication. Bangkok: Family Planning
Research Unit, Chulalongkorn University.

Fawcett, J. T., A. Somboonsuk, and S. Khaisang (1967)
Thailand: An analysis of time and distance factors
at an IUD clinic in Bangkok. Studies in Family
Planning 1:8-12.

Fisher, A. A. (1978) Family planning opinion leadership
in the United States. International Journal of
Health Education 21:98-106.

Foreit, J. R., M. E. Gorosh, D. G. Gillespie, and C. G.
Merritt (1978) Community-based and commercial
contraceptive distribution: An inventory and
appraisal. Population Reports, Series J:1-39.

Freedman, R. (1974) Community Level Data in Fertility
Surveys. WFS Occasional Papers No. 8. London:
World Fertility Survey.

Freedman, R. (1978) Summarized findings on Asian
population programs. Population Reports, Series
J:380-381.

Freedman, R. (1979) Theories of fertility decline: A
reappraisal. In P. M. Hauser, ed., World Population
and Development: Challenges and Prospects.
Syracuse, N.Y.: Syracuse University Press.

Freedman, R., and B. Berelson (1976) The record of
family planning programs. Studies in Family Planning
7:1-40.

Fuller, G. (1972) The Spatial Diffusion of Birth Control
in Chile. Unpublished Ph.D. dissertation.
Department of Geography, Pennsylvania State
University, University Park.

Gardner, J. S., R. J. Wolff, D. Gillespie, and G. W.
Duncan, eds. (1976) Village and Household
Availability of Contraceptives: Southeast Asia.
Seattle, Wash.: Battelle Memorial Institute.

Gille, H. (1977) Recent trends in international
population assistance. In Rockefeller Foundation,
ed., Bellagio IV Population Conference. New York:
Rockefeller Foundation.

Himes, N. E. (1936) Medical History of Contraception.
Baltimore, Md.: Williams and Wilkins.

Hong, S. (1976) Fertility and Fertility Limitation in
Korean Villages: Community and Individual Level
Effects. Unpublished Ph.D. dissertation. Department
of Sociology, University of Hawaii, Honolulu.

Inter Governmental Coordinating Committee (1974)  Family
    Planning Administrators and Commercial Marketing
    Executives.  Kuala Lumpur:  IGCC Secretariat.
Kee, P.-K. (1981)  Population Socialization Research:  A
    Review.  Working Paper No. 9.  Honolulu:  East-West
    Population Institute.
Keeney, S. M. (1975)  East Asia Shares Experience in
    Family Planning.  Taichung, Taiwan:  The Chinese
    Center for International Training in Family Planning.
Kim, J. I., and J. A. Palmore (1978)  Personal Networks
    and the Adoption of Family Planning in Rural Korea.
    Paper presented at the Fourth Annual Social Networks
    Colloquium, University of Hawaii, Honolulu.
Kim, T. I., J. A. Ross, and G. C. Worth (1972)  The
    Korean National Family Planning Program.  New York:
    Population Council.
Kinderman, C. R. (1969)  Perception and Source of
    Information:  Their Effect on Contraceptive Use in
    Taiwan.  Ph.D. dissertation, Department of Sociology,
    University of Michigan, Ann Arbor, Mich.
Kirk, D. (1971)  A new demographic transition?  Pp.
    123-147 in National Academy of Sciences, eds., Rapid
    Population Growth.  Baltimore, Md.:  The Johns
    Hopkins University Press.
Knodel, J. (1977)  Family limitation and the fertility
    transition:  Evidence from the age patterns of
    fertility in Europe and Asia.  Population Reports
    31:219-249.
Knodel, J. (1979)  From natural fertility to family
    limitation:  The onset of fertility transition in a
    sample of German villages.  Demography 16:493-521.
Knodel, J., and N. Debavalya (1978)  Thailand's
    reproductive revolution.  International Family
    Planning Perspectives and Digest 4:34-50.
Knodel, J., and E. van de Walle (1979)  Lessons from the
    past:  Policy implications of historical fertility
    studies.  Population and Development Review 5:217-245.
Korean Institute for Family Planning (1978)  Statistics
    on Population and Family Planning in Korea, Vol. 1.
    Seoul:  Korean Institute for Family Planning.
Laing, J. E. (1979)  Coordination of Outreach and Clinic
    Activities.  1978 Community Outreach Survey,
    Preliminary Report No. 2.  University of the
    Philippines Population Institute, Manila.
Lee, S.-B. (1977)  System Effects on Family Planning
    Innovativeness in Korean Villages.  Unpublished Ph.D.
    dissertation.  Department of Population Planning,
    University of Michigan, Ann Arbor, Mich.

Leibenstein, H. (1957) *Economic Backwardness and Economic Growth*. New Haven, Conn.: Yale University Press.

Lesthaeghe, R. (1977) *The Decline of Belgian Fertility, 1800-1970*. Princeton, N.J.: Princeton University Press.

Livi-Bacci, M. (1971) *A Century of Portuguese Fertility*. Princeton, N.J.: Princeton University Press.

Livi-Bacci, M. (1977) *A History of Italian Fertility during the Last Two Centuries*. Princeton, N.J.: Princeton University Press.

Mauldin, W. P. (1975) Assessment of national family planning programs in developing countries. *Studies in Family Planning* 6:30-31.

Mauldin, W. P. (1978) Patterns of fertility decline in developing countries, 1950-75. *Studies in Family Planning* 9:75-84.

Mauldin, W. P., and B. Berelson (1978) Conditions of fertility decline in developing countries, 1965-75. *Studies in Family Planning* 9:90-147.

Miller, W. B., and R. K. Godwin (1977) *Psyche and Demos: Individual Psychology and the Issues of Population*. New York: Oxford University Press.

Miller, W. B., and P. E. Hollerbach (1979) A Model for the Cross-Cultural Study for Marital Fertility Regulation. Paper presented at the annual meeting of the Population Association of America, Philadelphia, Pa.

Mosk, C. (1978) Rural-Urban Differentials in Swedish Fertility, 1880-1960. Working Papers in Economics, No. 123. Department of Economics, University of California, Berkeley.

Myers, G. D., and J. M. Roberts (1968) A technique for measuring preference for family size and composition. *Eugenics Quarterly* 15:164-172.

Nortman, D., and E. Hofstatter (1980) *Population and Family Planning Programs: A Compendium of Data through 1978*, 10th ed. New York: Population Council.

Palmore, J. A. (1967) The Chicago snowball: A study of the flow of influence and diffusion of family planning information. Pp. 272-363 in D. J. Bogue, eds., *Sociological Contributions to Family Planning Research*. Chicago: Community and Family Study Center, University of Chicago.

Palmore, J. A. (1968) Awareness sources and stages in the adoption of specific contraceptives. *Demography* 5:960-972.

Palmore, J. A. (1976)  The target that talks back: Personal communication and population research.  Pp. 51-55 in S. H. Newman and V. D. Thompson, eds., Population Psychology:  Research and Education Issues.  Washington, D.C.:  U.S. Government Printing Office.

Palmore, J. A., and R. Freedman (1969)  Perceptions of contraceptive practice by others:  Effects on acceptance.  Pp. 224-240 in R. Freedman and J. Y. Takeshita, eds., Family Planning in Taiwan:  An Experiment in Social Change.  Princeton, N.J.: Princeton University Press.

Palmore, J. A., P. M. Hirsch, and A. B. Marzuki (1971) Interpersonal communication and the diffusion of family planning in West Malaysia.  Demography 8:411-425.

Palmore, J. A., M. J. Furlong, F. X. Buchmeier, I. H. Park, and L. M. Souder (1976)  Family planning opinion leadership in Korea:  1971.  Studies in Family Planning 7:349-356.

Palmore, J. A., C. K. Cheong, K. C. Ahn, S. K. Park, and H. Y. Kwon (1977)  Interpersonal family planning communication in Korea 1976:  Opinion leadership, home visits by family planning workers, and population problem groups.  Pp. 79-105 in D. W. Han, C. K. Cheong, and K. C. Ahn, eds., Reducing Problem Groups in Family Planning IE&C Program.  Seoul: Korean Institute for Family Planning.

Pardthaisong, T. (1978)  The Recent Fertility Decline in the Chiang Mai Area in Thailand.  Paper No. 47. Honolulu:  East-West Population Institute.

Perkin, G., and L. Saunders (1979)  Extending Contraceptive Use.  PIACT Papers No. 5.  Seattle, Wash.:  Program for the Introduction and Adapation of Contraceptive Technology.

Placek, P. J. (1974-75)  Direct mail and information diffusion:  Family planning.  Public Opinion Quarterly 38:548-561.

Population Council (1978)  A Chronicle of the First Twenty-Five Years 1952-1977.  New York:  Population Council.

Preston, S. H. (1975)  The changing relation between mortality and level of development.  Population Studies 29:231-248.

Repetto, R. (1977)  Correlates of field-worker performance in the Indonesian family planning program:  A test of the homophily-heterophily hypothesis.  Studies in Family Planning 8:19-21.

Retherford, R. D. (1979) A theory of rapid fertility decline in homogeneous populations. Studies in Family Planning 10:61-67.

Retherford, R. D. (1980) Modeling Sudden and Rapid Fertility Decline. Working Paper No. 1. Honolulu: East-West Population Institute.

Richards, W. D., Jr. (1975) A Manual for Network Analysis (Using the NEGOPY Network Analysis Program). Mimeo. Institute for Communication Research, Stanford University, Stanford, Calif.

Roberto, E. L. (1975) Strategic Decision-Making in a Social Program: The Case of a Family Planning Diffusion. Lexington, Mass.: Lexington Books.

Rockefeller Foundation (1977) Bellagio IV Population Conference. New York: Rockefeller Foundation.

Rogers, E. M. (1962) Diffusion of Innovations. New York: The Free Press.

Rogers, E. M. (1973) Communication Strategies for Family Planning. New York: The Free Press.

Rogers, E. M., and D. L. Kincaid (1981) Communication Networks: Toward a New Paradigm for Research. New York: The Free Press.

Rogers, E. M., and F. F. Shoemaker (1971) Communication of Innovations: A Cross-Cultural Approach. New York: The Free Press.

Rogers, E. M., H. J. Park, K. K. Chung, S.-B. Lee, W. S. Puppa, and B. A. Doe (1976) Network analysis of the diffusion of family planning innovations over time in Korean villages: The role of Mothers' Clubs. Pp. 253-276 in G. C. Chu, S. A. Rahim, and D. L. Kincaid, eds., Communication for Group Transformation in Development. Honolulu: East-West Communication Institute, East-West Center.

Salas, R. M. (1979) International Population Assistance: The First Decade, A Look at the Concepts and Policies Which Have Guided the UNFPA in its First Ten Years. New York: Pergamon Press.

Schramm, W. (1971) Communication in Family Planning. Reports on Population/Family Planning, No. 7. New York: Population Council.

Schrimshaw, S. C. M. (1978) Infant mortality and behavior in the regulation of family size. Population and Development Review 4:383-403.

Shah, N. M., and J. A. Palmore (1979) Desired family size and contraceptive use in Pakistan. International Family Planning Perspectives 5:143-149.

Shannon, C. E., and W. Weaver (1949)  The Mathematical Theory of Communication. Urbana, Ill.: University of Illinois Press.

Sun, T. H., H. S. Lin, and R. Freedman (1978)  Trends in fertility, family size preferences, and family planning practice: Taiwan, 1961-76. Studies in Family Planning 9:54-70.

Terhune, K. W., and S. Kaufman (1973)  The family size utility function. Demography 10:399-418.

Thomas, W. I., and D. S. Thomas (1928)  The Child in America: Behavior Problems and Programs. New York: Alfred A. Knopf.

United Nations (1972)  The Role of Voluntary Organizations in National Family Planning Programmes. Asian Population Studies Series No. 13. Bangkok: Economic Commission for Asia and the Far East.

United Nations (1976)  Role of Surveys and Studies in Family Planning Programme Management and Development. Asian Population Studies Series No. 24.  Bangkok: Economic Commission for Asia and the Far East.

United Nations (1977)  Report on a Comparative Study on the Administration of Family Planning Programmes in the ESCAP Region:  Organizational Determinants of Performance in Family Planning Services.  Asian Population Studies Series No. 29.  Bangkok:  Economic and Social Commission for Asia and the Pacific.

United Nations Fund for Population Activities (UNFPA) (1979)  Consultation on Population Assistance Co-ordination, Geneva.  New York:  United Nations Fund for Population Activities.

van de Walle, E., and J. Knodel (1980)  Europe's fertility transition:  New evidence and lessons for today's developing world.  Population Bulletin 34(6).

Westoff, C. F. (1978)  The unmet need for birth control in five Asian countries.  Family Planning Perspectives 10:173-181.

Westoff, C. F., N. Goldman, S.-E. Khoo, and M. K. Choe (1980)  The recent demographic history of sterilization in Korea.  International Family Planning Perspectives 6:136-145.

World Bank (1972)  Population Planning:  Sector Working Paper.  Washington, D.C.:  World Bank.

Part II
# FERTILITY DECISION-MAKING PROCESSES

# Chapter 9

# Fertility Decision-Making Processes: A Critical Essay

PAULA E. HOLLERBACH

Previous chapters have examined the elements involved in fertility decisions--the demand for children, the supply of children, and the costs of fertility regulation. The assumption has been that these elements affect fertility because individuals somehow take all of them into account; however, the manner in which this actually transpires is a relatively new focus of inquiry. Individual percep- tions, motivations, and decision processes have been increasingly investigated because they are assumed to have predictive power in explaining fertility behavior. In developing nations, greater use of effective fertility regulation promotes a closer association between fertil- ity preferences and actual behavior; within various developed nations, a narrowing of demographic differen- tials in fertility also means that personal preferences have become more important.

This essay reviews insights on this issue provided in other chapters, and examines how these insights comple- ment one another. In addition, aspects of the fertility decision-making process not directly addressed elsewhere will be examined. The outline of the essay is as follows. Models of fertility decision making require that the individual, couple, or household first forms perceptions of the major elements in the decision. These perceptions of supply (fecundity, child survival), demand (the value of children, sex preferences), and fertility regulation costs (characteristics of contraceptive methods, conse- quences of use) may differ from objective assessments. The first section of the essay reviews information on these perceptions, providing more detail about supply and alternatives to fertility to complement the discussions of perceptions of demand and perceptions of regulation costs in other chapters. The second section identifies various decision types such as nonrational decisions, ambivalent decisions, and passive and active decisions. In the third section, various decision rules and decision-making models that represent the way individuals combine and weigh factors in decisions are examined. In connection with this discussion, limitations on rational models are covered. The fourth section discusses the more elaborate sequential model for fertility decisions. The fifth section discusses how the perspectives of the two spouses as well as those of other family and nonfamily members are weighed in a decision. The sixth section, finally, considers differences in the decision process between pretransition and posttransition societies.

## PERCEPTIONS OF SUPPLY, DEMAND, AND FERTILITY REGULATION COSTS

### Perceptions of Supply

The perceived supply of children depends on a woman's assessment of her fecundity and of the chances of infant and child survival. With regard to perceived fecundity, individuals may deny susceptibility to pregnancy, recognize it as a statistical possibility but not a personal probability, or perceive direct susceptibility. Women appear more likely to err on the side of perceiving higher rather than lower fecundity: in comparison with studies of sterility in natural fertility populations at various ages, self-reports in survey data appear to considerably understate the true proportions sterile (Nortman, 1982). For instance, in a recent analysis of nine Contraceptive Prevalence Surveys conducted by Westinghouse Health Systems in Bangladesh, Colombia, Costa Rica, the Republic of Korea, rural and urban sectors of Mexico, and Thailand, reported infecundity among married women of reproductive age ranged from 6 percent in Costa Rica to 9 percent in South Korea (Nortman, 1982). Summary reports from selected World Fertility Survey (WFS) countries indicate that the proportion of women in union reporting that they think themselves and their husbands physically incapable of having a child ranges from 5 percent to 15 percent and of course varies by the age composition of the sample. In a reinterview following the Indonesian WFS, the reliability of this measure was assessed. Given the total proportion of women who provided similar responses in both surveys, the question appears to be reliable. However, the relatively high proportions of women for whom no answer was available (17-22 percent), or who could not respond to the question (11 percent), indicate problems of validity or reluctance to acknowledge subfecundity (MacDonald et al., 1978).

Fecundity is difficult to measure; it is influenced by heredity, health, age, and regularity of the menstrual cycle, and assessments must also take account of the complicating effects of frequency and regularity of intercourse, duration of postpartum breastfeeding, spontaneous intrauterine mortality, induced abortion, postpartum infecundability, and sterilization. Women appear to base their judgments of fecundity on various criteria. In developed countries, the most significant criterion appears to be the time required to achieve conception. Other criteria include the pattern of the menstrual cycle and flow; the occurrence of a conception while using contraception, or the failure to conceive while not using contraception; maternal childbearing history; and current health conditions or medical tests (Miller, 1981b). In developing countries, there is very little research on the topic; one rural Mexican study suggests that two significant criteria are the time required to achieve conception and number of live births. In addition, variation in beliefs on the interrelationship between exposure to intercourse and the probability of pregnancy were also reported for this sample (Shedlin and Hollerbach, 1981). The pattern of the menstrual cycle also appears to be significant, since it offers regular reassurance of nonpregnancy and indicates that the body is eliminating "impure" blood, a condition perceived as necessary for the maintenance of health; the latter belief is more widespread among older, less-educated, and rural women in the ten-country investigation conducted by the World Health Organization (WHO Task Force, 1981).

The second component of perceived supply is perceived infant and child survival. If mortality is viewed as high, couples must have more births in order to have the expectation of attaining any desired family size; on the other hand, higher perceived mortality may reduce the demand for surviving children, e.g., through increasing the costs of attaining a particular surviving family size. Perceptions are typically measured by asking respondents to assess the number surviving to a specific age (such as 15) among a hypothetical number of births, sometimes the average for women in the area. Analyses relating perceptions to actual fertility behavior are scant and difficult to interpret. As Bongaarts and Menken note (in these volumes), it may also make sense to assess the number of surviving adult children (or sons specifically) when parents reach age 45 (indicating the supply of children as insurance against economic risks) and the number of surviving adult children when parents reach age 65 (indicating the supply of children for old age security). Respondents have not been asked such questions, however.

Perceptions of lower child survival have some positive effect on fertility preferences and behavior in Taiwanese townships (Heer and Wu, 1975, 1978), although research conducted in Guatemala, where mortality is higher, shows no association between perception of child survival and fertility desires (Pebley et al., 1979). It is difficult to separate the influence of this factor from that of many other influences on fertility desires and behavior, such as mother's age, parity, education, residence, and access to health services (see Heer, in these volumes). Moreover, assessments of general probabilities of survival may differ from personal assessments of risk.

It might be expected that perceptions of general survival levels would be greatly affected by the experience of losing a child. However, those who had and had not lost children showed no sharp differences in the perceived value of children or family-size preferences in a study conducted among Javanese and Sundanese parents in Indonesia (Darroch et al., 1981). Part of the reason may have been that relatively large numbers of couples had experienced child loss. Differentials in perceptions that may affect fertility may occur only as child loss becomes rarer within the society. That expectations of high mortality can be especially persistent despite change in actual probabilities is suggested by a study of Australian, Greek, and Italian parents in Sydney, Australia (Callan, 1980). Greek parents were the most concerned about the possible death of an only child and the concomitant loss of parental status; their fears about child loss were related to the high incidence of child mortality they had witnessed during their youth in rural Greece, rather than to their experiences in Australia.

## Perceptions of Demand

Perceptions are also important with regard to demand for children. Various approaches have been undertaken to measure perceptions of demand, including direct measures of fertility desires and preferences; unfolding theory, especially for assessment of family-size ranges and sex preferences; research on the value of children; and attitude scaling to measure the subjective utility or expected value of children.

Survey responses on these measures are available for a wide variety of less developed country settings, and the evidence available suggests that these measures of perceptions are related to fertility behavior. Fertility desires are related to actual fertility (see McClelland, in these volumes; Pullum, in these volumes); value-of-children indices predict fertility to some extent and vary according to the level of economic development and modernization within a country (Arnold et al., 1975; Fawcett, in these volumes). Perceptions of the value of children also differ by social class and parity, as do the weights parents attach to these costs and benefits in the process of decision making (Bulatao, 1979a, 1979b, 1981). Perceptions regarding the importance of sons and daughters also affect demand. Attitude scaling measures of the subjective utility or the expected value of children satisfactorily predict actual fertility behavior or intentions, although most of the research, to be reviewed in a later section of this chapter, has been conducted within developed-nation contexts. Finally, research has focused on a more difficult topic, estimation of the actual economic costs and benefits of children, primarily the labor contribution of children to parents within rural households.

Despite the varied research already undertaken on perceptions of demand, a few areas related to the perceived and objective utility of children require further clarification and evaluation. Investigation of perceptions of economic benefits and costs, especially educational costs, as well as socioemotional costs and benefits within economically homogeneous and heterogeneous settings, would be a useful complement to research on the actual economic contributions of children. Variation in perceptions among husbands and wives, and by parity and socioeconomic status, should be examined. Although couples in the least developed nations show strong awareness of the economic values of children and couples in developed-country settings stress socioemotional values, noneconomic benefits no doubt exist at all stages of development, and are associated with alternative sources of status for women (see Oppong, in these volumes).

Similarly, parental expectations of old age support
from surviving children in less developed nations have
been substantiated.  However, data are scant on the
salience of such concerns among couples during their
childbearing years, and on the actual contributions of
children to old age support, such as financial aid, social
exchange, and intergenerational coresidence.  The possible
associations between perceptions of old age support and
perceptions of spouse and child survival to various ages
should be investigated.  Institutional social security
systems, cooperatives, unions, and credit and savings
institutions, if implemented on a large scale, provide
couples with alternative investment strategies, and may
help to reduce but will not eliminate the economic value
of children as sources of old age security.  The impact
of such programs on changing perceptions of the economic
value of children needs to be examined (see Lindert, in
these volumes).  Finally, there is limited evidence on
actual parental reliance on children as a source of income
when usual earnings are reduced because of environmental
events, widowhood, or loss of land or employment, and the
extent to which perceptions of such risks influence fertility behavior (Cain, 1981; Potter, in these volumes).
The opposite situation--perceptions of improved living
conditions and of the probability of social mobility, and
their impact on fertility--also requires investigation.

## Perceptions of Fertility Regulation Costs

The motivation to space births or terminate childbearing
depends not only on perceptions of supply and demand but
also on the perceived characteristics and costs of fertility regulation methods.  Research on the costs of
fertility regulation includes both subjective costs
(normative and psychic costs, fears of serious and minor
side effects) and objective costs (time, distance, and
monetary costs involved in acquiring knowledge and access
to fertility regulation and actual side effects associated with methods).  Perceived costs of fertility
regulation are more salient within less developed nations
in decisions to initiate and continue contraception, but
are amenable to change.

Monetary, time, and health costs of contraception in
both developing and developed nations are examined by
Schearer (in these volumes).  Although monetary costs can
have a significant effect on levels of use in developing

nations, these should be offset by active public family planning programs, which considerably reduce the level of cost. Unfortunately however, data assessing this impact are extremely limited, inconclusive, and sometimes contradictory. Data on the impact of perceptions of costs are even more limited, but demonstrate that, in some societies, couples would prefer to pay moderate charges for contraceptives than receive them free (see Schearer, in these volumes).

Travel time, means of transport, and distance costs involved in the acquisition of supplies have recently been investigated through World Fertility Survey data measuring perceptions of these costs. Whereas assessments of time of travel can be obtained from most respondents, only a minority can estimate distance (Rodriguez, 1977). There is substantial evidence that limited availability of contraceptive supplies results in high fertility. Rodriguez (1978), analyzing the effect of perceived availability and accessibility of family planning services (i.e., knowledge of a nearby outlet), reported that current use of effective contraception among exposed women who desired no more children increased as perceived accessibility of services increased in Colombia, Korea, and Malaysia, but not in Costa Rica, where unmet need was uniformly low. However, for Colombia, Korea, and Malaysia, the effect of perceived accessibility was greatly reduced after controlling for various sociodemographic variables, especially place of residence.

With regard to health costs and benefits of contraception, all methods provide at least partial protection against pregnancy, thereby reducing the incidence of potential adverse effects of pregnancy and childbirth, especially in developing nations. However, these potential benefits must be weighed against the major and minor side effects associated with the methods available for use. In developing nations, objective information on serious side effects or health hazards appears very limited; however, fears and misconceptions regarding serious and especially minor side effects strongly affect contraceptive use, selection of particular methods, and therefore fertility. Approximately one-third of women in these countries who discontinue methods report minor side effects as the underlying reason, and drop-out rates far exceed those in developed nations. Attributes of contraceptives which are most significant in method selection are effectiveness, absence of side effects, desired duration of action, and length of time until return of fertility; convenience of use and route of administration are of far less importance (Marsella et al., 1979; WHO Task Force, 1980). Among a variety of contraceptive side effects, alterations in menstrual bleeding patterns are particularly significant, since they are associated with many different types of contraceptives. The impact of misinformation and fears associated with minor side effects is likely to decline with the diffusion of information and services, a topic which should be empirically investigated. However, the significance of serious objective health hazards is likely to increase as levels of information and education increase (see Schearer, in these volumes).

Frameworks relating to the various factors determining acceptability of fertility regulation methods have been formulated (Freedman and Berelson, 1976). Despite these categorizations, systematic integrative models of normative and psychic costs have not been devised and tested in cross-cultural investigations. In standard classifications, these factors are merely grouped together as personal reasons for method discontinuation, a category including personal, social, or cultural factors, as well as discontinuation for a desired pregnancy. The categorization does not provide sufficient data on the sociocultural and psychological reasons for termination.

Based on a variety of studies, Bogue (in these volumes) attempts to estimate the prevalence of a cost (proportion of the population of reproductive age that experiences a particular cost) and the impact of a cost (the degree of association between the cost and contraceptive use). He concludes that major normative and psychic costs of contraception include fears of major and minor side effects of methods, anxiety over contraceptive failure, and the need to discuss contraception with the spouse. Still other costs less well documented in the literature, such as the threat to moral and religious beliefs, questions about the legitimacy of contraceptive use, insecurity regarding family status, and fear of infant deaths are moderately important. Still other costs less well documented in the literature, such as the threat to harmony in the extended family, discord between spouses, interference with sexual relationships, shyness at a gynecological examination, and the perceived risks of contraceptive failure are comparatively minor, neither very prevalent nor very significant in affecting contraceptive practice.

However, in the absence of systematic data on psychic
and normative costs associated with contraceptive nonuse
and discontinuation, these conclusions must be considered
tentative. The prevalence and impact of normative and
psychic costs will differ widely among different sociodemographic groups and have important programmatic
implications for service delivery. The impact of these
costs should be assessed not only by comparing users and
nonusers but also, separately, among those who desire to
space or terminate fertility, but are not using or do not
intend to use a method; those who have previously used
but have discontinued methods, especially after a short
period of time; and those who are potential acceptors of
contraception but are not currently exposed due to pregnancy or breastfeeding. The impact of normative and
psychic costs of contraception should be higher within
these subgroups.

Data on the perceived costs of abortion are much more
limited and pertain to women who report previous use, or
small samples of abortion patients, rather than to all
women of reproductive age (David, in these volumes).
Although psychic costs are difficult to assess, U.S. data
demonstrate that, for the vast majority of women receiving abortions, feelings of guilt and depression, when
noted, are mild and transitory. In developing nations,
where abortion is typically illegal, use is seriously
underreported, but appears related to women's exaggerated
fears of contraceptive side effects, their knowledge of
service providers, the accessibility of these providers,
the methods they utilize in abortion procedures, and the
financial costs (David, in these volumes). Thus, accessibility, monetary, and health factors seem to be associated with abortion use in developing countries. Data
on normative and psychic costs of abortion in developing
nations are too scant to warrant even tentative conclusions, although the high level of underreporting is
indicative of the normative costs where abortion is not
legalized.


## Alternatives to Fertility

Fertility decisions, like all other decisions, involve
choices among alternative behaviors. Some psychosocial
models have incorporated perceptions of trade-offs between
perceived costs and benefits of children and perceived
costs and benefits of contraception and abortion, as well

as perceived fecundity (Hass, 1974; Luker, 1975; Steinhoff et al., 1971). But relatively few psychosocial models have examined perceptions of alternatives to fertility for the attainment of these values, especially in developing nations, in part due to the relative scarcity of such avenues. Psychosocial models which have included this dimension have been tested exclusively within the U.S.

One theoretical schema does incorporate alternatives: motivations for and against childbearing are seen as determined by the value of children, alternatives to children which fulfill the same values, the costs incurred (what must be lost or sacrificed) in order to obtain these values, and barriers and facilitators (Hoffman and Hoffman, 1973). Costs include factors like consumption expenditures (education, food, clothing, and medical care), the reduction in family savings and alternative investments, and foregone opportunities for female labor force participation. Barriers and facilitators include such factors as socioeconomic status, community norms, and work and time demands.

As noted by Oppong (in these volumes), high fertility is associated with the economic values provided by children for women. These benefits include child labor, household assistance, old age security, a guarantee of the husband's continued economic support, and strengthened ties with kin who contribute to labor-intensive production. Children also provide political status within the community: they ensure kinship ties, and may increase women's familial influence and power, including their control over their own labor, marital alliances, and future fertility. Children can provide social status because of the approval, prestige, and deference accorded to marriage and motherhood, leading to greater seniority within the domestic group and extended family. Finally, psychic satisfaction can be obtained through the companionship and love of children.

All of these maternal role rewards are hypothesized to be associated with pronatalist role expectations and behaviors. The expansion of alternative role rewards, or other opportunities for women, as well as men, to obtain economic, political, and social status and psychic satisfaction and pleasure, depend upon the level of economic development and the social constraints imposed by sex roles. These constraints in turn involve required allocations of time and material resources to different roles, imposing opportunity costs in time and money on childcare.

*occupation — status.*

   The shift of women's activities from domestic to public
spheres can be attained through the provision of a variety
of alternative sources of status. Employment opportunities, in particular, can provide alternative sources of
economic and political status (previously provided by
children and) increase motivation for fertility regulation.
The perceived opportunity costs of children at later
stages of development can also be raised by an increase
in female wage rates concomitant with rising educational
attainment; reduction in the labor substitutability of
children; and greater childcare constraints (due to
reduced reliance on the extended family and siblings for
childcare, the higher cost of childcare substitutes, and
greater equality in the division of domestic labor) (see
Standing, in these volumes).

   Aside from occupational opportunities, Oppong (in
these volumes) suggests that greater political and social
status and psychic satisfaction can be provided through
greater leisure time to pursue education, training, and
personal pleasure, possibilities for community and civic
participation, and opportunities for individual recrea-
tion outside the home. When childcare is incompatible
with them, these alternative sources of status will raise
the perceived opportunity costs of childcare and increase
motivation to regulate fertility. Finally, within the
home, relative freedom from the constraints of kin, relatives, and spouse; shifts in the division of labor between
husband and wife, with greater sharing of domestic labor;
and development of companionate marital relationships can
also reduce constraints on the selection of alternative
sources of status, and provide psychic satisfaction and
pleasure as well.

   The key concern is the alternatives couples perceive
for obtaining the rewards that children provide, or
aspects of modernization that make such alternatives more
attractive by stimulating perceptions of higher time and
money costs of children and childcare. The absence of
such alternatives within developing nations is both the
primary cause and an effect of high fertility. The impact
of such forces within communities can be assessed through
psychosocial studies which gather data on the perceived
costs and benefits of children, actual role behavior
(best gathered through time-budget studies), preferred
sex-role behavior, and perceived constraints to alternative sex roles.

   Psychosocial research on the topic is limited and
inferential, offering partial support for the relation-

ship between alternative sources of status, the value of
children, and fertility regulation. Using data from
Mexico City and Ankara, Turkey, Bagozzi and Van Loo
(1978) have tested with some success the proposition that
socioeconomic variables (normative social structure and
stratification) and economic constraints (income and
price) influence fertility through their impact on
social-psychological processes within the family. These
processes include the nature of husband-wife interaction
(power, conflict, decision making, and marital satisfaction), which in turn determines family size. Research by
Scanzoni (1975) in the urban United States also supports
the proposition that more modern egalitarian family attitudes and interaction are related to lower demand for
children. Another study using national survey data of
the value of children to American couples in the childbearing years (Hoffman et al., 1978) tested the hypothesis
that the presence of few alternative means for satisfying
a particular need would increase the value of children
for satisfying this need. This hypothesis did receive
some limited empirical support from an examination of
subgroup differences, although intensity of need was not
considered in the analysis. For instance, low socioeconomic groups with less access to economic resources
attached more importance to economic utility values than
did others. Women with traditional sex-role definitions
valued adult status more than others, and unemployed
women gave more importance to fun and stimulation as a
perceived value of children.

The complexity of perceptions of supply, demand, and
regulation costs, and the degree to which they often
differ from objective assessments and are influenced by
alternatives to fertility, suggest the importance of
considering the decision process as both psychological
and social, rather than simply a balancing of economic
utilities. Perceptions partly determine the types of
decisions that are made, a topic that is considered next.


## TYPES OF FERTILITY DECISIONS

One approach to studying fertility decisions is to create
typologies of decisions. The more important distinctions
are discussed here. Nondecisions may be said to occur
when a couple does not foresee that pregnancy results
from particular actions, misperceives their fecundity, or
lacks knowledge of fertility regulation. Passive

decisions take place when restricted perceptions and
particular habits or customs, institutionalized within
the culture, reinforce the childbearing behavior functional for group survival or growth and leave individuals
with little perceived choice (Hull, in these volumes).
An alternative characterization of both situations is to
say such couples are in a preawareness stage of decision
making (Miller and Godwin, 1977); though they make decisions relating to marriage, breastfeeding, sexual relations, and infant and childcare that indirectly affect
fertility, decisions directly relating to fertility goals
are precluded by lack of knowledge. Another interpretation of passive decision making posits a situation in
which individuals or couples act according to internalized
social norms regarding appropriate minimum family size or
act on the basis of their assumptions about partners'
fertility desires. In such situations, the benefits of
childbearing are socially reinforced, internalized and
recognized, but the relative costs and benefits of
childbearing and alternatives to childbearing are not
actively discussed and weighed until some later stage
(Hollerbach, 1980).

For more active decision making to take place, a
couple must be aware of a number of things: the probability of pregnancy, the possibility of regulating
fertility, and the fact that costs and benefits are
attached to the fertility outcome. Fertility may then be
said to be salient to the couple (Hass, 1974; Shedlin and
Hollerbach, 1981). Alternatively, the key factor in
active decision making may be seen as the weakness of
external incentives or internalized motivations to bear
children. Individual perceptions of child costs and
benefits may then be considered and weighed against one
another and against alternatives to childbearing (Fawcett
et al., 1972). Active consideration of the consequences
of fertility behavior may result in a decision to regulate
fertility or to have additional children; however, it may
also result in an implicit decision to do nothing. In
this case, through the process called behavioral drift, a
series of small decisions may lead by default to an
unintended major decision. For instance, a series of
decisions to have unprotected intercourse may eventually
produce an unintended pregnancy (Neal and Grote, 1980).
Such decisions are sometimes characterized as ambivalent.
Ambivalence is most noted among the high proportions of
women who state that they do not want additional children
but are not practicing contraception. High ambivalence

about the probability or desirability of pregnancy, about
a sexual partner and couple communication, and about the
medical, social, and psychological implications of contraceptive use have been found in studies of unwanted pregnancy among adolescents and abortion patients in the U.S.
(Kantner and Zelnik, 1973; Kellerhals and Wirth, 1972;
Kerenyi et al., 1973); similar observations have been
made for multiparous Mexican women considering contraception (Shedlin and Hollerbach, 1981) and for Colombian
women considering abortion (Browner, 1979). Women feeling such ambivalence are also more likely to experience
failure when they do practice contraception (Jones et
al., 1980).

Decisions may also be nonrational if individuals act
against their better interests; regret over previous
decisions may be seen as indicating irrationality. When
one individual has the power to enforce a decision on
another, decision making may be termed coercive, although
even this behavior involves elements of choice. Also,
decisions can be categorized as joint if reached by two
or more individuals on the basis of accommodation, compromise, compliance, or mutual agreement, or unilateral
if made by one or more individuals in conflict with the
desires of another, either openly or surreptitiously
(Hollerbach, 1980).

## RULES AND MODELS FOR FERTILITY DECISIONS

Research on how individuals choose among alternative fertility behaviors and how they weigh the different perceptions involved has led some to propose simple rules and
more complex psychosocial models. Leibenstein (1981) has
proposed a hierarchy of rules for fertility decisions:
choice may be based on some ethic, or on some definition
of conventional behavior, or on partial calculation, or
on full calculation. The first two of these alternatives
will be considered together briefly, and then the second
two. More complex decision models generally assume some
degree of calculation. Among these, the most frequently
applied to fertility behavior--though mainly in the United
States--are subjective expected utility, expectancy x
value, and judgment-value-integration-choice models.

## Choice by Ethic or Conventional Behavior

In Leibenstein's (1981) hierarchy of decision rules, the
first two strategies of choice--on the basis of some
ethic and on the basis of some definition of conventional
behavior--are influenced by cultural or normative factors.
Recourse to either of these rules involves following
precedent, and allows the individual to avoid the effort
of continual decision making and monitoring of consequences. Fertility decisions that arise repeatedly, such
as those related to coital frequency or contraceptive
use, are likely to follow one of these rules (Hull, in
these volumes); those that are unique (such as age at
first coitus), infrequent (marriage), or regarded as
serious (abortion or infanticide) are more likely to
involve one of the other rules to be discussed next.

## Maximization of Utility and Satisficing

These two strategies have received the greatest attention
in the theoretical literature. Maximization of utility,
or full calculation in Leibenstein's terms, involves
comparing alternative strategies and selecting the best.
Satisficing, or partial calculation, involves selecting
some satisfactory alternative that meets minimum expectations or demands, though it may not be the best among
all possible options (Demeny, 1970; Leibenstein, 1981;
Simon, 1979). The focus in satisficing is not on absolute rationality, but on rationality given constraints on
information, time, and perceptions. The range of options
considered in satisficing may be limited for various
reasons. The individual may not consider options that
violate his or her image of family life, may exclude the
consideration of alternatives because of social pressure,
or may perceive certain limitations to the possibility of
upward mobility (McNicoll, 1980).

Although theories abound, only limited research exists
on the degree to which these two strategies are used, and
none of this research pertains to fertility behavior. In
a small-scale study involving comparative ratings of
films, Mills et al. (1977) found a tendency to use a
maximizing strategy in situations offering few alternative choices; satisficing was more prevalent in situations offering a larger number of options, when the task
of comparing those options was thought to be arduous or
possibly to exceed the limits of information processing,
and when choices were presented in sequential order.

## The Subjective Expected Utility Model

More complex decision models all assume calculation by individuals of the costs and benefits associated with childbearing and fertility regulation. In the subjective expected utility (SEU) model, consequences of behavior are assumed to vary according to their desirability or utility (or the degree to which they are expected to be liked or disliked) and their subjective probability (the perceived probability that they will actually result from the particular behavior). The SEU of a particular behavior is the sum across all relevant consequences of the products of desirability and subjective probability. SEU and behavior are reciprocally related: SEU determines when behavior occurs, and the behavior itself produces modifications in SEU through the incorporation of new consequences that were not originally expected, or through changes, based on actual experience, in the subjective probability and desirability associated with particular consequences; a modified SEU would then influence subsequent behavior (Edwards, 1954; Lee, 1971).

The theory has not been applied in developing countries. It has been applied in assessing American husbands' and wives' positive and negative birth planning values at different parities and the ability of this hierarchy of values to predict actual fertility within limited time periods (Beach et al., 1976; Townes et al., 1977). In the small sample studied, there were few pregnancies or attempts to become pregnant within a year among couples for whom no pregnancy was predicted by the SEU measure; among those for whom maximum SEU would be derived from having a child, approximately half reported a pregnancy attempt. Another investigation of sexual behavior among American adolescents (Bauman and Udry, 1981) also generally confirmed the SEU model. SEU scores were related to sexual behavior among both men and women; however, SEU scores did not completely explain racial differences in sexual intercourse among males.

## The Expectancy x Value Model

The expectancy x value model was originally developed by Fishbein (1972; also see Fishbein and Jaccard, 1973). It posits that behavioral intentions are determined by both attitudinal and normative variables; in the equation $BI = (\sum B_i A_i)w_1 + (\sum NB_i MC_i)w_2$, an individual's intention to

perform some behavior (BI) is a function of that individual's beliefs about the consequences of performing the
behavior ($B_i$) and the evaluation of these consequences
($A_i$), as well as his beliefs about what others think he
should do ($NB_i$) and his motivation to comply with those
others ($MC_i$). Empirically determined weights $w_1$ and $w_2$
reflect the relative importance of each component in the
determination of BI.

In empirical studies, behavioral intentions may be
represented by intentions to use contraception in general,
to use a particular method, or to have a child. Rating-
scale measures of beliefs ($B_i$ and $NB_i$) and values ($A_i$
and $MC_i$) are generally obtained, combined, and correlated
with measures of intentions to test the model. The first
sum of products corresponds to individual utilities,
whereas the second corresponds to social norms (Jaccard
and Davidson, 1976).

The Fishbein model has important limitations. The
consequences to be evaluated are not specified by the
model (Adler, 1979). Moreover, since multiplication is
required, the model assumes that ratings are on ratio
scales, which is seldom in fact the case (Schmidt, 1973).
Furthermore, the model assumes rational decision making
and maximization of utility, thus imposing a decisional
framework that may not be accurate. One advantage of the
approach, nevertheless, is its incorporation of a normative component to constrain individual choices.

The model has been used repeatedly in U.S. studies to
explain various family planning practices as well as the
demand for children (Cohen et al., 1978; Davidson et al.,
1976; Fishbein and Jaccard, 1973; Fisher et al., 1976;
Jaccard and Davidson, 1975; Werner et al., 1975).
Behaviors or intentions predicted with some success by
the model over fairly limited time spans (two or three
years) include having another child or a two-child family, using birth control pills, contraceptive purchases,
types of contraceptives chosen, and the acceptability of
actual and hypothetical male contraceptives.

Cross-cultural research based on the Fishbein model is
extremely limited. Davidson et al. (1976) compared an
American sample with two Mexican samples: college students and low-status women in Mexico City. Intentions to
have a two-child family, to use birth control pills, and
to have a child in the next two years (among the married
women) were predicted as well in the Mexican samples as
in the U.S. sample, the multiple correlation coefficients
ranging from 0.66 to 0.87. Interestingly, the attitu-

dinal component was the better predictor of intentions
for the U.S. and Mexican college samples, whereas the
normative component was the better predictor of intentions among the low-status Mexican women.  Thus, the
appropriate weights of the components of the model vary
from sample to sample.

Finally, some research indicates that this model is
less effective in predicting a behavior when the individual has no prior experience with that behavior; when the
behavior is not directly within the individual's control;
when the measure of intention is more abstract; and when
the interval between measurement of intention and behavior
is longer (Jaccard and Davidson, 1975; Davidson and
Jaccard, 1979).

### The Judgment-Valuation-Integration-Choice Model

The final model of the fertility decision-making process
consists of four major stages:  judgment, during which
the decision maker identifies the possible consequences
of a behavior; valuation, in which each perceived consequence is assigned some subjective value according to its
desirability; integration, in which the values of the
consequences are combined to form an overall evaluation
of the behavior; and choice, in which the individual
compares the overall evaluations of a number of behaviors
and selects the optimal behavior.  Many decisions will be
suboptimal because of errors in judgment.  Moreover, since
individual differences can exist at each stage of the
decision sequence, the same choice can result from different sets of beliefs, values, and integration rules
(McClelland, 1980).

In particular, integration rules are allowed to vary
across individuals.  Three main types of rules are
posited:  additive, in which the overall evaluation of
each alternative is the sum of the values attached to
each of its consequences; conjunctive/additive, in which
an individual eliminates all alternatives with some
unacceptable consequence and then evaluates the remaining
alternatives according to an additive model; and one-
consequence, in which the comparisons across behaviors
are based on only one consequence and respondents are
indifferent to all other consequences.

In a first test of the model, the framework has been
applied to clients of a U.S. family planning clinic

(Nickerson et al., 1981), who were asked about their judgments of three characteristics of contraceptive methods;
their preference orderings of alternative behaviors (to
provide integration rules), from which their evaluations
of the consequences were inferred; and their actual
choices, represented in rankings of birth control methods
from most to least preferred. The framework accurately
described the contraceptive decision-making process of 56
percent of the respondents able to complete all required
tasks. The largest group used the additive integration
rule, fewer used the conjunctive/additive rule, and a few
used the one-consequence rule. Errors in response were
attributed to factors such as the restricted set of
consequences being considered, lack of prior thought or
low salience of the issue to respondents, and difficulty
in understanding the task.

## Limitations to Rationality

Except for decisions by ethic or conventional behavior,
all the rules and models described involve some degree of
rationality. It is important to note various impediments
to rational decision making that may make particular
models less applicable.

First, the consequences or outcomes of actions are not
always known and sometimes cannot be taken into account.
For instance, under environments of high mortality, a
decision to terminate childbearing must be weighed against
the unknown possibilities of future widowhood or child
mortality. Possible loss of income due to environmental
factors may also produce a situation of unknown future
risks, and fertility regulation may therefore seem inappropriate (Cain, 1981); the use of fertility regulation
itself may have unknown associated health risks. Fertility decisions which cannot take all consequences into
account may in retrospect appear irrational.

Second, individuals differ in their ability to acquire
accurate information on probabilities (Pitz, 1980; Pitz
et al., 1980) and may inaccurately judge the likelihood
of different consequences (Tversky and Kahneman, 1974).
For instance, cultural differences have been noted in the
probability parents attach to having a son or a daughter;
these perceived probabilities can systematically deviate
from the true ones. When gender preference affects
fertility, these cultural variations in perceptions can
have some effect (McClelland and Hackenberg, 1978).

Similarly, individuals differ in their assessments of the probability and severity of side effects of fertility regulation methods and the efficacy of methods in preventing pregnancy (Bardwick, 1973; Miller, 1975). For instance, contraceptive use in Egypt is comparatively low among respondents who are unsure of or fatalistic about their ability to control family size (see Bogue, in these volumes). Actual experience and knowledge of recent occurrences among acquaintances have the greatest effects on these perceptions (Tversky and Kahneman, 1974). When the probability of contraceptive failure or side effects is assessed from acquaintances' experiences or by analogy to other types of health risks, predictable biases can result.

Third, collecting information on consequences and probabilities is time-consuming, and the value of the information may be outweighed by the costs of its collection, especially in developing nations (Meeker, 1980). Better-educated individuals or those with greater exposure to the mass media can more easily obtain accurate information on the costs of contraception. The less-educated may bear higher information costs. Information costs have important effects: the kind of information available prior to use affects satisfaction with and later perceptions of contraceptive methods and therefore continuation of use (WHO, 1977). Balanced information on the advantages and disadvantages of contraceptive methods and free choice among them also lead to different choices than when decisions are influenced by the preferences of clinic personnel (WHO Task Force, 1980).

Fourth, the decision-making process itself has other associated normative and psychic costs, such as the acknowledgment it requires of sexual activity, shyness associated with medical examination, the need to discuss family planning with the partner or with others, and fear of disclosure. These costs, discussed by Bogue (in these volumes), may also lead to suboptimal decisions, and are assumed to be a major psychic costs of fertility regulation in developing nations.

Fifth, fertility decisions may involve a mix of consequences, costs, and benefits that produces a situation of ambivalence. For instance, decisions to regulate fertility may be weighed against fears of abandonment, community censure, or familial discord (Shedlin and Hollerbach, 1981). Even when such consequences do not determine the decision, they can increase the individual's insecurity about it. Ambivalence and the absence of

clear-cut decisions may mean a failure to maximize utility
or may lead to the surreptitious practice of contraception, which also involves psychic costs associated with
risk taking.

Finally, the degree of rationality may depend on whose
perspective is being considered. Meeker (1980) contends
that marital fertility decisions generally attempt to
maximize the total reward to all members of the household.
Caldwell (in these volumes) cautions, however, that it
may be the living standard of the older generation or the
satisfaction of one member of the nuclear family, such as
the husband, that dominates decision making. The consequences of having several people involved in a decision
will be discussed further after consideration of another
complication in the application of the preceding rules
and models--the possibility that decisions on ultimate
fertility are made sequentially and are subject to
revision.

## SEQUENTIAL FERTILITY DECISIONS

Fertility decisions are linked to the life course. Each
birth may be influenced by a different set of motivational, cultural, and family conditions, and fertility
decision making therefore involves a complex series of
decisions over the life cycle. The sequential or successive decisions approach investigates this premise and
attempts to determine whether and how influences on fertility decisions change (Namboodiri, in these volumes).
In principle, the rules and models just described could
be applied sequentially to a series of fertility decisions, but the focus in that research has been on confirming the models rather than on using them to understand
changing decision patterns.

One critical way in which decision patterns may change
in the life course is in the impact of norms. Empirical
evidence indicates that there is widespread agreement
within and across societies on norms prescribing minimum
family size, but far less agreement on maximum norms
(Mason, in these volumes). Fertility plans and behavior
before a couple attains the norm may be determined
primarily by normative pressures; for those above the
floor, however, the absence of a maximum norm may mean
much greater individual discretion and more recourse to
specific cost-benefit calculations. For instance, middle-
class couples in a longitudinal U.S. study reported feel-

ing under pressure from family and friends in decisions to remain childless or to have only one child, but not in decisions about a second child (Miller, 1981b). There is conflicting evidence about this proposition, however (Bulatao and Fawcett, 1981), possibly because normative pressures are subtle and may not be recognized as such by those being influenced, or such pressures may simply be internalized and expressed as personal motivations; the institutional contexts of such pressures are complex and difficult to measure through survey interviews; and subgroups within a society may differ in their normative family-size thresholds (Namboodiri, in these volumes).

Changes in the influence of socioeconomic character- istics on fertility decisions across parities have been studied mainly with cross-sectional data from the United States. A number of these studies have consistently shown that permanent income has a positive effect on the propen- sity to have additional children at lower parities, but a negative effect at higher parities (Bulatao and Fawcett, 1981). The changing influence of other characteristics has also been investigated, with somewhat less consistent results (Namboodiri, in these volumes).

The revision of fertility plans is also of concern in the sequential approach. Namboodiri (in these volumes) suggests that implementation failures are the main cause, and attributes these largely to fecundity impairment, marital disruption, child loss, and differences between sex preferences and actual family composition. In addi- tion, he suggests, plan revision may be due to changes in the extrafamilial and familial contexts of reproduction. The former pertains to social and geographic mobility, and the latter to family living arrangements, the wife's extrafamilial involvements, and the marital power struc- ture. With few exceptions (Bulatao, 1981; Bulatao and Arnold, 1977), the research on sequential decision making has been undertaken in developed nations, and has not used longitudinal data.

## COMMUNICATION AND POWER IN DECISIONS

Having children requires two people, but they are not always equally involved in the fertility decision. This section examines how communication and the relative power of the spouses affect decisions. The most frequently investigated question in this area is how these factors affect decisions on family size; also considered in the

literature are the effects of communication and power on
contraception and abortion decisions (Beckman, in these
volumes). This section considers, finally, the roles
other people besides the couple play in fertility
decisions.

## Couple Communication and Fertility

The research on couple communication and fertility has
been handicapped by two problems: the measurement of
communication and the treatment of communication as
static (Beckman, in these volumes). First, within the
typical fertility survey, complex concepts such as
marital communication, communication on fertility-related
issues, and social power generally receive only cursory
attention. Research on communication has relied on
responses, usually the wife's, about general communication, previous discussion of family-size preferences or
fertility regulation, the frequency of discussion, or the
initiation of discussion. Spouse agreement on family-
size and family planning preferences, as reported in
various studies, may be based on discussion, simple
coincidence, or projection of individual preferences.
Research comparing husbands' and wives' responses is
limited, but studies using this approach indicate that
discussion is not used that extensively and that joint
fertility decisions do not predominate (Coombs and Chang,
1981; Coombs and Fernandez, 1978; Gadalla, 1978; Hill et
al., 1959; Yaukey et al., 1967).

On the second problem, the examination of the relationship between communication and fertility at one point in
time presents communication as static, rather than as a
dynamic process subject to change. Communication has
different meanings depending on its timing: in certain
situations, casual discussion may indicate the expectation of a large family or a lack of knowledge or inaccurate knowledge about fertility regulation and the
monetary and health costs of contraception. Communication may be difficult because of the sensitivity of the
topic, feelings of shyness or modesty, and fear of
infidelity or of challenging the husband's authority;
unilateral fertility regulation may then be more likely.
Unilateral use of fertility regulation is dependent in
part upon the relative autonomy of partners (number and
stability of relationships), the degree of economic
dependency in the relationship, and the availability of
such methods.

Communication may be absent for several reasons, but even in its absence there may still be agreement on fertility behavior. This may be the case, for instance, where unquestioned power is vested in one person and issues are therefore not discussed (Caldwell, in these volumes). Apparent agreement may actually mean that few family members are in a position to challenge the decision maker. If the decision is made not to control fertility, it may be very difficult to identify the decision maker in pretransition settings or in the early childbearing stage in transitional settings.

Where communication is present, on the other hand, the evidence supports the conclusion that it is positively related to contraceptive use and duration and effectiveness of use, and negatively related to the demand for children and fertility preferences (Beckman, in these volumes; Bogue, in these volumes). A few studies do suggest, however, that discussion follows rather than leads to contraceptive use, which may initially result from a unilateral decision making. Communication is assumed to lead to greater empathy and increase a couple's ability to act together to achieve goals. Thus it is not the mere occurrence of the communication, but the quantity, quality, content, and timing that are significant. The two most important determinants of the frequency of fertility discussions, in a U.S. study, are the length of time since the birth of the last child and how soon the next child is expected (Miller 1981b).

## Marital Power, Dominance, and Fertility

Studies of power and dominance are similarly handicapped by the superficiality of the measures employed; these typically rely on the wife's assessment of final decision-making power over aspects of family life, including finances, childrearing, and leisure time pursuits. The research on this topic may be reviewed from two perspectives: the effects of egalitarian decision making on fertility and the resolution of disgreement or conflict.

### Egalitarianism

One general hypothesis has been that egalitarian decision making, which allows the costs women bear to be weighed more heavily, influences fertility negatively through lowered demand for children and earlier and more effective use of contraception. As Hull notes (in these volumes), younger couples in developing nations tend to have more egalitarian decision styles than their elders (Coombs and Chang, 1981; Fox, 1975; Gupta, 1979). However, studying this relationship is complicated by possible reverse effects: having many children, particularly sons, may increase the wife's or the husband's authority (Beckman, in these volumes; Oppong, in these volumes). Another complication is that changes in power may occur over the life cycle that do not relate to fertility. Thus as age and marital duration may affect power distribution in ways that cloud the relationship between power and fertility.

Weak or nonsignificant relationships between decision-making power and contraceptive use are generally reported (Beckman, in these volumes). Even those studies reporting some relationship between male dominance and cumulative fertility, such as Hill et al. (1959), show only small correlations. However, much of the research to date (Hass, 1971; Hill et al., 1959; Liu and Hutchinson, 1974; Weller, 1968) refers to developing countries in which, at the time of the survey, coitus-dependent methods, requiring greater motivation and cooperation for use, were still comparatively common. Furthermore, the questions used to measure decision-making power are not highly correlated with one another (Hass, 1971), suggesting that negative findings may be due to inappropriate measures.

Another approach in this area is to determine the relative contributions of husbands' and wives' attributes in predicting specific reproductive behaviors; this has typically been done with cross-sectional U.S. data. Neal and Grote (1977) report that using both husbands' and wives' alienation scores predicted fertility better than using scores for each spouse alone, and that husbands' scores often predicted as well as wives'. Two-sex models are usually better predictors than one-sex models, but the differences are not great. Thus the majority of studies, although few, do not support the conclusion that adding data from husbands is worthwhile for investigations of fertility in the United States. It is typically reported that female-only models are better predictors than male-only models, especially for white U.S. couples (Fried and Udry, 1979; Fried et al., 1980). Townes et al. (1977), comparing the ability of wives', husbands', and both spouses' SEU scores to predict the occurrence of a pregnancy among well-educated white couples, reported

that a model using an average of wives' and husbands'
scores predicted about as well as wives' scores alone,
and that husbands' scores alone did not predict as well.
The influence and dominance of husbands and wives in
fertility decisions may also differ within subgroups of a
population, and be masked in aggregate comparisons (Fried
and Udry, 1979).

Namboodiri (in these volumes) also notes that there is
disagreement on whether marriages begin on an egalitarian
footing and evolve until each spouse is dominant in
selected domains, or whether most marriages begin as wife-
dominant but become egalitarian or husband-dominant later
in the life cycle. If either speculation is correct in a
given society, it is plausible to expect fertility decisions to be monopolized by the husband or the wife at
different stages in the life cycle. Fried and Udry (1979)
report that, among a sample of U.S. couples, wives'
preferences better predicted fertility outcomes than
husbands' preferences at parity one. At parities two and
over, wives' and husbands' preferences were about equally
important in predicting attempts to become pregnant.
Although this particular study indicates that parity-
specific models are somewhat better than all-parity
models, other research shows conflicting results (Fried
et al., 1980; Miller, 1981b).


Resolution of Disagreement and Conflict

Research in developing countries generally supports the
view that contraceptive use is more prevalent and continuous when the husband approves, particularly within
lower-class or less-educated subgroups (Beckman, in these
volumes). Husbands' approval is also related to communication between spouses about family planning and accounts
for discrepancies between wives' motivation for fertility
control and couples' contraceptive behavior (Card, 1978).
In the absence of disagreement or conflict, however, it
is difficult to tell whether approval by either spouse is
the determining factor in fertility decisions. Some
research therefore focuses specifically on conflict
situations.

The evidence reviewed by Beckman (in these volumes)
regarding whether husbands' or wives' views prevail in
situations of disagreement is contradictory. Beckman
attempts to reconcile the contradictions by hypothesizing
that profertility decisions are controlled by the husband

in high-fertility societies, and antinatal decisions are
dominated by the wife, who controls most methods of contraception, in lower-fertility settings.

By contrast, other research in transition and posttransition societies supports the influence of wives in
both pronatal and antinatal decisions. For instance,
Coombs and Chang (1981), analyzing follow-up data on
fertility over a four-year period, concluded that, in
cases of disagreement, the wife's attitude prevails,
especially if she holds stronger beliefs about the future
security and status to be derived from a large family and
from sons. A small-scale study of U.S. couples (Miller,
1981a) noted that, in situations of strong disagreement,
decisions were commonly postponed until the dissenting
spouse was ready for childbearing or a decision was made
against childbearing. Women were more influential than
men, tending to take a strong position with regard to
childbearing, either for it or against it; men tended to
be more analytic, more inclined to consider the costs and
benefits of children and the general effect that childbearing would have on their lives, thereby tending toward
greater neutrality or ambivalence. Men were also less
affected emotionally by failure to achieve conception. A
larger longitudinal U.S. study of reproductive decision
making, which showed that initial disagreement on decisions to have a first or second child was relatively
common, also found the majority of wives reporting that
they had been more influential than their husbands in the
decision to have children (Miller, 1981b).

Substantial disagreement about childbearing may be
settled in several ways. Using a recent theoretical
paradigm on bases of power (Hollerbach, 1980), Miller
(1981a) suggests that acquiescence by one spouse may be
justified as an attempt to avoid major marital problems
or avert divorce, or as an exercise in altruism, or as
acceptance of the legitimacy of the spouse's reasons; it
may also be rooted in emotional dependency on the partner.
Less frequently, Miller (1981a) notes, neither spouse
acquiesces, and one spouse may take unilateral action
(such as having a vasectomy or an abortion) or deliberately take risks while contracepting in order to have a
child.

Which spouse wins a disagreement may depend partly on
status differentials between the spouses. Differences in
age, education, and actual or potential earning power may
affect the influence the husband and the wife have over
fertility decisions. The research on the effects of

education, income, and female employment on fertility is
discussed in other chapters (Cochrane, in these volumes;
Mueller and Short, in these volumes; Standing, in these
volumes). However, there is little developing-country
research on the implications of status differentials
between spouses for relative power and for fertility
decisions.

## The Influence of Kin and Nonkin

Fertility decision making in pretransition societies need
not be the monopoly of the biological parents. Caldwell
(in these volumes) argues, in fact, that in such societies
the biological parents have little say; the older generation, who control patterns of production, the consumption
of food, medical care, and other items, and exchanges of
goods within the household, also control fertility. If
fertility is advantageous to these people, the interests
of the biological parents may be overridden, according to
Caldwell. However, little research exists to confirm the
applicability of Caldwell's view to different societies.

The influence of the elderly on fertility decisions
depends, obviously, on whether they survive. In pretransition societies, female survival is lower at all ages,
and elderly males are more likely to have influence. In
transitional societies, female survival is more likely
than male survival among the elderly, and the wife's
mother or mother-in-law may be more likely to exert influence. The influence of the elderly, which may be assumed
to be pronatalist, should be greater in rural areas, among
the landless or land poor, where patrilocal rather than
neolocal residence and patrilineality prevail, and when
the surviving children are few.

Decisions may also be influenced by other relatives or
by extrafamilial sources, including neighbors, peers,
community leaders, health professionals, and state authorities. Hull (in these volumes) notes three ways in which
such sources influence decisional style: by social consensus transmitted to the individual through socialization; by shared value judgments on the propriety of
fertility-related behavior and the imposition of sanctions; and by advice and counsel.

The influence of other individuals in fertility
decision making is difficult to corroborate through
survey research. As previously noted, social pressures
may simply become internalized and expressed as personal

motivations or preferences for minimum family sizes. In
addition, individuals may be reluctant to admit social
influence, especially pronatalist pressure or opposition
to fertility regulation; such admissions may reveal
familial conflict. Some urban studies indicate cases in
which kin as well as nonkin appear to exert minimal
influence; however, complementary data from rural areas
are unavailable. For instance, in a large-scale study of
urban Mexican men and women, nine out of ten men and three
out of four women who had discussed family planning with
their spouses reported no outside influence on the decision to use contraception (PROFAM-PIACT de Mexico, 1979).
The Value of Children study also reported that the majority of respondents in each country considered social pressure and the influence of moral and religious prescriptions as unimportant in relation to their fertility
preferences (Arnold et al., 1975; Bulatao, 1979a).

## THE FERTILITY TRANSITION AND DECISION MAKING

Much of the foregoing discussion has been based on
research in developed countries; comparable research on
fertility decision making in developing countries is
often lacking. Not surprisingly, there is little evidence on which to base a discussion of changes in fertility decision making in the course of the demographic
transition.

Hull (in these volumes) argues that the nature of the
decision process is related to the individual's interactions within his or her social setting. Societies
undergoing cultural change, particularly in family
relations, necessarily change in the way fertility
decisions are made. The resultant changes in fertility
behavior may be far greater than those expected as a
specific consequence of economic change. Conversely, it
is possible that fertility decision-making processes and
behavior remain relatively stable despite substantial
economic change.

Despite the lack of hard evidence, alternative views
of pretransition and posttransition fertility decisions
may be reviewed. These perspectives are contrasting and
highly generalized; their application to any specific
case requires much more elaboration than can be provided
here.

The first view is that there is no basic change in
decision making: in both settings, couples are conscious

of the economic consequences of childbearing and respond
essentially to these. Family-size preferences reflect
calculations of the potential exchanges between parents
and children, including costs and benefits that are not
strictly economic. Some degree of economic rationality
is applicable both before and after the transition. Caldwell (in these volumes) adopts this view in essence, in
his argument that the direction of the net transfers
between parents and children is primary, both before and
after the transition, in determining fertility. There
are further complications to Caldwell's view, however,
which will be discussed below. Also consistent in principle with the view that the basic features of decisions
do not change is Lindert's (in these volumes) review of
the empirical evidence on the economic value of children. Lindert focuses on the shift from time-supplying
to time-intensive children, and on the effects of rising
prices of staples and declining prices of luxury goods in
producing an initial increase and a subsequent decline in
the demand for children.

A second view is that there is some threshold before
which attitudinal inertia prevents any conscious individual control of family size and after which calculation
comes to underlie most fertility decisions. Until this
threshold has been passed, couples only regulate their
fertility in conformance with traditional rules of marriage, sexual relations, and breastfeeding, and do not
perceive the costs and benefits of children. In this
situation, fertility is affected by supply factors rather
than by explicit decisions. The threshold might be a
supply-demand crossroads (Easterlin, 1975), at which the
determinants of fertility change from the supply of
children to the demand for children. This threshold is
reached when the desired number of children declines
below the attainable number. Alternatively, the threshold might be seen as the point at which fertility regulation becomes salient (Hass, 1974; Shedlin and Hollerbach, 1981). Once couples are aware of the possibilities
for controlling fertility, fertility decisions may change
in character. Decisions before the threshold might be
characterized as nondecisions or passive decisions, or,
following Liebenstein (1981), as decisions governed by
ethic or conventional behavior. After the threshold,
more calculation may be involved.

Empirical research on this view is limited. For
traditional societies, some literature supports the
hypothesis that norms regarding family-size preferences

are less significant in regulating fertility than those regarding the proximate fertility variables, such as age at marriage and postpartum sexual taboos (Mason, in these volumes; Lee, 1977; Lesthaeghe, 1980). However, even in the least developed societies, couples show strong awareness of the economic and noneconomic benefits and costs of children (Fawcett, in these volumes), calling into question the assumption that decisions are entirely passive.

Part of Caldwell's argument (in these volumes) deserves elaboration as a third alternative view. Although Caldwell sees the basic nature of fertility calculations, rooted as they are in net transfers, as essentially unchanging, he also argues for other changes in the decision process. He sees change as taking place in the social relations underlying the economic transfers: family relations change in the direction of reduced age and sex differentiation, lowering the economic value of children and encouraging fertility regulation. In developing nations, he sees such changes in family relations as occurring through the direct influence of Western missionaries and Westernized administrators, new elites, media, and education systems. He argues further that the identity of the decision makers changes, from the older generation to the couple themselves.

None of these views of the linkage between the transition and decision processes has much empirical support so far.


CONCLUSION


Empirical research on fertility decision-making processes offers alternative perspectives on how the supply of children, demand for children, and costs of fertility regulation are perceived and weighed by individuals. However, few studies have examined these perceptions simultaneously or included perceptions of alternative sources of the economic, political, status, and psychic satisfactions provided by large families. Research on the supply of children (perceived fecundity and child survival) is extremely limited, especially in developing nations. Similarly, systematic data collection on the prevalence and impact of normative and psychic costs of contraception and abortion has not been undertaken. In contrast, there is much more research on the costs and benefits of children and the monetary, time, and health costs of fertility regulation.

Analysis of the rules of decision making, or the way individuals combine and weigh the consequences of alternative behaviors, has relied quite heavily on theoretical schemas of nondecisions, passive or irrational decisions, ambivalent decisions, and decision making guided by conventional behavior or ethic. More careful consideration of consequences by the individual may promote selection of that action which maximizes overall utility or satisfices. Empirical application of statistical models of decision making to fertility or fertility regulation behavior has also been attempted. A recent model, the judgment-integration-valuation-choice model, which specifies a variety of rules by which individuals integrate the perceived probability and desirability of the consequences of alternative actions, is an improvement over previous models that do not allow variation across individuals in decision rules. Nevertheless, the utility and applicability of this more recent model is reduced by its complexity. Moreover, with the exception of expectancy x value theory, there is little recognition in the various models of the influence of extrafamilial or normative factors, which are more significant in pretransition and transitional societies. Finally, all the models assume that decision making is a rational process in which individuals select the action with the highest expected value. Various impediments to rationality that have been discussed call this assumption into question. Thus, the greatest utility of all of these models may be that, when they are applied empirically, they lead to identification of those consequences which are perceived as probable and evaluated as strongly desirable or undesirable by individuals considering alternative fertility choices.

Research on sequential decision making focuses primarily on changes in the decision-making process below and above the normative family-size floor and changes in the determinants of fertility at different parities. Differences in normative family-size thresholds within subgroups, variation in maximum family-size norms, and plan revisions and plan-implementation failures complicate the study of factors influencing decisions at each birth order.

Research on communication and power has been handicapped by measurement problems and the lack of longitudinal data, although recent formulations of the concept of relative power or dominance should advance this area of study. The relationship between egalitarian decision

making and fertility is complicated by the likelihood
that these variables have reciprocal effects:  greater
egalitarianism may influence fertility negatively,
whereas having many children, particularly sons, may
increase the wife's or husband's authority in the family.
In transitional societies, attempts to measure the influence of relative power on fertility are more useful if
they focus on the point at which a couple first considers
fertility regulation or on situations of disagreement
about fertility goals and regulation.  Research has consistently shown that contraceptive use is more prevalent
and continuous when the husband approves of it, particularly among the lower class or the less educated; husband's approval is also related to communication about
family planning between spouses.  Within posttransition
societies, the dominance of wives in both pronatal and
antinatal decisions has been noted.  However, differences
in relative power and influence may exist within different subgroups.  Within-couple status differentials in
age, educational attainment, and income may also affect
marital power patterns in situations of disagreement over
fertility goals and regulation in both transitional and
posttransition societies.

Various views exist on changes in fertility decision
making in connection with the demographic transition from
high to low fertility.  The decision process may not
change in essentials, or may change radically from passive to active decisions when a threshold of economic
consciousness is reached, or may change in a number of
other ways, such as in the identity of the primary
decision makers.

Research on fertility decision making requires data,
ideally longitudinal, to trace shifts in content and
process within different cohorts, as well as across the
life cycle.  However, cross-sectional studies can still
be useful in focusing on decisions with apparently
irrational outcomes, such as unwanted births or unregu-
lated fertility when regulation seems called for.
Emphasizing the perceived rather than the objective
consequences of behavior, the subjective rather than the
actual probabilities of their occurrence, and the way
competing preferences among family and nonfamily members
constrain decision making or must be reconciled may help
explain fertility behavior that is nonrational from the
community perspective, but may well be rational for the
individual.  Investigation of changing decisional styles
within communities can provide insight into the institu-

tional and situational factors which stimulate a shift
from passivity or ambivalence to active decision making
on the basis of personally defined goals.

## BIBLIOGRAPHY

Adler, N. (1979)  Decision models in population
   research. Journal of Population 2:187-202.
Arnold, F., R. A. Bulatao, C. Buripakdi, B. J. Chung, J.
   T. Fawcett, T. Iritani, S. J. Lee, and T.-S. Wu
   (1975)  The Value of Children: Introduction and
   Comparative Analysis, Vol. 1.  Honolulu: East-West
   Population Institute.
Bagozzi, R. P., and M. F. Van Loo (1978)  Toward a
   general theory of fertility:  A causal modelling
   approach. Demography 15:301-320.
Bardwick, J. M. (1973)  Psychological factors in the
   acceptance and use of oral contraceptives.  In J. T.
   Fawcett, ed., Psychological Perspectives on
   Population.  New York:  Basic Books.
Bauman, K. E., and J. R. Udry (1981)  Subjective expected
   utility and adolescent sexual behavior. Adolescence
   16:527-535.
Beach, L. R., B. D. Townes, F. L. Campbell, and G. W.
   Keating (1976)  Developing and testing a decision aid
   for birth planning decisions. Organizational Behavior
   and Human Performance 15:99-116.
Browner, C. (1979) Abortion decision-making:  Some
   findings from Colombia. Studies in Family Planning
   10:96-106.
Bulatao, R. A. (1979a)  On the Nature of the Transition
   in the Value of Children.  Paper No. 60-A.  Honolulu:
   East-West Population Institute.
Bulatao, R. A. (1979b)  Further Evidence of the
   Transition in the Value of Children.  Paper No. 60-B.
   Honolulu:  East-West Population Institute.
Bulatao, R. A. (1981)  Values and disvalues of children
   in successive childbearing decisions. Demography
   18:1-25.
Bulatao, R. A., and F. S. Arnold (1977)  Relationships
   between the value and cost of children and fertility:
   Cross-cultural evidence.  In International Population
   Conference, Mexico, 1977, Vol. 1.  Liege:  Inter-
   national Union for the Scientific Study of Population.
Bulatao, R. A., and J. T. Fawcett (1981)  Dynamic
   perspectives in the study of fertility decision-

making:   Successive decisions within a fertility
career.   Pp. 433-499 in <u>International Population
Conference, Manila, 1981</u>, Vol. 1.   Liege:
International Union for the Scientific Study of
Population.

Cain, M. (1981)   Risk and insurance:   Perspectives on
fertility and agrarian change in India and
Bangladesh.   <u>Population and Development Review</u>
7:435-474.

Callan, V. J. (1980)   <u>The Value of Children to
Australian, Greek, and Italian Parents in Sydney</u>.
Paper No. 60-C.   Honolulu:   East-West Population
Institute.

Card, J. J. (1978)   The correspondence of data gathered
from husband and wife:   Implications for family
planning studies.   <u>Social Biology</u> 25:196-204.

Cohen, J. B., L. Severy, and O. T. Ahtola (1978)   An
extended expectancy-value approach to contraceptive
alternatives.   <u>Journal of Population</u> 1:22-41.

Coombs, L. C., and M. C. Chang (1981)   Do husbands and
wives agree?   Fertility attitudes and later behavior.
<u>Population and Environment</u> 4:109-127.

Coombs, L. C., and D. Fernandez (1978)   Husband-wife
agreement about reproductive goals.   <u>Demography</u>
15:57-73.

Darroch, R. K., P. A. Meyer, and M. Singarimbun (1981)
<u>Two Are Not Enough:   The Value of Children to Javanese
and Sundanese Parents</u>.   Paper No. 60-D.   Honolulu:
East-West Population Institute.

Davidson, A. R., and J. J. Jaccard (1979)   Variables that
moderate the attitude-behavior relation:   Results of a
longitudinal survey.   <u>Journal of Personality and
Social Psychology</u> 37:1364-1376.

Davidson, A. R., J. J. Jaccard, H. C. Triandis, M.
Morales, and R. Diaz-Guererro (1976)   Cross-cultural
model-making.   Towards a solution of the emic-etic
dilemma.   <u>International Journal of Psychology</u> 11:1-13.

Demeny, P. (1970)   Causes and consequences of excess
fertility.   <u>A Report on a Family Planning Conference</u>.
Monograph No. 7, Carolina Population Center.   Chapel
Hill, N.C.:   University of North Carolina.

Easterlin, R. A. (1975)   An economic framework for
fertility analysis.   <u>Studies in Family Planning</u>
6:54-63.

Edwards, W. (1954)   The theory of decision making.
<u>Psychological Bulletin</u> 51:380-417.

Fawcett, J. T., S. Albores, and F. Arnold (1972) The value of children among ethnic groups in Hawaii: Exploratory measurements. In J. T. Fawcett, ed., The Satisfactions and Costs of Children: Theories, Concepts, Methods. Honolulu: East West Population Institute.

Fishbein, M. (1972) Toward an understanding of family planning behavior. Journal of Applied Social Psychology 2:214-227.

Fishbein, M., and J. J. Jaccard (1973) Theoretical and methodological considerations in the prediction of family planning intentions and behaviour. Representative Research in Social Psychology 4:37-51.

Fisher, W. A., J. D. Fisher, and D. Byrne (1976) Situational and Personality Determinants of Reactions to Contraceptive Purchasing. Paper presented at the meeting of the American Psychological Association, Washington, D.C.

Fox, G. L. (1975) Love match and arranged marriage in a modernizing nation: Mate selection in Ankara, Turkey. Journal of Marriage and the Family 37:180-193.

Freedman, R., and B. Berelson (1976) The record of family planning programs. Studies in Family Planning 7:1-40.

Fried, E. S., and J. R. Udry (1979) Wives' and husbands' expected costs and benefits of childbearing as predictors of pregnancy. Social Biology 26:265-274.

Fried, E. S., S. L. Hofferth, and J. R. Udry (1980) Parity-specific and two-sex utility models of reproductive intentions. Demography 17:1-12.

Gadalla, S. M. (1978) Is There Hope? Fertility and Family Planning in a Rural Egyptian Community. Cairo, Egypt: American University in Cairo Press.

Gupta, G. R. (1979) Love, arranged marriage and the Indian social structure. In G. Kurian, ed., Cross-Cultural Perspectives of Mate-Selection and Marriage. Westport, Conn.: Greenwood Press.

Hass, P. H. (1971) Maternal Employment and Fertility in Metropolitan Latin America. Unpublished Ph.D. dissertation. Duke University, Durham, N. C.

Hass, P. H. (1974) Wanted and unwanted pregnancies: A fertility decision-making model. Journal of Social Issues 30:125-165.

Heer, D. M., and H.-Y. Wu (1975) The effect of infant and child mortality and preference for sons upon fertility and family planning behavior and attitudes in Taiwan. In J. F. Kantner and L. McCaffrey, eds.,

Population and Development in Southeast Asia.
Lexington, Mass.:  Lexington Books.
Heer, D. M., and H.-Y. Wu (1978) Effects in rural Taiwan
and urban Morocco:  Combining individual and aggregate
data.  In S. H. Preston, ed., The Effects of Infant
and Child Mortality on Fertility. New York:  Academic
Press.
Hill, R., J. M. Stycos, and K. W. Back (1959)  The Family
and Population Control:  A Puerto Rican Experiment in
Social Change. Chapel Hill, N.C.:  University of
North Carolina Press.
Hoffman, L. W., and M. L. Hoffman (1973)  The value of
children to parents.  Pp. 19-76 in J. T. Fawcett, ed.,
Psychological Perspectives on Population. New York:
Basic Books.
Hoffman, L. W., A. Thornton, and J. D. Manis (1978)  The
value of children to parents in the United States.
Journal of Population 1:91-131.
Hollerbach, P. E. (1980)  Power in families, communica-
tion, and fertility decision making.  Population and
Environment 3:146-173.
Jaccard, J. J., and A. R. Davidson (1975)  A comparison
of two models of social behavior:  Results of a survey
sample.  Sociometry 34:497-517.
Jaccard, J. J., and A. R. Davidson (1976)  The relation
of psychological, social, and economic variables to
fertility-related decisions.  Demography 13:329-338.
Jones, E. F., L. Paul, and C. F. Westoff (1980)
Contraceptive efficacy:  The significance of method
and motivation.  Studies in Family Planning 11:39-50.
Kantner, J. F., and M. Zelnick (1973)  Contraception and
pregnancy:  Experience of young unmarried women in the
United States.  Family Planning Perspectives 5:21-35.
Kellerhals, J., and G. Wirth (1972)  Social dynamics of
abortion requests:  Some considerations and
preliminary results.  International Mental Health
Research Newsletter 14:1.
Kerenyi, T. D., E. L. Glascock, and M. L. Horowitz
(1973)  Reasons for delayed abortion:  Results of 400
interviews.  American Journal of Obstetrics and
Gynecology 117:299-311.
Lee, R. D., ed. (1977)  Population Patterns in the Past.
New York:  Academic Press.
Lee, W. (1971)  Decision Theory and Human Behavior. New
York:  John Wiley and Sons, Inc.
Leibenstein, H. (1981)  Economic decision theory and
human fertility behavior.  Population and Development
Review 7:381-400.

Lesthaeghe, R. (1980)  On the control of human reproduction. _Population and Development Review_ 6:527-548.

Liu, W. T., and I. W. Hutchinson (1974)  Conjugal interaction and fertility behavior:  Some conceptual problems in research. In H. Y. Tien and F. D. Bean, eds., _Comparative Family and Fertility Research_. Leiden: E. J. Brill.

Luker, K. (1975)  _Taking Chances:  Abortion and the Decision Not To Contracept_. Berkeley, Calif.: University of California Press.

MacDonald, A. L., P. M. Simpson, and A. M. Whitfield (1978)  _An Assessment of the Reliability of the Indonesian Fertility Survey Data_. WFS Scientific Reports No. 3.  London:  World Fertility Survey.

Marsella, A. J., C. S. Chin, R. Haditono, and C. E. Santiago (1979)  The Acceptability of Alternative Routes of Administration of Fertility Regulating Methods among Rural Indonesian, Korean and Filipino Women.  Unpublished manuscript.  Human Reproduction Unit, World Health Organization, Geneva.

McClelland, G. H. (1980)  A psychological and measurement theory approach to fertility decision-making.  In T. K. Burch, ed., _Demographic Behavior:  Interdisciplinary Perspectives on Decision-Making_.  Boulder, Colo.:  Westview Press.

McClelland, G. H., and B. H. Hackenberg (1978)  Subjective probabilities for sex of next child:  U.S. college students and Philippine villagers.  _Journal of Population_ 1:132-147.

McNicoll, G. (1980)  Institutional determinants of fertility change.  _Population and Development Review_ 6:441-462.

Meeker, B. (1980)  Rational decision-making models in interpersonal behavior.  In T. K. Burch, ed., _Demographic Behavior:  Interdisciplinary Perspectives on Decision-Making_.  Boulder, Colo.:  Westview Press.

Miller, W. B. (1975)  Psychiatry and physician illness: The psychosomatic interface.  In C. P. Rosenbaum and J. E. Beebe, eds., _Psychiatric Treatment:  Crisis, Clinic, and Consultation_.  New York:  McGraw-Hill.

Miller, W. B. (1981a)  The Personal Meanings of Voluntary and Involuntary Childlessness.  Center for Population Research Contract N01-HD-82853.  National Institute of Child Health and Human Development, Bethesda, Md.

Miller, W. B. (1981b)  _The Psychology of Reproduction_. Washington, D.C.:  National Technical Information Service.

Miller, W. B., and R. K. Godwin (1977)  Psyche and Demos:  Individual Psychology and the Issues of Population.  New York:  Oxford University Press.

Mills, J., R. Meltzer, and M. Clark (1977)  Effect on number of options on recall of information supporting different decision strategies.  Personality and Social Psychology Bulletin 3:213-218.

Neal, A. G., and H. T. Grote (1977)  Alienation and fertility in the marital dyad.  Societal Forces 56:77-85.

Neal, A. G., and H. T. Grote (1980)  Fertility decision making, unintended births and the social drift hypothesis:  A longitudinal study.  Population and Environment 3:221-236.

Nickerson, C. A., G. H. McClelland, and S. M. Kegeles (1981)  A Decision-Making Approach to Contraceptive Choice.  Center for Research on Judgment and Policy Report No. 234.  Institute of Behavioral Science, University of Colorado, Boulder, Colo.

Nortman, D. (1982)  Estimating Potential Contraceptive Demand:  An Improved Method of Measurement.  Center for Policy Studies Working Paper No. 82.  Population Council, New York.

Pebley, A. R., H. Delgado, and E. Brinemann (1979)  Fertility desires and child mortality experience among Guatemalan women.  Studies in Family Planning 10:129-136.

Pitz, G. F. (1980)  Sensitivity of direct and derived judgments to probabilistic information.  Journal of Applied Psychology 65:531-540.

Pitz, G. F., N. J. Sachs, and J. Heerboth (1980)  Assessing the utility of multiattribute utility assessments.  Organizational Behavior and Human Performance 26:65-80.

PROFAM-PIACT de Mexico  (1979)  Family Planning in Mexico--PROFAM-PIACT de Mexico 1979.  Mexico, D.F.:  PROFAM-PIACT de Mexico.

Rodriguez, G. (1977)  Assessing the Availability of Fertility Regulation Methods:  Report on a Methodological Study.  WFS Scientific Reports No. 1.  London:  World Fertility Survey.

Rodriguez, G. (1978)  Family planning availability and contraceptive practice.  International Family Planning Perspectives 4:100-115.

Scanzoni, J. H. (1975)  Sex Roles, Life Styles, and Childbearing:  Changing Patterns in Marriage and the Family.  New York:  The Free Press.

Schmidt, F. L. (1973)  Implications of a measurement problem for expectancy theory research. Organizational Behavior and Human Performance 10:243-251.

Shedlin, M. G., and P. E. Hollerbach (1981)  Modern and traditional fertility regulation in a Mexican community: Factors in the process of decision-making. Studies in Family Planning 12:278-296.

Simon, H. A. (1979) Models of Thought. New Haven, Conn.: Yale University Press.

Steinhoff, P. G., R. G. Smith, and M. Diamond (1971)  The Hawaii pregnancy, birth control and abortion study: Social-psychological aspects. In Proceedings of a Conference on Psychological Measurement in the Study of Population Problems. Berkeley, Calif.: Institute of Personality Assessment and Research, University of California.

Townes, B. D., L. R. Beach, F. L. Campbell, and D. C. Martin (1977)  Birth planning values and decisions: The prediction of fertility. Journal of Applied Social Psychology 7:73-88.

Tversky, A., and D. Kahneman (1974)  Judgement under uncertainty: Heuristics and biases. Science 185:1124-1131.

Weller, R. H. (1968)  The employment of wives, dominance and fertility. Journal of Marriage and the Family 30:437-442.

Werner, P. D., S. E. Middlestadt-Carter, and T. J. Crawford (1975)  Having a third child: Predicting behavioral intentions. Journal of Marriage and the Family 37:348-358.

World Health Organization (1977)  Special Programme of Research, Development and Research Training in Human Reproduction Sixth Annual Report. Geneva: WHO.

World Health Organization Task Force on Psychosocial Research in Family Planning and the Task Force on Service Research in Family Planning (1980)  A study of user preferences of fertility regulating methods in India, Korea, the Philippines, and Turkey. Studies in Family Planning 11:267-273.

World Health Organization Task Force on Psychosocial Research in Family Planning (1981)  A cross-cultural study of menstruation. Implications for contraceptive development and use. Studies in Family Planning 12:3-16.

Yaukey, D., W. Griffiths, and B. J. Roberts (1967) Couple concurrence and empathy on birth control motivation in Dacca, East Pakistan. <u>American Sociological Review</u> 32:716-726.

# Chapter 10
# Cultural Influences on Fertility Decision Styles

TERENCE H. HULL*

In the framework for these volumes, fertility is seen as
determined by a number of proximate variables that control, for example, the exposure to coitus, the likelihood
of conception, and the process of parturition. Within
this framework, ideational cultural variables--norms,
beliefs, values, and so on--can only affect fertility to
the extent that they influence behavior associated with
these proximate variables. Such effects can be direct,
as when nuptiality patterns are molded by norms concerning the proper timing of marriage; they can also be
indirect, as when behaviors such as schooling or migration that in turn influence the proximate determinants
are affected.

Although this framework can be used to analyze fertility at either the individual or social level, it is not
as useful for dynamic analysis of the complex interactions
between the individual life cycle and the process of
social change. In particular, it does not lend itself
well to analysis of fertility decision making by people
confronted with a variety of constraints and opportunities, a subject on which there is relatively little in
the literature generally. Thus, although the framework
provides a comprehensive--if not exhaustive--categoriza-
tion of how socioeconomic variables may affect fertility
decision making, it falls short of specifying how and by
whom such decisions are made. To address this issue, it
is necessary to ask a number of key questions. First, do
individuals make conscious decisions about fertility, or
is fertility behavior externally determined? Second, if
they do make such decisions, to what extent can these be

*I would like to thank John Casterline and Lincoln Day in
addition to the reviewers and editors.

381

considered "rational"?  To what extent do decisions about
the proximate variables affect fertility indirectly?  How
much conscious control over their own fertility do individuals feel they have, and how much fatalism is involved
in their perceptions?  To what extent and under what circumstances are fertility decisions based on precedent or
habit?  How does the decision-making process change with
changes in the life cycle and in the sociocultural environment?  How do couples make fertility decisions?  To
what extent do those outside the conjugal relationship
influence such decisions?  The sections below address
these questions.

## DO INDIVIDUALS MAKE FERTILITY DECISIONS?

The theoretical and empirical literature contains many
assumptions about the nature of fertility decision making.
In some cases, the notion of individual decision making
is ignored, and the focus is on societal "decisions" in
the form of codes of conduct, norms, and values formulated to achieve behavior that is "functional" for the
survival or growth of a group.  Alternatively, the
emphasis is on the individual as decision maker carefully
weighing costs and benefits, and making choices to satisfy
personally defined objectives.

An examination of classic fertility theories offers
interesting insights into this issue of decisional
"style."  Carr-Saunders (1922:222-223) argued that primitive societies regulate fertility levels by prescribing
customs and actions designed to achieve an "optimum"
population for the environment.  He noted that, because
the self-sufficient compact nature of tribal life made
pressure on resources or expansion opportunities
"obvious," there could be "some semi-conscious adjustment
of numbers" by resort to abstinence, abortion, or infanticide.  However, exactly how this fine-tuning of numbers
might work in practice was not explained.  Notestein
(1945:39-40) offered an alternative view of primitive
societies.  Rather than adjusting their numbers to
changing fortunes, they were chronically faced with the
burden of high, though variable, mortality.  As a result,
these societies were "ingeniously arranged [with] . . .
religious doctrines, moral codes, laws, education, community customs, [etc.] . . . focused toward maintaining
high fertility."  Thus, whereas Carr-Saunders saw the
possibility of selective invocation of cultural variables,

Notestein argued that the weight of culture pressed individuals to reproduce at high rates, and that antinatalist ideas and behavior were exceptions to the general rule. This conceptualization fitted well with his theory of demographic transition, which posited certain socioeconomic determinants of the shift from high to low rates of fertility and mortality.

Neither of these writers offered an account of individual perceptions or motivations; in describing the process of population control, they attributed to society such anthropomorphic qualities as "semi-conscious deliberations" and "ingenious" designs. In contrast, Ford (1945: 86-87), summarizing a review of hundreds of ethnographies, saw fertility as resulting from a balance of pressures acting on individuals: "Promises of security, approval, and prestige accorded to parents are weighed up against perceptions of pain and possibly death in childbearing, and the impositions of child care." This description (though not the case studies offered by Ford) sounds like a model economizer: a person consciously collecting information and comparing costs and benefits before taking action. However, even this notion of balance of pressures does little to describe whether individuals think much about their fertility, or even whether they consider behavior associated with the proximate determinants as it affects fertility. Instead, this and other classic depictions of fertility control emphasize culture and ecology as interacting determinants of fertility decisions.

This emphasis on social and economic factors in discussions of primitive population control also underlies many analyses of high and low fertility regimes. High fertility, it is sometimes argued, occurs where the pronatalist factors identified by Notestein predominate (see Benedict, 1972:82, for a concise presentation of this argument). Individual decision making is irrelevant in such circumstances because the full weight of custom reinforces behavior conducive to childbearing. Variations in fertility, then, are the result of external factors, such as the environment or biology, or actions of individuals that have only an indirect, and presumably unintended, impact on fertility. In fact, many early anthropological studies of culture and fertility made no specific mention of individual decision making (e.g., Marshall et al., 1972). The contrasting argument is that low fertility developed when individuals began to make decisions. Economic models (Becker, 1960) and early

fertility surveys (Hill et al., 1959) reflected this
perspective on individual decision making.

## ARE FERTILITY DECISIONS RATIONAL?

Much of the debate about the applicability of economic
models to fertility analysis has swung between the extreme
views that individuals make no real fertility decisions,
or that all fertility behavior implies important decisions
(Duesenberry, 1960). Often the issue of whether decisions
are made is couched in terms of whether people are behaving rationally (see, e.g., Lorimer, 1954). However, the
term "rational" can be interpreted in different ways.
Instead of simplistically dividing fertility behavior
into rational and nonrational depending on whether or not
conscious deliberation takes place, recent writers have
suggested that it may be more useful to consider decision
making ubiquitous. The way that behavior is shaped
through interaction between the individual and the social
setting can then be examined (see especially Leibenstein,
1981). Demeny (1970:35) contends that "the word 'rationality' should not be interpreted as suggesting some
explicit and careful confrontation of pluses and minuses
associated with pregnancy, childbirth, and having a
child." Rather, it is "simply behavior that represents a
best accommodation of individual desires to the impositions of the environment." The focus is therefore not on
absolute rationality, such as the maximization principle,
but on different types of rationality that take account
of informational, political, time, and perceptual constraints. Cultures are seen as representing a wide range
of such constraints or "impositions," since they constitute the cognitive apparatus through which people perceive, reflect upon, and understand their social and
physical environment.[1]
An example from anthropology may clarify this point.
Malinowski (1929) presented evidence showing that the
Trobrianders did not believe that the male had any
necessary role in reproduction, but that conception
occurred when a spirit entered the womb. Clearly, such a
belief would have important implications for decision
making related to a wide range of proximate variables.
However, later ethnographers showed that, although this
belief was an important part of the Trobrianders' explanation of the nature of life, it did not constitute their
full understanding of reproduction; rather, they under-

stood but did not attach much symbolic importance to the biological facts (Leach, 1969). Thus overlapping spiritual, social, and physical realities together define the position of the individual within the culture and the context within which decisions are made.

However, this conception of rationality can become a tautology. If decision making is ubiquitous and always surrounded by a complex web of cultural knowledge and symbolism, and if the efficiency of decisions is defined according to the individual's own perceptions, then all behavior is "rational" by definition unless individuals choose to act against their own interests. Even then the sophist might argue that such a choice reveals higher interests, and hence the behavior is still rational. There are two ways to avoid this tautology. First, the criteria for judging the efficiency of decisions can be seen as external to the individual's immediate perceptions. This lies at the heart of Demeny's (1970) depiction of the externalities involved in fertility behavior, in which high fertility may be rational for the individual but against the interests of the community as a whole, and hence from one perspective irrational. Also, when decisions are seen within a time dimension, an action may be observed to contravene an individual's own a priori and a posteriori perceptions of his or her interests; in this sense, regret is the acknowledgement of a form of irrationality. Second, Herbert Simon and others have introduced the concept of bounded rationality, whereby decision making is depicted not as an exhaustive process of sifting data, but as making the best choice under the circumstances (Simon, 1957; Adler, 1979). It is argued that people limit the number of alternatives they consider, and also avoid the effort of constant decision making by recourse to precedents.

This restriction of perceptions and the development of habits (or customs) also constitute elements of culture which can be institutionalized. One function of culture is to structure the decision-making framework. People think (or do not think) about fertility options in accordance with the language, concepts, and symbols of their cultures. Beliefs about the natural and supernatural worlds condition perceptions about the wisdom of alternative actions. Interactions with and observation of other people provide examples of the opportunities and constraints prevailing in the society. Repetitive, or at least understandable, experiences suggest a basis for habitual behavior, and belief in the predictability of the consequences of actions makes planning possible.

It should be noted, however, that expressing the issue
in this form does damage to the concept of culture.  For
many anthropologists (Keesing, 1974:73-97) and institutional economists (Samuels, 1966:237-288), the argument
that culture--or the economy--provides a framework for
decision making misses the point that cultures and economies themselves exist as complex patterns of decisions
(or choices, or ideas).  Thus the framework both
influences and is shaped by decision making.

## LEVELS OF FERTILITY DECISION MAKING

Once the basic questions have been addresssed of whether
decisions are made and, if so, whether they are rational,
it becomes important to ask at what levels decision making
takes place.  What is the nature of individual decision
making?  How do couples make fertility decisions?  And
what role do other people have in the decision making of
a married couple?  In decision making related to marital
fertility, decisions are not informed by the principle of
"might makes right," or by the simple rule of "optimization," or even by more sophisticated models of interpersonal behavior such as that described by Meeker (1980).
Rather, the levels of decision making vary widely according to specific situations and differ across cultures.
The subsections below examine this complex issue at three
levels:  the individual, the couple, and extraconjugal
groups.

### Individual-Level Decision Making

A number of issues need to be examined at the level of
individual decision making.  First, individual decisions
may affect fertility indirectly through their effects on
the proximate variables.  Second, it can be asked to what
extent an individual's decisions are conscious, and to
what extent determined by either external constaints or
habit and precedent.  Finally, it is important to address
the question of individual decision making over the life
cycle.

### Decisions Affecting the Proximate Variables

An important, but often overlooked, distinction is that
between decisions about fertility per se and those about

the proximate variables that determine fertility.  The
decisional styles involved in each are likely to be
different both within and between cultures.

An example is provided by the argument that the demographic transition involves the development of "rational,"
conscious decision making by individuals who were previously unaware of fertility control issues or methods.
It is possible to provide empirical support for the
contention that some people do not explicitly plan their
family sizes; however, it is still clear that they make
carefully considered decisions about marriage, sexual
relations, and infant care that have the indirect effect
of determining family size, and that these decisions are
made within the constraints of a complex set of norms,
values, and social rules.  (Such cultural influences on
behavior related to each of the proximate variables were
reviewed systematically by Freedman [1961-62], Nag [1968],
and Hawthorn [1970].)

Failure to recognize the importance of decisions like
these that are not consciously concerned with fertility
has led to an unfortunate tendency to see the problem of
fertility decision making simply as a balancing between
the demand for and the supply of children.  It is sometimes argued, for instance, that, as long as an individual wants as many children as possible, it is irrelevant
to study fertility decision making; the supply constraint
alone determines the fertility level.  This argument
ignores the fact that the supply constraint is itself a
product of decision-making processes.  Thus it is inadequate to depict fertility decline as the attainment of
rationality in family-size decision making; a more
complete explanation is needed that includes a description of these more indirect decisional procedures.


Conscious Decisions, External Constraints, and Habit

A central question that needs to be addressed is how
conscious individual fertility decisions are, and to what
degree they are determined by external constraints or
habit.  It is difficult to find satisfying answers to
these questions in the literature; it is more difficult
still to find them in the field.  Even where language,
social status, race, and relative income are not barriers
between researcher and informant, explanations of specific
decisions are often vague, contradictory, confused, or,
at times, withheld.

One of the most detailed examinations of this problem
has been done by Cicourel (1967, 1974), who advocates the
use of in-depth interviewing to uncover the specifics of
decision making. Such research, he contends, must aim at
understanding the contexts in which decisions are made;
decision-making processes are truly complex behaviors and
retrospective reports of fertility behavior are difficult
to interpret without knowledge of their context. In a
related effort, Rainwater (1960:177-178) records the
fatalism of lower-class Americans who saw no alternative
to continued childbearing because of the constraints of
their religion and a general lack of knowledge and awareness of alternatives. Also, Shedlin and Hollerbach
(1981:294) find that Mexican culture creates a climate in
which many "couples proceed through the lifecycle . . .
accepting pregnancies with ambivalence or regret and
feeling powerless to remedy the situation in an acceptable, understandable manner." Neal and Groat (1980:221)
refer to such a situation as "social drift," Day (1979:
284) as "behavioral drift"; they stress the social and
psychological factors constraining ranges of individual
choice and leading to acceptance of fate rather than the
assertive consideration of alternatives. "If couples
perceive no alternatives to pregnancy and childbearing,
they cannot consciously <u>decide</u> to influence the probability of pregnancy and childbearing" since this is determined by biology alone, say Shedlin and Hollerbach
(1981:282).

This view of the decision maker as victim does not
square well with the concept of culture and decision
making presented above. Fatalism, in particular, implies
that the external culture or society determines individual
behavior. If culture itself consists of patterns of
individual decisions and perceptions of the meaning of
those decisions, then cultural influences on the individual are not one-way, but are interactive. Two recent
studies of women's roles in Africa illustrate this distinction. Joseph (1979:191-201) challenges the formalist
model of Berber social structure, which implies strict
boundaries to female decision making. Seen from an
interactive perspective, "the experiential life of
Berbers . . . allows for a considerable amount of
individualistic manipulation and a resulting fluidity of
social relations." Women have a "set of means [to]
pursue their own interests," even though these are
neither codified nor formally acknowledged. Little
(1979) develops a similar theme with regard to West

African women, who, he says, "have their own goals" and a
substantial scope of potential actions for achieving
them, despite the formal structure of implied male
dominance.

This interaction between individuals and external
constraints is complicated by the fact that people must
make multiple decisions about different types of behavior
often involving contradictory consequences. Unhappiness
over one result must be weighed against benefits gained
from other results. If the background is one of poverty,
then the challenge for the decision maker is to do the
best under bad conditions. The statement "I had no other
choice" is thus not a denial of decision making, but a
confirmation that alternatives were unacceptable, or that
the contradictions inherent in the decision problem could
not be overcome. In these circumstances, acceptance may
be the best decision. "Aberrant" behaviors, such as
abortion, suicide, homicide, abstinence, celibacy, and
flight, are available alternatives in most societies;
when such behaviors are rejected, decisions are being
made.

Like external constraints, habit is sometimes seen as
the basis for rejecting notions of individual decision
making and straightforward utility models of behavior.
Leibenstein has recently explored this topic in detail,
suggesting that repetitious behavior "may account for
most of the fertility behavior that takes place" (1981:
396-397). He is concerned with what he calls "passive"
decision making, which arises when individuals "choose"
to repeat previous behavior rather than invest time and
energy in continually calculating the costs and benefits
involved in particular decisions.

Repetitive decision making involves two considerations.
First, if the decision problem arises routinely, an individual is likely to behave according to habit in making
decisions related to both the proximate determinants and
fertility itself. For example, frequency of coitus is
more likely to involve personal habits than is divorce or
abortion; abstinence may perhaps become a habit, but
infanticide is too rare and abhorrent to become routine
for most mothers. Thus habitual behavior depends very
much on the particular fertility decision problem.
Second, habitual behaviors can occur not only at the
individual but also at the social level. Individuals who
refer to and follow precedents may be behaving routinely
at the social level even though they have never experienced the particular decision problem before. In this

sense it is meaningful to speak of a group of people routinely marrying in early adolescence even though no individual repeats this behavior. The literature on norms, customs, and traditions is relevant here (Freedman, 1961-62): the culture provides a guide for analyzing the decision problem and suggests solutions to the decision maker, in lieu of personal trial and error.

Another factor is involved in habitual responses to decision problems. For those living in environments of capricious productivity, high mortality, and widespread poverty, fertility decisions can lead directly or indirectly to economic difficulty. Moreover, it is usually impossible to predict accurately the consequences of such decisions (Namboodiri, 1980:87-88). These problems of risk and uncertainty dominate the decision-making process, inhibiting innovation while encouraging social conformity and repetitive individual behavior (Hull, 1975:377; Neher, 1971; Cain, 1981).

Decision Sequences Over the Life Cycle

Routine or habitual behavior can be observed not only in simple individual decisions but also in patterns of decision making over the life cycle (see Bulatao and Fawcett, 1981; Namboodiri, 1973:87-92; Namboodiri, 1980:76-80). Many of these decision patterns related to fertility and the proximate variables are logically consistent and common, although others are inconsistent and rare (see also Kyriazis, 1979; Miller and Godwin, 1977:86-89, 119-131).

The various routine choices that are made over time help to define the individual's decisional style. Ethnographers commonly record observations on rites of passage and family cycles in this way. An implication of this conceptualization is that systematic patterns of decision-making behavior contain an inner logic whose meaning transcends the functional relations between specific decisions. Caldwell (1981) and Lesthaeghe (1980:543) make a similar point by arguing that fertility decline in Africa depends on more than a shift in economic parameters. The decision-making process is changing, as seen in greater individual choice and concern for personal welfare; this change is likely to proceed systematically and sequentially as young people use new strategies to address classic decision problems. The working out of these overlapping sequences of decisional

styles varies widely across cultures, according to the
socioeconomic processes involved. "Development" is a
radically different thing in China and Brazil, in Saudi
Arabia and Singapore. Consequently, even if fertility
does fall as incomes rise--and this is by no means
vouchsafed--it will do so through different decision-
making processes and patterns that vary from those that
prevailed in the past (see Hull Hull, 1977; Hull, 1977).

As has been noted, many fertility decision sequences
are routine, and many decisional styles can therefore be
characterized as culture-specific. Examples have been
cited in which women seem to "drift" semiconsciously
through a series of decisions that produce large families.
However, some individuals break out of such cycles, and
it is interesting to ask why.

One obvious hypothesis is that economic changes
eventually challenge the reasonableness of following
established patterns, causing women to abandon the
security of culturally supported decisions in favor of
innovative behavior (Hull, 1977). This is basically an
argument describing the gradual evolution of cultural
styles. It is the argument used, for example, to explain
the development of abstinence, divorce, and traditional
birth control in poor, densely settled Java.

Another hypothesis is that the decision problems
themselves change. New methods of fertility control, new
ideas about marital relations, or alternative infant
feeding practices competing with breastfeeding offer
women a range of choices, making innovation possible.
Two aspects of this hypothesis are important. First, it
can help to explain stability. The overall decision
sequence can act to counterbalance change resulting from
the introduction of new alternatives. The changing
patterns of abstinence and breastfeeding in Africa have
been found by Lesthaeghe et al. (1981) to have balanced
each other, so that fertility remains relatively stable.
This may be interpreted as reflecting a general stability
in the logic of the overall decision sequence. Second,
the impact of innovation on an established sequence may
also be used to explain radical change. As economic or
social pressures against a particular set of decisions
grows, tension develops in the decision-making pattern.
Women may continue to behave in accordance with the
common pattern in spite of this tension, because of the
strength of the overall logic of the sequence. When a
major new factor like safe, efficient contraception is
introduced, this tension is stressed, and the whole

structure of decision making can change rapidly.  This
kind of explanation has been advanced to explain Bali's
rapid fertility decline (Hull, 1980).

Finally, decision sequences can be altered as relationships change between individuals and others involved in
the decision problems.  Such changes can take place in
three basic ways.  First, the decision sequence can be
altered by events in the middle of a woman's reproductive
years:  a life crisis, such as desertion; a social change
affecting male-female relations or employment patterns;
or an ideological change such as the reassertion of some
form of religious fundamentalism.  Such changes can alter
the locus of fertility decision making.  Second, young
women may be raised very differently from older women,
perhaps enough so to challenge the whole logic of traditional relations and shift the locus of decision making
(for a case study see Pool, 1972).  Third, women may be
either liberated or subjugated as a result of an overt
social movement; such changes, even if located primarily
in the political or economic sphere, again may have
important effects on the locus of fertility decision
making.  The issue here centers specifically on whose
decision is to prevail.  This issue is discussed in the
subsections below.


### Couples as Decision-Making Units

Fertility decisions can be analyzed from the viewpoint of
an individual woman, treating the influence of all other
people (including the husband) as a set of psychic "costs
and benefits"; however, it is more realistic to think of
a couple--usually a married couple--as forming the
decision-making unit (Miller and Godwin, 1977:76ff.).
Conjugal relationships are largely defined in cultural
terms; the relative power of spouses in the making of
fertility decisions involves both their socialization to
specific roles and their interaction over the reproductive life span.[2]

The nature of conjugal relations varies widely.  Firth
(1936, 1957:434) reports that, for Tikopian women,
marriage implies "emancipation because it enables [her]
to exercise authority in a sphere of her own.  Since
there is mutual deference between husband and wife,
marriage by explicit social custom means freedom not
servitude for her."  Halfway round the world, in
Tepoztlan, Mexico, Lewis (1949:603) found a different
situation:

Pregnancy and childbearing are viewed without
enthusiasm by women.  These attitudes are . . . in
sharp contrast to those of men.  The general reaction
of women to pressure to conform is one of a sense of
frustration and deprivation. . . .  The question of
authority in husband-wife relations is very much in
the minds of men and women in Tepoztlan.  There is an
awareness on the part of both of the growing asser-
tiveness of wives and the continual struggle of
husbands to keep them under control.

Harmony and partnership or distrust and conflict are
the two poles of conjugal style.  Which is more characteristic of contemporary cultures?  According to
Michaelson and Goldschmidt (1971:330), the male dominance
of Tepoztlan is at least overtly the norm in most peasant
societies.  However, this is a complex issue.  Although
men have strong authority in economic matters, including
such areas as the marriage of children that affect the
household economy, their personal ties with other family
members tend to be weak.  In this sphere, the woman exerts
strong influence.  Furthermore, the authors attribute the
widespread occurrence of this pattern among otherwise
disparate cultures to "recurrent structural responses to
the common organizational problems of peasant family life
[and] also recurrent structuring of social sentiments."
This theme of separate conjugal roles with constant
problems of authority is widespread in the literature.
In Sri Lanka, "although women can exert influence in many
situations, decisions are ultimately those of the husband-
father.  Rarely a rigid disciplinarian, the father is
still master in a society where that concept has a living
feudal memory" (Ryan, 1952:366).  In Botswana, among the
Kgatla, "a woman is explicitly instructed at marriage to
submit to her husband's attentions . . . quarrels owing
to a husband's failure to consider his wife's wishes are
commonplace . . ." (Schapera, 1940, 1971:161-162).  Evans-
Pritchard (1951:133) noted the latent hostility between
Nuer spouses:  "When a man has begotten several children
by his wife he wants her to die. . . ."  This feeling has
its roots in the inheritance system, but the tension is
not manifest in daily relations because the "authority of
the husband in the home" is unchallenged.  Nor is role
conflict between spouses limited to the tropics.  In
Shoreditch, near London, in the nineteenth century, a
similar though more overtly violent and cruel situation
prevailed.  As described by Young and Willmott (1957:18),

husbands were "mean with money," "callous in sex," and "violent when drunk," as well as harsh and secretive. This situation, they report, had been moderated but not eliminated by the time of their study in the mid-1950s.

Seen across cultures, then, a common pattern of male dominance and segregated conjugal roles is associated with many different cultural settings (Whyte, 1980: 341-343). Of course, the quality of the relationship depends on the local moral code, the religion, and the general pattern of social roles. The Sri Lankan "master" exercises authority very differently from a Nuer "chief" or a Tepoztlan "patron." Nonetheless, the important point is that inequality of relationships is widespread, and usually characterized by male dominance (see also Whyte, 1980; Davis, 1955; Back and Hass, 1963; for exceptions to this generalization see Kunstadter, 1963.)

How do fertility-related decisions take place in such contexts? To Blood and Wolfe (1960), the nub of the issue is the concept of relative conjugal power (see also Beckman, 1978:68-75). They note that each type of decision problem presents a couple with the need to establish a balance of interests, and that cultural and personal factors interact to determine the outcome. Hollerbach (1980) has applied this perspective to fertility research and suggests a categorization of typical conjugal power relationships according to the following qualities or characteristics:

    a.  coercive--threat of punishment;
    b.  reward--promise of reward;
    c.  legitimate--appeal to normative bases;
    d.  referent--identification with role model;
    e.  expert-oriented--claim of greater knowledge; and
    f.  informational--manipulation of knowledge.

These relationships are further related to different types of decision making--whether active or passive, joint or unilateral--and to particular cultural circumstances. In another characterization, patterns of power relationships have been classified according to their relative equality, concurrence, segregation, and openness (see Piepmeier and Adkins, 1973:513-514; Rosario, 1970; Hull, 1975; Pohlman, 1969:348-350).

These elements of decisional style are obviously related in subtle ways to the cultural setting. Westoff et al. (1963:243) contend that "effective family planning is based on accommodation, compromise or agreement" in

the American setting, and they relate these qualities to
social status and education. Back and Hass (1963:86)
have summarized a number of Latin American studies in
defining the relationship between "machismo" and
fertility (see also Beckman, these volumes); and Hull
(1975) analyzed the class differences in conjugal
relations in Java in an attempt to interpret fertility
differentials (see also Chamie, 1981:204-207). There is
clearly room for a great deal more of such work, which
could build usefully on the concepts and categorizations
proposed by Hollerbach (1980). Although a major purpose
would be to define differences between cultures, more
innovative work might focus on differences within cultures, comparing couples in different classes, castes,
educational groups, generations, and occupations. As
Berardo (1980:725) notes, although the issue of marital
power has received growing attention in the sixties and
seventies, "conceptual refinement remains a task for the
eighties," and this will only be achieved through more
detailed and diverse empirical studies (Hill, 1965:
126-128; Blood and Wolfe, 1960; Rodman, 1979:164-166;
Goldberg, 1975:101-102; Bagozzi and van Loo, 1980).

Although the dynamics of power relationships obviously
have a direct bearing on decision-making sequences,
communication and empathy are also dimensions of the
conjugal bond that influence fertility behavior. Husbands
and wives frequently do not communicate very freely about
fertility-related behavior, and empathy tends to be low
where interests and activities are segregated. Mukherjee
(1975) found "a marked absence of husband-wife communication" in India (see also Bhatia and Neumann, 1980;
Rosario, 1970). Similar results are found in Bangladesh
(Yaukey et al., 1967:716). In Egypt, most people studied
by Gadalla (1978:88) had not discussed family-size
desires, largely because three-quarters of respondents
had never thought about the issue. In Java, communication is strongly related to social class and generation.
One third of poor older women in a village survey had
discussed family planning with their spouses, compared to
two-thirds of poor young women and 84 percent of
well-to-do young women. Culture, class, and generation
are important considerations in studies of conjugal
relations.

If communication does take place, it is often assumed
that this will cause spouses to empathize with each
other's position and therefore act more efficiently to
achieve jointly defined goals. Studies addressing this

issue in developing countries are rare (Hill et al.,
1959; Stycos and Back, 1964; Yaukey et al., 1967).
However, in developed countries, empathy does appear to
be related to successful use of fertility control and
efficient limitation of family size.  Even in cases of
conflict, the result may be similar.  Townes et al.
(1980:219), Coombs and Chang (1979:21-22), and Fried and
Udry (1979:265) have shown that, in cases of disagreement, the woman's views on fertility behavior can
predominate because the issue may be considered part of
her "domain."  Although this clearly defines a power
relationship, it may also suggest a form of empathy
deserving more detailed consideration.

If male dominance, lack of communication, and segregated roles are common in contemporary cultures, can
these patterns of conjugal behavior be expected to
continue in the future?  The answer is probably no.  In
much of the developing world, arranged marriages are on
the wane.  Young people are being more innovative in
their fertility decision making (Hull and Hull, 1977;
Gupta, 1979; Coombs and Chang, 1979; Fox, 1975).  Moreover, changes toward more egalitarian decisional styles
can generate fertility effects quickly.  As Young and
Willmott (1957:26-27) found, even where the "old segregation of man and woman has not ended yet," a change in
decisional style can result in lower fertility.


The Influence of Other People on Decisional Style

As individuals or couples consider alternatives concerning marriage, sexual relations, contraception, gestation,
and parturition, they are strongly influenced by others
around them (Miller and Godwin, 1977:171-178; Beckman, in
these volumes).  Hollerbach's (1980) categories of power
relationships apply easily to the way women interact with
kin, neighbors, peers, community leaders, health professionals, and state authorities.  These extraconjugal
influences are important in shaping decisional style in a
number of ways:

a.  The meaning and nature of decision problems are
largely defined by social consensus and passed on to each
member of the culture in the process of socialization, as
well as in daily interaction and discussion.

b.  Value judgments about the propriety of fertility-
related behavior are shared; these can be expressed as
religious teaching, secular laws, or personal opinions.

c. Advice is sought from people who are regarded as generally wise, even though they may not have information directly related to the decision problem.

Consideration of extraconjugal influences thus returns analysis of fertility decision making back to basic questions about cultural and social influences (see Freedman, 1961-62; Burch and Gendell, 1970; Hill, 1962; Smith, 1963). On a practical level, these influences are thought to be undergoing substantial change in most areas of the world. Shorter (1975:15) sees this as a shift in the "boundary line between the family and the surrounding community" (see also Goode, 1963; Liu, 1977:54-57). The circle of people influential in decision-making sequences is changing (for a contrasting view see Laslett, 1972: 1-23). Whereas the traditional family is a productive and reproductive unit sharing strong economic interests among members of an extended kin group, innovative conjugal relations based on emotion modify this family structure. In her love for her husband, a wife may grow to resent his family's claim on his time, property, and loyalty. On the other hand, the extended family may be strengthened (as in Java) in an economy that encourages the growth of corporate units in industrial and commercial enterprise (Berardo, 1980; Hull and Hull, 1977). At issue is how kin relationships influence an individual's approach to particular fertility-related decisions. As Shah (1974:80) points out, "Every person in a household is involved in a complex pattern of behavior with every other member," and the meaning of these relationships may extend far beyond the economic or social activities that define them functionally. In appreciation of this, Cicourel (1974:21-26), Geertz (1960), and Jay (1969) counsel analysts to look for the "layers" of meaning in interactions.

Answers to questions about social change are not always simple. For example, although many writers see the trend toward individually arranged marriage as an aspect of personal liberation, Young and Willmott (1957:194) cite a different implication. "Affection, for its part, helps to make duty not so much the nicely balanced correlative of rights as a more or less unlimited liability beyond the bounds of self-interest and rational calculation." More public marriage arrangements tend to legitimize the involvement of extensive networks of people in the couple's affairs; although this can involve "meddling," it also offers possibilities of support and protection for individuals

facing difficult decision problems.  Because of such
complexities, Berardo (1980) concluded that "studies
which attempt to explain individual associations with kin
and how kin ties affect individuals and families might
very well predominate in the coming decade."  To be
useful, these will have to go beyond the rather narrow
analysis of "extended family and fertility" to probe
deeply the contexts of kin interactions.

Although the literature offers many examples of how
kin, neighbors, and peers can influence decisional style,
two relationships have so far received little attention
in the context of changing cultural settings:  the relationship of the decision-making couple to their children
and to the State.  Looking at developing countries over
the past 40 years, particularly in Asia and Africa, the
single most important force for change in society has
been nationalism.  With this have come strong demands for
mass education and medical and other services.  Governments, as personified by administrators, professionals,
fieldworkers, and local leaders, have usurped many functions formerly left to families and small communities.
This has radically changed the nature of decision-making
environments, and is an important factor in the innovative fertility decision making described above.  Schools
are in the vanguard of these changes.  They clearly alter
parent-child relationships in the economic sphere:  they
command the child's time, impose costs of attendance, and
change the child's perceptions of family roles and life
expectations.  Gaps grow between the parent and the child.
In this context, the parent at midpoint in a fertility
decision sequence is faced with not only a changing balance of costs and benefits but often also a different view
of what behavior associated with the proximate determinants is possible and proper.  The child, in Aries'
terms (1980), has a role in the family's plan and an
"affective" role in the family.  While the role of other
kin in fertility decisions is decreasing, the role and
influence of first-born children may be increasing.

## PROPOSITIONS

As this paper has suggested, fertility decision making is
far more complex than is suggested by the assumptions of
simple utility models.  An analysis of fertility decisions
must consider whether or not such decisions are conscious,
and, if so, whether they are rational; the extent to which

they involve external constraints or habitual responses;
how couples interact in the decision-making process; and
the extent of involvement of people other than the couple.
The propositions below summarize the major conclusions of
this paper on these topics. However, one major conclusion
that can be drawn is that further research is needed.
Tables 1 to 4 suggest a frame for such research. These
tables present some limited data gathered in a series of
studies in Java in the 1970s, and are followed by a number
of more specific propositions drawn from these data that
might be investigated by future research.

## Summary Propositions

1.  The decision-making environment is cultural, including
language, belief systems, technology, social institutions,
and individual environment. Decision making is both a
product and a determinant of this framework. Societies
undergoing cultural change are likely to be changing with
regard to the way fertility decisions are made.
    2.  Irrationality is a relative concept that must be
defined as a conflict between behavior and objectives in
specific situations. Irrationality in decision making
can take four forms:
        a. lack of adequate deliberation--although the
outcome may be reasonable, the process of decision making
may be regarded as "irrational" because the decision
maker did not use reason in achieving the result;
        b. conflict of an individual's decision with
objectives set by another individual or group;
        c. conflict of an individual's decision with
objectives professed by that individual at a different
time or level of consideration; and
        d. conflict of an individual's decision with
objectives attached to a particular decision problem, as
opposed to objectives implied in the logic of a decision
sequence.
    3.  Whether habitual or considered, most fertility
decision-making behavior involves purposes, benefits,
costs, and consequences that are unrelated to childbearing. Marriage serves a variety of social functions,
and sexual activity provides personal pleasures that are
often considered irrelevant to the number and spacing of
births.
    4.1.  Habitual decision making is most frequent with
decision problems that arise frequently and uniformly

TABLE 1   Is the Decision Problem Normally a Matter of Conscious Choice?

| Decision Problem | Is Individual Aware of Choices: | | Does Individual Usually See Choice as Related to: | |
| --- | --- | --- | --- | --- |
| | Ever? | Usually? | Birth Spacing | Family Size |
| **Fertility Decisions** | | | | |
| Number of children | Yes | Yes | Yes | Yes |
| Gender of children | Yes | No | No | Sometimes |
| Spacing of births | Yes | Yes | Yes | Yes |
| Termination norm | Yes | ? | No | Yes |
| **Proximate Behavior Decisions** | | | | |
| Celibacy | -- | -- | -- | -- |
| Initiation of sexual activity | Yes | Yes | No | No |
| Legitimation of sexual union | Yes | Yes | No | No |
| Establishment of coresidence | Yes | Yes | No | No |
| Temporary separation | Yes | Yes | No | No |
| Dissolution of sexual union | | | | |
|   Permanent separation | Yes | Yes | No | No |
|   Divorce (legal) | Yes | Yes | No | Sometimes |
|   Widowhood/death | Yes | No | No | No |
| Sexual activity within union | | | | |
|   Average frequency | Yes | Yes | No? | No? |
|   Periodic abstinence | Yes | Yes | No | Yes? |
|   Postpartum abstinence | Yes | Yes | Yes | No |
|   Other voluntary abstinence | Yes | Yes | No | No |
|   Physical incapacity | Yes | No | No | No |
|   Other involuntary abstinence | -- | -- | -- | -- |
| Fecundity of union | | | | |
|   Natural fecundity | -- | -- | -- | -- |
|   Sterilization | Yes | No | -- | -- |
| Use of contraceptives | | | | |
|   Barrier methods | Yes | Yes | Yes | Yes |
|   Chemical methods | Yes | Yes | Yes | Yes |
|   Pill, injection | Yes | Yes | Yes | Yes |
|   IUD | Yes | Yes | Yes | Yes |
| Parturition behavior | | | | |
|   Involuntary abortion | -- | -- | -- | -- |
|   Voluntary abortion | Yes | Yes | No | No |
| Postpartum behavior | | | | |
|   Breastfeeding behavior | Yes | Yes | Yes | No |
|   Infant care | Yes | Yes | No? | No? |

Note:   The answers in each cell are speculations based on field research and survey results.   Dash indicates rare, inapplicable, or indeterminate situations.

Source:   Maguwoharjo (Indonesia) survey, 1972-73, reported in various publications by Hull and Hull.

TABLE 2    Habit and Precedent in Fertility Decision Making

| Decision Problem | Arises Frequently from the Viewpoint of: | | Routine Because of: | |
|---|---|---|---|---|
| | Individuals | Society | Habit | Custom |
| **Fertility Decisions** | | | | |
| Number of children | At high parities | Yes | No | Yes |
| Gender of children | No | No | -- | -- |
| Spacing of births | 3-6 times | Yes | Yes | Yes |
| Termination norm | No | Yes | No | Yes |
| **Proximate Behavior Decisions** | | | | |
| Celibacy | Rarely | Rarely | Rarely | No |
| Initiation of sexual activity | In adolescence | Yes | No | Yes |
| Legitimation of sexual union[a] | No | No | No | Yes |
| Establishment of coresidence | Upon marriage | Yes | No | Yes |
| Temporary separation | Possibly | Yes | Possibly | Possibly |
| Dissolution of sexual union | | | | |
|   Permanent separation | Rarely | Rarely | -- | -- |
|   Divorce (legal) | Commonly | Commonly | No | Yes |
|   Widowhood/death | -- | -- | -- | -- |
| Sexual activity within union | | | | |
|   Average frequency | Yes | Yes | Yes | No? |
|   Periodic abstinence | Possibly | No | Yes | Sometimes |
|   Postpartum abstinence | 3-4 times | Yes | Yes | Yes |
|   Other voluntary abstinence | Possibly | No | No | Yes |
|   Physical incapacity | -- | -- | -- | -- |
|   Other involuntary abstinence | -- | -- | -- | -- |
| Fecundity of union | | | | |
|   Natural fecundity | -- | -- | -- | -- |
|   Sterilization | No | No | -- | -- |
| Use of contraceptives | | | | |
|   Barrier methods | Rarely | Rarely | Yes | No |
|   Chemical methods | Rarely | Rarely | Yes | No |
|   Pill, injection | Yes | Yes | Yes | No |
|   IUD | No | Yes | No | No |
| Parturition behavior | | | | |
|   Involuntary abortion | -- | -- | -- | -- |
|   Voluntary abortion | Rarely | Yes | No | Yes |
| Postpartum behavior | | | | |
|   Breastfeeding behavior | Yes | Yes | Yes | Yes |
|   Infant care | Yes | Yes | Yes | Yes |

Note:   Dash indicates inapplicable or indeterminate situations.

[a]Involves question of marriage, legal, religious, and customary.

Source:   Maguwoharjo survey, 1972-73.

## TABLE 3   Conjugal Interaction in Decision Making

| Decision Problem | Unilateral Decisions by Either Partner: | | Requires Both Partners': | | |
|---|---|---|---|---|---|
| | Possible | Common | Knowledge | Approval | Cooperation |
| **Fertility Decisions** | | | | | |
| Number of children | Yes | No | No | No | Yes |
| Gender of children | -- | -- | ? | ? | ? |
| Spacing of births | Yes | No | Yes | ? | Yes |
| Termination norm | Yes | No | Yes | ? | Yes |
| **Proximate Behavior Decisions** | | | | | |
| Celibacy | -- | -- | -- | -- | -- |
| Initiation of sexual activity | Yes | No | Yes | Yes | Yes |
| Legitimation of sexual union | No | No | Yes | Yes | Yes |
| Establishment of coresidence | No | No | Yes | Yes | Yes |
| Temporary separation | Yes | No | Yes | ? | -- |
| Dissolution of sexual union | | | | | |
|   Permanent separation | Yes | Yes | Yes | No | -- |
|   Divorce (legal) | Yes | Yes | Yes | No | Yes |
|   Widowhood/death[a] | -- | -- | -- | -- | -- |
| Sexual activity within union | | | | | |
|   Average frequency | Yes | No | Yes | No | Yes |
|   Periodic abstinence | Yes | No | Yes | No | Yes |
|   Postpartum abstinence | Yes | No | Yes | No | Yes |
|   Other voluntary abstinence | Yes | No | Yes | No | Yes |
|   Physical incapacity | -- | -- | -- | -- | -- |
|   Other involuntary abstinence | -- | -- | -- | -- | -- |
| Fecundity of union | | | | | |
|   Natural fecundity | -- | -- | -- | -- | -- |
|   Sterilization | Yes | No | Yes | Yes | Yes |
| Use of contraceptives | | | | | |
|   Barrier methods | Yes | No | Yes | Yes | No |
|   Chemical methods | Yes | No | Yes | Yes | No |
|   Pill, injection | Yes | No | No | No | No |
|   IUD | Yes | No | Yes | Yes | No |
| Parturition behavior | | | | | |
|   Involuntary abortion | -- | -- | -- | -- | -- |
|   Voluntary abortion | Yes | No | No | No | No |
| Postpartum behavior | | | | | |
|   Breastfeeding behavior | Yes | Yes | No | No | No |
|   Infant care | Yes | No | No | No | No |

Note:  Dash indicates inapplicable or indeterminate situations.

[a]Applicable only to murder, suicide.

Source:  Maguwoharjo survey, 1972-73.

TABLE 4   Influence of Kin and Community in Fertility Decision Making

| Decision Problem | Morally Sensitive | Requires Someone Else's: | | |
|---|---|---|---|---|
| | | Knowledge | Approval | Cooperation |
| **Fertility Decisions** | | | | |
| Number of children | No | No | No | No |
| Gender of children | No | No | No | No |
| Spacing of births | No | No | No | No |
| Termination norm | No | No | No | No |
| **Proximate Behavior Decisions** | | | | |
| Celibacy | No | No | No | No |
| Initiation of sexual activity | Yes | No | No | No |
| Legitimation of sexual union | Yes | Yes | Yes | Yes |
| Establishment of coresidence | No | Yes | Yes | Yes |
| Temporary separation | No | Yes | No | No |
| Dissolution of sexual union | | | | |
|   Permanent separation | Yes | Yes | No | No |
|   Divorce (legal) | Yes | Yes | Yes | Yes |
|   Widowhood/death | -- | -- | -- | -- |
| Sexual activity within union | | | | |
|   Average frequency | No | No | No | No |
|   Periodic abstinence | No | No | No | No |
|   Postpartum abstinence | No | No | No | No |
|   Other voluntary abstinence | No | No | No | No |
|   Physical incapacity | -- | -- | -- | -- |
|   Other involuntary abstinence | -- | -- | -- | -- |
| Fecundity of union | | | | |
|   Natural fecundity | -- | -- | -- | -- |
|   Sterilization | Sometimes | Yes | Yes | Yes |
| Use of contraceptives | | | | |
|   Barrier methods | No | Yes | Yes | Yes |
|   Chemical methods | No | Yes | Yes | Yes |
|   Pill, injection | No | Yes | Yes | Yes |
|   IUD | Sometimes | Yes | Yes | Yes |
| Parturition behavior | | | | |
|   Involuntary abortion | -- | -- | -- | -- |
|   Voluntary abortion | Yes | Yes | Yes | Yes |
| Postpartum behavior | | | | |
|   Breastfeeding behavior | No | No | No | No |
|   Infant care | No | No | No | No |

Note:  Dash indicates not applicable or indeterminate.

Source:  Maguwoharjo survey, 1972-73.

(especially with the proximate variables of coitus, abstinence, and contraceptive use), and often develops into unconscious reactions to regular stimuli.

4.2. Nonhabitual decision making is most prominent with decision problems that are unique (age at first coitus), infrequent (marriage, periodic abstinence), or regarded as involving serious consequences (abortion, divorce).

4.3. Decision making is likely to follow social precedent under conditions of general uncertainty and risk.

5. Fertility decision making involves a complex sequence of decision problems over the lifetime of individuals. Fertility is best seen as determined by the combined effects of numerous decisions, rather than as the product of a single decision.

5.1. Decision sequences consist of individual decisions and the logical links that bind them together.

5.2. Given the strength of the logic of decision sequences and established habits and patterns of relationships, the way to induce change is not to provide information about alternative behaviors, but to promote systematic challenges to the power structures involved in the decision-making process.

6. Generally, decision making related to fertility involves the conjugal pair. The nature of the relationship between spouses depends on their relative power to communicate, negotiate, and enforce their desires. Commonly, males dominate in this process, although females can often exert their will informally, or within specific domains.

7.1. Kin influence on decisional style is reciprocal rather than directive. An understanding of this reciprocal relationship is important in distinguishing apparently coerced from more complex, mutually determined behavior.

7.2. The power of individuals other than the couple to influence decisional style is defined by social institutions such as the family, the community, and the state. The nature of the extended family is changing in many areas, with the result that its influence is being modified. Of particular interest is the growing role of the state and children in defining decisional styles.

8. Whatever the aspirations of those attempting to induce fertility change, evidence from most of the developing world indicates that autonomous social changes are currently transforming the style of fertility decision making. Fertility may be modified by shifts in family

relations resulting from these changes much more than by changes in economic conditions. Conversely, in the case of some decision-making frameworks, it is possible that fertility behavior may remain relatively stable despite substantial economic changes.

## Specific Propositions

As noted above, specific data on the issues raised in this paper are generally lacking. Further research is needed to provide such data, and thereby to permit a more thorough investigation of the general propositions offered above. The data in Tables 1-4 were collected in Java in the 1970s, and are presented here as a frame for the further work needed. The propositions that follow are based on these tables and should be worth further empirical testing.

1. Decision making concerned directly with issues of fertility (number, gender, spacing, and termination) varies in style, both across and within cultures.

2. There may be a lack of congruence between fertility objectives and behaviors related to the proximate variables. Thus, for example, high proportions of women saying they "want no more children" may not indicate a practical desire for birth control.

3. Decisions about celibacy are usually related primarily to personal (often physical) characteristics of individuals, and to social roles developed within specific religious or economic institutions.

4. The formation of sexual unions varies across cultures, being based on the timing of initiation of sexual activity, the practices related to the legitimizing of liaisons, and residence patterns.

5. Decisions about sexual behavior, including regularity and style of coitus, patterns of abstinence, and suspension of normal sexual relations, involve complex and often contradictory motivations on the parts of husbands and wives. In settings where conjugal roles are distinct, communication on these matters will be limited, and behavior is likely to be determined by coercion or reward power, rather than by appeals to information, norms, or expert opinion.

6. Power relationships among families reflect those of the broader society.

7. Involuntary behaviors (or conditions, such as infecundity) form part of decision-making sequences.

Even an involuntary condition is frequently surrounded by
decisions that directly condition or flow from it.
    8.  Decision making relating to gestation and the
postpartum period focuses on the welfare of the infant
rather than on that of older or future children.
    9.  Innovative contraceptive behavior can be evaluated
according to its degree of adaptation to the prevailing
decision-making sequence; both the method and the delivery
system must be seen in the context of how individuals,
couples, and others currently view reproductive decisions.
However, adaptation does not always demand accomodation.
Such innovations may require--and promote--changes in the
way decisions are made.  Therefore, whereas current
research is directed at modifying methods or educating
individuals, a more crucial question in some cases is how
particular styles of family relationships can be altered
to facilitate acceptance of contraception.

NOTES

1. A very good review of the concept of rationality as
   used by social scientists is Benn and Mortimore
   (1976).  See especially Chapters 3, 6, 8, and 14.
2. Conjugal relationships take many forms.  Although this
   discussion focuses on marriage, other mating patterns
   are also important (see Burch, in these volumes).  The
   literature on the Caribbean family offers many
   insights into decision-making sequences in the context
   of relatively fluid relationships (see Slater,
   1977:154-189).

BIBLIOGRAPHY

Adler, N. E. (1979)  Decision models in population
    research.  Journal of Population 2:187-202.
Aries, P. (1980)  Two successive motivations for the
    declining birth rate in the West.  Population and
    Development Review 6:645-650.
Back, K. W., and P. H. Hass (1963)  Family structure and
    fertility control.  In J. T. Fawcett, ed.,
    Psychological Perspectives on Population.  New York:
    Basic Books.
Bagozzi, R. P., and M. F. Van Loo (1980)  Decision-making
    and fertility: A theory of exchange in the family.
    Pp. 91-134 in J. K. Burch, ed., Demographic Behavior:

Interdisciplinary Perspectives on Decision-Making.
Boulder, Colo.: Westview Press.
Becker, G. (1960) An economic analysis of fertility.
Pp. 209-231 in National Bureau of Economic Research,
Demographic and Economic Change in Developed
Countries. Princeton, N.J.: Princeton University
Press.
Beckman, L. J. (1978) Couples' decision-making processes
regarding fertility. Pp. 57-81 in K. E. Taeuber, L.
L. Bumpass, and J. A. Sweet, eds., Social Demography.
New York: Academic Press.
Benedict, B. (1972) Social regulation of fertility. Pp.
73-89 in G. A. Harrison and A. J. Boyce, eds., The
Structure of Human Populations. Oxford: Clarendon
Press.
Benn, S. I., and G. W. Mortimore, eds. (1976)
Rationality and the Social Sciences. London:
Routledge and Kegan Paul.
Benn, S. I., and G. W. Mortimore (1976) Rationality and
the Social Sciences: Contributions to the Philosophy
and Methodology of the Social Sciences. London:
Routledge and Kegan Paul.
Berardo, F. M. (1980) Decade preview: Some trends and
directions for family research and theory in the
1980s. Journal of Marriage and the Family 42:723-728.
Bhatia, J. C., and A. K. Neumann (1980) Inter-spousal
communication and practice of contraception in India.
Journal of Family Welfare 26(4):18-30.
Blood, R. O., and D. M. Wolfe (1960) Husbands and
Wives: The Dynamics of Married Living. New York:
The Free Press.
Bongaarts, J. (1978) A framework for analyzing the
proximate determinants of fertility. Population and
Development Review 4:105-132.
Bulatao, R. A., and J. T. Fawcett (1981) Dynamic
perspectives in the study of fertility
decision-making: Successive decisions within a
fertility career. Pp. 433-449 in International
Population Conference, Manila, 1981, Vol 1. Liege:
International Union for the Scientific Study of
Population.
Burch, T. K. (1980) Decision-making theories in
demography: An introduction. Pp. 1-22 in T. K.
Burch, ed., Demographic Behavior: Interdisciplinary
Perspectives on Decision-Making. Boulder, Colo.:
Westview Press.

Burch, T. K., and M. Gendell (1970) Extended family
    structure and fertility: Some conceptual and
    methodological issues. Journal of Marriage and the
    Family 32:227-236.
Cain, M. (1981) Risk and insurance: Perspectives on
    fertility and agrarian change in India and
    Bangladesh. Population and Development Review
    7:435-474.
Caldwell, J. C. (1981) The mechanisms of demographic
    change in historical perspective. Population Studies
    35:5-27.
Carr-Saunders, A. M. (1922) The Population Problem: A
    Study in Human Evolution. Oxford: Clarendon Press.
Chamie, M. (1981) Marital relations and fertility
    control decisions among Lebanese couples. Population
    and Environment 4:189-208.
Cicourel, A. V. (1967) Fertility, family planning and
    the social organization of family life: Some
    methodological issues. Journal of Social Issues
    23(4):57-81.
Cicourel, A. V. (1974) Theory and Method in a Study of
    Argentine Fertility. New York: John Wiley and Sons.
Coombs, L. C., and M.-C. Chang (1979) Consistency of
    Fertility Attitudes Between Marital Partners and its
    Role in Subsequent Fertility. Taiwan Population
    Studies, Working Paper No. 43. University of Michigan
    Population Studies Center and Taiwan Provincial
    Institute of Family Planning.
Davis, K. (1955) Institutional patterns favoring high
    fertility in underdeveloped areas. Eugenics Quarterly
    2(1):33-9.
Davis, K., and J. Blake (1956) Social structure and
    fertility: An analytic framework. Economic
    Development and Cultural Change 4:211-235.
Day, L. H. (1979) Demographic concerns of the 1980s and
    the applicability of economic and sociological frames
    of reference to their analysis. Pp. 277-287 in
    Proceedings of the Conference on Economic and
    Demographic Change: Issues for the 1980s. Liege:
    International Union for the Scientific Study of
    Population.
Demeny, P. (1970) Causes and consequences of excess
    fertility. Pp. 33-44 in A Report on a Family Planning
    Conference. Monograph 7, Carolina Population Center.
    Chapel Hill, N.C.: University of North Carolina.
De Tray, D. (1979) The demand for children in a "natural
    fertility" population. Pakistan Development Review
    18:55-65.

Duesenberry, J. S. (1960) Comment. Pp. 231–234 in National Bureau of Economic Research, Demographic and Economic Change in Developed Countries. Princeton, N.J.: Princeton University Press.

Evans-Pritchard, E. E. (1951) Kinship and Marriage among the Nuer. Oxford, Eng.: Clarendon Press.

Firth, R. (1936, 1957) We, the Tikopia. Boston: Beacon Press.

Ford, C. S. (1945) A Comparative Study of Human Reproduction. New Haven, Conn.: Yale University Press.

Fox, G. L. (1975) Love match and arranged marriage in a modernizing nation: Mate selection in Ankara, Turkey. Journal of Marriage and the Family 37:180–193.

Freedman, R. (1961-62) The sociology of human fertility: A trend report and bibliography. Current Sociology 10/11:35–121.

Freedman, R. (1967) Applications of the behavioral sciences to family planning programs. Studies in Family Planning 23:5–9.

Fried, E. S., and J. R. Udry (1979) Wives' and husbands' expected costs and benefits of childbearing as predictors of pregnancy. Social Biology 26:265–274.

Gadalla, S. M. (1978) Is There Hope? Fertility and Family Planning in a Rural Egyptian Community. Cairo, Egypt: American University in Cairo Press.

Geertz, C. (1960) The Religion of Java. Glencoe, Ill.: The Free Press.

Goldberg, D. (1975) Socioeconomic theory and differential fertility: The case of the LDC's. Social Forces 54:84–106.

Goode, W. J. (1963) World Revolution and Family Patterns. New York: The Free Press.

Gupta, G. R. (1979) Love, arranged marriage and the Indian social structure. Pp. 169–179 in G. Kurian, ed., Cross-Cultural Perspectives of Mate-Selection and Marriage. Westport, Conn.: Greenwood Press

Hawthorn, G. (1970) The Sociology of Fertility. London: Collier-MacMillian.

Hill, R. (1962) Cross-national family research: Attempts and prospects. International Social Science Journal 4:425–451.

Hill, R. (1965) Decision-making and the family life cycle. Pp. 113–139 in E. Shanas and G. F. Streib, eds., Social Structure and the Family: Generational Relations. Englewood Cliffs, N.J.: Prentice-Hall.

Hill, R., Stycos, J. M., and Back, K. W. (1959) The Family and Population Control. Chapel Hill, N.C.: University of North Carolina Press.

Hollerbach, P. E. (1980) Power in families, communication and fertility decision-making. Journal of Population 3(2).

Hull, T. H. (1975) Each Child Brings Its Own Fortune: An Enquiry into the Value of Children in a Javanese Village. Unpublished Ph.D. dissertation. Australian National University, Canberra.

Hull, T. H. (1977) A Review of Research on the Price, Cost, and Value of Children in Indonesia. Paper prepared for the Workshop on the Costs of Children, Pattaya, Thailand. Working Paper No. 12, Population Institute, Gadjah Mada University, Yogyakarta.

Hull, T. H. (1980) Fertility decline in Indonesia: A review of recent evidence. Bulletin of Indonesian Economic Studies 16:104-112.

Hull, T. H., and V. J. Hull (1977) Indonesia. Pp. 827-894 in J. C. Caldwell, ed., The Persistence of High Fertility: Population Prospects in the Third World. Monograph 1, Family and Fertility Change Series. Canberra: Department of Demography, Australian National University.

Jay, R. R. (1969) Javanese Villagers: Social Relations in Rural Modjokuto. Cambridge, Mass.: MIT Press.

Joseph, R. (1979) Sexual dialectics and strategy in Berber marriage. Pp. 191-201 in G. Kurian, ed., Cross-Cultural Perspectives of Mate-Selection and Marriage. Westport, Conn.: Greenwood Press.

Keesing, R. M. (1974) Theories of culture. Annual Review of Anthropology 3:73-97.

Kunstadter, P. (1963) A survey of the consanguine or matrifocal family. American Anthropologist 65:56-66.

Kyriazis, N. (1979) Sequential fertility decision making: Catholics and Protestants in Canada. Canadian Review of Sociology and Anthropology 16:275-286.

Laslett, P., ed. (1972) Household and Family in Past Time. Cambridge, Eng.: Cambridge University Press.

Leach, E. (1969) Genesis as Myth and Other Essays. London: Jonathan Cape.

Leibenstein, H. (1981) Economic decision theory and human fertility behavior: A speculative essay. Population and Development Review 7:381-400.

Lesthaeghe, R. (1980) On the social control of human reproduction. Population and Development Review 6:527-548.

Lesthaeghe, R., I. H. Shah, and H. Page (1981)
Compensating changes in intermediate fertility
variables and the onset of marital fertility
transition. Pp. 71-94 in International Population
Conference, Manila, 1981, Vol 1. Liege:
International Union for the Scientific Study of
Population.

Lewis, O. (1949) Husbands and wives in a Mexican
village: A study of role conflict. American
Anthropologist 51:602-610.

Little, K. (1969) Women's strategies in modern marriage
in Anglophone West Africa: An ideological and
sociological appraisal. Pp. 202-217 in G. Kurian,
ed., Cross-Cultural Perspectives of Mate-Selection and
Marriage. Westport, Conn.: Greenwood Press.

Liu, W. T. (1977) The myths of the nuclear family and
fertility in Central Philippines. Pp. 35-62 in L.
Lenero-Otero, ed., Beyond the Nuclear Family Model:
Cross-Cultural Perspectives. London: Sage
Publications Ltd.

Lorimer, F. (1954) Notes on human fertility in Central
Africa. Pp. 130-135 in The Interrelations of
Demographic, Economic and Social Problems in Selected
Underdeveloped Areas. New York: Milbank Memorial
Fund.

Malinowski, B. (1929) The Sexual Life of Savages.
London: Routledge and Kegan Paul.

Marshall, J. F., S. Morris, and S. Polgar (1972) Culture
and natality: A preliminary classified bibliography.
Current Anthropology 13:268-278.

Meeker, B. F. (1980) Rational decision-making models in
interpersonal behavior. Pp. 23-42 in T. K. Burch,
ed., Demographic Behavior: Interdisciplinary
Perspectives on Decision-Making. Boulder, Colo.:
Westview Press.

Michaelson, E. J., and W. Goldschmidt (1971) Female
roles and male dominance among peasants. Southwestern
Journal of Anthropology 27:330-352.

Miller, W. B., and R. K. Godwin (1977) Psyche and
Demos. New York: Oxford University Press.

Mukherjee, B. N. (1975) The role of husband-wife
communication in family planning. Journal of Marriage
and the Family 37:655-667.

Nag, M. (1962, 1968) Factors Affecting Human Fertility
in Nonindustrial Societies: A Cross-Cultural Study.
Yale University Publications in Anthropology No. 66.
Reprinted by Human Relations Area Files Press.

Namboodiri, N. K. (1973)  Some observations on the economic analysis of human fertility. Pp. 78-95 in I. Z. Husain, ed., Population Analysis and Studies. Kent: Abacus Press.

Namboodiri, N. K. (1980)  A look at fertility model-building from different perspectives. Pp. 71-90 in T. K. Burch, ed., Demographic Behavior: Interdisciplinary Perspectives on Decision-Making. Boulder, Colo.: Westview Press.

Neal, A. G., and H. T. Groat (1980)  Fertility decision-making, unintended births, and the social drift hypothesis: A longitudinal study. Population and Environment 3:221-236.

Neher, P. A. (1971)  Peasants, procreation, and pensions. American Economic Review 61(3,1):380-189.

Notestein, F. W. (1945)  Population--The long view. In T. W. Schultz, ed., Food for the World. Chicago: University of Chicago Press.

Piepmeier, K. B., and T. S. Adkins (1973)  The status of women and fertility. Journal of Biosocial Science 5:507-520.

Pohlman, E. H. (1969)  The Psychology of Birth Planning. Cambridge, Mass.: Schenkman Publishing Co.

Pool, J. E. (1972)  A cross-comparative study of aspects of conjugal behavior among women of three West African countries. Canadian Journal of African Studies 6:233-259.

Rainwater, L. (1960)  And the Poor Get Children: Sex, Contraception and Family Planning in the Working Class. Chicago: Quadrangle Books.

Repetto, R. (1977)  Correlates of field-worker performance in the Indonesian family planning program: A test of the homophily-hererophily hypothesis. Studies in Family Planning 8:19-21.

Rodman, H. (1979)  Marital power and the theory of resources in cultural context. Pp. 149-168 in G. Kurian, ed., Cross-Cultural Perspectives of Mate-Selection and Marriage. Westport, Conn.: Greenwood Press.

Rogers, E. M. (1973)  Communication Strategies for Family Planning. New York: The Free Press.

Rosario, F. Z. (1970)  Husband-Wife Interaction and Family Planning Acceptance: A Survey of the Literature. Working Paper No. 3. Honolulu: East-West Population Institute.

Ryan, B. (1952)  Institutional factors in Sinhalese fertility. Milbank Memorial Fund Quarterly 30:359-381.

Samuels, W. J. (1966)  The Classical Theory of Economic Policy. New York: World Publishing Company.

Schapera, I. (1940)  Married Life in an African Tribe. Middlesex, Eng.:  Pelican Books.

Shah, A. M. (1974)  The Household Dimension of the Family in India: A Field Study in a Gujarat Village and a Review of Other Studies. Berkeley, Calif.: University of California Press.

Shedlin, M. G., and P. E. Hollerbach (1981)  Modern and traditional fertility regulation in a Mexican community:  The process of decision making.  Studies in Family Planning 12(6/7).

Shorter, E. (1975)  The Making of the Modern Family. Glasgow:  William Collins and Sons.

Simon, H. A. (1957)  Models of Man. New York:  John Wiley.

Slater, M. K. (1977)  The Caribbean Family. New York: St. Martin's Press.

Smith, R. T. (1963)  Culture and social structure in the Caribbean:  Some recent work on family and kinship studies. Comparative Studies in Society and History 6:24-46.

Stycos, J. M., and K. W. Back (1964)  The Control of Human Fertility in Jamaica. New York:  Cornell University Press.

Tien, H. Y. (1968)  The intermediate variables, social structure and fertility change:  A critique. Demography 5:138-157.

Townes, B. D., L. R. Beach, F. L. Campbell, and R. L. Wood (1980)  Family building:  A social psychological study of fertility decisions. Population and Environment 3:210-220.

Trussell, T. J., R. Faden, and R. A. Hatcher (1976) Efficacy information in contraceptive counselling: Those little white lies. American Journal of Public Health 66:761-767.

Valentine, C. H., and J. E. Revson (1979)  Cultural traditions, social change, and fertility in sub-Saharan Africa. Journal of Modern African Studies 17:453-472.

Westoff, C. F., R. G. Potter, and P. C. Sagi (1963)  The Third Child: A Study in the Prediction of Fertility. Princeton, N.J.:  Princeton University Press.

Whyte, M. K. (1980)  Cross-cultural codes dealing with the relative status of women. Pp. 335-361 in H. Barry and A. Schlegel, eds., Cross-Cultural Samples and Codes. Pittsburgh, Pa.:  University of Pittsburgh Press.

Yaukey, D. (1979)  On theorizing about fertility. American Sociologist 4:100-104.

Yaukey, D., W. Griffiths, and B. Roberts (1967)  Couple concurrence and empathy on birth control motivation in Dacca, East Pakistan. American Sociological Review 32(5):716-726.

Young, M., and P. Willmott (1957)  Family and Kinship in East London. Harmondsworth:  Penguin Books Ltd.

Chapter 11

# Communication, Power, and the Influence of Social Networks in Couple Decisions on Fertility

LINDA J. BECKMAN

Fertility decisions are highly complex. First, they are dyadic or group decisions, usually involving at least one man and one woman, and, where family and social ties are strong, a number of other persons as well. Moreover, these decisions do not represent a simple averaging of the participants' intentions; rather, "the decision is made in the total context of the particular dyadic relationship and is influenced by all aspects of that relationship [especially] communication and dominance" (Miller and Godwin, 1977:77). Additionally, fertility decisions involve a wide range of psychological and interpersonal influences, causing variations in strength, style, and specificity. Such decisions may even vary in their degree of explicitness: some couples become parents without making any conscious decision, while others care- fully plan the timing of each birth.

This complexity helps to explain the limited research on fertility decision making. The present paper reviews the literature that does exist on how couple decision making influences fertility, focusing on how communication and dominance or social power affect the demand for chil- dren, contraceptive use, and fertility levels. Although most research has focused on the first of these areas-- the demand for children--it is important to note that a couple's fertility decision making can also influence the psychic costs of contraception and abortion, and, indi- rectly, the supply of children. For present purposes, communication can be defined as the verbalization of information, ideas, attitudes, and beliefs to another person, implying, though not requiring, a two-way or multi-way flow of information. Social power or dominance is the ability to influence another person or group. The discussion here generally refers to married couples;

however, it applies equally to stable nonmarital sexual unions.

The first section of this paper examines agreement between spouses on fertility intentions and preferences, focusing on the possible effects of such agreement and on the relative importance of the husband's and the wife's attitudes. The second section considers the role of husband-wife communication in the decision process; the relationship between communication and agreement is also examined. The third section explores the role of power in structuring communication and resolving disagreement. The fourth section examines the conditions under which unilateral, usually surreptitious, fertility decisions are made in stable sexual unions. The fifth section discusses the conditions under which kin or social networks affect couple communication, relative power, and fertility behavior. Finally, the sixth section explores the relationship of macro-level variables to fertility behavior, focusing on how conjugal communication and power mediate the effects of these variables.

## PARTNER AGREEMENT

### Concurrence, Consensus, and Concordance

The extent to which spouses have similar preferences regarding family size and family planning is called concurrence (e.g., Yaukey et al., 1967; Hill et al., 1959). The concept of concurrence involves both mutually recognized agreement based on discussion (consensus) and coincidentally similar preferences (concordance). Presumably, concurrence is important because it is linked to husband-wife discussion and may influence actual fertility by reducing the psychic costs of fertility regulation.

Yaukey et al. (1967) reported that those successful in guessing their partners' family planning goals most often were projecting their own preferences. Only 21 percent of nonconcurring couples correctly guessed their spouses' responses, as compared to over 70 percent of concurring couples. The authors also concluded that much concurrence between spouses was essentially concordance, i.e., could be attributed to coincidentally similar views. Studies in four other countries comparing husbands' and wives' responses support this conclusion (Coombs and Chang, 1981, for Taiwan; Coombs and Fernandez, 1978, for Malaysia; Hill et al., 1959, for Puerto Rico; United Nations, 1961, for

India).  Such findings question the predominance of joint
fertility decisions.  In particular, there may be little
need for such decisions in countries where strong shared
social norms support certain levels of fertility.  In such
cases, individuals base behavior on these internalized
norms or on assumptions about their partners' attitudes.
This pattern, which Hollerbach (1980) labels passive
decision making, is more likely to occur in the early
stages of the family cycle, when couples still desire more
children, or when partners lack contraceptive knowledge.
Moreover, since societies with strong pronatalist norms
tend to be more traditional and less developed, it follows
that concordance between partners is probably associated
with high demand for children, low levels of family planning, and high fertility.

High levels of couple concurrence will affect fertility
differently if consensus is involved.  Although no studies
directly compare the effects of concordance and consensus
on demand for children, it may be argued that couples who
have reached consensus should be more effective in achieving their fertility desires because their decision making
is more explicit.  Consensus may also be more characteristic of couples who desire no more children.  However,
agreement to have no more children must be translated
into consistent behavior; if the partners do not practice
regulation, agreement alone will not lead to lower
fertility.

## Female Versus Male Approval of Family Planning

Use of birth control usually requires both the husband's
and the wife's approval.  Male approval can follow rather
than precede contraceptive use; however, research around
the world supports the conclusion that contraceptive use
is more prevalent and continuous when the husband approves
of it, particularly among the lower classes (Latin America:  Brody et al., 1974; DESAL, 1968; Hall, 1971; Hass,
1971; Hollerbach, 1980; Kar and Talbot, 1980; Mundigo,
1973; Requena, 1965; Simmons and Culagovski, 1975; Stycos,
1968; Africa:  Kar and Talbot, 1980; Asia:  ESCAP, 1974;
Kim and Lee, 1973; the Middle East:  Chamie, 1978).  For
instance, Chamie (1978) reported that over 40 percent of
women who did not return to a clinic for a tubal ligation
cited their husbands' objections as a reason.  Kim and
Lee (1973), analyzing data from a national probability
sample of South Korean married women, found that the

husband's perceived support for family planning was significantly related to the wife's contraceptive practices:
women who did not themselves support family planning but
believed their husbands strongly supported it had higher
contraceptive adoption rates than women who were favorable toward family planning but perceived their husbands
as less supportive. The husband's approval was also
related to communication about family planning between
the spouses. Less educated women depended more on their
husband's support for use of family planning than those
with more education.

Abortion decisions are likewise influenced by men's
desires, although sometimes indirectly. Kim and Lee's
(1973) findings also applied to abortion. Among Colombian
women, the man's acceptance or rejection of economic
responsibility for the child was the most important
single factor in determining whether a woman sought
abortion (Browner, 1976). However, surreptitious,
unilateral decisions on abortion by women may also be
common in some settings, as discussed below.

It should be noted that the biases inherent in the
survey questionnaire method of data collection used in
most of the above studies may lead to underestimation of
the husband's influence on contraceptive use. The majority of respondents to a Mexican survey characterized
contraceptive decisions as joint ones, with the remainder
stating that they themselves were the final decision
makers (PROFAM-PIACT de Mexico, 1979). In contrast, in
open-ended same-sex group discussions, although both men
and women said the decision should be joint, respondents
almost invariably reported that the husband actually made
the decision.

These findings do not show conclusively that male attitudes are dominant in contraceptive use; they do present
strong evidence that, in cases of disagreement, the male
view frequently prevails. On the other hand, two longitudinal studies in the U.S. and in Taiwan provide evidence
that the wife's views are most likely to prevail when
partners disagree about additional births (Beckman and
Bardsley, 1981; Coombs and Chang, 1981). One possible
explanation for these contradictory findings is that,
although profertility decisions are controlled by the
husband, in lower-fertility countries antinatal decisions
are dominated by the wife, who controls most methods of
contraception. The distribution of power in the marital
dyad is also obviously a factor, as discussed below.

## COUPLE COMMUNICATION

Communication in the marital dyad is generally defined as
the frequency (or occasionally "openness") of discussion
between spouses, as reported by one or both partners.
Attempts to measure communication vary in specificity:
some researchers note general spouse interaction (e.g.,
Hill et al., 1959; Mitchell, 1972), whereas others measure communication specific to fertility.  For instance,
Mitchell (1972) asked how often spouses discussed amusing
or interesting incidents, conversations with their
friends, and problems or worries; the general communication index consisted of a simple sum of item scores.
More specific measures have covered communication on
family size and sex preferences (e.g., Coombs and
Fernandez, 1978; Rainwater, 1965), use of contraception
(Koenig, 1980; Mukherjee, 1975; Rainwater, 1965), and
sexuality (Beckman and Bardsley, 1981; Chamie, 1978).
Some researchers contend that such fertility-related
topics, especially sexuality, are not subject to the same
channels and patterns of communication as are more impersonal and instrumental issues (Coombs and Fernandez, 1978;
Hollerbach, 1980; Liu and Hutchison, 1974).

It is difficult to evaluate the validity and reliability of retrospective measures of frequency and patterns
of communication.  The literature on concurrence reveals
that spouses do not always agree on the quality and content of communication.  Couples frequently disagree about
the extent to which family planning has been discussed
(Beckman and Bardsley, 1981; Coombs and Chang, 1981;
Coombs and Fernandez, 1978; Hill et al., 1959).  This may
indicate that communication has been of insufficient
clarity, duration, or intensity to impress both spouses
in the same way (Hill et al., 1959), or it could indicate
measurement error.

The majority of studies of couple communication and
power have included only wives (Brody et al., 1974;
Browner, 1976; Chamie, 1978; Hartford, 1971; Johnson,
1971; Kar and Talbot, 1980; Mukherjee, 1975; Ramakumar
and Gopal, 1972; Rosen and Simmons, 1971; Shedlin and
Hollerbach, 1981); a few studies consider only men (e.g.,
Hall, 1971).  Some recent surveys have collected information from both men and women (e.g., Coombs and Fernandez, 1978; Koenig, 1980; Liu and Hutchison, 1974).  Such
studies allow gender comparisons, although, unfortunately,
the data are frequently based on samples of unrelated
individuals rather than paired couples.  Among the find-

ings in these studies, males in Asia reported more spouse communication than did females (ESCAP, 1974); and Mexican men and women (not paired couples) frequently disagreed on who initiated discussion of family planning (PROFAM-PIACT de Mexico, 1979). These data, however, are too limited to permit firm conclusions about partner differences in perceptions of communication patterns.

## Communication and Fertility Behavior

Research on the fertility decision-making process suggests that couple discussion is positively related to contraception and current fertility; conversely, communication is negatively related to demand for children.

Higher levels of family planning discussion have been associated with greater fertility regulation in many studies (Asia: ESCAP, 1974; Kim and Lee, 1973; Lee, 1979; Mukherjee, 1975; Shah, 1974; Africa:  Kar and Talbot, 1980; Latin America:  Brody et al., 1976; Hill et al., 1959; Kar and Talbot, 1980; PROFAM-PIACT de Mexico, 1979; Simmons and Culagovski, 1975; Stycos and Back, 1964). These studies assessed past and current contraceptive practices, as well as duration and effectiveness of use. The relationship between more general communication and birth control is less well documented, though a similar positive association has been reported in Puerto Rico and Jamaica (Hill et al., 1959; Stycos and Back, 1964), and in several Asian countries (ESCAP, 1974; Jolly, 1976; Mitchell, 1972). On the other hand, Liu and Hutchison (1974), using observational rather than survey measures, found no relationship between general communication and contraception or fertility in the Philippines.

Decisions about specific fertility regulation methods have also been investigated. Latin American data show that the wife is less likely to initiate discussion about abortion than about other types of family planning (Browner, 1976; Scrimshaw, 1978; Shedlin and Hollerbach, 1981); in such cases, decision making may in fact be surreptitious, and the man may be unaware of the pregnancy. Chamie (1978) found that Lebanese women who chose to have a tubal ligation reported higher rates of discussion with their spouses than did women who decided against the procedure. Shah's (1974) data from Pakistan show a strong positive association between spouse communication and use of the IUD. Methods with permanent or long-term effects like these may require more discussion.

The relationship between family planning discussion and fertility is problematic, some studies showing a positive association (ESCAP, 1974; Jolly, 1976), and others no or a negative association (Johnson, 1971; Stycos and Back, 1964). However, lower fertility preferences are related to more family planning discussion, particularly among husbands (Coombs and Fernandez, 1978). Moreover, when preferences and actual fertility are compared, it is found that family planning communication is higher among couples who have reached or exceeded their desired family size (Chamie, 1978; ESCAP, 1974, Jolly, 1976; Koenig, 1980; PROFAM-PIACT de Mexico, 1979; Shedlin and Hollerbach, 1981).

In the majority of countries in the nine-nation Value of Children study, wives saw being tied down as a greater cost of children than did husbands (Bulatao, 1979a). As a consequence, women may initiate discussions of family planning more often than men; this is confirmed by data from Mexico (PROFAM-PIACT de Mexico, 1979; Shedlin and Hollerbach, 1981). Women also may have greater access to family planning information. On the other hand, Koenig (1980) reported that, in rural India, initiative for discussing family planning rests primarily with the husband. Whether or not males initiate the discussion of family planning may be related to the extent of male dominance in family-size preferences, discussed below.

In some cases, the need for communication itself may increase the psychic cost of fertility regulation. Family planning may be perceived as a sensitive or emotionally loaded issue (PROFAM-PIACT de Mexico, 1979). Communication may also be inhibited by feelings of shyness or modesty on the part of the wife (ESCAP, 1974; Rao, 1959), resulting in unilateral or no fertility regulation.

## Communication and Concurrence

One way that communication may affect fertility is through its effect on concurrence. The limited evidence suggests that communication is related to less concurrence; however, communication is associated with greater awareness of the other person's attitudes and views (Hill et al., 1959). Coombs and Fernandez's (1978) Malaysian study suggests that couple discussion brings disagreements about fertility desires into the open. They found that the degree of concurrence was greater among couples who had never discussed the number of children they wanted.

Since concordance between partners has been associated with high levels of demand for children, the effect of communication could be to lower demand. Given the popular belief that men desire large families (see Hollerbach, 1980), ignorance about each other's preferences may lead to higher fertility. In addition, a study of young couples in the United States found that the person who did not want an additional child was likely to prevail in cases of disagreement, especially if that person was the wife (Beckman and Bardsley, 1981). If these results hold more generally, exposing such disagreements through discussion should lead to lower fertility without necessarily affecting the preferences of each spouse.


## Possible Causal Connections

Most of the research evidence supports a negative relationship between the desire for children and couple communication, and a positive relationship between communication and the practice of birth control. It might be assumed that a desire to limit childbearing encourages discussion of family planning, which in turn leads to contraception, although whether communication is really a necessary link in this process remains an unanswered question.

Some contend that husband-wife communication is a correlate or consequence, rather than a determinant, of birth control practice. Hartford (1971) found that in Colombia a "high proportion" began discussing birth control only after initiating it. Other studies suggest that surreptitious use of birth control by the wife is fairly common in cultures where fertility regulation is not widespread (Brody et al., 1974; Shedlin and Hollerbach, 1981). In a qualitative analysis of life in a rural Indian village, Poffenberger (1968) maintains that effective husband-wife communication is not always necessary for birth control adoption; a decision for sterilization or an IUD may involve the whole extended family, but entail little discussion between the husband and wife themselves. On the other hand, if more communication were solely a consequence of birth control practice, it would be difficult to explain the positive association between general communication and contraception. It appears probable that communication is partly a cause and partly a consequence of birth control use, although evidence to support this view is difficult to obtain.

## POWER AND EQUALITY IN THE DYAD

Relative social power in the marital dyad is generally measured by asking respondents who makes the "decision" or the "final decision" about family issues (e.g., finances, wife's employment, family planning). This approach, concerned only with the outcome of group choice, relies on the individual's beliefs about what was important in the choice process. The process itself, "how families come to do what they do" (Turk, 1975), has rarely been studied. Perhaps this is because processes are momentary, changeable, and difficult to observe.

The usual approach to measuring power is problematic in several ways. Power does not necessarily reside in the person who wins in a disagreement (Beckman, 1978; Safilios-Rothschild, 1970). Moreover, it is necessary to know not only who makes a decision, but also who delegates the authority to do so. Additionally, in measuring over-all decision making, the outcome obviously depends on the particular decisions sampled (Centers et al., 1971; Douglas and Wind, 1978; Safilios-Rothschild, 1970). When specific areas are not clearly defined, or when the decisions sampled happen infrequently (e.g., choice of housing), some disagreement occurs; when specific decision areas are defined, husbands and wives still frequently disagree about their relative influence (Beckman, 1979; Cochrane and Bean, 1976; Coombs and Fernandez, 1978). There are many reasons for such disagreement. It may be difficult for respondents to identify the person who exercises power in the family because they may have to recall experiences occurring months before, and may not be used to conceptualizing family interactions in power terms. Various types of perceptual and reporting biases may also exist.

The problems involved in describing marital power in relation to decision outcomes are illustrated by a study of 104 Japanese-American wives living in Honolulu (Johnson, 1975). When assessment of marital power was based on structured questions about decision-making outcomes, the women reported that their marriages exhibited egalitarian patterns. However, in open-ended discussions, wives saw themselves as clearly subordinate in the family hierarchy, with half reporting that their husbands were dominant. These inconsistencies indicate that husbands may delegate routine decisions to their wives, reserving more important, infrequent decisions for themselves (Salfilios-Rothschild, 1970, 1975). Thus, the wives' presumed "power" may actually be based on their husbands' desires and prerogatives. Despite these problems, most studies in developing countries use couple self-reports to measure and describe family power patterns.

The status of women in the family and society is important in any consideration of relative power in the marital dyad. Generally, the higher the status of women and the more egalitarian the roles of husband and wife, the more social power the wife is believed to have vis-a-vis her husband. Although power and couple communication are not necessarily associated, research demonstrates a positive correlation between egalitarian relationships and couple communication (e.g., ESCAP, 1974). It is generally believed that the wife's power positively influences husband-wife communication, rather than the reverse.

## Decision-Making Power

It is frequently hypothesized that more egalitarian decision making, or reduced husband dominance, in developing countries is associated with lower demand for children, more effective contraceptive use, and lower fertility. However, research has not provided consistent empirical support for this hypothesis.

Hass (1971) found a relationship between style of decision making and demand for children in only one of seven Latin American cities studied. Contrary to prediction, the more egalitarian the wife reported family decision making to be, the larger her family-size preference.

Research results vary as to the effects of egalitarian decision making on birth control practice. Confirming the hypothesis, Mitchell (1972) found a positive relationship between greater wife influence and contraception among Hong Kong couples. Also, Hill et al. (1959) observed that traditional male-dominated family patterns in Puerto Rico correlated negatively with birth control, although male dominance in decision making by itself was not significantly related to use of birth control. Other data also reveal weak or nonsignificant relationships between decision-making outcomes and contraception, perhaps because husbands see family planning decisions as a female domain (Hass, 1971; Kar and Talbot, 1980; Liu and Hutchison, 1974; Lozare, 1976; Weller, 1968). Kar and

Talbot (1980) found that conjugal communication was a much more important predictor of current contraceptive use than was joint conjugal power, as indexed by decision making. The one study (Liu and Hutchison, 1974) that used observational techniques to measure power processes did not find any significant relationships between power or communicativeness, as measured by a revealed difference technique (Strodtbeck, 1951), and current use of contraception among a small sample of couples in the Philippines. According to one small study, power specific to sexual relations may indirectly influence acceptance of at least one method of contraception--tubal ligation. Lebanese women who chose this method did not differ from those who rejected it in reported equality in sexual relations; however, wives' attitudes toward the value of marital equality in sexual relations were strongly related to the tubal ligation decision (Chamie, 1978).

The relation of egalitarian decision making to actual fertility is complicated by the likelihood that these variables have reciprocal effects: wife equality in decision making may influence fertility negatively through lowered demand and earlier initiation and more effective use of contraception; on the other hand, having many children, particularly sons, may increase the wife's authority in the family in some traditional societies. Most research in developing countries has shown no or only a weak negative relationship between fertility and egalitarian decision making. Rosen and Simmons (1971) do report a negative relationship between family size and equality in conjugal decision making in Brazilian data after industrialization and social status are controlled; Hill et al. (1959) also conclude that less restrictive family types in Puerto Rico have lower fertility. However, less supportive studies also exist (Hass, 1971; Weller, 1968).

Relative power, one might assume, would be most important in cases of disagreement or conflict between spouses. In such cases, the more powerful member of the marital dyad should be able to impose his or her will upon the partner. However, so far there is little support for this assumption in the limited U.S. data examining fertility demand from a conflict-resolution perspective (Beckman and Bardsley, 1981). Most studies of power and fertility do not consider the spouses' respective levels of fertility demand.

## Conjugal Role Relationships

Family power and equality should be reflected in relationships between the spouses. Rainwater (1965) sought to
assess these relationships from intensive interview data
rather than from the brief self-reports usually used to
measure power. He developed a three-fold classification
of relationships: joint-role relationships, in which
husbands and wives share activities, tasks, and decisions;
segregated-role relationships, which emphasize a formal
division of labor and activities within the family; and
intermediate-role relationships, which fall between joint
and segregated relationships in the degree to which activities and tasks in the family are formally prescribed.
Research using this typology has been done mainly in the
United States. Most of the work indicates that less segregated role relationships are related to earlier and more
frequent use of birth control among some population subgroups. The Rainwater (1965) study shows that joint-role
relationships are most strongly correlated with coitus-
related contraception among lower-class couples after the
birth of their last wanted child. Conjugal role relationships were not related to effective contraception among
the middle class. However, other studies show that, when
age is controlled, women in joint-role relationships have
lower fertility than those in segregated-role relationships (Polgar and Rothstein, 1970; Stokes and Dudley,
1972).

Two types of linkages are possible between joint-role
relationships and lower fertility: couples in such relationships may want smaller families and, therefore, be
more likely to use contraception; or these couples might
be more effective at limiting family size (Back and Hass,
1973). Evidence discussed above supports the first of
these linkages, while the second is supported by the finding that spouses with more segregated role relationships
communicate less on birth control matters and are less
effective in limiting family size (Hill et al., 1959;
Rainwater, 1965).

## Machismo

Power inequality and segregated role relationships may be
reinforced by the cultural complex called machismo, which
may be defined as exaggerated masculinity reinforced by
sex-role stereotypes (Nicassio, 1977). Important facets

include exercise of authority over women, sexual prowess, and fatherhood. Machismo, as both a set of prescribed cultural expectations and a personal trait, may be of particular importance in Latin American countries in keeping women's status low. Machismo is demonstrated in a PROFAM-PIACT de Mexico (1979) study revealing sharply different, conflicting cultural perspectives among men and women in Mexico: most women thought it was all right to work outside the home and rejected the notion that women who have many children are better wives; men tended to believe the reverse and supported autocratic attitudes toward women.

Although Hollerbach's (1980) review concluded that there is little evidence that men high on machismo prefer more children, the belief exists, especially among women, that men want larger families (e.g., Nicassio, 1977; PROFAM-PIACT de Mexico, 1979; Van Keep and Rice-Wray, 1973). Regardless of desire for children, however, men in cultures characterized by machismo are more likely than women to disapprove of birth control. About one-third of a sample of Indian and mestizo women in Mexico reported negative attitudes toward birth control among their husbands (Shedlin and Hollerbach, 1981). Other Latin American men objected to women's use of contraception because they feared loss of authority and possible infidelity (PROFAM-PIACT de Mexico, 1979; Stycos, 1968).

## UNILATERAL AND SURREPTITIOUS DECISIONS

Under certain conditions, one partner may make a unilateral and frequently surreptitious decision on fertility regulation. This is expecially true for the wife, given the prevalence of female-controlled methods. However, surreptitious fertility regulation is also possible for the husband, primarily through vasectomy, although no data exist on male behavior in this area.

It is difficult to ascertain the prevalence of women's unilateral or surreptitious use of contraception or abortion. However, limited information from Latin America indicates that, when satisfactory methods are available, surreptitious fertility regulation may represent up to 25 percent of users (Brody et al., 1974; Shedlin and Hollerbach, 1981). As mentioned above, studies in Latin America imply more widespread approval of contraception among women than men, which may result in unrevealed use of contraception or abortion.

The determinants of surreptitious fertility regulation by women have rarely been explored.  Small-scale studies have found an association between instability of the relationship and unilateral contraception and abortion (Brody et al., 1974; Browner, 1976).  Modesty or shyness, making it difficult for the wife to discuss family planning or sexuality with her spouse, may also be a factor (ESCAP, 1974; PROFAM-PIACT de Mexico, 1979).  Anxiety about a mate's loyalty during pregnancy may be an important reason for an abortion, frequently a hidden one (Brody et al., 1974; Browner, 1976).  In a Jamaican study (Brody et al., 1974), unilateral decision makers reported having experienced less stable sexual relationships, earlier age at initiation of coitus, and more sexual partners; they were also less likely to be currently living with their partners.  Their greater economic autonomy and their distrust of men probably resulted in their unilateral decisions.

Hollerbach (1980) has tried to provide a theoretical framework for predicting unilateral versus joint decisions.  She argues that the basis on which power is allocated between spouses affects the frequency and quality of discussion between them, and that these two factors together lead to either unilateral or joint decisions:  coercive and reward power can lead to passive or unilateral decisions, which can become surreptitious if spouse interaction is inadequate to resolve conflicts; informational, expert, and referent power (distinctions owed to French and Raven, 1959) are more likely to produce negotiation between the partners and to lead to joint decisions.  However, no direct empirical support for this formulation has been provided to date.


## INFLUENCE OF KIN AND SOCIAL NETWORKS

Sometimes those outside the marital dyad participate in fertility decisions.  Extended family and friends may affect fertility decision making by providing information or exerting influence (Dubey and Choldin, 1967; Hill et al., 1959; Kar and Talbot, 1980; Mani, 1970).  Although couples sometimes deny such influences (PROFAM-PIACT de Mexico, 1979), careful probing generally reveals them.

In many traditional cultures, members of the extended family can play an important role in contraceptive decisions.  In rural India, for example, the wife is usually brought into the coresidential extended family to benefit

the larger family group. In such circumstances, the
decision to use birth control is often made by the entire
family and is heavily influenced by the husband's mother
(Poffenberger, 1968). Mexican wives also reported that
one reason for their husbands' disapproval of birth control was their mother-in-law's resistance (PROFAM-PIACT
de Mexico, 1979; Shedlin and Hollerbach, 1981). Moreover, mothers often affect their adolescent daughters'
contraceptive behavior (Fox and Inazu, 1979 [U.S. data]).
Other Latin American data support such influences of kin
on contraceptive decisions (Hill et al., 1959).

Besides kin, others close to the couple may affect
fertility decisions. Hill et al. (1959) reported friends
and neighbors (mentioned by 40 percent of men and 28 percent of women) as the most frequent sources of information
and influence regarding contraception; in these data,
Puerto Rican women were more vulnerable to influence than
were men. Mani's (1970) anthropological study of an
Indian village found that the husband's friends and the
wife's friends and relatives were the most important
influences. In fact, these persons were much more likely
to be consulted regarding family planning than was the
spouse, although husband-wife communication was stimulated by informal discussions with friends and neighbors
(ESCAP, 1974).

Peer groups and confidants may play an especially
important role in the adoption and continuation of
contraception (Cheong and Suh, 1979), and may be more
effective in promoting family planning than the mass
media (Cheong and Suh, 1979; Lee, 1979; Mani, 1970;
Rogers, 1974; Rogers et al., 1976). Lee (1979) has shown
that a woman is more likely to adopt family planning if
women in her social network have already done so. Peer
contacts provide women not only with information but also
with emotional support. Most studies of peer influence
concentrate on female groups; male groups are largely
ignored, despite their possible role in sustaining norms
of machismo (DeHoyas and DeHoyas, 1966; Nicassio, 1977).

Deliberately created groups can also be important.
Mothers' Clubs, created partly to distribute oral contraceptives to village women, play an important role in
facilitating family planning in South Korean villages
(Rogers et al., 1976). At the structured end of the
spectrum, the village production brigades in China make
collective decisions on which couples should have a child
in the next year (Rogers, 1974).

Contact with medical and paramedical personnel can facilitate decisions to adopt or continue using family planning. In data from Mexico (PROFAM-PIACT de Mexico, 1979), doctors were mentioned as influential by half of the respondents who admitted being influenced by external sources. Koenig (1980) reported that contact with family planning workers, especially by husbands, was strongly correlated with both husband-wife communication and contraceptive use in his Indian sample. Rogers and Solomon (1979) analyzed the role of traditional midwives as family planning communicators in six Asian countries, and concluded that midwives can make an important and unique contribution to adoption of family planning by rural, more traditional women.

These various sources of influence can outweigh the influence spouses have on each other, as Mani's (1970) study suggests. In analyzing influences on contraceptive practices in Venezuela and Kenya, Kar and Talbot (1980) derived findings partly similar to Mani's by using a general measure of social support which combined approval of spouses, friends, and relatives. However, separate examination of the variables showed that, in Venezuela, the approval of relatives and friends was about as important as that of the spouse in determining contraceptive use, whereas in less developed Kenya, approval of spouse was most important. Among external influences, specific communication with individuals outside the marital dyad was a stronger influence in Kenya, and overall social support in Venezuela. In contrast to decisions on contraception, limited data show that abortion decisions tend to be made solely by the couple. In Browner's (1976) study of Colombian women, 91 percent did not tell extraconjugal kin that they were considering an abortion because they feared disapproval. Intensity of interaction with kin was not related to the abortion decision, and only the husband had a role in the decision making process.

## SOCIOECONOMIC AND MODERNIZING INFLUENCES

The socioeconomic characteristics that usually change with economic development are related to couple communication and relative power in the dyad. Greater discussion of family planning has been associated with higher education for wives (Caldwell, 1968; ESCAP, 1974; Jolly, 1976; Mitchell, 1972; Ramakumar and Gopal, 1972), higher socioeconomic status (Brody et al., 1976; Caldwell, 1968;

ESCAP, 1974; Jolly, 1976; Mitchell, 1972), and urban
rather than rural residence (Caldwell, 1968; Kim and Lee,
1973), although the relationship between communication
and wife's age and length of marriage is inconsistent
across samples (Hill et al., 1959; Kim and Lee, 1973;
Koenig, 1980; Mukherjee, 1975). Greater decision-making
authority on the part of the wife is likewise associated
with her having higher education (Buric and Zecevic, 1967;
Rosen and Simmons, 1971; Safilios-Rothschild, 1969). However, a resource theory analysis of power indicates that
it is the relative education (or occupation) of the wife
vis-a-vis the husband, rather than absolute status, that
is significant (Bahr, 1972). In addition, the relative
power of the wife is higher if she is employed outside
the home, particularly in more prestigious occupations
(Kagitcibasi, 1979; Rosen and Simmons, 1971; Weller,
1968).


## Modernization and Equality

Changes in both communication and relative dominance
within the marital dyad are likely to occur as a by-
product of economic development; however, there is only
scattered evidence on the effects of such changes on
fertility and fertility regulation. The ESCAP (1974)
study and Hass (1971) have investigated husband-wife
communication cross-culturally, but have not directly
related development, communication, and fertility.

Kar and Talbot (1980), comparing data from Kenya and
Venezuela, showed a more positive relationship between
spouse discussion of family planning and current contraceptive use in Venezuela, which has a higher level of
modernization than Kenya. This suggests that couple
communication may play a more important role as societies
modernize. Rosen and Simmons (1971) found that, among
currently mated women in Brazil, smaller family size was
associated with higher status levels for women and greater
equality in family decision making. Their data indicate
that the egalitarian family structure associated with
industrial development influences fertility. New educational and employment opportunities accompanying industrialization promote modern conceptions of the woman's
role, and thus foster more egalitarian decision making.
Moreover, since women tend to want fewer children, shared
decision making leads to lower fertility. Bagozzi and
Van Loo (1978) suggest that, among wives in Turkey and

Mexico, modernization (including increases in a wife's power and authority in the home) is a direct cause of lower fertility.

This is very limited evidence for the intervening role of couple communication and egalitarian conjugal decision making in the relationship between modernization and fertility. Other studies have shown that modernization, higher socioeconomic status, and employment do not always provide women with greater autonomy and freedom, nor do they necessarily lead to lower fertility (Blumberg, 1976; Mernissi, 1976; Piepmeier and Adkins, 1973; Tinker, 1976). The hypothesis that modernization reduces demand for children and fertility through improvements in the status of women in both home and community therefore requires further investigation.

## PROPOSITIONS

### Partner Agreement

1. Consensus (i.e., mutually recognized agreement) between partners is associated with lower fertility than is concordance (i.e., coincidentally similar preferences). Since consensus requires discussion, the evidence that discussion leads to lower fertility is relevant (Brody et al., 1976; ESCAP, 1974; Hill et al., 1959; Kar and Talbot, 1980; Kim and Lee; 1973; Lee, 1979; Mukherjee, 1975; PROFAM-PIACT de Mexico, 1979; Shah, 1974; Simmons and Culagovski, 1975; Stycos and Back, 1964).

2. In many developing societies, the husband's approval of contraception is critical to the wife's initiation and continuation of use; on average, the husband's view is more important than the wife's. This is strongly supported by Brody et al. (1974), Browner (1976), Chamie (1978), Hall (1971), Hollerbach (1980), and PROFAM-PIACT de Mexico (1979).

### Couple Communication

3. Frequency of husband-wife discussion of birth control and family size (a) is negatively affected by demand for children, (b) positively influences use of contraception, and (c) negatively influences fertility. Support for the three parts of this proposition varies. Research confirms the demand-discussion relationship: discussion tends to

increase as the desire to prevent pregnancies becomes stronger (Chamie, 1978; ESCAP, 1974; Jolly, 1976; Koenig, 1980; PROFAM-PIACT de Mexico, 1979; Shedlin and Hollerbach, 1981). The association between couple discussion and contraceptive use in developing countries has even stronger support (e.g., Chamie, 1978; ESCAP, 1974; Hill et al., 1959; Kar and Talbot, 1980; Kim and Lee, 1973; Lee, 1979; PROFAM-PIACT de Mexico, 1979; Shah, 1974; Simmons and Culagovski, 1975), although some studies suggest that husband-wife discussion is a correlate rather than a determinant of birth control use (Brody et al., 1976; Browner, 1976; Hartford, 1971; Koenig, 1980; Shedlin and Hollerbach, 1981). The association between discussion and actual fertility is less strongly substantiated: some studies have found high fertility associated with husband-wife discussion (ESCAP, 1974; Jolly, 1976); other studies have found no relationship (Johnson, 1971) or a negative relationship (Stycos and Back, 1964).

4. Frequency (or openness) of general husband-wife communication (a) negatively influences demand for children, (b) positively influences use of contraception, and (c) negatively influences actual fertility. No direct evidence exists for the relationship to demand for children; however, such findings as Rosen and Simmons's (1971) that egalitarian family structures are linked with lower demand imply this relationship. The influence of general communication on contraceptive use is confirmed by the findings of ESCAP (1974), Hill et al. (1959), Jolly (1976), Mitchell (1972), and Stycos and Back (1974). The relationship of general communication to actual fertility is supported by ESCAP (1974) and Jolly (1976).

5. Women initiate discussion of family planning more often than men because they (a) are more affected by the consequences of unplanned pregnancies, and (b) have more access to family planning information. Data on the female initiation of family planning discussions conflict (e.g., Koenig, 1980; PROFAM-PIACT de Mexico, 1979; Shedlin and Hollerbach, 1981). Family planning programs tend to focus on women, who also receive more contraception information from peers than men (Cheong and Suh, 1979; Rogers and Solomon, 1979; Rogers et al., 1976). Women's apparently greater concern about contraception reflects the heavier childcare responsibilities imposed on them in most societies. On the other hand, male prerogatives regarding contraception are still strong, particularly in traditional cultures (PROFAM-PIACT de Mexico, 1979; Shedlin and Hollerbach, 1981; Stycos, 1968).

6.  Couple communication about family planning involves a psychic cost in cultures where birth control is a sensitive issue or where the wife is expected to be shy and modest.  Findings from Asia and Mexico tend to bear out this proposition (ESCAP, 1974; PROFAM-PIACT de Mexico, 1979; Shedlin and Hollerbach, 1981; Rao, 1959).

7.  Some birth control techniques are more likely to require couple discussion than others.  Data from Pakistan and Lebanon indicate that permanent or long-term methods are linked more than others to couple communication (Chamie, 1978; Shah, 1974).  Abortion is linked with low levels of couple communication, possibly because, in a relatively large number of cases, the decision is unilateral and surreptitious (Browner, 1976; Scrimshaw, 1978; Shedlin and Hollerbach, 1981).

## Power in the Dyad

8.  Egalitarian couple authority in the marital dyad (a) negatively influences demand for children, (b) positively influences use of contraception, and (c) lowers fertility. The research does not support the relationship between joint couple authority and demand for children.  In only one Latin American country of seven studied was there a correlation between decision making and demand, and there the results contradicted expectations (Hass, 1971).  Data on relative dominance and birth control use are conflicting and on balance only weakly support the proposition (Chamie, 1978; Hass, 1971; Hill et al., 1959; Kar and Talbot, 1980; Liu and Hutchison, 1974; Lozare, 1976). The relationship between fertility and power is also not clearly documented by the studies (Hass, 1971; Rosen and Simmons, 1971; Weller, 1968), although the insignificant associations may be due to difficulties in adequately measuring power.

9.  Fertility increases the wife's power in the marital dyad, even after the effects of her age have been controlled.  Data suggest a progression from enforced dependence to greater independence for wives over time; this change in status is linked to fertility (Chulasai, 1975; Hollerbach, 1980; Poffenberger, 1968; Scrimshaw, 1978).

10.  Joint-role relationships among lower-class couples are associated with (a) lower demand for children, (b) greater birth control use, and (c) lower fertility. Rainwater (1965) found a negative relationship between

these relationships and number of children among lower-class couples in the United States, but the results did not hold for middle-class families (see also Polgar and Rothstein, 1970; Stokes and Dudley, 1972).

11.  Machismo is related to disapproval of birth control on the part of Latin American men.  Limited evidence suggests that lower-class and rural Latin American men are more negative toward birth control than their wives (Shedlin and Hollerbach, 1981).  This is explained by aspects of machismo specifying male authority over the wife, fatherhood, and female fidelity (PROFAM-PIACT de Mexico, 1979; Shedlin and Hollerbach, 1981; Stycos, 1968).

12.  In cases of disagreement over fertility preferences, the views of the more powerful spouse will prevail.  This hypothesis is largely speculative.  The limited U.S. data examining fertility demand from a conflict-resolution point of view provide little support (Beckman and Bardsley, 1981).

13.  Egalitarian couple relationships are related positively to couple communication, as demonstrated by the ESCAP (1974) study.


## Unilateral Decisions

14.  A significant minority of persons, mainly women, use fertility regulation without their partners' knowledge.  The exact proportion of women who contracept or abort surreptitiously is unknown and difficult to estimate.  Those who do so may never tell their partners (Brody et al., 1974; Browner, 1976; Shedlin and Hollerbach, 1981).  An important determinant of surreptitious regulation may be the woman's expectation that she can successfully hide her behavior.

15.  Unilateral and surreptitious use of fertility control is more likely to occur in unstable relationships.  The studies of Brody et al. (1974) and Browner (1976) support this contention.

16.  Reward and coercive power are associated with (a) passive decision making in which no communication occurs and persons act in accordance with internalized social norms, and (b) unilateral decision making; expert, informational, and referent power are associated with joint decision making.  These propositions are based on a theoretical rationale recently advanced by Hollerbach (1980) for which empirical support is unavailable.

Influence of Kin and Social Networks

17.  Communication with friends, other family members, confidants, and opinion leaders influences the initiation and continuation of contraception. This is supported by numerous studies (Cheong and Suh, 1979; Dubey and Choldin, 1967; ESCAP, 1974; Hill et al., 1959; Hollerbach, 1980; Kar and Talbot, 1980; Koenig, 1980; Lee, 1979; Fox and Inazu, 1979; Mani, 1970; Poffenberger, 1968; PROFAM-PIACT de Mexico, 1979; Rogers, 1974; Rogers and Solomon, 1979; Rogers et al., 1976; Shedlin and Hollerbach, 1981).

18.  Communication with friends, other family members, confidants, and opinion leaders is associated with initiation of contraception because it stimulates husband-wife discussion. The ESCAP (1974) study suggests this hypothesis. However, supporting data from the couple-interaction literature specific to developing countries are slim. Of course, it is possible for communication with peers, kin, and opinion leaders to be associated with birth control use without any increase in husband-wife discussion of family planning.

19.  Female peer groups provide women with informational or expert bases of power to use in communicating with their partners. The studies done to date have not examined peer influence in these terms. However, Cheong and Suh (1979) have shown that peers can play an important role in providing information on contraception. Moreover, the ESCAP (1974) study suggests that husband-wife communication is stimulated by informal discussion with friends and neighbors.

20.  In traditional societies, demand for children on the part of the husband's mother or other kin may block birth control use by the couple. Limited supporting data on the role of the mother-in-law are available for India (Poffenberger, 1968) and Mexico (PROFAM-PIACT de Mexico, 1979; Shedlin and Hollerbach, 1981).

21.  Extended kin usually play no role in abortion decisions. This conclusion is based on retrospective data from a small sample of women in Cali, Colombia (Browner, 1976). To the degree to which abortion is approved in other societies, information flow, family structure, and decision-making patterns might produce different findings.

## Socioeconomic Determinants

22.  Both general and family planning-specific communication are greater among couples (a) of higher socioeconomic status, (b) with more highly educated wives, and (c) with urban rather than rural residence. A moderate amount of data supports these propositions (Brody et al., 1976; Caldwell, 1968; ESCAP, 1974; Jolly, 1976; Kim and Lee, 1973; Mitchell, 1972; Ramakumar and Gopal, 1972).

23.  Greater wife decision-making authority is associated with (a) higher family socioeconomic status, (b) a higher educational level for the wife, (c) greater employment opportunities for the wife, and (d) the wife's age. The first two of these factors are associated with a more egalitarian division of decision-making authority (e.g., Buric and Zecevic, 1967; Rosen and Simmons, 1971; Safilios-Rothschild, 1969); there is also evidence of a similar association for the third (Kagitcibasi, 1979; Rosen and Simmons, 1971; Weller, 1968) and fourth (Chulasai, 1975; Poffenberger, 1968; Scrimshaw, 1978). Support also exists for the alternative proposition that equality of couple education rather than the wife's absolute level of education is predictive of egalitarian decision making (Bahr, 1972).

24.  Husband-wife discussion and more egalitarian power relations are intervening variables through which demographic and socioeconomic factors affect fertility. Higher levels of education and wider employment opportunities for wives, as well as higher family socioeconomic status, may directly influence discussion and egalitarian decision making in the marital dyad, leading in turn to more effective contraceptive use. This is indicated by the preceding propositions, and partly supported by Rosen and Simmons (1971) and Bagozzi and Van Loo (1978). Some contrary evidence indicates, however, that modernization, higher socioeconomic status, and employment do not necessarily grant women greater autonomy, power, or freedom (Blumberg, 1976; Mernissi, 1976; Piepmeier and Adkins, 1973; Tinker, 1976), nor are these factors always associated with lower fertility.

## BIBLIOGRAPHY

Armijo, R., and T. Monreal (1965)  Epidemiology of provoked abortion in Santiago, Chile. Journal of Sex Research 1:143-159.

Back, K. W., and P. H. Hass (1973)  Family structure and fertility control.  In J. T. Fawcett, ed., Psychological Perspectives on Population.  New York: Basic Books.

Bagozzi, R. P., and M. F. Van Loo (1978)  Toward a general theory of fertility:  A causal modeling approach.  Demography 15:301-320.

Bahr, S. J. (1972)  Comment on "The study of family power structure: A review 1960-1969."  Journal of Marriage and the Family 34:239-243.

Beckman, L. J. (1978)  Couples' decision-making processes regarding fertility.  In K. Taeuber, L. Bumpass, and J. Sweet, eds., Social Demography.  New York: Academic Press.

Beckman, L. J. (1979)  The Process of Couples' Fertility Decision-Making.  Paper presented at the Family Planning, Contraception and Abortion Symposium of the American Psychological Association, New York.

Beckman, L. J. (in press)  Measuring the decision-making process regarding fertility.  In G. L. Fox, ed., Decision-Making, Family Planning and Child-Bearing.  Beverly Hills, Calif.:  Sage Publications.

Beckman, L. J., and P. E. Bardsley (1981)  Couples' Motivation for Parenthood, Decision-Making and Fertility Regulation.  Final Report (contract HD-52807) prepared for Center for Population Research, National Institute of Child Health and Human Development.  Washington, D.C.:  U.S. Department of Health and Human Services.

Blumberg, R. L. (1976)  Fairy tales and facts: Economy, family, fertility, and the female.  In I. Tinker, M. B. Bramsen, and M. Buvinic, eds., Women and World Development.  New York: Praeger Press.

Brody, E. B., F. Ottey, and J. LaGranade (1974)  Couple communication in the contraceptive decision-making of Jamaican women.  The Journal of Nervous and Mental Disease 159:407-412.

Brody, E. G., F. Ottey, and J. LaGranade (1976)  Fertility-related behavior in Jamaica.  In Cultural Factors and Population in Developing Countries, ICP Work Agreement Reports, Occasional Monograph Series, No. 6.  Washington, D.C.:  Smithsonian Institution.

Browner, C. (1976)  Poor Women's Fertility Decisions: Illegal Abortion in Cali, Colombia.  Unpublished Ph.D. dissertation.  University of California, Berkeley.

Bulatao, R. A. (1979a)  On the Nature of the Transition in the Value of Children.  Paper No. 60-A.  Honolulu: East-West Population Institute.

Bulatao, R. A. (1979b)  Further Evidence of the Transition in the Value of Children. Paper No. 60-B.  Honolulu: East-West Population Institute.

Buric, O., and A. Zecevic (1967)  Family authority, marital satisfaction and the social network in Yugoslavia.  Journal of Marriage and the Family 29:325-336.

Caldwell, J. C. (1968)  The control of family size in tropical Africa.  Demography 5:598-619.

Centers, R., B. H. Raven, and A. Rodrigues (1971)  Conjugal power structure:  A reexamination.  American Sociological Review 31:1073-1082.

Chamie, M. J. W. (1978)  Middle Eastern Marriages and Contraceptive Decisions:  Toward a Sociopsychological Understanding of Fertility Behavior.  Unpublished Ph.D. dissertation.  University of Michigan, Ann Arbor, Mich.

Cheong, C. K., and M. H. Suh (1979)  Intra Village Communication Networks and Family Planning Acceptance in Rural Korea.  Seoul:  Korean Institute for Family Planning.

Chulasai, L. (1975)  The Roles of Husbands and Fathers in Family Planning in Rural Chiang Mai.  SEAPRAP Research Report, No. 3.  Chiang Mai, Thailand:  Chiang Mai University.

Cochrane, S. H., and F. D. Bean (1976)  Husband-wife differences in the demand for children.  Journal of Marriage and the Family 38:297-307.

Coombs, L. C., and M. C. Chang (1981)  Do husbands and wives agree?  Fertility attitudes and later behavior.  Population and Environment 4:109-127.

Coombs, L. C., and D. Fernandez (1978)  Husband-wife agreement about reproductive goals.  Demography 15:57-73.

DeHoyas, A., and G. DeHoyas (1966)  The amigo system and alienation of the wife in the conjugal Mexican family.  In B. Farber, ed., Kinship and Family Organization.  New York:  John Wiley and Sons.

DESAL (Center for the Social and Economic Development of Latin America) (1968)  Comportamientos Anticonceptivos en la Familia Marginal.  Cuadernos de Discusion #1. Santiago:  DESAL.

Douglas, S. P., and Y. Wind (1978)  Examining family role and authority patterns:  Two methodological cases.  Journal of Marriage and the Family 40:35-47.

Dubey, D. C., and H. M. Choldin (1967)  Communication and diffusion of the IUD:  A case study in urban India.  Demography 4:601-614.

ESCAP (1974)  Husband-Wife Communication and Practice of
    Family Planning. Bangkok Asian Population Studies
    Series, No. 16. New York:  United Nations.
Fox, G. L., and J. K. Inazu (1979)  The Effect of Mother-
    Daughter Communication on Daughter's Sexual and
    Contraceptive Knowledge and Behavior.  Paper presented
    at the annual meeting of the Population Association of
    America, Philadelphia, Pa.
French, J. R. P., Jr., and B. H. Raven (1959)  The bases
    of social power. In D. Cartwright, ed., Studies in
    Social Power. Ann Arbor, Mich.:  University of
    Michigan Press.
Hall, F. (1971)  Family planning in Santiago, Chile:  The
    male viewpoint. Studies in Family Planning 2:143-147.
Hartford, R. B. (1971)  Attitudes, information, and
    fertility in Medellin, Colombia. In J. M. Stycos,
    ed., Ideology, Faith and Family Planning in Latin
    America. New York:  McGraw Hill.
Hass, P. H. (1971)  Maternal Employment and Fertility in
    Metropolitan Latin America. Unpublished Ph.D.
    dissertation. Duke University, Durham, N.C.
Hill, R., J. M. Stycos, and K. W. Back (1959)  The Family
    and Population Control. Chapel Hill, N.C.:
    University of North Carolina Press.
Hollerbach, P. E. (1980)  Power in families, communica-
    tion, and fertility decision-making. Population and
    Environment 3:146-173.
Johnson, C. (1975)  Authority and power in Japanese-
    American marriages. In R. E. Cromwell and D. H.
    Olson, eds., Power in Families. New York:  Sage
    Publications.
Johnson, E. J. (1971)  Lower-income mothers in Bogota.
    In J. M. Stycos, ed., Ideology, Faith and Family
    Planning in Latin America. New York:  McGraw Hill.
Jolly, S. K. G. (1976)  Impact of inter-spouse
    communication on family planning adoption. Journal of
    Family Welfare 23:38-44.
Kagitcibasi, C. (1979)  Effects of Employment and
    Children on Women's Status and Fertility Decisions.
    Paper presented at the International Development
    Research Center Workshop on Women's Roles and
    Fertility, Ottawa, Canada.
Kar, S. B., and J. M. Talbot (1980)  Attitudinal and
    non-attitudinal determinants of contraception:  A
    cross-cultural study. Studies in Family Planning
    11:51-64.

Kim, C. H., and S. J. Lee (1973)   Role of husband in family planning behavior. Psychological Studies in Population/Family Planning 1(5).   Seoul:   Korean Institute for Research in the Behavioral Sciences.

Koenig, M. (1980)   Husband-Wife Interaction and Contraceptive Adoption in Rural India.   Paper presented at the Workshop on Psychosocial Factors in Population Research, Denver, Colo.

Lee, S. B. (1979)   Communication Networks and Family Planning in Korean Villages.   Seoul:   Korean Institute for Family Planning.

Liu, W. T., and I. W. Hutchison (1974)   Conjugal interaction and fertility behavior:   Some conceptual problems in research.   In H. Y. Lien and F. D. Bean, eds., Comparative Family and Fertility Research. Leiden:   E. J. Brill.

Lozare, B. V. (1976)   Communication between couples and decision-making in relation to family planning.   In R. A. Bulatao, ed., Philippine Population Research. Makati, Rizal:   Population Center Foundation.

Mani, S. B. (1970)   Family Planning Communication in Rural India.   Unpublised Ph.D. dissertation, Syracuse University, Syracuse, N.Y.

Mernissi, F. (1976)   The Moslem world:   Women excluded from development.   In I. Tinker, M. B. Bramsen, and M. Buvinic, eds., Women and World Development.   New York:   Praeger.

Miller, W. B., and R. K. Godwin (1977)   Psyche and Demos.   New York:   Oxford University Press.

Mitchell, R. E. (1972)   Husband-wife relations and family-planning practices in urban Hong Kong.   Journal of Marriage and the Family 34:139-146.

Mukherjee, B. N. (1975)   The role of husband-wife communication in family planning.   Journal of Marriage and the Family 37:655-667.

Mundigo, A. I. (1973)   Honduras revisited:   The clinic and its clientele.   In J. M. Stycos, ed., Clinics, Contraception, and Communication.   New York:   Appleton-Century-Crofts.

Nicassio, P. M. (1977)   Social class and family size as determinants of attributed machismo, femininity, and family planning:   A field study in two South American communities.   Sex Roles 3:577-598.

Piepmeier, K. B., and T. S. Adkins (1973)   The status of women and fertility.   Journal of Biosocial Science 5:507-520.

Poffenberger, T. (1968)   Motivational aspects of resistance to family planning in an Indian village. Demography 5:757-766.

Polgar, S., and F. Rothstein (1970)   Family planning and conjugal roles in New York City poverty areas. Social Science and Medicine 4:135-139.

PROFAM-PIACT de Mexico (1979)   Family Planning in Mexico. New York:  Population Council.

Rainwater, L. (1965)   Family Design:  Marital Sexuality, Family Size and Contraception. Chicago:  Aldine Publishing Co.

Ramakumar, S. R., and S. Y. S. Gopal (1972)   Husband-wife communication and fertility in a suburban community exposed to family planning. Journal of Family Welfare 18:30-36.

Rao, K. (1959)   Progress in family planning in Bangalore. Journal of Family Welfare 6:16-23.

Requena, B. M. (1965)   Studies of family planning in the Quinta normal district of Santiago:  The use of contraceptives. Milbank Memorial Fund Quarterly 43:69-99.

Rogers, E. M. (1974)   Communication for Development in China and India:  The Case of Health and Family Planning at the Village Level.  Paper presented at the Summer Program of Advanced Study on Communication and Development, East-West Communication Institute, Honolulu.

Rogers, E. M., and D. S. Solomon (1979)   Traditional Midwives as Family Planning Communicators in Asia, Case Study 1. Honolulu:  East-West Communication Institute.

Rogers, E. M., H. J. Park, K.-K. Chung, S. B. Lee, W. S. Puppa, and B. A. Doe (1976)   Network analysis of the diffusion of family planning innovations over time in Korean villages:  The role of Mothers' clubs.  In G. C. Chu, S. A. Rahim, and K. L. Kincaid, eds., Communication Monographs, No. 2.  Honolulu:  East-West Communication Institute.

Rosen, B. C., and A. B. Simmons (1971)   Industrialization, family and fertility:  A structural-psychological analysis of the Brazilian case. Demography 8:49-69.

Safilios-Rothschild, C. (1969)   Patterns of familial power and influence. Sociological Focus 2:7-19.

Safilios-Rothschild, C. (1970)   The study of family power structure:  A review 1960-1969. Journal of Marriage and the Family 32:539-552.

Safilios-Rothschild, C. (1975)  A Macro- and Micro-
Examination of Family Power and Love:  An Exchange
Model.  Paper presented at the Dynamics of Family
Ecology session of the ISSBD Symposium, Surrey,
England.

Scrimshaw, S. C. M. (1978)  Stages in women's lives and
reproductive decision-making in Latin America.
Medical Anthropology 2:41-58.

Shah, N. M. (1974)  The role of interspousal communication
in adoption of family planning methods:  A couple
approach.  Pakistan Development Review 13:454-469.

Shedlin, M. G., and P. E. Hollerbach (1981)  Modern and
traditional fertility regulation in a Mexican
community:  Factors in the process of decision-
making.  Studies in Family Planning 12:278-296.

Simmons, A. B., and M. Culagovski (1975)  If They Know,
Why Don't They Use?  Selected Factors Influencing
Contraceptive Adoption in Rural Latin America.  Paper
presented at the annual meeting of the Population
Association of America, Seattle, Wash.

Stokes, C. S., and C. J. Dudley (1972)  Family planning
and conjugal roles:  Some further evidence.  Social
Science and Medicine 6:157-161.

Strodtbeck, F. L. (1951)  Husband-wife interaction over
revealed differences.  American Sociological Review
16:468-473.

Stycos, J. M. (1968)  Human Fertility in Latin America.
Ithaca, N.Y.:  Cornell University Press.

Stycos, J. M., and K. W. Back (1964)  The Control of
Human Fertility in Jamaica.  Ithaca, N.Y.:  Cornell
University Press.

Tinker, I. (1976)  The adverse impact of development on
women.  In I. Tinker, M. B. Bransen, and M. Buvinic,
eds., Women and World Development. New York:  Praeger.

Turk, J. L. (1975)  Users and abusers of family power.
In R. E. Cromwell and D. H. Olson, eds., Power in
Families.  New York:  Sage Publications.

United Nations, Department of Economic and Social Affairs
(1961)  The Mysore Population Study.  Population
Studies, No. 34.  New York:  United Nations.

Van Keep, P. A., and E. Rice-Wray (1973)  Attitudes
towards family planning and contraception in Mexico
City.  Studies in Family Planning 4:305-309.

Weller, R. H. (1968)  The employment of wives, dominance
and fertility.  Journal of Marriage and the Family
30:437-442.

Yaukey, D., W. Griffiths, and B. J. Roberts (1967)
Couple concurrence and empathy on birth control
motivation in Dacca, East Pakistan.  American
Sociological Review 32:716-726.

# Chapter 12

# Sequential Fertility Decision Making and the Life Course

N. KRISHNAN NAMBOODIRI*

Over the past 25 years, fertility analysis has increasingly emphasized the importance of sequential decision
making.[1] According to this perspective, each birth is
influenced by a different set of motivational, cultural,
and family conditions.[2] Among these changing conditions
are the individual births themselves: each birth changes
family circumstances and so affects the probability and
timing of subsequent births (Mishler and Westoff, 1955).
    The subsections that follow address 15 specific propo-
sitions having roots in the sequential perspective.[3]
Three of these relate to characteristics of fertility
plans and behavior linked to the life course; six to plan
revisions and plan-implementation failures; two to the
extrafamilial context of reproduction and three to the
familial context; and one to the statistical interaction
between the life course and the reproduction context.
The empirical support, if any, available for each proposition is examined, though no attempt is made to give an
exhaustive review of the relevant data.

## PROPOSITIONS

### Characteristics of Fertility Plans and Behavior Linked to the Life Course

The following three hypotheses relate to the general idea
that fertility plans and behavior are influenced by dif-

*The author wishes to express his gratitude to Professors
R. R. Rindfuss, R. Udry, and E. K. Wilson for their
comments on earlier versions of the paper.

ferent factors, or differently influenced by the same
factor, at different stages of life.

Proposition 1   A couple's reasons for having the nth
child are different from those for having other children.
Another way to say this is that children of different
birth orders have different values and disvalues.
This hypothesis is based on the considerations that
the first child confers the unalterable state of parenthood on a couple, and probably cements the relationship
between the parents in a unique way; the second child
brings companionship to the first; and so on.  It is, of
course, the subjective perception of these alterations
that is relevant to the proposition.  The most ambitious
attempts to examine this idea used data from the Value of
Children study (Arnold et al., 1975).  For wives and
husbands from the Philippines, Korea, and the United
States, Bulatao (1981) reports the following predominant
values placed on various birth orders:  for the first
child, bringing the spouses closer, having someone to
love and care for, and carrying on the family name; for
the second to fifth child, sibling companionship, gender
preference, and the pleasure of watching children grow;
for the sixth and higher-order births, economic benefits.
As for disvalues, the one most prominantly mentioned in
connection with the first few births is loss of time to
spend with one's spouse; for higher births, most prominent
is the financial burden.  Similar patterns are reported
in Bulatao and Arnold (1977), Beckman (1976), and Fawcett
(1978).
It would be interesting to see whether such patterns
prevail in longitudinal data.  Such studies could also
show whether a couple's reasons for having the nth child
change as they move from one parity to the next.  For
example, it might be determined whether the reasons for
having a third child are the same when a couple are at
zero parity as when they move up to first or second
parity.

Proposition 2   (a) In any given population,[4] there
exists a normative family-size floor.  (b) Fertility
plans and behavior of couples below that floor are primarily determined by normative pressures; above the floor,
cost-benefit calculations and similar considerations are
primary (Fawcett et al., 1972; Kammeyer, 1972:117; Blake,
1968).[5]

The empirical support for the first part of this hypothesis--the existence of a normative family-size floor--is examined in detail by Mason (in these volumes). Three observations are relevant. First, childlessness is preferred by only a small minority of couples in every population, and then generally because of pregnancy problems and the like. Second, final parity preferences, determined according to psychological measurement theory, show a great distance between very low parities (0 and 1) and middle-level parities (2 and 3); moreover, the middle-level ones are bunched together (see, e.g., Goldberg and Coombs, 1963). Finally, some studies have shown that reinforcing sanctions are associated with pronatalist norms do exist, and are especially strong in cases of extreme deviance (Ory, 1978; Miller and Newman, 1978).

The second part of the hypothesis--that fertility behavior and plans are influenced by different sets of factors below and above the normative family-size floor--can be examined empirically in light of studies on factors affecting successive-parity progressions. These studies offer conflicting evidence. Namboodiri (1974) found that only at higher parities do such variables as wife's education, husband's income, and wife's religion have significant influence on couples' decisions to have additional children. However, when the same data were analyzed by Rosenzweig and Seiver (1975), using a different specification, socioeconomic predictors were found to have significant impact on expected parity progressions of women at lower parities as well. Hout (1978) found that wife's "potential earnings" had significant negative effects on fertility only at parities above 2. Kyriazis (1979), using a different data set, could not confirm Hout's results, however. With reference to the hypothesized primacy of social pressures as determinants of progressions below the normative family-size floor, Bulatao (1981:21,3) remarks that, in the Value of Children study, "rather than pleading social necessity, respondents considering low-parity births provided a cogent hierarchy of emotional gains from children" and that "social influences were very seldom cited" among the advantages of having children.

These inconsistencies might suggest that the second part of Proposition 2 has no solid empirical foundation (Bulatao and Fawcett, 1981). However, this conclusion seems to be premature in view of the difficulties involved in empirically testing this hypothesis: normative pressures operate subtly and may not even be recognized as

such by those being influenced; moreover, the institutional pathways of such pressures are so complex that
they are difficult to trace through survey interviews.

It should also be noted that all norms pertain to
specific occasions and social positions; thus subgroups
within a society may differ in their normative family-
size thresholds. For example, childlessness may not be
regarded as so terrible by all population subgroups in a
society; an only child may be "allowable" in some status
groups in some time periods. Thus if an analyst is only
partially successful in using a social or economic variable to distinguish between those who stay at a given low
parity and those who move up, this does not mean that
normative pressures are either nonexistent or inoperative.
A fair test of the present hypothesis would therefore
involve establishing the normative family-size threshold,
if any, characteristic of specified population subgroups,
and then examining whether parity progressions below the
subgroup threshold are primarily governed by generalized
disapproval of and sanctions against alternative behavior.
In such a study, the survey interview may not be the best
method of data collection.

Proposition 3   The effect of individual factors on
fertility plans and behavior changes with parity.  (This
is a more general version of the second part of
Proposition 2.)

A number of studies have empirically examined this
hypothesis.[6]  These studies generally use cross-
sectional data, mostly from the United States, and
differences in the methods they employ make comparisons
difficult.[7]  However, they typically show that the
effects of selected independent variables on fertility
plans and behavior change with increasing parity. For
example, Snyder (1978) reports that, for a United States
sample, permanent household income affects parity progressions positively at low parities but negatively at higher
parities. Goldberg (1960b) reports for a Detroit sample
that the degree to which the wife's leisure pursuits are
home-centered has a significant (positive) effect on
expectations about future reproduction only for women at
low (0 or 1) parities. Hout (1978) reports for the
United States that the effects of a number of variables
on the propensity to increase the size of the family
during a given period vary substantially across parities.

Thus, cross-sectional studies have provided some
empirical support for this hypothesis; however, it has

not yet been tested with longitudinal data.  Also, the
differences in the effects of particular independent
variables on different parities need to be satisfactorily
explained.  For example, although many studies have
reported a negative permanent income effect on the propensity to have additional children at higher parities,
there is no consensus on why this is so.[8]


### Plan Revisions and Failures

The following six hypotheses relate to the idea that fertility plans are revised according to changing circumstances, and that plans can fail to be implemented because
of various unpredictable factors.

   **Proposition 4**  Reformulations of fertility plans and
plan-implementation failures do occur.
   Data in support of this hypothesis come from longitudinal studies recording fertility plans at successive
points in time; from panel studies comparing plans at one
point in time to subsequent plans; and from cross-
sectional studies comparing current and past plans, with
the latter determined through retrospective questions.[9]
Data from several United States studies provide general
empirical support (Goldberg et al., 1959; Freedman et
al., 1980; Westoff et al., 1957, 1961; Westoff and Ryder,
1977a), and comparable data are reported in two Taiwan
studies (Hermalin et al., 1979; Nair and Cho, 1980).
However, Taiwanese women appear to be less successful
than their U.S. counterparts in preventing unwanted
births, but more likely to carry out intentions to have
more children.
   The data therefore indicate that intentions are not
always translated into behavior.  Along with some measurement error (between-interview instability, test-retest
unreliability) associated with the preference indicator,[10]
three other factors, discussed in the hypotheses below,
can be seen as responsible for the inconsistencies
between intentions and behavior:  the general tendency to
revise preferences to suit changing circumstances (Propositions 8 and 9); accidental or unplanned pregnancies
(Proposition 7); and the onset of infecundity and other
involuntary phenomena (Proposition 5).

   **Proposition 5**  Fecundity impairment is one of the
unpredictable causes of plan-implementation failures.

The risk of permanent sterility increases with age, as
Bongaarts (in these volumes) reports, but there is no way
to predict at what age a particular woman will become
sterile.  This unpredictability is intensified by the
possibility of pathological damage to the reproductive
system.  The role of fecundity impairments in changing
fertility plans is supported by a number of empirical
studies (United Nations, 1976, 1980; Westoff and Ryder,
1977a; Whelpton et al., 1966).  However, there is a need
for more systematic data on this hypothesis.[11]

Proposition 6  Marital disruption is associated with
reformulation of fertility plans and plan-implementation
failures.[12]

A number of factors are involved in this association
(see Burch, in these volumes).  First, divorce, separation, and widowhood involve a period outside the married
state, which reduces lifetime exposure to fertility.
This loss of exposure time is, of course, a function of
the probability of remarriage (Henry, 1956; Nag, 1962;
Davis, 1946; Dandekar, 1961) and the length of the waiting time outside the married state.  Second, divorce may
be preceded by a period of separation, and separation by
an interval of low frequency of coitus within marriage
(Thornton, 1978; Caldwell et al., 1980).  Third, sterility
or low fertility may be a direct cause of a divorce or
may facilitate it (Caldwell et al., 1980); conversely,
the presence of children, particularly young ones, often
deters separation and divorce (Cherlin, 1977; Glick, 1967;
see, however, Veevers, 1973).  Finally, when divorced or
widowed persons enter new unions, they may make up for
lost reproduction time by adopting a relatively older age
pattern of childbearing (Thornton, 1978).  Many people
tend to want at least one additional child in each marital
union.

Empirical data in support of this proposition are
rather sparse, perhaps because it is considered obvious.
However, some support is provided by Coombs (1979), who
reported that when the preference goal stated at an
initial interview was used to predict final parity, the
relationship was weaker in the total group than in the
subgroup consisting only of continuous marriages.  The
greatest difference was observed among women who had just
been married at the time of the first interview--the group
that also had the highest incidence of interrupted marriages.  Similarly, cross-sectional data, such as those
from the World Fertility Survey, show a clear association

between termination of marriage and low fertility (e.g.,
Caldwell et al., 1980). Again, however, these data are
not sufficient to provide clear insight into the subtle-
ties of the hypothesis.

Proposition 7  Unintended pregnancies occur with some
frequency, and are traceable to inadequacies in the
couple's fertility decision-making process or the
ineffectiveness of their implementation strategies.

Specifically, the causes of unintended pregnancies may
consist of the following:  (a) inability to understand
fertility options or their implications; (b) limited
information; (c) conflicts, such as those between individual desires and social norms; (d) crises at the personal, familial, or higher levels, creating stress and
preventing clear and decisive thinking; and (e) uncertainty about the outcome of a contemplated course of
action (e.g., even sterility may not be 100 percent
effective) (Miller and Godwin, 1977:103-109).

Data on unintended pregnancies come from various
sources.  In several cross-sectional surveys, the number
of children wanted or planned by respondents at the time
of their marriage was ascertained through retrospective
questions; these responses were then compared with current statements about ideal or expected family size
(e.g., United Nations, 1976:142-146; Hill et al., 1959).
If current expectations exceed the number wanted at the
time of marriage, the inference can sometimes be drawn
that unintended births have occurred (United Nations,
1976:147).  On the other hand, the discrepancies could
also be due to revised fertility goals since marriage, or
to measurement errors associated with responses to retrospective questions on family-size preferences (United
Nations, 1976, 1980).  Another question often included in
cross-sectional surveys is whether the last birth was
wanted:  "Thinking back to the time before you became
pregnant with your (last) child, had you wanted to have
any more children?"  The World Fertility Survey included
this question in the optional fertility regulation module,
which approximately two-thirds of the participating countries elected to use.  Primarily from responses to this
question, and secondarily from desired and ideal family
sizes, Westoff (1980) estimated that substantial proportions of births in Indonesia, Korea, Sri Lanka, Colombia,
Panama, and Peru could be classified as unwanted (see
also Udry et al., 1973).

A number of longitudinal studies also support the hypothesis. These include the 1970-75 rounds of the U.S. National Fertility Survey (Jones et al., 1980); the Princeton Study (Bumpass and Westoff, 1970); the National Longitudinal Study of Social, Economic, and Demographic Change in Thailand (Knodel and Pitaktepsombati, 1975); and longitudinal studies in Taiwan (Hermalin et al., 1979).

Analysis of the empirical data also leads to a number of generalizations.

7.1. Delaying conception for a long time may lead to the unintended consequence of delaying conceptions forever (Freedman et al., 1975:267). This may be explained in part by the unpredictable intervention of infecundity (see Proposition 5). However, it is also true that some couples change their plans from later to never as they become committed to nonchild-centered activities (Rindfuss and Bumpass, 1978).

7.2. The higher the age at marriage, the fewer the number of unwanted births and the lower the likelihood of contraceptive failure. This may be primarily due to the selectivity of who marries at what age: better-educated persons capable of making sound decisions and effectively carrying them out may marry at disproportionately higher ages (Westoff, 1980; Jones et al., 1980).

7.3. The probability of contraceptive failure is higher for couples who aim to delay a pregnancy than for those who want to prevent further childbearing altogether (Westoff et al., 1963; Jones et al., 1980).[13]

Proposition 8  Fertility plans change according to the couple's experience with infant deaths. Some couples may include extra births in their plans to insure against potential losses. However, such forecasts may and do go wrong, and hence even these couples often revise their plans in accordance with actual experience.

Heer's paper (in these volumes) contains an extensive review of the empirical data on this hypothesis. Some studies have found no support for it; others have claimed some, but many such claims are questionable on methodological grounds. Some more or less defensible support is provided by cross-sectional studies showing that, at any given parity, there is a significant negative association between experience with child deaths and readiness to cease childbearing, this association vanishing when number of living children, instead of parity, is used as the control (United Nations, 1980).

Proposition 9 Fertility plans are adjusted if the preferred and actual sex compositions of children are incongruent. Because the sex of each child is randomly determined,[14] a discrepancy may develop between what a couple prefer and what they get. Fertility plans are usually revised upward to counteract a less-preferred sex composition of offspring. On the other hand, couples may decide to terminate childbearing without having achieved the preferred composition (McClelland, 1979), depending on the perceived likelihood of the next birth yielding the desired sex; the values and disvalues attached to the status quo; and the perceived costs and benefits of success or failure in achieving the desired sex at the next birth. Some couples may prefer the status quo to risking a less desirable alternative; in that case, sex preference may lead to a downward revision of fertility plans.

Empirical data related to this hypothesis receive treatment elsewhere (McClelland, in these volumes). Generally, however, sex preference for children varies widely among populations, sometimes being associated with the propensity to have larger families (Williamson, 1976; Freedman and Coombs, 1974; United Nations, 1980). It may also be noted that, in cross-sectional surveys, it has been found that gender preference as a reason for wanting additional children is mentioned more often by couples at medium parities (e.g., 3 or 4) than by those at either end of the parity range (Bulatao, 1981).


## The Extrafamilial and the Familial
## Contexts of Reproduction

This section addresses shifts in the reproduction context. Two general points are relevant. First, when this context changes, the previous context will have a carry-over and the new context a current influence. Second, a couple's fertility plans and behavior themselves may be partly responsible for changes in the reproduction context.


## The Extrafamilial Context

Proposition 10 Social mobility and fertility are recip-rocally related. A mobile couple's class of origin has a carry-over effect and their class of destination a current effect on their postmobility fertility plans and behavior.[15]

The term mobility is used broadly to include movement from one occupational class to another, from below to above the poverty line, from being a landless laborer to being an owner-cultivator, etc. It should also be noted that mobility may be reckoned in terms of a time interval starting either before or after the beginning of a couple's reproductive career. Thus, for example, if a woman brought up in a landless laborer's household marries a landowner, she is regarded as mobile, as is one whose husband experiences mobility after marriage.[16] Finally, the hypothesis is of primary interest only if intrinsic class differences exist in family-building patterns.

This hypothesis has received empirical support from a number of studies in developed countries (Andorka, 1978; Berent, 1951; Blau and Duncan, 1967; Bumpass and Westoff, 1970; Duncan, 1966; Duncan et al., 1972; Hope, 1972; Zimmer, 1979). As for less developed countries, more data are needed. Opportunities for gathering such data are offered by the social experimentation now underway in many of these countries (Murdock, 1980). Specific research questions worth investigating concern the effect on fertility of upward mobility from being a landless laborer or tenant farmer to being a landowner, and of downward mobility from being a landlord of a relatively large estate to being the owner-cultivator of a small parcel of land.[17]

Proposition 11  Geographic mobility and fertility are reciprocally related. A migrant couple's place of origin has a carry-over effect and their place of destination a current effect on their postmigration fertility plans and behavior.

There is a vast literature on the relationship between migration and fertility (see Macisco et al., 1969, for an extensive bibliography). It is generally believed that the relationship runs in both directions. However, most of the empirical work to date has treated migration as an antecedent and fertility as a consequence; moreover, the results of such studies have not been conclusive (Macisco et al., 1969; United Nations, 1973:182–183).

Empirical material relevant to the second part of the hypothesis comes mostly from studies in the United States. Blau and Duncan (1967) found in their 1962 U.S. Occupational Change in a Generation Survey that women who moved away from a farm background had an average terminal parity intermediate between that of women remaining on farms and that of women with a nonfarm background. Similar patterns were observed earlier in other sets of data (Goldberg, 1959, 1960a; Freedman and Slesinger, 1961; see also Duncan, 1965; Ritchey and Stokes, 1972), although Kiser (1959) observed a different pattern.[18]

## The Familial Context

The familial context comprises a number of complex elements, including, for example, the influence of the extended family on a couple, the availability of mother surrogates, and the degree of independence of the generations. Changes in any of those elements will affect the familial context as a whole; moreover, changes in one element may well be dependent on changes in the others. In general, it should also be noted that, when such changes do occur, a couple's behavior may continue for some time to be influenced by past conditions; thus, for example, the extended family's hold on a couple may prevail even after the couple move into a separate residence.

The following three hypotheses relate to three dimensions of the family context: the family living arrangements, the wife's extrafamilial involvement, and the marital power structure.

Proposition 12   The fertility plans and behavior of a couple who move from one living arrangement (or household composition) to another are influenced by the original as well as by the new arrangement. There is fertility selectivity in the move from one arrangement to another.

Very little empirical research has been done on the second part of this hypothesis. Even on the first part, most research has merely compared the average fertility of couples in different living arrangements. Moreover, the results of this research have been inconclusive (Freedman, 1961/62), mainly because of inconsistencies in the concepts and methodology used (Burch and Gendell, 1970). Only recently have scholars begun to realize that misleading inferences can be drawn from a classification based exclusively on living arrangements. Several studies do report data on living arrangements over the life course (e.g., Bebarta, 1977; Karim, 1974; Palmore, 1972), but the relationship between these data and fertility has not been systematically explored.

Bebarta's (1977) study indicates that those who change living arrangements during the childbearing years have a higher final parity than those who do not, the latter group (nonchangers) showing no marked difference in fertility by the type of family unit involved. Thus the data imply that type of household does not influence fertility, but any change in household composition does; in other words, there may be a special mobility effect. If such data are to be useful in testing the hypothesis, one must know: (a) in which setting the couple received socialization and training; (b) at what stages in life any changes in living arrangements took place; and (c) whether selectivity (in fertility level) was operating on those who changed living arrangements.

Proposition 13    (a) A woman's plans for and actual participation in extrafamilial activities (such as work outside the home) affect and are affected by her fertility plans and behavior, and the influences in both directions have long-term as well as short-term components. (b) The effects in question are conditional on the various dimensions of the familial context.

Standing (in these volumes) and Oppong (in these volumes) review a number of studies bearing on one aspect or another of this hypothesis. In general, however, a number of points may be noted.

First, relatively little empirical data exist on the reciprocal relationship between women's work and fertility in developed countries; even less exist for the developing countries. Most of the research to date has been concerned with whether the two variables (work and fertility) are associated at all. Although a negative relationship between the two variables has been observed in the developed countries, the corresponding results for developing country populations have been inconsistent, sometimes showing a positive relationship between the variables, sometimes a negative relationship, and sometimes none at all. In theory, it is recognized that the familial context of childbearing and rearing has a conditioning influence on the work-fertility relationship; however, the specific components of this influence have not yet been systematically studied. It is known that, in the developed countries, the recent occurrence of a live birth has a short-term depressant effect on the mother's propensity to participate in the labor force (Cramer, 1980; Smith-Lovin and Tickamyer, 1978; Hout, 1978). It should be noted, however, that this pattern is conditional on such factors as the separation of the work place from the home, the unavailability of socially acceptable mother surrogates, and the unconventionality of caring for the child at the work place. Because such conditions are not the rule in the developing countries, the applicability of this depressant effect to those countries is questionable.

Finally, the long-term effect of each birth on the mother's work participation will not be clear until longitudinal data covering relatively long segments of the couple's life course are available. On the other hand, a woman's work participation, especially before marriage and early in the marriage, is taken to affect her fertility in both the short and long term via her work commitment and the delay of marriage and first birth (Standing, in these volumes; Cramer, 1980). A careful analysis of the work-history data in the World Fertility Survey might shed light on these effects.

Proposition 14  (a) The marital power structure is affected by and affects the couple's fertility plans and behavior.  (b) The effects in both directions are conditional on the various dimensions of the familial context of reproduction.  It should be noted that very little attention has been given to the reciprocal aspect of this relationship; most of the research has treated fertility as a consequence and the marital power structure as an antecedent.

In the empirical research, the marital power structure has been measured in a number of different ways (see Bagozzi and Van Loo, 1978b, following Goldberg, 1975; Blood and Wolfe, 1960; Cromwell and Olsen, 1975; Hill et al., 1959; Ridley, 1968; Safilios-Rothschild, 1970; Scanzoni and Scanzoni, 1981). Because of these differences in operational definitions, it is inevitable that the results of these studies will not be entirely comparable. However, even taking this into account, the empirical evidence for the hypothesis is at present sketchy. For example, the Hill et al. (1959) study in Puerto Rico reports virtually no association between a husband-dominance index and any of these measures of contraceptive use:  ever-use, length of use, and contraceptive success. On the other hand, their couple communication index, which in a sense may be regarded as including husband-wife power relations, is reported to have been one of the better predictors of fertility control behavior. Similar inconsistencies exist on whether the marital power structure changes over the life course, and, if so, in what pattern. There are those who believe that, in industrialized societies, most marriages begin on a more or less egalitarian footing, only to change eventually into a pattern where each spouse is dominant in selected domains (Miller and Godwin, 1977:76). Then there are those who speculate that most marriages, at least in the developed world, are in the beginning characteristically wife-dominant, as far as fertility behavior is concerned, but become egalitarian or husband-dominant later in the life course (Goldberg, 1960a, 1960b). If such speculations are correct, it seems plausible that fertility decisions are monopolized by one spouse at one stage in the life course, and by the other at another stage. However, the data are simply not sufficient to test this empirically. It may also be noted that the data on the work-fertility relationship (see Proposition 13) are also pertinent to the present discussion insofar as that relationship is mediated by marital power structures, as some scholars believe (Ridley, 1968; Weller, 1968; see also Namboodiri, 1966).

## Interaction Between the Life Course and the Reproduction Context

The following hypothesis addresses the interactional effect of the life course and the reproduction context on fertility plans and behavior.

Proposition 15    The impact on the couple's fertility plans and behavior of a change in the reproduction context depends on the life-course stage at which that change occurs.

This hypothesis has one of its roots in the primitive notion of the cohort approach to the study of social phenomena, which holds that "transformations of the social world modify people of different ages in different ways" (Ryder, 1965:859). The hypothesis may also be viewed from the commonplace perspective that reproduction tends to be concentrated in certain age groups. Although this is partly due to the age pattern of fecundity, it is also due to social and economic factors, such as the belief that grandparents are not supposed to give birth. With the age concentration of childbearing, it is reasonable to expect a stimulus to have the greatest impact on reproduction when childbearing activity is at its peak.

Obviously, the greater the age concentration, the more relevant this observation will be. Proposition 15 may also be viewed according to the underlying theme of Propositions 1, 2, and 3--that fertility plans and behavior are affected by different sets of factors or differently affected by particular factors at different stages of the life course. Thus, for example, it is logical to expect that couples below a normative family-size floor are less likely than those above the floor to respond to a family-planning program that emphasizes sterilization.

The empirical data relevant to Propositions 1, 2, and 3 are also relevant to the present hypothesis. Other pertinent data include those on differentials by life-course stage in the receptivity of couples to organized family planning programs. Also worth mentioning is Namboodiri's (1981) analysis of the U.S. cohort fertility data; this study indicates a heavy concentration of age-period interactions in the age group 20 to 24, reflecting extra sensitivity in this group to environmental shifts.

## CONCLUSIONS

Although the sequential approach to fertility decision making is intuitively more appealing than the single-decision approach, its much greater complexity generates tremendous data needs (Heckman and Willis, 1976). Data are especially needed on changes over the life course (by age, parity, or length of the reproductive career) in the following areas:

a.  the familial and extrafamilial contexts of reproduction (e.g., shifts in the marital power structure, work history, mobility and migration history, and changes in economic conditions),
b.  the proximate determinants of fertility (e.g., coital frequency, onset of infecundity due to various causes, and fetal wastage), and
c.  contraceptive and noncontraceptive behavior.

Such longitudinal panel data, together with detailed fertility histories, would permit comparisons of the adequacy of the sequential approach against other, more easily implemented, approaches. These would answer the question whether the sequential model is capable of delivering explanatory or predictive power commensurate with the conceptual complexity it introduces and the magnitude of its data requirements.

The form these data should take, the design of their collection, and the methods for their analysis are equally important considerations. New methodology may need to be developed to handle such longitudinal data, as well as some existing longitudinal data from fertility surveys.

The hypotheses presented in this paper offer a number of opportunities to apply the sequential approach through collection of the necessary empirical data. The following are examples of topics needing further research:

a. What are the changes in parents' reasons for having their nth child as they move from 0 to n-1 parity? For example, are the reasons for having the third child the same before and after the second child is born?

b. What explains the parity differences in the effects of various factors on the probability of parity progression?

c. What is the precise relationship between a woman's work history and her fertility history?

Another question to be answered empirically is whether the sequential approach is universally applicable. For example, can it be applied where families are not planned? Because the sequential model includes factors that are not deliberately manipulated, its application to populations in which large-family or "supply-side" norms prevail cannot be dismissed.

## NOTES

1. Recently, some scholars (e.g., Bulatao, 1981) have begun to use the term successive decisions to refer to what used to be called sequential decisions. Because the latter term has been in use for a long time, it has been adopted in the present paper. It should be noted, however, that scholars have used the term sequential decisions in more than one sense: it has been applied to the hierarchical arrangement of lower-level decisions within higher-level ones, as well as to the horizontal sequencing of a number of decisions of the same level. An example of the former is the following: a teenager decides to seek contraceptive protection; she (he) is then faced with

deciding what contraception to use, where to go for the needed supplies or services, where to store the supplies (if necessary), and so on. An example of the latter type is the decision to have the first birth, followed by the decision to have the second, and then to have the third, and so on. This paper is concerned with this latter type.

2. A number of studies have focused on sequential decision-making, or used this theory as their point of departure. These include the following: Bulatao (1981), Bulatao and Arnold (1977), Bumpass and Westoff (1970), Coombs (1979), Freedman et al. (1965, 1980), Fried et al. (1980), Goldberg (1960b), Hout (1978), Khan and Sirageldin (1977), Kyriazis (1979), Lee and Khan (1978), Miller and Newman (1978), Mishler and Westoff (1955), Namboodiri (1974), Park (1978), Rosenzweig (1976), Rosenzweig and Seiver (1975), Seiver (1978), Simon (1975a, 1975b), Snyder (1978), Terhune (1974), West (1980), and Westoff et al. (1961). Theoretical expositions of the sequential perspective can be found in Cochrane (1979), Hass (1974), Heckman and Willis (1976), and Namboodiri (1972a, 1980). Relevant discussions can also be found in Bagozzi and Van Loo (1978a), Leibenstein (1979), Turchi (1975, 1979), and Lee (1980).

3. See Namboodiri (1980) for a development of the sequential perspective based on some of the ideas of temporary equilibrium theory in economics (Grandmont, 1977).

4. The term population is used advisedly here: the reference is not always to a society or a country as a whole, but includes any aggregate of humans having a unit character, in the sense of an interdependence, resulting in a separate identity.

5. This notion of a normative family-size floor parallels the stipulation in economics that, for the consumer, there is a "subsistence level" for certain items in the consumption basket, and that there are trade-offs between consumption programs only if that subsistence level is equalled or exceeded in each program (see, e.g., Hakansson [1972] also see Namboodiri [1980:79], for a discussion of the relationship between this notion and Maslow's [1954] postulate of a hierachy of human needs; and Georgescu-Roegen [1968] for a discussion of the roots of the subsistence-level notion and needs hierarchies in early economic thought).

6. See, for example, Bernhardt (1972), Fried et al. (1980), Goldberg (1960b), Hout (1978), Khan and Sirageldin (1977), Kyriazis (1979), Lee and Khan (1978), Namboodiri (1974), Rosenzweig (1976), Rosenzweig and Seiver (1975), Seiver (1978), Simon (1975a, 1975b), Synder (1978), and West (1980).

7. To give an example, in some studies, wife's education has been used as a proxy for the value of the wife's time. However, in other studies where the latter variable has been exogenously estimated using instrumental variables, it has been found that wife's education and the value of her time exert opposite influences on the decision to have additional children (see, e.g., Snyder, 1978). Those who have used instrumental variables to estimate the value of the wife's time have, however, ignored the potential problems stemming from selectivity bias (Heckman, 1980).

8. To explain this empirical regularity, some authors have pointed to the higher contraceptive efficacy among higher-income couples; some have invoked the idea that high-income groups invest more in quality than in quantity of children; some have proposed that high-income couples have different tastes; and some believe that the observed income effect reflects the interaction of income with some other variable such as education (see Simon, 1975a; Hout, 1978; Bulatao and Fawcett, 1981).

9. For example, the fertility regulation module of the World Fertility Survey includes the following question: "Thinking back to the time before you became pregnant [with your (last) child], had you wanted to have any (more) children?" Another example is the following: "Before you had your first child, did you think a great deal about how many children you wanted to have, or didn't you think about it? [If yes] How many children did you want to have?" (Hill et al., 1959).

10. Better measures of preferences, such as those based on psychological measurement theory, have been shown to have greater predictive power as far as subsequent behavior is concerned (Coombs, 1979).

11. There is ample evidence for the prevalence of sterility due to both pathological and nonpathological causes; what is lacking is the classification of sterile women according to their fertility plans before they became aware of their sterility.

12. Marital unions are understood broadly here to include all sexual unions, regardless of whether they have been legally recognized as marriages.
13. This was first observed as an empirical regularity in the Princeton Fertility Study, and has since then been noted in all major investigations of contraceptive efficacy.
14. Current medical technology permits ascertaining the sex of the fetus early in the pregnancy. It is therefore possible through sex-selective abortion to prevent the birth of infants of the undesired sex. Similarly, it is possible through sex-selective infanticide to ensure that only infants of the desired sex survive. Both of these possibilities are ignored in the present context on the grounds that very few parents currently adopt either of these strategies.
15. In early formulations of the mobility-fertility relationship, fertility was seen as the antecedent and mobility the consequence (Fisher, 1929; Dumont, 1890); however, in many later formulations, fertility has been treated as the consequence and mobility the antecedent.
16. Defined in this broad fashion, mobility is becoming very common in less developed countries. The fact that this is occurring when fertility levels are also changing offers an opportunity to investigate the applicability of this hypothesis.
17. Similarly, the relationship between fertility as an antecedent and fragmentation of landholdings as a consequence in these countries remains to be carefully examined (Merrick, 1978).
18. It may be noted that the extrafamilial context may include other components besides those covered in Propositions 10 and 11. It has often been held, for example, that, when times are good economically, people feel freer to have children (Easterlin, 1978). This would suggest that, if a shift occurs in a couple's economic state, the old economic conditions will have a carry-over and the new ones a current effect on their subsequent fertility plans and behavior.

BIBLIOGRAPHY

Andorka, R. (1978) Determinants of Fertility in Advanced Societies. New York: The Free Press.

Arnold, F., R. A., Bulatao, C. Buripakdi, B. J. Chung, J. T. Fawcett, T. Iritani, S. J. Lee, and T.-S. Wu (1975) The Value of Children: Introduction and Comparative Analysis, Vol. I. Honolulu: East-West Population Institute.

Bagozzi, R. P., and M. F. Van Loo (1978a) Fertility as consumption: Theories from the behavioral sciences. Journal of Consumer Research 4:199-288.

Bagozzi, R. P., and M. F. Van Loo (1978b) Toward a general theory of fertility: A causal model approach. Demography 15:301-319.

Bebarta, P. C. (1977) Family Type and Fertility in India. North Quincy, Mass.: Christopher Publishing.

Beckman, L. J. (1976) Values of Parenthood among Women Who Want an Only Child. Paper presented at the annual meeting of the American Psychological Association, Washington, D.C.

Berent, J. (1951) Fertility and social mobility. Population Studies 5:244-260.

Bernhardt, E. M. (1972) Fertility and economic status-- Some recent findings on differentials in Sweden. Population Studies 26:175-184.

Blake, J. (1968) Are babies consumer durables? A critique of the economic theory of reproductive motivation. Population Studies 22:5-25.

Blau, P. M., and O. D. Duncan (1967) The American Occupational Structure. New York: Wiley.

Blood, R. O., Jr., and D. M. Wolfe (1960) Husbands and Wives. New York: The Free Press.

Bulatao, R. A. (1981) Values and disvalues of children in sequential childbearing decisions. Demography 18:1-26.

Bulatao, R. A., and F. Arnold (1977) Relationships between the value and cost of children and fertility: Cross-cultural evidence. Pp. 141-156 in International Population Conference, Mexico, 1977, Vol. I. Liege: International Union for the Scientific Study of Population.

Bulatao, R. A., and J. T. Fawcett (1981) Dynamic perspectives in the study of fertility decision-making: Successive decisions within a fertility career. Pp. 433-449 in International Population Conference, Manila, 1981, Vol. 1. Liege:

International Union for the Scientific Study of Population.

Bumpass, L. L., and C. F. Westoff (1970) The Later Years of Childbearing. Princeton, N.J.: Princeton University Press.

Burch, T. K., and M. Gendell (1970) Extended family structure and fertility: Some conceptual and methodological issues. Journal of Marriage and the Family 32:227-236.

Caldwell, J. C., P. F. McDonald, and L. T. Ruzicka (1980) Interrelationships between Nuptiality and Fertility: The Evidence from the World Fertility Survey. Paper presented at the World Fertility Survey Conference, London.

Cherlin, A. (1977) The effect of children on marital dissolution. Demography 14:265-272.

Cochrane, S. H. (1979) Fertility and Education: What Do We Really Know? World Bank Staff Occasional Papers, Number 26. Baltimore, Md.: The Johns Hopkins University Press.

Coombs, L. C. (1976) Are Cross-Cultural Preference Comparisons Possible?: A Measurement-Theoretic Approach. IUSSP, No. 5. Liege: International Union for the Scientific Study of Population.

Coombs, L. C. (1979) Reproductive goals and achieved fertility: A fifteen-year perspective. Demography 16:523-534.

Cramer, J. C. (1980) Fertility and female employment. American Sociological Review 45:167-190.

Cromwell, R. C., and D. H. Olsen (1975) Power in Families. New York: Wiley.

Dandekar, K. (1961) Widow remarriage in six rural communities in western India. Pp. 191-207 in International Population Conference, New York, Vol. 2. Liege: International Union for the Scientific Study of Population.

Davis, K. (1946) Human fertility in India. American Journal of Sociology 52:243-254.

Dumont, A. (1890) Depopulation et Civilisation. Paris: Lecrosnier-Babe.

Duncan, O. D. (1965) Farm background and differential fertility. Demography 2:240-249.

Duncan, O. D. (1966) Methodological issues in the analysis of social mobility. Pp. 51-97 in J. J. Smelser and S. M. Lipset, eds., Social Structure and Social Mobility in Economic Development. Chicago: Aldine.

Duncan, O. D., D. L. Featherman, and B. Duncan (1972)
Socioeconomic Background and Achievement. New York:
Seminar Press.

Easterlin, R. A. (1978) The economics and sociology of
fertility: A synthesis. Pp. 57-133 in C. Tilly, ed.,
Historical Studies of Changing Fertility. Princeton,
N.J.: Princeton University Press.

Fawcett, J. T. (1978) The value and cost of the first
child. Pp. 244-265 in W. B. Miller and L. F. Newman,
eds., The First Child and Family Formation. Chapel
Hill, N.C.: Carolina Population Center, University of
North Carolina.

Fawcett, J. T., S. Albores, and F. Arnold (1972) The
value of children among ethnic groups in Hawaii:
Exploratory measurements. Pp. 234-257 in J. T.
Fawcett, ed., The Satisfactions and Costs of
Children: Theories, Concepts, Methods. Honolulu:
East-West Population Institute.

Fisher, R. A. (1929) The General Theory of Natural
Selection. New York: Dover.

Freedman, D. (1963) The relation of economic status to
fertility. American Economic Review 53:414-426.

Freedman, R. (1961/62) The sociology of human
fertility: A trend report and bibliography. Current
Sociology X/XI:35-121.

Freedman, R. (1963) Norms for family size in underdeveloped areas. Proceedings of the Royal Statistical
Society 159:220-234.

Freedman, R. (1975) The Sociology of Human Fertility:
An Annotated Bibliography. New York: Irvington
Publishers.

Freedman, R., and L. Coombs (1974) Cross-Cultural
Comparisons: Data on Two Factors in Fertility
Behavior. New York: Population Council.

Freedman, R., and D. P. Slesinger (1961) Fertility
differentials for the indigenous non-farm population
of the United States. Population Studies 15:161-173.

Freedman, R., L. C. Coombs, and L. Bumpass (1965)
Stability and change in expectations about family
size: A longitudinal study. Demography 2:250-275.

Freedman, R., A. J. Hermalin, and M. C. Chang (1975) Do
statements about desired family size predict
fertility? The case of Taiwan 1967-1970. Demography
12:407-416.

Freedman, R., D. S. Freedman, and A. D. Thornton (1980)
Changes in fertility expectations and preferences
between 1962 and 1977: Their relation to final
parity. Demography 17:365-378.

Fried, E. S., S. L. Hofferth, and J. R. Udry (1980)
Parity-specific and two-sex utility models of
reproductive intentions. Demography 17:1-11.

Georgescu-Roegen, N. (1968) Utility. In D. Sils, ed.,
International Encyclopedia of the Social Sciences.
New York: MacMillan and The Free Press.

Glick, P. (1967) Marriage and family variables related
to fertility. Pp. 210-213 in Proceedings of the World
Population Conference, Belgrade, Vol. II. New York:
United Nations.

Goldberg, D. (1959) The fertility of two-generation
urbanites. Population Studies 12-214-222.

Goldberg, D. (1960a) Another look at the Indianapolis
study fertility data. Milbank Memorial Fund Quarterly
38:23-36.

Goldberg, D. (1960b) Some recent developments in
American fertility research. In National Bureau of
Economic Research, Demographic and Economic Change in
Developed Countries: A Conference of the Universities-
Committee for Economic Research. Princeton, N.J.:
Princeton University Press.

Goldberg, D. (1975) Socioeconomic theory and
differential fertility: The case of the LDCs. Social
Forces 54:84-106.

Goldberg, D., and C. H. Coombs (1963) Some applications
of unfolding theory to fertility analysis. Pp.
105-129 in Emerging Techniques in Population
Research. New York: Proceedings of the 1962 Annual
Conference of the Milbank Memorial Fund.

Goldberg, D., H. Sharp, and R. Freedman (1959) The
stability of expected family size. Milbank Memorial
Fund Quarterly 37:369-385.

Goldberger, A. S. (1971) Econometrics and psychometrics:
A survey of communalities. Psychometrika 36:83-105.

Goldscheider, C. (1967) Fertility of the Jews.
Demography 4:196-209.

Grandmont, J. M. (1977) Temporary general equilibrium
theory. Econometrika 45:535-573.

Hakansson, N. H. (1972) Sequential investment-
consumption strategies for individuals and endowment
funds. In J. L. Bicksler, ed., Methodology in
Finance-Investments. Lexington, Mass.: D. C. Heath
and Company.

Hass, P. H. (1974) Wanted and unwanted pregnancies: A
fertility decision-making model. The Journal of
Social Issues 30:125-165.

Heckman, J. J. (1980)  Sample selection bias as a specification error with an application to the estimation of labor supply functions.  Pp. 206-248 in J. P. Smith, ed., Female Labor Supply:  Theory and Estimation.  Princeton, N.J.:  Princeton University Press.

Heckman, J. J., and R. J. Willis (1976)  Estimation of a stochastic model of reproduction:  An econometric approach.  Pp. 99-138 in N. Terleckyj, ed., Household Production and Consumption.  New York:  Columbia University Press.

Henry, L. (1956)  Caracteristiques demographiques des pays sousdeveloppes:  Natalite, nuptialite, fecondite.  Pp. 149-173 in G. Balandier, ed., Le "Tiers Monde": Sous-developpement et Development.  Institut National d'Etudies Demographiques Travaus et Documents Cahier No. 27.

Hermalin, A. I., R. Freedman, T.-H. Sun, and M. C. Chang (1979)  Do intentions predict fertility:  The experience in Taiwan, 1967-74.  Studies in Family Planning 10:75-95.

Hill, R., J. M. Stycos, and K. W. Back (1959)  The Family and Population Control.  Chapel Hill, N.C.: University of North Carolina Press.

Hope, K., ed. (1972)  The Analysis of Social Mobility: Methods and Approaches.  Oxford, Eng.:  Clarendon Press.

Hout, M. (1978)  The determinants of marital fertility in the United States, 1968-1970:  Inferences from a dynamic model.  Demography 15:139-159.

Jones, E. F., L. Paul, and C. F. Westoff (1980)  Contraceptive efficacy:  The significance of method and motivation.  Studies in Family Planning 11:39-50.

Kammayer, K. C. (1972)  An Introduction to Population. London:  International Textbook Co.

Karim, M. S. (1974)  Fertility differentials by family type.  Pakistan Development Review 13:129-144.

Khan, M. A., and I. Sirageldin (1977)  Son preference and the demand for additional children in Pakistan. Demography 14:481-495.

Kiser, C. V. (1959)  Fertility rates by residence and migration.  Pp. 273-286 in International Population Conference, Vienna.  Liege:  International Union for the Scientific Study of Population.

Knodel, J., and P. Pitaktepsombati (1975)  Fertility and family planning in Thailand:  Results from two rounds of a national study.  Studies in Family Planning 6:402-413.

Kyriazis, N. (1979) Sequential fertility decision
making:  Catholics and Protestants in Canada.
Canadian Review of Sociology and Anthropology
16:275-286.

Lee, C. F., and M. M. Khan (1978) Factors related to the
intention to have additional children in the United
States:  A reanalysis of data from the 1965 and 1970
National Fertility Studies. Demography 15:337-344.

Lee, R. D. (1980) Aiming at a moving target:  Period
fertility and changing reproductive goals. Population
Studies 34:205-226.

Leibenstein, H. (1979) Comments on "Fertility as
consumption:  Theories from the behavioral sciences."
Journal of Consumer Research 5:287-290.

Lenski, G., and J. Lenski (1978) Human Societies:  An
Introduction to Macrosociology, 3rd ed. New York:
McGraw Hill.

MacDonald, M. M., and R. R. Rindfuss (1980) Earnings,
Relative Income, and Family Formation. Chapel Hill,
N.C.: Carolina Population Center, University of North
Carolina.

Macisco, J. J., L. F. Bouvier, and M. J. Renzi (1969)
Migration status, education and fertility in Puerto
Rico, 1960. Milbank Memorial Fund Quarterly
47:167-187.

Maslow, A. H. (1954) Motivation and Personality. New
York:  Harper and Row.

McClelland, G. (1979) Determining the impact of sex
preference on fertility:  A consideration of parity
progression ratio, dominance, and stopping rule
measures. Demography 16:377-388.

Merrick, T. W. (1978) Fertility and land availability in
rural Brazil. Demography 15:321-336.

Miller, W. B., and R. K. Godwin (1977) Psyche and
Demos. New York:  Oxford University Press.

Miller, W. B., and L. F. Newman, eds. (1978) The First
Child and Family Formation. Chapel Hill, N.C.:
Carolina Population Center, University of North
Carolina.

Mishler, E. G., and C. F. Westoff (1955) A proposal for
research on social psychological factors affecting
fertility:  Concepts and hypotheses. In Current
Research in Human Fertility. New York:  Milbank
Memorial Fund.

Murdoch, W. W. (1980) The Poverty of Nations:  The
Political Economy of Hunger and Population.
Baltimore, Md.: The Johns Hopkins University Press.

Nag, M. (1962)  Factors Affecting Human Fertility:  A
    Cross-Cultural Study.  Yale University Publication in
    Anthropology No. 66.  New Haven, Conn.:  Yale
    University.
Nair, N. K., and L. P. Cho (1980)  Fertility intentions
    and behavior:  Some findings from Taiwan.  Studies in
    Family Planning 11:255-263.
Namboodiri, N. K. (1966)  Another look at structural-
    functional analysis:  An exercise in axiomatic theory
    construction.  Sociological Bulletin 15:75-89.
Namboodiri, N. K. (1972a)  Some observations on the
    economic framework for fertility analysis.  Population
    Studies 26:185-206.
Namboodiri, N. K. (1972b)  The integrative potential of a
    fertility model:  An analytic test.  Population
    Studies 26:465-485.
Namboodiri, N. K. (1974)  Which couples at given parities
    expect to have additional births?  An exercise in
    discriminant analysis.  Demography 11:45-56.
Namboodiri, N. K. (1975)  Review symposium on "Economics
    of the Family:  Marriage, Children, and Human
    Capital," T. W. Schultz, ed.  Demography 14:561-569.
Namboodiri, N. K. (1980)  A look at fertility model
    building from different perspectives.  Pp. 71-90 in T.
    K. Burch, ed., Demographic Behavior:  Interdisciplinary
    Perspectives on Decision-Making.  AAAS Selected
    Symposium, 45.  Boulder, Colo.:  Westview Press.
Namboodiri, N. K. (1981)  On factors affecting fertility
    at different stages in the reproduction history:  An
    exercise in cohort analysis.  Social Forces
    59:1114-1129.
Ory, M. G. (1978)  The decision to parent or not:
    Normative and structural components.  Journal of
    Marriage and the Family 40:531-539.
Palmore, J. A. (1972)  Population change, conjugal status
    and the family.  In Population Aspects of Social
    Development.  Asian Population Studies, Series No.
    11.  Bangkok:  United Nations.
Palmore, J. A., and M. B. Concepcion (1980)  Desired
    Family Size and Contraceptive Use.  Paper presented at
    the World Fertility Survey Conference, London.
Park, C. B. (1978)  The fourth Korean child.  The effect
    of son preference on subsequent fertility.  Journal of
    Biosocial Science 10:95-106.
Ridley, J. C. (1968)  Demographic change and the roles
    and status of women.  The Annals of the American
    Academy of Political and Social Sciences 375:15-25.

Rindfuss, R. R., and L. L. Bumpass (1978)  Age and the sociology of fertility:  How old is too old?  Pp. 43-56 in K. Taeuber et al., eds., Social Demography. New York: Academic Press.

Ritchey, P. N., and C. S. Stokes (1972)  Residence background, migration, and fertility. Demography 9:217-230.

Rosenzweig, M. (1976)  Female work experience, employment status, and birth expectations:  Sequential decision-making in the Philippines. Demography 13:339-356.

Rosenzweig, M., and D. A. Seiver (1975)  Comment on Namboodiri's "Which couples at given parities expect to have additional births?" Demography 12:665-668.

Ryder, N. B. (1965)  The cohort as a concept in the study of social change. American Sociological Review 30:843-886.

Safilios-Rothschild, C. (1970)  The study of family power structure:  A review, 1960-1969. Journal of Marriage and the Family 32:539-552.

Scanzoni, L. D., and J. Scanzoni (1981)  Men, Women, and Change:  A Sociology of Marriage and Family, 2nd ed. New York:  McGraw-Hill.

Seiver, D. A. (1978)  Which couples at given parities have additional births. Research in Population Economics 1:309-319.

Simon, J. A. (1975a)  Puzzles and further explorations in the interrelationship of successive births with the husband's income, spouse's education and race. Demography 12:259-274.

Simon, J. A. (1975b)  The effect of income and education upon successive births. Population Studies 29:109-122.

Smith-Lovin, L., and A. R. Tickamyer (1978)  Labor force participation, fertility behavior, and sex-role attitudes. American Sociological Review 43:541-556.

Snyder, D. (1978)  Economic variables and the decisions to have additional children:  Evidence from the Survey of Economic Opportunities. American Economics 22:12-16.

Terhune, K. W. (1974)  Rationality and Rationalization in the Perceived Consequences of Family Size.  Paper presented at the 82nd Annual Convention of the American Psychological Association, New Orleans.

Thornton, A. (1978)  Marital dissolution, remarriage, and childbearing. Demography 15:361-380.

Turchi, B. A. (1975)  The Demand for Children:  The Economics of Fertility in the United States. Cambridge, Mass.:  Ballinger.

Turchi, B. A. (1979)  Comments on "Fertility as consumption:  Theories from the behavioral sciences." Journal of Consumer Research 5:293-296.

Udry, J. R. (1980)  Do Couples Make Fertility Decisions One at a Time?  Unpublished paper presented at a seminar organized by the Carolina Population Center, University of North Carolina, Chapel Hill.

Udry, J. R., K. E. Bauman, and C. L. Chase (1973) Population growth rates in perfect contraceptive populations. Population Studies 27:365-371.

United Nations (1961)  The Mysore Population Study. Population Studies No. 34 (ST/SOA/Ser. A/34).  New York:  United Nations.

United Nations (1973)  The Determinants and Consequences of Population Trends. New York:  United Nations.

United Nations (1976)  Fertility and Family Planning in Europe Around 1970:  A Comparative Study of Twelve National Surveys. (ST/ESA/SER A/58).  New York: United Nations.

United Nations (1980)  Selected Factors Affecting Fertility Preferences in Developing Countries: Evidence from the First Fifteen WFS Country Reports. Paper prepared by the Population Division and presented at the World Fertility Survey Conference, London.

Veevers, J. E. (1973)  The child-free alternative: Rejection of the motherhood mystique.  Pp. 183-199 in M. Stephenson, ed., Women in Canada. Toronto:  New Press.

Weller, R. H. (1968)  The employment of wives, dominance and fertility. Journal of Marriage and the Family 30:437-442.

West, K. (1980)  Sequential Fertility Behavior:  Study of Socio-Economic and Demographic Determinants of Parity Transitions.  Unpublished Ph.D. dissertation, University of North Carolina, Chapel Hill, N.C.

Westoff, C. F. (1980)  Unwanted Fertility in Six Developing Countries.  Paper presented at the World Fertility Survey Conference, London.

Westoff, C. F., and N. B. Ryder (1977a)  The predictive validity of reproductive intentions. Demography 14:431-453.

Westoff, C. F., and N. B. Ryder (1977b)  The Contraceptive Revolution. Princeton, N.J.:  Princeton University Press.

Westoff, C. F., E. G. Mishler, and E. L. Kelly (1957) Preferences in size of family and eventual fertility twenty years later. American Journal of Sociology 62:491–497.

Westoff, C. F., R. G. Potter, Jr., P. C. Sagi, and E. G. Mishler (1961) Family Growth in Metropolitan America. Princeton, N.J.: Princeton University Press.

Westoff, C. F., R. G. Potter, Jr., and P. C. Sagi (1963) The Third Child. Princeton, N.J.: Princeton University Press.

Whelpton, P. K., G. A. Campbell, and J. E. Patterson (1966) Fertility and Family Planning in the United States. Princeton, N.J.: Princeton University Press.

Williamson, N. E. (1976) Sons or Daughters: A Cross-Cultural Survey of Parental Preferences. Beverly Hills, Calif.: Sage Publications.

Willis, R. J. (1973) A new approach to the economic theory of fertility behavior. Journal of Political Economy 81:S14–S64.

Zimmer, B. G. (1979) Urban Family Building Patterns: The Social Mobility-Fertility Hypothesis Re-Examined. Bethesda, Md.: National Institute of Child Health and Human Development.

Part III
# NUPTIALITY AND FERTILITY

Chapter 13

# The Impact of Age at Marriage and Proportions Marrying on Fertility

PETER C. SMITH

## INTRODUCTION

The importance of marriage and family institutions to both individuals and social groups is unmistakable. For individuals, marriage marks maturity and permits a range of adult behavior, including childbearing; it is a crucial rite of passage. At the societal level, marriage creates new family nuclei and realigns households as units of consumption, savings, labor use, and production. Marriage both creates and satisfies intergenerational responsibilities and alliances.

Marriage systems--the sets of social arrangements surrounding and defining sexual unions--can be studied from many perspectives. This paper focuses on research concerned with two demographic features of marriage that are directly relevant to the study of fertility: variations and trends in the timing of first marriage within individual lives, and differences in the chances that individuals will ever enter marriage. Viewed as characteristics describing whole societies, these can be expressed as the average age at marriage and the proportions every marrying, or the timing and prevalence of marriage. Throughout this paper, the phrase "marriage pattern" refers to these two features of any marriage system.

This review is limited to first marriages; marital dissolution and remarriage patterns are considered by Burch in the next chapter. The phrase "marital structure" as used here thus refers to percentages ever or never married by age. The discussion concentrates on female marriage patterns, though male patterns are not entirely ignored, and has little to say about nonmarital fertility except where it has a direct bearing on the first marriage pattern. At both the individual and societal

DETERMINANTS OF FERTILITY
IN DEVELOPING COUNTRIES
Volume 2

473

levels of analysis, researchers from numerous disciplines have worked to disentangle the various sociocultural and economic influences on marriage patterns. This review addresses a wide range of possible social and economic determinants of marriage timing and prevalence; in so doing, it draws on literature whose focus ranges from pretransition to modern settings and spans a variety of cultures. This literature is voluminous, and is based on a broad spectrum of evidence: historical materials, largely from Europe since about 1700, encompassing aggregate statistics and various other kinds of documents; contemporary national data, including both census materials for subareas and survey data for individuals or couples; and various specialized studies, including sample surveys and geographically focused field investigations. The present review must therefore be selective, particularly for topics that have been examined in numerous settings with similar results.

The discussion is organized around a series of propositions expressing relationships between marriage patterns and various determinants, and between marriage and fertility. To avoid excessive interruption, these propositions are presented within the discussion, but are identified by numbers given in brackets, from [1] to [69]. Assertions that are only weakly supported by research are sometimes mentioned, but are not numbered. These propositions do not form an exhaustive list, nor are they axiomatically or hierarchically organized. Instead, they vary in specificity and geographic scope, and are often used only to illustrate larger groups of propositions. The discussion here draws on an extensive listing of propositions on family patterns provided by Goode et al. (1971); other listings have also been consulted, including those of Bartz and Nye (1970) and Otto (1979).

This paper is organized as follows. The first section discusses areal variations in the levels of marriage timing and prevalence, and the next considers national trends. The third section examines the fertility implications of these national levels and trends. The fourth section summarizes what is known about the demographic and socioeconomic determinants of levels and changes in marriage timing. Though much of this material bears on the prevalence of marriage as well, findings related to prevalence are considered separately in the next section. The final section presents concluding observations.

AREAL VARIATION

There are systematic variations in marriage patterns
across the world's regions, and areas of pronounced
homogeneity within those regions.  A variety of patterns
has been documented on the basis of various sources:
worldwide data (Bogue, 1969; Bourgeois-Pichat, 1965;
Dixon, 1971; Henry and Piotrow, 1979; International
Center for Research on Women [ICRW], 1979a; United
Nations, 1973, 1976b, 1980:104-107; Whiting et al., 1982);
data for specific regions such as Asia (Agarwala, 1969;
Blayo, 1978; D'Souza, 1979; P. Smith, 1980), the West
Indies (Roberts, 1979), Africa (van de Walle, 1968), Latin
America (Arretx, 1969; Henriques, 1979), the Pacific
(McArthur, 1961), and Europe (Hajnal, 1965; Watkins,
1981); or data from a particular source, such as the
World Fertility Survey (Durch, 1980; Caldwell et al.,
1980; D. Smith, 1980).  With the percentage ever married
among women aged 15-19 serving as an indicator of marriage timing, Henry and Piotrow (1979:M106) presented
data for world regions ranging from a negligible two
percent in late-marrying East Asia to 58 percent on the
early-marrying Indian subcontinent.  The ICRW compilation
(1979a:Table 3) includes countries with mean ages at
marriage ranging from below 16 to well above 22.

A few authors have advanced beyond simple description
to regional classification of populations along an
early/late dimension.  For example, examining the percentages currently married for 51 populations between
1926 and 1961, Bourgeois-Pichat (1965) identified five
levels of age at marriage, ranging from early in sub-
Saharan Africa, through intermediate in North Africa,
Asia, and Latin America, to late in Europe.  Following
Hajnal (1965), Dixon (1971) looked at percentages never
married for 57 countries around 1960 and distinguished
"European" and "traditional" populations:  the former,
located northwest of his infamous imaginary line from
Trieste to Leningrad, have ages at marriage several years
older than those of populations southeast of the line.
ICRW (1979a) examined 43 countries around 1970, also
distinguishing geographic regions, whereas analysis by
the United Nations (1980:104-107) distinguished Europe,
Latin America, and North America as a group from Africa
and Asia.  Focusing on the Western European countries,
Lesthaeghe (1977) distinguished three nuptiality regions:
France; Belgium, the Netherlands, and Germany; and the
remainder of Western Europe.  Sklar (1974) described two

patterns within Eastern Europe. In another regional
study, P. Smith (1980) distinguished three zones within
Asia, finding variations of more than seven years for
females and five years for males. Similar analyses have
been carried out with data on geographic areas within
individual countries. For example, Chojnacka (1976)
distinguished northern, central, and southern regions of
European Russia in 1897 (also see Coale et al., 1979a);
Knodel (1974) found three nuptiality zones in Germany;
Livi-Bacci (1971) found distinct northern and southern
zones in Portugal; and P. Smith (1980) found geographic
patterns within each of ten Asian countries examined.

These contributions are useful because they organize
an array of data that demonstrates the considerable
variation that exists in marriage patterns. However, few
studies test for homogeneity statistically, and without
statistical controls it is often unclear whether cultural
or developmental factors underlie the variations observed.
Some authors stress sociocultural determinants of nuptiality differences (ICRW, 1979a, and Dixon, 1971, both stress
family systems, for example), and others the level or
pattern of economic development. The most prominent
global difference--that between traditional late marriage
in northwestern Europe and marriage several years earlier
in most other populations--can clearly be traced to both.
This issue is never resolved, and leads to a first proposition: that geographic regions tend to have internally
homogeneous marriage patterns, and that this reflects
both common cultural features and common developmental
levels [1]. It should be noted that the stock of cross-
national data on marital status has expanded rapidly in
recent years; it now provides sufficient coverage and
comparability to support the multivariate analysis that
is needed to disentangle sources of global variation in
marriage patterns.

Most of the literature on areal variations in nuptiality is concerned with marriage timing and only by inference with marriage prevalence or the relationship between
the two. It is generally assumed that early marriage is
associated with a high proportion eventually marrying.
The implicit assumption here--that marriage timing and
prevalence have common determinants--is taken up later in
this discussion.

A set of observations on the relationship between
female and male marriage patterns can also be noted [2].
That age at marriage for males exceeds that for females
is virtually always true on average, but is not the case

for at least a minority of couples within any population. Variation in the mean age gap between spouses has been shown to be an important aspect of family systems (Cox, 1970; Laslett, 1977; Drake, 1969b; Wrigley, n.d.). It may also be stated that the timing of marriage for females and males is positively associated across populations, as is the prevalence of marriage for each sex; the only exceptions to these patterns are found in settings dominated by sex-ratio distortions, a point discussed further below.

## TRENDS

### The Historical European Transitions

There are many studies of historical changes in Europe, some very rich in detail, that address marriage patterns. These include well-known studies of particular countries (e.g., Connell, 1950, on Ireland; Drake, 1969b, on Norway), or even of regions or localities within countries (Chambers, 1957 on the Vale of Trent); they also include analyses with broader coverage, such as the series of country volumes resulting from the Princeton European Fertility Study (Livi-Bacci, 1971, 1977; Knodel, 1974; van de Walle, 1974; Lesthaeghe, 1977; Coale et al., 1979a). The overall comparative findings have been summarized by Coale and Treadway (1979) and the comparative results on marriage by Watkins (1981). The Princeton European Fertility Study reports, based on local-area census data, necessarily emphasize areal patterns. Pretransition European marriage patterns have been interpreted by Hajnal (1965), while further descriptive material has been assembled by Gaskin (1978) and D. Smith (1977) from reconstitution studies. Many studies of nuptiality change in eighteenth- and nineteenth-century Europe have posited that much of the rapid population growth during the Industrial Revolution resulted from a shift to earlier marriage. It has generally been concluded, however, that a decline in age at marriage did indeed contribute, but not significantly--certainly not enough to account for much of the increase in the population growth rate, as discussed further below (Crafts and Ireland, 1976; Drake, 1969a; McKeown et al., 1972; Outhwaite, 1973; Razzell, 1965; Wrigley and Schofield, 1981).

From these historical studies, a series of assertions about areal patterns of nuptiality change can be drawn [3]. Both across and within European countries, a progressive diminution of areal variations is observed as the extremes of early and late marriage disappear. The Watkins (1981) and Coale and Treadway (1979) summaries suggest a two-stage process: first, the industrial areas ceased to be early-marrying outliers as other areas caught up with them; then the late-marrying outliers disappeared as the transition process was completed (also see Coale et al., 1979a). Similar results are reported for twentieth-century Japan (Kobayashi and Tsubouchi, 1979; Mosk, 1980a). In general, though, studies like these indicate very little restructuring of subarea differentials as the changes occurred; areas of relatively early and late marriage maintained these relative positions even as their absolute levels shifted.

## Recent Trends in LDCs

Although less developed countries (LDCs) are quite diverse in their current levels of nuptiality, they are remarkably similar in their recent trend toward later marriage. Both global studies (Durch, 1980; Caldwell et al., 1980; Henry and Piotrow, 1979; ICRW, 1979a) and those that focus on specific regions (e.g., Chamie and Weller, 1982, on the Middle East and North Africa; P. Smith, 1980, for Asia) show upward trends in national percentages single in the younger age groups and in mean ages at marriage for virtually all the countries studied. Numerous countries have experienced marriage delays of two or three years over as many decades among females; in a few countries, such as Korea, the shift to later marriage has been extremely rapid (Coale et al., 1979b). Whenever geographic subareas are considered (e.g., P. Smith, 1980), uniform changes across them are found as well.

The data for LDCs also support the findings summarized earlier concerning the convergence of areal patterns over time. For those LDCs where very early marriage prevails, it may also be observed that, when marriage is initially very early, a rise in the mean age at marriage is just as likely to accompany modernization as is a decline in marital fertility [4] and may well occur first (Coale et al., 1979a:146).

The universality of marriage delays across countries varying widely in sociocultural features and development levels is a remarkable aspect of the observed pattern in LDCs. Another puzzle is the absence of any indication of accompanying declines in marriage prevalence. Both of these issues are considered below.

## MARRIAGE AND FERTILITY

The links between marriage and fertility are at least superficially obvious. Rising mean ages at marriage and rising percentages single are associated with declines in period measures of fertility such as the birth rate; the women who marry latest in any population ultimately have the fewest children on average. However, even at the aggregate level, a closer look reveals contrary evidence, and at the individual level the mechanisms linking marriage timing and fertility are not always obvious.

There are serious problems associated with assessing the impacts of marriage patterns on fertility. Definitions of marriage, in contrast to those related to childbearing, are not entirely clear or consistent across societies, though de facto concepts generally prevail. Moreover, definitions of marriage sometimes subtly involve parenthood; thus, youth may more readily define themselves as married when they are parents. Even apart from these definitional and conceptual problems, the direction of causal influence is frequently elusive. It is often argued, at least implicitly, that marriage timing is guided by fertility intentions [5]. Certainly, normative systems create a "fundamental complementarity" between marriage and childrearing (Schultz, 1981:26ff.), and the cultural pressure toward parenthood, whatever its origins or functions, may influence marriage patterns. It is claimed, for example, that marriage timing will be later and prevalence lower when social penalties for childlessness are low, whereas concern over the number of surviving sons--greatest when mortality is high or natural fertility low--is thought to motivate early marriage (e.g., Mosk, 1981a, on Japan). Of course, these arguments assume an exceptionally distant planning horizon, and direct evidence that this kind of planning actually occurs is scant.

The reasons for an association between marriage timing and fertility were catalogued some time ago by Coale and Tye (1961), Ryder (1960), and others. Later marriage reduces the total duration of fecund exposure to sexual activity, and shifts it to the older ages of lower fecundity [6]. Moreover, when marriage is later, a greater fraction of each cohort will not survive to marry [7]. Delay also reduces the tempo of population change as the mean length of a generation is extended [8]. Finally, there is a temporary "translation" effect on period fertility as any shift in marriage timing occurs [9].

Analytic problems arise in efforts to measure these influences, mainly because of the very strong selectivities that can operate to create spurious associations between marriage timing and fertility. Another complication is the need to sort out deliberate volitional aspects from nonvolitional exposure effects of marriage timing on fertility. These and other issues arise in research findings at both the aggregate and micro levels.

## Aggregate-level Relationships

Several techniques are used to study aggregate marriage-fertility links. One straightforward approach is to examine correlations between marriage timing and fertility across countries or other areal units. These correlations generally indicate an association of late marriage and low birth rates [10]. One rule of thumb states that a threshold level of 80 percent single among women aged 15-19 is associated with a crude birth rate below 35 per thousand (Mauldin and Berelson, 1978). Another common approach involves attributing changes in fertility over time to changes in marriage patterns and marital fertility. This literature is concerned not only with simple decomposition (e.g., Wunsch, 1979), but also with a much broader set of questions concerning the interplay of nuptiality and fertility in an equilibrium or homeostasis model of society, discussed in further detail below. Decomposition into marriage pattern and marital fertility components is also used to examine recent fertility declines in LDCs (Cho and Retherford, 1973; Lee and Chao, 1973), generally for the purpose of assessing the direct effects of family planning programs. "Extraneous" changes in fertility due to delayed marriage have been found to be quite important; for example, Mauldin and Berelson found that among the ten countries with major fertility declines over the 1962-77 period, delayed marriage accounted for about 40 percent of the fertility change. Another approach involves aggregate

simulation or projection. Simulation has been employed
in the debate over eighteenth- and nineteenth-century
England (Crafts and Ireland, 1976; Mendels, 1978); in
projecting the marriage and marital fertility components
of future LDC fertility levels (Lesthaeghe, 1971, 1973);
and in sorting out the various impacts of nuptiality
change on fertility (Trussell et al., 1979).

This research has produced a series of assertions.
The projections of Lesthaeghe and others disaggregating
assumed nuptiality and marital fertility changes indicate
that the effects of the two components are cumulative (an
arithmetic result), and that, when they change at the
same time, the impact of nuptiality changes is felt
sooner [11]. Some research has distinguished components
of nuptiality change. Projecting alternate changes in
the age at which the marriage process begins for a cohort
and the tempo or time required for the process to be
completed, Lesthaeghe (1971, 1973) found that the impact
of changes in marriage tempo is greatest, but also that
upward movement in the age at which the process begins
may be compensated by an accelerating tempo [12].

Various other complex interactions of aggregate
marriage and fertility levels are also noted [13]. Some
relate to compensating changes between age at marriage
and marital fertility (Matras, 1965; McDonald, 1981).
Others suggest institutional changes as nuptiality delay
occurs, for example, changing linkages between formal
union and cohabitation, resulting in a shorter interval
between the two (Wyon and Gordon, 1971).


## Individual-level Relationships

The aggregate-level connection between marriage timing
and fertility levels must ultimately reflect an association at the individual level. At this level, direct
effects are clear. Ceteris paribus, less total exposure
will reduce completed fertility [14]. Lower fecundity
during that exposure will create greater spacing of births
and further reduce completed fertility [15]. For another
fraction of persons, delaying marriage will increase the
probability of never marrying and thus eliminate some
fertility [16]. The factors held constant here include
several proximate determinants, including probabilities
of intercourse, conception, successful gestation, and
live birth.

It is widely held that in natural-fertility popula-
tions--those in which there is no deliberate (parity-
dependent) fertility control behavior--exposure times and
fecundity levels alone determine the association between
marriage timing and fertility [17]. Likewise, it is held
that, when fertility control is widespread in a population, exposure times and fecundity levels are irrelevant;
that is, there need be no direct connection between marriage timing and fertility at all, only spurious correlations resulting from the association of both marriage
timing and fertility with other variables [18]. However,
the growing body of research on these relationships suggests a number of complications and caveats. Research on
natural-fertility populations shows that the later
marriage-lower fertility relationship frequently persists
even after exposure time is controlled (e.g., Caldwell et
al., 1980). Just as unexpectedly, a marriage timing-
fertility association is sometimes found in populations
practicing fertility control (Busfield, 1972; Bumpass and
Mburugu, 1977; Day, 1979).

It is obviously necessary to consider additional connections between marriage timing and fertility in both
kinds of society. Several speculative catalogs of such
connections have been compiled, motivated mainly by the
surprising persistence of fertility differentials with
age at marriage in contracepting societies, but often
relevant to LDCs as well. Busfield (1972) distinguishes
"social causation" and "social selection" models. The
former encompasses "genuine" linkages operating through
one or another of the exposure schedules for rates of
intercourse, conception, or fetal wastage; each of these
has a regular schedule with age, such that late marriage
generally prevents exposure when the probabilities of
outcomes leading to births are highest. The "social
selection" model identifies factors that link marriage
timing and fertility through their associations with
other variables. Bumpass and Mburugu (1977) distinguish
"demographic" components, essentially the same as
Busfield's exposure factors, and "social" components,
which include factors governing the chances of contraceptive failure, selective marriage patterns, and two
sociological elements involving life-cycle and age-norm
considerations. Day (1979) proposes a more exhaustive
list of 20 possible factors.

Although these three schema are useful, they are not
easily synthesized. However, the core exposure variables
appear in each. One of these is the age-curve of inter-

course frequencies. Though there is little supporting
evidence, frequencies probably decline with age as well
as with marriage duration, but may not vary much within
the usual range of marriage ages. Second is the age-curve
of fecundity, which is well documented (Henry, 1961) and
peaks at above the prevailing age at marriage in most
societies. The Coale and Trussell (1974) model of
marriage-pattern impacts on marital fertility incorporates this age-fecundity relationship, and Page (1977)
has shown an equally close relationship between duration
of marriage and marital fertility. These relationships
are widely evident in survey data (e.g., Caldwell et al.,
1980, with WFS data; P. Smith, 1982, on Indonesia and the
Philippines). Third is the age-curve of fetal wastage,
which is U-shaped. Since fecundity is curvilinear with
age, the effect of marriage delay on marital fertility
via these exposure variables is indeterminate and governed by the range involved. A small upward shift from a
very young age at marriage may well increase marital
fertility, while an upward shift toward a very late age
at marriage should reduce marital fertility [19].

Also common to all societies is a series of possible
selectivities involving the core exposure variables that
can create an association between fertility levels and
marriage timing. It is commonly suggested that early
adolescent fecundity (e.g., resulting from early menarche)
leads to early marriage [20]. For many societies, this
link may involve premarital conception (Lowrie, 1965),
which would also produce a short or negative first birth
interval, though fear of conception (by inference from
the experience of others) might be a sufficient motivation
to marry early. Though the opposite claim is also made
(Freedman and Casterline, 1979), it is sometimes speculated that a high coital frequency is associated with
early marriage [21]. Evidence for this is lacking, but
it might occur because premarital coital behavior accelerates entrance into marriage (due either to pregnancy or
fear of pregnancy) and in turn is associated with high
coital frequencies and thus higher fertility within marriage. Also, high coital frequencies might be associated
with other background characteristics, such as social
class, that are associated with early marriage, thus
leading to a link between early marriage and high fertility. Another suggestion, though as yet with little
supporting evidence, is that early marriers have relatively low contraceptive efficiencies. Inefficient
contraceptive use might lead to premarital pregnancy and

thus to early marriage; by persisting during marriage, inefficient use would lead to higher marital fertility and hence an association between early marriage and fertility despite the use of contraception. Further, a set of such associations might be generated by a background connection with a variable like social class.

Another set of possibilities has to do with indirect causal links between delayed marriage and fertility. It is argued that a period of adolescent or adult status before marriage can permit the formation of role definitions antithetical to high fertility within marriage (Call and Otto, 1977; see also Oppong, in these volumes) [22]. More generally, later marriage may be associated with relaxation of the cultural pressure for high fertility (McDonald, 1981). Other life-cycle arguments involve age norms for appropriate parities [23] (Bumpass and Mburugu, 1977). For example, late marriage may lead to the perception that parities in the early years of marriage are too low, and thus to "catching up" behavior through shorter birth intervals. At longer marriage durations (and therefore at older ages), age norms may dictate termination of childbearing at relatively low parities; it has been suggested, for instance, that norms may press for an end to a woman's childbearing once one of her daughters has married or borne a grandchild.

For a variety of reasons, the relationship between marriage timing and fertility can be weak or complex. Because the fecundity age pattern is curvilinear, upward movement from early and intermediate levels of marriage timing can have opposite effects on early childbearing and even on completed fertility. Moreover, the causal connection may be reversed; that is, high pregnancy wastage and even childlessness might be direct physiological consequences of early childbearing due to early marriage.

Marriage timing can affect other social patterns bearing on fertility in ways that obscure the timing-fertility relationship [24]. Thus, early marriage is generally associated with higher divorce rates and with widowhood (Moore and Waite, 1981), especially when the age gap between spouses is greatest among early marriers. Also, in some settings (see Wyon and Gordon, 1971, on India), a rise in marriage timing from a very early age may not indicate a commensurate rise in the age at cohabitation. Similarly, late marriage may be associated with shorter periods of breastfeeding and thus with higher fertility (Coale et al., 1979b; Freedman and

Casterline, 1979). As noted previously, shorter birth
intervals may be found among late marriers trying to
"catch up" with the fertility of others in their age
group. Premarital pregnancy may be most common when
marriage is either very early or very late relative to
the societal norm, though most investigators suggest that
the dominant association is with early marriage. Finally,
childhood coresidence associated with very early marriage
may reduce intercourse frequencies and thus fertility,
though the evidence for this claim is especially weak
(see Wolf, 1974, on Taiwan).

In principle, the associations and selectivities discussed here can account for both the association of
marriage timing and fertility net of exposure times in
LDCs and the association of marriage timing and fertility
despite contraceptive use in MDCs. However, there is
insufficient research on these selectivities for developed countries. The principal problems are a lack of
understanding of how selectivities operate in different
settings and poor measurement of key variables such as
frequencies of intercourse. Few efforts have been made
to adjust for components of exposure time, or to document
specific selectivities that might link marriage timing
and fertility. There is still less empirical attention
to these issues in developing countries, other than descriptions of differentials.

## DETERMINANTS OF MARRIAGE TIMING

Levels and trends in nuptiality have been examined from
every disciplinary and topical perspective, at levels of
aggregation from the individual to the global; studies
range from the purely descriptive to those focused on
explicit testing of theoretical propositions. The review
of the literature in this section proceeds from the
societal to the individual level of marriage patterns,
focusing in particular on marriage timing; findings
related specifically to marriage prevalence will be
discussed in the next section. First, this section
examines the complex of interdependencies known as the
"demographic system," and the influences of demographic
structure, specifically sex ratios. Next, the discussion
turns to the impact on nuptiality patterns of the major
institutional changes associated with socioeconomic
development: changes in family, household, and kinship
institutions; in urbanization; in education; and in labor

markets and occupations, including the influences of wage
levels and accumulated wealth.


## Demographic Determinants

### Nuptiality in the Demographic System

Analysts have found it useful to view populations as
socioeconomic systems that depend on homeostatic or
feedback mechanisms, institutional or biological, to hold
the rate of population growth near zero and thus preserve
living standards (Davis, 1963; Lee, 1977, 1978; Lesthaeghe, 1980; D. Smith, 1977). Nearly all of the research
based on this framework relates to Europe or Japan,
although some pertain to very high mortality settings in
general without regard to specific institutional arrangements, whereas some focus on the "European Demographic
System" in the context of European social arrangements.

In pretransitional settings, where mortality is at a
level very close to the level of fertility and population
growth is difficult to maintain, fluctuations in mortality
can generate alternating periods of population growth and
decline. In these settings, it is argued, early marriage
occurs because it is necessary to maintain long-run population equilibrium [25] (Ohlin, 1961; Lee, 1977; Mosk,
1980a; Wrigley, 1978). Long-run equilibrium and short-
run adjustment arguments can be distinguished (R. Smith,
1981), but their basic ideas are common. Support for
this putative marriage-mortality linkage is provided by
ethnographic evidence on pretransition populations (Nag,
1962); by time-series information for specific localities
(e.g., Herlihy, 1977, on Tuscany); and by cross-sectional
evidence (D. Smith, 1977).

One major objective for empirical research in this area
is to establish plausible connections between needs and
goals at the societal level and the behavior of individuals (McNicoll, 1980; Lesthaeghe, 1980). The negative
association across populations between marriage timing
and mortality levels (all high-mortality, primitive
populations have early marriage) does not establish a
necessary connection between group needs and individual
behavior, since the association could be caused by the
disappearance from observation of any high-mortality
populations where marriage was typically late. The
theoretical literature on this topic is diverse, and much
of it figurative or otherwise unclear (see the comments

in Lesthaeghe, 1980). Two examples illustrate. Davis
(1963) argues strongly that the linkage is fundamentally
at the micro level: that individuals are motivated by a
desire to seize upon perceived opportunities provided by
the surrounding society. However, he does not address
the question of how the sum of individual self-interested
actions meets the aggregate needs of society. Wrigley
(1978) unabashedly calls on something he labels "unconscious rationality" to link individuals and the group; he
stresses "heirship strategies"--behaviors aimed at maximizing outcomes for families and households that somehow
achieve society's aggregate goals.

Most of the arguments made about the link between individuals and the group involve institutional or structural
arrangements, particularly family systems and inheritance
patterns. The general view, discussed further in a later
section, is that mortality decline places strains on
traditional family institutions and thus not only allows
but even motivates later marriage. Much of this discussion focuses on the particular institutional context
provided by northwestern Europe. The model of the European demographic system that emerges (Flinn, 1980; D.
Smith, 1977; Lee, 1977, 1978; Lesthaeghe, 1977) involves
a natural-fertility regime combined with Malthusian
control over population growth--high and fluctuating
mortality associated with fluctuations in economic
conditions, combined with a marriage institution governed
by the principle of economic viability. This "establishment" view of marriage is crucial because it links
the timing of marriage and the availability of resources,
creating a "nuptiality valve" that compensates for high
mortality by tapping a "reproductive reserve" through
declining ages at marriage (Lesthaeghe, 1977).

The long-run European population equilibrium was
thrown into imbalance in the seventeenth and eighteenth
centuries, and quite rapid rates of population growth
(relative to the general European experience) were common
in the nineteenth century. There has been considerable
argument over whether this burst of population growth was
due mainly to the elimination of crisis mortality or to
increases in fertility. There is also dispute over
whether increases in fertility were due to a decline in
the age at marriage or to increases in age-specific
marital fertility. Much of the argument is over how
inheritance systems (a) link marriage timing and economic
conditions; (b) link marriage and mortality; and (c)
determine whether control of marriage or control of

fertility within marriage is the major mechanism employed. These arguments are taken up in greater detail below, but some findings on the last of these issues can be summarized here.

One viewpoint is that control of marriage timing and control of marital fertility are alternatives (Demeny, 1968), especially when one or the other is proscribed by culture (Easterlin, 1978); another view is that increased control over population growth by one mechanism permits a relaxation in use of the other mechanism, provided that fertility is under some cultural control initially. Both of these arguments suggest a negative association between marriage timing and the level of marital fertility [26]. On the other hand, as noted earlier, a positive association between earlier marriage and higher marital fertility is predicted by the supposed connections between both of these factors and high mortality. A combination of cross-sectional and over-time evidence has been brought to bear on this issue, with inconsistent results: a negative association between marital fertility levels and marriage timing is found in industrializing Austria-Hungary (Demeny, 1968) and Italy (Livi-Bacci, 1977), but positive correlations are found for Russia (Chojnacka, 1976) and Belgium (Lesthaeghe, 1977). Recent over-time evidence for developing countries suggests negative associations (e.g., Coale et al., 1979b, on Korea; Kobayashi and Tsubouchi, 1979 and Mosk, 1981a, on Japan).

Many points in this literature remain to be clarified, for example, the distinction between short- and long-run interactions, and the problem of sorting out homeostatic control via nuptiality versus control by means of limits on marital fertility. Most critical, though, is how relevant these analyses and the European model are to contemporary developing countries. In some of the latter populations, substantial rates of population growth have prevailed for some time, and in many cases land has been abundantly available until very recently. Also, in many of these societies, the "establishment" characteristic of the European marriage institution is essentially absent because of the existence of joint family systems or other mechanisms for sharing the costs of marriage. There is as yet virtually no research on homeostatic mechanisms involving marriage in societies outside Europe and Japan.

The Impact of Demographic Structure on Marriage Timing:
Sex Ratios

One of the most obvious of the possible determinants of
marriage timing is the sheer availability of potential
spouses. The effects of sex ratios are sometimes explicit
in theoretical models (e.g., Dixon, 1971) and sometimes
only implicit. In empirical work, sex ratios sometimes
appear as independent variables, but sex composition is
most often entered as a control, an extraneous factor to
be adjusted for before other effects can be interpreted
properly. This section summarizes literature on the
cross-sectional and over-time associations between sex
ratios and marriage timing. Research has uncovered weak
or even unexpected associations in cross-section analyses,
but stronger and more plausible associations between
changes in sex ratios and age at marriage over time.
Some general propositions are given here, along with
propositions that illustrate aspects of the marriage
market structure and the marriage decision process that
might influence outcomes.

   Under stringent stable population assumptions, the
effects of birth and death rates on the sex ratios at
marriageable ages in a population are given by a formal
relationship:

$$\frac{M_x}{F_y} = 1.05 \; \frac{l_x^m \; e^{-rx}}{l_y^f \; e^{-ry}} \; ,$$

where $F_y$ and $M_x$ are numbers of marriageable women and
men at their prevailing ages at marriage y and x (we suppose that everyone of each sex marries at the same age;
so that d = x - y, the age gap between husband and wife
is constant); $l_y$ and $l_x$ are probabilities of survival
to the various ages at marriage; and r is the intrinsic
rate of population change. Under these assumptions, and
given a sex ratio at birth of 1.05, males are in shortest
supply relative to females when d and r are large and
positive.

   A more realistic model would incorporate recent
changes or fluctuations in r and in survivorship, and
there is of course the further problem of defining the
level of aggregation that best approximates true marriage
markets--the arenas within which options are considered
and choices made. This in turn raises some vexing issues
of marriage rules based on proximity, social class, and

the like.  There is also the complication raised by movements from one marriage market to another.

Some general points may be made here about the major kinds of variation in age-sex structure likely to be found that bear on nuptiality.  In historical Europe, population growth rate (r) and the age gap between spouses (d) were both relatively slight.  Because these are often considerable in today's LDCs, the potential for an impact on marriage timing in these countries clearly exists.  As discussed further below, rural-to-urban population transfers were substantial in Europe, involving single youth of both sexes, but females disproportionately (Weber, 1899).  Although single youth also predominate in urban-bound migration streams in contemporary LDCs, the sex composition of the migration varies considerably, along cultural lines for the most part:  rural-to-urban migration is heavily male in South and East Asia, the Muslim world, and Africa, but disproportionately female in Southeast Asia and Latin America (ICRW, 1979b).  Another source of sex-ratio variations in LDCs results from rapid post-World War II improvements in survivorship combined with the sometimes substantial traditional age gap between spouses, creating temporary marriage squeezes among females.  Finally, there are many historical instances of one-time but massive sex ratio distortions due to sex-selective migration--as with the overseas Chinese throughout Southeast Asia (Barclay, 1954; Caldwell, 1963), and, more recently, the temporary migration overseas of large numbers of male workers from countries like Pakistan and the Philippines.

The general proposition from all of this is that the availability of potential spouses (the sex ratio) will be important in marriage trends when the age gap between spouses is great; when fluctuations in fertility and (to a lesser degree) mortality have occurred in the past; and, in the stable case, when the underlying population growth rate is positive and substantial [27].  The basic proposition relating sex ratios and marriage patterns is, of course, that when one sex is in relative oversupply, timing will be later and prevalence lower than otherwise [28].

Research has uncovered many instances of cross-sectional association between sex-ratio differences and variations in marriage timing; as a rule, however, these associations are weak or even in unexpected directions, indicating the simultaneous influence of other factors.  Dixon's (1971) analysis of data for 57 countries around

1960 produced very weak correlations:   0.25 among Western countries; 0.16 among the remaining countries; and 0.11 for all the countries combined.   Moreover, among the Western countries, the directions of correlation are, unexpectedly, the same for males and females.   P. Smith's (1980) analysis of data from 523 Asian states and provinces around 1970 produced generally stronger correlations, although, again, the signs within each country are the same for males and females.   On the other hand, the cross-sectional relationship across the counties of England and Wales in 1861 (Anderson, 1976) is both strong and in the expected direction.

Because male marriage patterns in LDCs have received relatively little attention, there is scant basis for evaluating the expectation, based on sex-ratio considerations, that changes in female and male ages at marriage move in opposite directions.   Though few supporting examples can be cited (e.g., Wrigley, 1966, for Colyton during some time periods), the evidence available from LDCs suggests that male ages at marriage have in fact moved upward along with female ages.

The effects of sex-ratio changes on marriage patterns within a given population have been studied ever since Sundt's (1980) nineteenth-century analysis of Norway (e.g., Akers, 1967).   One focus of interest is on the potential impacts of the combined rapid mortality decline and baby boom immediately following World War II in developing countries.   The suggestion here is that the availability effect of the postwar mortality decline has been to temporarily encourage later female marriage (Fernando, 1975).   Although such postwar marriage-squeeze effects are likely, it is improbable that these account for the near-universal shift in marriage timing around the world, particularly since, as noted above, male ages at marriage are also shifting upward.

Three general observations seem warranted.   First, the availability of prospective spouses is apparently a significant factor in research only when operative marriage markets have been properly identified; that is, the closer researchers come to identifying actual marriage markets by disaggregating the society into large endogamous cultural or class groups, the stronger their correlations will be (McFarland, 1970, 1972).   Second, the availability of potential spouses can be important for marriage trends, even when unimportant in cross-sectional patterns.   Third, the sex-ratio effect is usually overwhelmed by other aspects of social change that influence both sex ratios and marriage timing, often creating spurious correlations.

Two areas need to be explored much more thoroughly if sex-ratio effects are to be more clearly understood: the effects of structures within marriage markets, and the ways in which the marriage decision process can be flexible in the face of marriage-market characteristics. As an example of the first of these issues, for a given sex ratio, more heterogeneous populations may have later marriage because greater sex-ratio variations within the smaller marriage markets in such populations result in less efficient marriage markets overall. Similarly, for a given sex ratio, more dispersed populations may have later marriage because of the high search costs associated with dispersed marriage markets; this may be one of the factors underlying the later marriage found in heterogeneous LDC urban areas, for example.

Studies of mate selection make it clear that decision criteria in marriage markets can be quite flexible in the face of market characteristics, creating a variety of social adjustments along with or even in place of change in marriage timing. As one illustration of these possible social adjustments, when a sex is in oversupply, the range of acceptable ages for spouses may shift (Hirschman and Matras, 1971), though perhaps only temporarily. The work of Henry (1972, 1975) in modeling "marriage circles" and related work by McFarland (1975) are examples of theoretical development along these lines. Another possibility is that marriage squeezes (for example, due to postwar population growth) result in a reduction of the age gap between spouses. Reductions in the age gap seem to be a general feature of modernizing societies (Presser, 1975); this may have important further ramifications, for example, for couple fertility decision making. Finally, flexibility in individual decision making can be matched by variation in decision rules across cultures. Polygyny, for example (Chojnacka, 1980), is found to be associated with early marriage for females and late marriage for males, and to promote universal marriage among women [29].

## Socioeconomic Determinants

### Family Institutional Changes

Implicit in much of this literature is the claim that the traditional spectrum of subsistence-based family systems worldwide is rapidly being homogenized, first by intrusion of the cash nexus into agriculture, followed by industrialization. At best, this theme is a useful way to organize a disparate body of materials; at worst, the claim that homogenization is occurring has served constructively as a foil for those wishing to argue otherwise. The aggregate results reviewed earlier seem to provide some initial support for a convergence view.

Arguments for the convergence of family systems under the force of industrialization were advanced forcefully in functionalist terms two decades ago. Goode (1963) described a narrowing of family functions as economy and state take over various roles and increasingly dominate the decisions of individuals about work, residence, marriage, and the like (see also Aries, 1977; Lasch, 1977). More recently, and with more explicit reference to demographic behavior, Caldwell (1981; in these volumes) has written of changing "modes of production" and their role in eroding the "cultural superstructure," including family systems. For present purposes, the key transformation is from the subsistence household mode of production to production in and for the market; the central features of importance here include the separation of work from family activities and the rise of wage-based relative to family-based labor markets. Other transformations include a trend toward "emotional nucleation"; more intensive dyadic bonding within nuclear units (Aries, 1977; Shorter, 1975; Caldwell, 1976); the related separation of family units from other kin (Goode, 1963; Shorter, 1975); and important changes in intergenerational relations within families as parental control diminishes (Goode, 1963) and the resource transfers across generations begin to favor children (Caldwell, 1976). These changes can clearly affect the timing of the marriage of offspring, since marriage can mark a significant change in resource distribution and in the supply and allocation of household labor. This section examines these potential effects, focusing first on peasant marriage systems and the protoindustrial family, and then on some additional findings about family background and certain intrafamily influences on marriage timing.

The "cultural superstructure" of any agricultural system includes such social arrangements as family types, residence rules, inheritance systems, and, at least indirectly, marriage patterns. Research on this complex topic frequently focuses on particular issues and variables while leaving others in the background. One emphasis has been on the labor strategies of agricultural households as they relate to marriage patterns. The household developmental cycle is said to create cyclical fluctuations in both consumption needs and labor supply. Since the two cycles often are not synchronized with each other or with changes in the availability of key resources such as land or other capital, much of the demography of agricultural households reflects strategies for cyclically redistributing labor in relation to other inputs. Along with permanent and circular migration, servanthood, and adjustments in the intensity of agricultural labor use (e.g., redistributing land instead of labor; see Ankarloo, 1979), marriage is a significant tool for such redistribution. For example, the importance of household labor strategies for the marriage timing of offspring under stem family conditions in Japan is highlighted by T. Smith (1977). A daughter's marriage is described as a "complex and dangerous transition in the life of families"; one daughter-in-law is added when a son is married, but all other offspring depart before the marriage or soon thereafter. It is generally thought that the offspring of large agricultural households marry relatively late [30], though evidence on this point is sparse; moreover, Smith's study, for example, illustrates the case where labor needs in small families with few working members encourage late marriage. It may also be noted that, since marriage involves exchanges and transfers across generations as well as across households, a persistent dilemma of household strategy is a conflict between current consumption and accumulation for transmission to the next generation.

Relationships between farm household resources and household size and composition are expected to be clearest in societies in which individual family farms are operated independently. Thus it is commonly claimed that, where the nuclear or conjugal family type prevails, marriages will occur later than in extended family systems [31] (Sklar, 1974); the well-documented European marriage pattern illustrates this proposition (Hajnal, 1965; Habakkuk, 1955). The argument that the extended family encourages early marriage is commonly, but not easily, made. First, it is necessary to distinguish "patriarchal/extended," "joint," and "stem" family types since they can have quite different impacts on marriage timing (Timur, 1977). The former two types are said to encourage early marriage because in both there is only the weakest of connections between marriage and material independence. In sharp contrast, the stem family incorporates the principle of

impartible inheritance.  The European example generally
takes the form of primogeniture, in which the male heir
delays marriage until his father's death or serious illness, whereas other sons and perhaps even daughters are
placed in wage labor in the community or are expected to
migrate elsewhere.  It is argued that, in a single-heir
system such as this, male marriage is quite late on average; male celibacy is relatively likely among nonheirs,
and is most likely among the sons of farmers with the
least resources.  There is considerable evidence to support these propositions in Europe, but little research
elsewhere.  Apparent counterexamples deserve further
study:  Korea before 1930 was characterized by early
marriage and low celibacy despite its stem family system,
while contemporary Korea is characterized by late marriage
and low celibacy (Coale et al., 1979b); stem family
arrangements in Thailand have also generated low levels
of celibacy (Foster, 1977).

Much of the literature on family systems addresses
issues involving inheritance.  It is generally argued
that resource scarcity is associated with impartible
inheritance systems and thus with both late marriage and
high celibacy; conversely, land abundance is associated
with bilateral kinship and early marriage [32] (see e.g.,
Wolf, 1966:73).  Others have associated bilateral/nuclear
family systems with relatively high status for women and
thus with late marriage (Goldschmidt and Kunkel, 1971).
Two features of inheritance systems are frequently
stressed:  the degree of partibility of land, and the
degree to which independent household formation with its
accompanying economic requirements is an integral aspect
of marriage.

The study of inheritance systems in relation to population behavior has suffered from an early and influential
statement by Davis (1963) asserting its unimportance (see
also Davis and Blake, 1956).  More recently, others have
properly emphasized the remarkable flexibility of inheritance systems, presenting an image not of an irrelevant
institution, but one that is used imaginatively to achieve
family goals.  The classic European example of impartibil-
ity and its impact on marriage patterns is Ireland
(Arensberg and Kimball, 1968; Kennedy, 1973), but much of
the literature discusses less clearcut situations revealing a good deal of subtlety in the application of inheritance rules (Berkner, 1977; Berkner and Mendels, 1978;
Hammel and Wachter, 1977; Hermalin and van de Walle,
1977; Chojnacka, 1976).  Studying Japan, for example,

Mosk (1981a) argues that a link between marriage and inheritance affects males directly; it affects females only indirectly through the competing goals of old age insurance and dowry accumulation, with the former pressing for early marriage of daughters and the latter for later marriage. As noted earlier, inheritance arrangements lie at the base of Hajnal's (1965) classic distinction between European and Eastern European marriage patterns, and at the heart of the "European Demographic System" (Lee, 1977:3).

Another closely related issue involves the direct costs of marriage, that are defined by prevailing social arrangements: it is asserted that age at marriage is late where the direct costs of marriage (both ceremonial and transfer costs) are high [33]. This relationship can involve institutionalized payments of any kind, such as bridewealth and dowry. The marriage delay associated with high costs is generally attributed to the time needed to accumulate resources (e.g., Mosk, 1981a, on Japan); it is also argued, however, in apparent contradiction, that marriage is earliest among nobilities and other elites for whom direct marriage costs can be very high, and that the highest payments go for the youngest brides.

The impingement of markets on traditional family systems is more fully considered below in relation to specific aspects of urbanization and industrialization. The discussion here briefly summarizes work on marriage patterns under the historical conditions labeled "proto-industrialization" (Braun, 1978; Levine, 1977; Mednick, 1976; Thadani, 1980; Tilly, 1978); this work is limited entirely to Europe in the eighteenth and nineteenth centuries.

The rise of manufacturing activity outside the factory system in many of the agricultural regions of Europe removed traditional land-based constraints on marriage and thus led to both earlier marriage and higher fertility. Wage earning based on labor power alone fulfilled the economic requirements for marriage, even among those for whom an adequate land inheritance was impossible, enabling men and women who would have been forced to delay their marriages to marry relatively early. The argument is sometimes carried further to suggest that very low protoindustrial wage rates necessitated an overall labor-intensive strategy for households. In essence, the traditional family system is said to have generated new marriage and fertility behavior by pursuing traditional goals under new labor market conditions; the

result was early marriage and an expansive labor strategy
involving full-time employment for both husband and wife
(Thadani, 1980). A further argument relates protoindustry
to higher fertility, motivated by the need to create an
ever-larger family labor force. This is seen as a
destabilizing influence: earlier marriage resulted in
population growth, which in turn encouraged the creation
of a rural proletariat and "eroded the European marriage
pattern and its sense of social stability" (Gutman and
Laboutte, 1980). There is some empirical support for
these ideas (Levine, 1977; Anderson, 1976; Mendels, 1968).
In contrast, Gutman and Laboutte (1980) found that in
eastern Belgium, the age at marriage remained high despite
the rise of rural industry. However, this apparent exception is thought only to prove the rule: the rural industry prevalent in eastern Belgium required substantial
at-home training; the result was continued family control
over offspring, and an expectation that young couples
would acquire property before they married.

A few additional relationships between marriage timing
and various facets of family background may be noted.
One claim frequently made is that parental levels of
living are positively associated with the ages at marriage
of offspring [34]. According to this variant on the
relative income hypothesis (Easterlin, 1971), at any
level of parental education or income, the high material
aspirations passed on by parents make marriage seem costly
(see Lee, 1977). However, intergenerational linkages like
these have not been studied sufficiently, and there is
also some contrary evidence (e.g., MacDonald and Rindfuss,
1980).

Another common observation is that unsatisfactory
family situations lead to early marriage [35]. For
example, it is claimed that those whose parents were
unhappy, whose mothers worked when they were adolescents,
and whose families were disrupted by mortality or marriage dissolution marry earlier (Carlson, 1979).

A third set of findings relates to intrafamily differences in marriage timing. For example, in single-heir
inheritance systems, the brothers and sisters of the
inheritor tend to remain single [36]. It has also been
observed that only sons marry early, and that first-borns
marry earlier than their siblings [37] (Prothero and
Diab, 1968). Such intrafamily differences have not been
examined systematically across cultures; moreover, competing claims are made, such as that sibling position
affects age at marriage for females, but not for males

(Altus, 1970; but see Walsh, 1973, for a clear relationship among Irish males).

One variable discussed in much of the literature on
family systems and marriage patterns is the degree of
parental control over marriage decisions. The general
view is that strong parental control over marriage nego-
tiations leads to early marriage [38]. Parental preferences are said to dominate when their resources are great
or when much is at stake in the marriage for other family
or kin group members, conditions that of course tend to
occur together. Some results, if confirmed, would serve
to specify this relationship. For example, Lesthaeghe
(1977) suggests that parental control mainly increases
the tempo of marriage (reduces variation in marriage
timing). Another claim is that family control focusing
on unmarried females leads to later marriage for men as
they seek to better their positions in the marriage market; this implies a wider age gap between spouses when
parental control is great. On balance, the evidence for
propositions about parental control is mixed. Clear
support comes from settings like the People's Republic of
China, where parental controls have been weakened and
marriage is now much later than in the past, although
there as elsewhere numerous other changes are occurring
that might also influence marriage timing. Then there
are settings like northwestern Europe, where a shift to
earlier marriage accompanied reduced parental control.

Another important element of change in family systems
has been the degree of parental control over sexual
access. Relaxation of that control seems to be a universal feature of modernization. The general assertion
in this area is that, comparing societies, late marriage
and premarital sexual relations tend to occur together
[39]. Some of these claims distinguish the sexes: it is
said that male marriage is late where social arrangements
permit common law liaisons or prostitution, and that a
decline in the double standard will increase the female
age at marriage, reduce the age range of marriages, and,
especially, reduce teenage marriage among women.

Finally, it is important to note a biological factor
in marriage behavior that is closely associated with
family background--the age at menarche. Because of its
dependence on nutritional levels, the age at onset of
menarche declines with economic development. Since the
age at marriage among LDCs is rising with development,
the cross-national correlation between ages at menarche
and marriage is probably negative. However, at the

individual level within societies, a positive association
is often observed and a causal connection suggested,
though the specific linkages are disputed (Buck and
Stavrasky, 1967; Chowdhury et al., 1977; Kiernan, 1977;
Udry and Cliquet, 1982). The appropriate proposition
based on this literature seems to be that early menarche
hastens marriage, but only (or at least particularly) in
traditional settings, where marriage is relatively early
and female virginity at marriage is a concern [40].


Urbanization and Urban Residence

Most descriptive studies of marriage patterns include a
classification by place of residence and often one by
birthplace; occasionally, information is presented on
urban areas by size or type as well. Research on LDCs
almost always covers only recent periods of time, but
studies of Europe and Japan often include time series
depicting rural-urban differences over the course of
demographic transition. Most notable in these studies is
the contrast between LDCs today and Europe in its period
of rapid development: urban marriage came earlier than
rural marriage in most nineteenth-century European populations; in today's LDCs, urban residence is all but
universally associated with marriage delay [41]. Contemporary urban-rural differences across world regions
are also interesting (United Nations, 1973, 1976b,
1980:104-107). Urban percentages single exceed rural
percentages single for each of the sexes by a substantial
margin in Asia and Africa, but this is true only for
females in Europe, Northern America, and Latin America.
Also, the age gap between spouses is smaller in urban
than in rural sectors.
    It has been suggested that urban-rural differences in
marriage timing are only derivative patterns; that is,
they are explained not by urban versus rural residence as
such, but by differences in the composition of urban and
rural populations. Efforts to account for urban-rural
differences by controlling for population characteristics
such as levels of schooling generally do reduce observed
urban-rural differences, but rarely eliminate them
entirely (although see Rindfuss et al., 1981). There are
many features of urban versus rural life that may account
for observed urban-rural differences; however, most cannot
be explored with existing census or survey data. Urban
institutional arrangements need to be studied, including,

notably, the workings of the urban family in different cultural settings. For example, it is argued that one important element in later female marriage in urban Hong Kong is a loss of familial control over the marriage choices of daughters (Mitchell, 1971). Another important institution is the urban marriage market. It seems likely that marriage will be delayed wherever institutional arrangements for meeting and evaluating potential spouses are weak or inefficient (Hirsch, 1978; Keeley, 1977, 1979; Wessels, 1976); this may be especially important for recent migrants from rural areas (e.g., Salaff, 1976, on Hong Kong). Other institutions in need of study are urban labor markets and educational institutions, both of which are considered below.

The pattern of empirical findings on this topic strongly suggests the need for a more systemic view of urban-rural differentials and their relationship to marriage patterns. For example, the claim that women in industrial societies have a higher mean age at marriage and a higher proportion never marrying is not supported. Instead, whether industrialization leads to a rise or a fall in the age at marriage may depend upon the traditional agrarian system, a possibility supported by the differing marriage patterns of Europe and the LDCs. As noted earlier, delayed marriage is an important part of the European Demographic System, holding down rural population growth; in contrast, rural systems in most LDCs do not achieve significant control over either marital timing or population growth.

One feature of agrarian systems that relates directly to urban-rural marriage (as well as other) differentials is the pattern of migration (Chambers, 1972:44-50). An important element here is local and longer-distance marriage migration, and the nature of rural marriage markets generally. There are important variations in marriage migration that need to be studied (see Hugo, 1978:146ff., on Java, for example); the contrast between village-exogamous northern India and village-endogamous southern India illustrates the possibilities (Libbee and Sopher, 1975). Also of importance are rural-to-urban migration streams that need to be examined from both rural and urban standpoints. It is apparent that the age and sex structures of contemporary (ICRW, 1979b; United Nations, 1980) and historical (Weber, 1899) urban and rural populations largely reflect age and sex selectivities in rural-to-urban population transfers: in all countries, it is disproportionately youth who move to the cities.

Since youth are disproportionately single, this in turn
affects rural and urban marital status distributions
(Moch, 1981).  There is also a close association globally
between rural-urban marital status differences and resulting differences in rural and urban age-sex structures
(United Nations, 1973, 197___ ___pecially for males
(United Nations, 1980).  A_                      ____s among
urban females in Africa an  _no clear link._     _ sex
ratios do not result in lc                       _ted
Nations, 1980:105).

One illustration of th                           gra-
tion on marriage patterns                         e,
including conscription.                           _lves
young single males almos_                         ary
bases are quite often in                          ,
large militaries reduce rurai ___ _              _trol
over personnel is rigid, military service may eriectively
lower urban sex ratios as well, at least temporarily.  On
the other hand, urban exposure through the military can
lead former soldiers to take up urban residence.  The
role of "military migration" has been considered only
occasionally in the European literature (Knodel and
Maynes, 1976; Weber, 1899) and needs careful study in
today's LDCs, where military establishments are often of
large but unknown size and may be having dramatic but
unmeasured effects on marriage patterns.


Education

The rise of mass literacy and the spread of basic education are central features of the development process in
LDCs today, just as they were important in Europe.  In
LDCs, the educational revolution is notable for its rapid
pace, for its starting point near total illiteracy in many
societies, and for its inclusion of women, which has
resulted in the rapid decline of educational sex differentials in many societies.  It has also had a distinctly
secular and even a western flavor, not only resulting
from colonial rule, but also reflecting the global
Westernization that is so much a part of twentieth-
century economic change.

Research on the impacts of education on marriage and
fertility emphasizes education's complex character as an
independent variable (Caldwell, 1980; Cochrane, 1979, in
these volumes; Holsinger and Kasarda, 1976; Jain, 1981;
Kasarda, 1979).  Underlying much of this research is the

assumption that marriage follows school leaving in the
life cycle, with the timing of the latter influencing the
timing of the former. Although this assumption is probably appropriate for most LDCs, it has not been examined
carefully; in fact, research on the United States shows
that this chronology is often reversed (Davis and Bumpass,
1976; Modell et al., 1976) and that the causality is
unclear (Alexander and Reilly, 1981).

Much of the research on education and marriage has
been done within a causal life-cycle modeling framework
in which age at marriage is one of several status attainment variables (Bayer, 1969b; Elder and Rockwell, 1976;
Modell et al., 1978). These studies indicate that the
educational attainments of both parents are important
determinants of the status attainments of their offspring, and that an individual's schooling influences his
or her marriage timing both directly and by transmitting
parental and other background influences [42] (Bayer,
1969a, 1969b; Carlson, 1978, 1979; Marini, 1978; Voss,
1977; Call and Otto, 1977). The most direct effect of
education occurs mainly at the highest attainment levels,
where it acts as a competing use of time [43]. College
attendance has been associated with late marriage in the
United States for this reason (Hogan, 1978a), and college-
going elites in LDCs marry late as well. The average
difference in age at marriage between those with no
schooling and those with a college education is sometimes
six years or more.

Another kind of explanation emphasizes the labor market
value of the years spent in school, which of course rises
with educational attainment. This labor market impact on
marriage timing is predicted to be positive for women, but
negative for men [44] (Becker, 1975; Cochrane, 1979).
Among females, more education is seen to raise the opportunity cost of marrying and remaining outside the labor
force; it also reduces the pool of eligible males with
similar or higher educational attainments. Since males
are expected to utilize their labor power fully whether
single or married, more schooling increases their earning
capacity without creating any opportunity cost of marrying; the income effect of education is expected to predominate and push age at marriage downward, other things
being equal. However, these assumptions about the effects
of education on marriage timing need to be examined more
closely.

Comparative analysis of World Fertility Survey data
from the 1970s in a number of countries, as well as

numerous studies of individual countries, does show positive relationships between schooling and marriage timing
among females. However, in these cross-sectional surveys, the most highly educated women are disproportionately in the younger cohorts and have characteristics
other than education which might also influence marriage
timing. Still, multivariate analysis has shown common
positive net effects of schooling on marriage timing for
females (e.g., Rindfuss et al., 1981). Nevertheless, even
where the overall association is clearly positive, a further look suggests more complex patterns. In many societies, those in the lowest educational category (especially those with no schooling at all) marry somewhat later
than do those in the next higher educational group (Cochrane, 1979:83ff; Preston and Richards, 1975). Cochrane
observes that the effect of a small amount of schooling
versus no schooling at all is small, but that a similar
increment higher on the educational ladder has greater
effects on marriage timing. She also notes that urban-
rural interactions with education in relation to marriage
timing are inconsistent.

The assumption that male age at marriage declines with
educational attainment also requires further examination.
For one thing, it has not been adequately explored in
LDCs, partly because so much analysis for these countries
is based on samples of women. Country-level correlations
introduce further complications. Examining data for the
period around 1960, Dixon (1971) found that, worldwide,
the correlations between percentages single and literate
were positive for both sexes, except in Western Europe.
Dixon attributes this latter result to a connection
between poverty (indexed by years of schooling) and late
marriage in nuclear-family cultures.

Other findings in the literature relate to aspects of
the educational process itself. Marriage is said to be
later among those with higher academic performances [45]
(Call and Otto, 1977). Other things being equal, interruptions in education are said to lead to earlier marriage [46], and it is claimed by Alexander and Reilly
(1981) that, in the U.S., marriage generally terminates
schooling for women, but not for men [47]. For any level
of female schooling, the greater the educational advantage of males, the lower the female age at marriage [48].
Finally, across societies, a high level of education is
said to be associated with a reduction in variations in
age at marriage [49].

## The Labor Market

Historically, transformations in economic activity have been associated with widespread social changes, including transformations in marriage patterns. Since societies differ in their urbanization processes and in the structure of their labor markets, there are corresponding variations in the timing and quantity of marriage among countries at similar development levels. There are also substantial within-country variations in nuptiality across occupational categories, whether these are defined according to home or class background or immediate work setting.

It is necessary to distinguish several kinds of occupational effect. Social and economic background is defined in part by parental occupational status, which may influence marriage timing by determining the quantity of resources available for marriage, defining the cultural milieu in which attitudes about marriage are formed, and providing the social networks in which spouses are sought. An individual's own occupation or occupational prospects define (especially for women) the opportunity costs of marrying. The individual's occupational setting can also be instrumental in defining available resources, fixing attitudes toward marriage, and creating marriage opportunities. It is also necessary to consider indirect effects resulting from associations between occupational status and such personal characteristics as education, as well as such group characteristics as local sex ratios. Finally, occupational changes can create other changes in opportunity structures, which can in turn lead to new nuptiality patterns. Such links between historical occupational transformations and nuptiality change are not readily captured by simple propositions. Certainly, the common idea that, across countries, industrialization is associated with later marriage needs to be qualified. Though this is true for today's LDCs, the occupational transformation of Europe was associated with steady or sometimes declining rather than rising marriage ages.

Researchers have addressed three basic areas in exploring the effects of occupation on nuptiality: links between marriage timing and work force participation; marriage patterns in specific occupational settings; and income, wealth, and other effects of occupation that may relate to individuals, families, or households.

Important empirical differences in female labor force participation rates are evident across as well as within societies (Durand, 1975). Although there is little variation in these rates for single and currently married men in any age group, there are two notable patterns among women:  in some societies, labor force participation rates are relatively high among adolescent and young adult single women but are much lower among married women of the same age; in other societies, labor force participation rates are exceptionally low among single women but may rise substantially after marriage (United Nations, 1962, 1976a).  The issues of relevance here are the structure of social and economic opportunities inside versus outside of marriage, and the tradeoff between utility from personal earnings and husband's earnings (Santos, 1975).

It is difficult to sort out economic need versus equal or desirable work opportunities as determinants of female labor force participation; it is equally difficult to determine how each of these factors might influence marriage timing.  Conceptual and measurement problems with assessing labor force participation help make successful cross-national generalization difficult.  One claim is that easy access to equal or desirable work opportunities leads women to marry later [50].  Although some research supports this claim, in many other settings, high labor force participation rates indicate economic need rather than opportunity and are associated with early marriage (on the Javanese, see Hull and Hull, 1977).  On the other hand, when over-time fluctuations in labor force participation are related to marriage rates within a given population, a positive relationship is found consistently: work opportunities for women delay their marriages [51] (see Preston and Richards, 1975; Freiden, 1972; Tella, 1960; Becker, 1975; Basavarajappa, 1971; Walsh, 1970; but also see White, 1981).

Turning to the effects of occupational setting, European urbanization involved occupational changes that had varying impacts on marriage timing (Outhwaite, 1973; Ogle, 1980).  Some urban centers grew up around mineral resources and their associated heavy industries; these cities attracted primarily male workers, and the resulting high sex ratios resulted in early marriage for women. Other cities featured lighter industrial development. Those dominated by clerical-administrative employment or by domestic service attracted disproportionate numbers of female migrants, who tended to marry late.  Domestic service for females (Tilly and Scott, 1978; Laslett, 1977) and military service for males (Hogan, 1978b) have been shown to have significant impacts on marriage pat-

terns; these occupations involve a substantial fraction
of the youth in LDCs, and their nuptiality effects may
therefore be considerable.

Some generalizations relate to certain socioeconomic
characteristics of occupations rather than to specific
occupational settings. It is argued, for example, that
those in occupations with the lowest schooling and other
requirements marry earliest; it is also argued that
occupations with the highest socioeconomic characteristics contain a high percentage of single females, but a
low percentage of single males [52].

Nearly all of the empirical literature on occupations
and marriage is focused on Europe. There are remarkably
few data for LDCs on the marriage patterns of specific
occupations, and there is relatively little analysis of
the data that do exist. Thus, LDC censuses and surveys
rarely tabulate the marital status distributions of
occupational groups (United Nations, 1962, shows data for
only 11 countries); the sample sizes of surveys allow
only the broadest occupational groups to be tabulated in
this way. Even easily obtained census tabulations of
current labor force participation or current occupation
against current marital status are rare.

Finally, as for the impact of wages and wealth on
marriage timing, a number of propositions derive from a
household production model of marriage and labor force
decisions (Becker, 1975, 1981b; Santos, 1975; Nerlove,
1974; Manser and Brown, 1980). Among these are the claim
that a high wage rate for single relative to married
women is associated with late marriage, and that a low
female wage relative to the male wage is associated with
early marriage [53]. However, other institutions can
intervene. In Bangladesh, for example, it is found that
relative decreases in the female wage have shifted the
burden of marriage payments toward the daughters' parents
and thus have led to later marriage (Lindenbaum, 1981).
Another proposition is that female marriage is delayed as
women's real absolute wage rises, regardless of its
relationship to male wages [54] (Ermisch, 1981). It is
claimed that this association is frequently concealed by
certain other effects of real wage increases, including
reduced financial constraints on household formation,
which would cause earlier marriage. On the other hand,
the increased time costs of searching for a spouse and of
providing a family life style associated with rising real
wages would delay marriage and reinforce the relationship.
A related proposition associates male unemployment and

late marriage for females [55]; an important LDC example
is Sri Lanka (Weekes-Vagliani, 1979).

Income and accumulated wealth are broader concepts
related to standard and style of living as determinants
of marriage behavior.  Here the dominant proposition
posits an association between wealth level or level of
living and early marriage (e.g., Waite and Spitze, 1981),
and includes the ability of wealthier populations to
handle the transaction costs of marriage [56].  This
relationship is thought to be clearest in neolocal
societies where new household formation is a part of
marriage.  However, the comparative evidence is very
mixed, ranging from traditional China and Tokugawa Japan,
where the children of wealthy farmers married earliest
(Gamble, 1954; Goode, 1963:286ff; Hayami, 1980), to an
association between poverty and earlier female marriage
in contemporary Latin America (Yaukey, 1973).

The relationship between wealth and marriage timing is
complicated by a number of factors.  First, it is found
to differ by sex, within families, or between urban and
rural settings.  Another complicating factor is the transfer of wealth from traditional to modern forms, such as
investments in human capital; these different forms of
wealth may have different effects on marriage timing.
Finally, the wealth of an individual woman is thought to
increase her age at marriage, but a more complete statement suggests the reverse relationship for men (e.g.,
Anderson, 1981, on Malaysia).

Other propositions relate more directly to the income
and wealth implications of choice of spouse.  It is argued
that the upwardly mobile marry relatively late and the
downwardly mobile relatively early, and, similarly, that
heterogeneous marriages tend to be later than homogeneous
ones [57].  The propositions in Goode et al. (1971)
include racial/ethnic and religious cases of this kind.
However, marriage delay associated with heterogeneous
unions may reflect the higher search costs in a heterogeneous population, or simply a relaxation of search
goals as time passes.


## DETERMINANTS OF MARRIAGE PREVALENCE

The timing and prevalence of marriage are distinct
features that share many determinants, but frequently
relate to those determinants in different ways.  With
regard to fertility, the prevalence of marriage is

certainly less important than its timing; however, from a broader perspective, prevalence can be a significant indicator of social organization. This section reviews some of the literature on marriage prevalence and its determinants, beginning with some findings and propositions about the aggregate, cross-sectional associations between marriage timing and prevalence, and some observations about the relationship between changes in these two features of the marriage pattern. This is followed by some propositions concerning marriage prevalence at the individual level.

### Aggregate, Cross-sectional Patterns

It is widely held that wherever marriage is late, its prevalence is low [58]. Although the reasoning behind this proposition is rarely elaborated, the assumption seems to be that similar causal influences operate on each. Dixon (1970, 1978) offers four explicit arguments for a close relationship between marriage timing and prevalence. First, where the economic feasibility of marriage is high, both the prevalence and timing of marriage will be affected [59]. As was noted earlier, economic feasibility is thought to be high in extended family systems, and marriage is thus expected to be both early and universal in those systems. Second, where marriage is highly desirable—in part due to the absence of attractive social or economic alternatives, particularly for females—it will not only be earlier for females, but also more prevalent [60]. Third, where the opposite sex has been in short supply for a substantial period of time, the prevalence of marriage will be low [61]. Fourth, wherever marriage decisions are controlled by parents, marriage will be more prevalent [62].

Some additional aggregate-level patterns and differentials in the prevalence of marriage are worth noting. It is frequently observed, for example, that levels of celibacy are at least slightly higher in urban than in rural areas [63] (Livi-Bacci, 1977). It has also been noted that celibacy levels are relatively high in certain occupational categories, including, for example, domestic service and secondary-school teaching. It is an unresolved issue whether such patterns are causal in nature or only reflect the selectivity of individuals into the particular residential or occupational categories. A relatively low prevalence of marriage has been linked to a variety of societal features [64], including corporate village allocation of land, sex equality, and the existence of socially approved adult single roles. As noted earlier, there is also a substantial body of literature on agricultural populations linking inheritance systems and celibacy. The general claim is that the nonheirs in a sibling set are least likely to marry [65]; thus in partible heirship systems, the celibacy level can be quite low, whereas in impartible systems of various kinds, it may be intermediate or even fairly high [66].

Some research has examined the relationship between changes in marriage timing and in marriage prevalence over time. Closely related to the presumed association between marriage timing and prevalence discussed above (as proposition 58) is the proposition that a shift towards later marriage is accompanied by a shift towards a lower prevalence of marriage [67] (e.g., Caldwell et al., 1980). Although this seems intuitively straight-forward, the evidence is mixed. It is supported by the historical shift throughout Europe from late marriage and high celibacy toward a pattern of earlier and more universal marriage. From this European evidence, Hajnal (1965) has drawn the general conclusion that modernization reduces the level of celibacy, although this is of course a historically limited observation. Contrary evidence includes, for example, trends in Japan over roughly the same period of time (Dixon, 1978). As a late-marriage pattern shifted toward an early one and then back again, there was a steady decline in the percent celibate toward the modern very low celibacy level. Ireland is another counterexample: although that country has seen substantial fluctuations in the prevalence of marriage, marriage timing has remained essentially constant (Dixon, 1978). Finally, and of greatest practical significance, the proposition is not supported by recent patterns in LDCs, where a shift to later marriage is very widespread, but rarely associated with a shift towards a lower prevalence of marriage. It is true, however, that the evidence is not yet in for the most recent cohorts (P. Smith et al., 1982).

Research is needed to investigate under what conditions changes in marriage timing and in marriage prevalence are alternative responses (Davis, 1963), and when they are complementary, multiphasic responses. Dixon (1978), for example, has argued that marriage timing and prevalence can be affected in the same or in opposite directions, depending upon the institutional setting.

## Individual-level Studies

At the individual level, research on marriage prevalence
explores what sorts of individuals never marry, distinguishing males from females, positive from negative
influences, and voluntary from involuntary determinants.
One set of propositions deals with the low marriage
chances of those with extreme or noticeable physical
impairments, mental illness, or low intelligence [68].
Psychological correlates of celibacy have also been
suggested (Najmi, 1980), along with various characteristics of the family of orientation (Spreitzer and Riley,
1974). Other propositions relate low marriage chances to
poverty backgrounds [69]. Personal socioeconomic characteristics are thought to relate to celibacy differently
for men and women; thus, for example, women's marriage
chances are said to decline with schooling, whereas men's
chances rise. Other propositions pertain to the institutional settings that more or less mandate fixed levels of
celibacy. This research tries to identify who the
celibates in these settings are likely to be; for example,
in the patriarchal, patrilocal system of Taiwan (Wolf,
1974, 1976), girls without older brothers in their sibling
sets have a significant chance of remaining celibate.

## CONCLUDING OBSERVATIONS

This section highlights some weaknesses in the field of
nuptiality research, traces a few implications for policy
making in developing countries, and suggests some promising new research directions.

Some weaknesses in the field stem from its heavy focus
on the fertility implications of nuptiality patterns.
Because female marriage timing bears upon fertility so
directly, it is often treated as a linchpin in the set of
arrangements surrounding marriage rather than as a product
of those arrangements. There is insufficient attention
paid to other aspects of marriage, including, for example,
male patterns and the connections between male and female
nuptiality.

A second problem, growing in part out of the first, is
the inadequacy of the data base available. The surveys
of knowledge, attitudes, and practices in family planning
(KAP) and other fertility surveys commonly available
generally fail to provide information for males or for
persons of either sex who are not yet married. Complete

data for birth cohorts are needed if determinants of
decisions to marry are to be examined (Weekes-Vagliani,
1979). Moreover, the independent variables available in
most fertility surveys limit the scope of nuptiality
studies: rarely do they describe the time in life when
marriage decisions were being made. Finally, the areal
focus of much of the available census data often leads
researchers to ignore important class differentials in
marriage.

A third problem is the lack of a unifying theoretical
framework. As with other fields, it is difficult to judge
at what point in the evolution of knowledge a conceptual
framework would serve to encourage rather than suppress
significant insight. Although the disparate character of
nuptiality research to date has probably had some benefits, it is now time to introduce some order. Vigorous
pursuit of several models is probably preferable to the
imposition of a single model at this stage. Just as with
fertility theory, the task is to understand both micro-
level patterns--marriage decision making--and relationships between marriage patterns and other societal
changes at the macro level. The elements of a promising
theoretical framework are contained in the household
decision-making perspective of Becker (1975, 1981b) and
others. The time allocation perspective (Birdsall et
al., 1979; Gronau, 1970; Grossbard, 1978; Grossbard-
Shechtman, 1981) encourages consideration of marriage,
labor, and other decisions as jointly determined. Other
contributions that may be especially useful for conceptualizing nuptiality decisions include efforts to address
intergenerational issues (Willis, 1981; Ben-Porath, 1980);
work on risk sharing and social control on the family
level (Lesthaeghe, 1980); the incorporation of intrafamily
exchanges (Ben-Porath, 1980; Becker, 1981a); and the
introduction of passive and segmented decision making
into the framework (Leibenstein, 1981; McNicoll, 1980).
Leibenstein singles out marriage decision making as a
realm in which models of passive decision making may well
be especially appropriate; the Leibenstein and McNicoll
perspectives are notable because they admit social norms
and structures into individual-level models of marriage
decisions.

Research directly related to policy is sparse, but
ranges widely from studies of elite perceptions of
marriage patterns and legislative possibilities (Duza and
Baldwin, 1977; Baldwin, 1977) to models of the impact
upon fertility of induced nuptiality changes. The views

expressed range from pessimistic (De Tray, 1977) to
optimistic (Lesthaeghe, 1971, 1973). However, there is
widespread agreement that policies will not have major
influences "unless institutional structures surrounding
behavior are changed" (Sklar, 1974:247). For example,
Blake (1965) urges weakening parental controls and
encouraging an instrumental view of marriage. Dixon
(1970) proposes the removal of disadvantages associated
with nonmarriage. Lesthaeghe (1973) argues that marriage
legislation can influence only the age at onset of marriage, while only social change can affect the tempo of
nuptiality. Direct legislative change to increase the
legal age at marriage has been the policy alternative
most commonly implemented (Peipmeir and Hellyer, 1977).
However, research assessing the impact of legislative
changes has been limited, and that which has been done
generally suggests that legislative change follows rather
than promotes changes in marriage patterns (see Parish
and Whyte, 1978; Potter, 1981; Croll, 1981; Duza and
Baldwin, 1977; Katz and Katz, 1978; McDonald and Kasto,
1978).

Numerous topics are in need of study in LDCs. Many
are analogous to topics already explored for Western
countries and Japan, and need not be listed here; others
are of special revelance for contemporary LDCs. A few
illustrations will suffice. The implications of stem
family systems for nuptiality are well understood;
however, there is a need to focus on the workings of
joint, bilateral, and other family systems since these
are common in LDCs, while the stem system, with its
characteristic rules of behavior (R. Smith, 1981), is
not. It is likely that the important cross-national
differences in the relationship between family systems
and nuptiality reflect not only differing levels of
development, but also distinct sociocultural features of
European societies bearing on nuptiality. Studies of
marriage in agricultural populations must address the
exceptionally small farm sizes typical in many LDCs, as
well as the rise of landlessness as a historically
unprecedented condition in many LDC settings. In the
European setting, proletarianization "dissolved the nexus
among employment, household position, marriage, procreation, inheritance, and the maintenance of household
continuity" (Tilly, 1978:40); the effects of landlessness
on marriage in LDCs have not yet been examined.
Twentieth-century demographic transitions are occurring
in the context of a highly developed world economic

system; the implications of this for nuptiality have not been examined. Thus, the exceptionally large tertiary sectors in many contemporary LDCs--a distinct feature of twentieth-century development--may exhibit distinct nuptiality patterns. Educational systems in LDCs generally convey global or even Western values and aspirations (Caldwell, 1980; Freedman, 1979), perhaps leading to a distinct role for education in LDC nuptiality patterns. These topics illustrate the range of issues that might be explored.

Researchers in the field of nuptiality face real difficulties. Marriage behavior and living arrangements are growing more diverse in all regions of the world, and our concepts and data for monitoring these changes are becoming less and less satifactory. Moreover, experience shows that, unlike the fertility and mortality transitions, a nuptiality transition can reverse itself. For LDCs, more marriage delay seems likely in the short run, but a long-run projection would be foolhardy. World nuptiality patterns may well present a very complex reality in the future.

## BIBLIOGRAPHY

Abelson, A. (1978)  Inheritance and population control in a Basque Valley before 1900.  Peasant Studies 7:1-10.

Agarwala, S. N. (1969)  Pattern of marriage in some ESCAP countries.  International Population Conference, Vol. 3.  Liege:  International Union for the Scientific Study of Population.

Akers, D. S. (1967)  On measuring the marriage squeeze.  Demography 4:907-924.

Alexander, C. L., and T. W. Reilly (1981)  Estimating the effects of marriage timing on educational attainment: Some procedural issues and substantive clarifications.  American Journal of Sociology 87:143-156.

Altus, W. D. (1970)  Marriage and order of birth.  Pp. 361-362 in Proceedings, 78th Annual Convention of the American Psychological Association.  Washington, D.C.:  American Psychological Association.

Anderson, K. (1981)  Age at Marriage in Malaysia.  Paper presented at the annual meeting of the Population Association of America, Washington, D.C.

Anderson, M. (1976)  Marriage patterns in Victorian Britain:  An analysis based on registration district

514    Peter C. Smith

data for England and Wales 1861. _Journal of Family History_ 1:55–78.

Ankarloo, B. (1979) Agriculture and women's work: Directions of change in the West, 1700–1900. _Journal of Family History_ 4:111–120.

Arensberg, C. M., and S. T. Kimball (1968) _Family and Community in Ireland_, 2nd ed. Cambridge, Mass.: Harvard University Press.

Aries, P. (1977) The family and the city. _Daedalus_ 106:227–235.

Arretx, C. (1969) Nuptiality in Latin America. Pp. 2127–2153 in _International Population Conference_, Vol. 3. Liege: International Union for the Scientific Study of Population.

Baldwin, C. S. (1977) Policies and realities of delayed marriage. _PBS Report_ 1(4).

Barclay, G. W. (1954) _Colonial Development and Population in Taiwan_. Princeton, N.J.: Princeton University Press.

Bartz, K. W., and F. I. Nye (1970) Early marriage: A propositional formulation. _Journal of Marriage and the Family_ 32:258–268.

Basavarajappa, K. G. (1971) The influence of fluctuations in economic conditions on fertility and marriage rates, Australia, 1920–21 to 1937–38 and 1946–47 to 1966–67. _Population Studies_ 25:39–53.

Bayer, A. E. (1969a) Life plans and marriage age: An application of path analysis. _Journal of Marriage and the Family_ 31:551–558.

Bayer, A. E. (1969b) Marriage plans and educational aspirations. _American Journal of Sociology_ 75:239–244.

Becker, G. (1975) A theory of marriage. In T. W. Schultz, ed., _Economics of the Family: Marriage, Children, and Human Capital_. Chicago: University of Chicago Press.

Becker, G. (1981a) Altruism in the family and selfishness in the market place. _Economics_ 48:1–15.

Becker, G. (1981b) _A Treatise on the Family_. Cambridge, Mass: Harvard University Press.

Ben-Porath, Y. (1980) The F-connection: Families, friends, and firms and the organization of exchange. _Population and Development Review_ 6:1–30.

Berkner, L. K. (1977) Peasant household organization and demographic change in lower Saxony (1689–1766). In R. D. Lee et al., eds., _Population Patterns in the Past_. New York: Academic Press.

Berkner, L. K., and F. S. Mendels (1978)  Inheritance systems, family structure, and demographic patterns in western Europe, 1700–1900. In C. Tilly, ed., Historical Studies of Changing Fertility. Princeton, N.J.: Princeton University Press.

Birdsall, N., J. Fei, S. Kuznets, G. Ranis, and T. P. Schultz (1979)  Demography and development in the 1980s. In P. M. Hauser, ed., World Population and Development. Syracuse, N.Y.: Syracuse University Press.

Blake, J. (1965)  Parental control, delayed marriage and population policy. Pp. 132–136 in World Population Conference, Vol. 2. New York: United Nations.

Blayo, Y. (1978)  First marriages of women in Asia. Population 33(4–5).

Bogue, D. (1969)  Families, households, and housing conditions. Pp. 367–391 in Principles of Demography. New York: John Wiley & Sons.

Bourgeois-Pichat, J. (1965)  Les facteurs de la fecondite non dirigee. Population 20:383–424.

Brandes, S. H. (1976)  La solteria, or why people remain single in rural Spain. Journal of Anthropological Research 32:205–233.

Braun, R. (1978)  Proto-industrialization and demographic changes in the Canton of Zurich. Pp. 289–334 in C. Tilly, ed., Historical Studies of Changing Fertility. Princeton, N.J.: Princeton University Press.

Buck, C., and K. Stavrasky (1967)  The relationship between age at menarche and age at marriage among childbearing women. Human Biology 39:93–102.

Bumpass, L. (1969)  Age at marriage as a variable in socio-economic differentials in fertility. Demography 6:45–54.

Bumpass, L., and E. K. Mburugu (1977)  Age at marriage and completed family size. Social Biology 24:31–37.

Busfield, J. (1972)  Age at marriage and family size: Social causation and social selection hypotheses. Journal of Biosocial Science 4:117–134.

Caldwell, J. C. (1963)  Fertility decline and female chances of marriage in Malaya. Population Studies 17:20–32.

Caldwell, J. C. (1976)  Toward a restatement of demographic transition theory. Population and Development Review 2:321–366.

Caldwell, J. C. (1980)  Mass education as a determinant of the timing of fertility decline. Population and Development Review 6:225–255.

Caldwell, J. C. (1981)  The mechanisms of demographic
    change in historical perspective.  Population Studies
    35:5-27.
Caldwell, J. C., P. F. McDonald, and L. C. Ruzicka
    (1980)  Interrelationships Between Nuptiality and
    Fertility:  The Evidence from the World Fertility
    Survey.  Paper prepared for the World Fertility Survey
    Conference, London.
Call, V. R. A., and L. B. Otto (1977)  Age at marriage as
    a mobility contingency:  Estimates for the Nye-Berardo
    Model.  Journal of Marriage and the Family 39:67-79.
Carlson, E. (1978)  Social Influences on the Timing of
    Marriage for American Women.  Unpublished Ph.D.
    dissertation, University of California, Berkeley.
Carlson, E. (1979)  Family background, school and early
    marriage.  Journal of Marriage and the Family
    41:341-353.
Chambers, J. D. (1957)  The Vale of Trent, 1670-1800:  A
    regional study of economic change.  Economic History
    Review, Supplement 3:44-46.
Chambers, J. D. (1972)  Population, Economy and Society
    in Pre-Industrial England.  Oxford, Eng.:  Oxford
    University Press.
Chamie, J., and R. Weller (1982)  Levels, Trends and
    Differentials in Nuptiality in the Middle East and
    North Africa.  Paper presented at the annual meeting
    of the Population Association of America, San Diego,
    Calif.
Cho, L.-J., and R. D. Retherford (1973)  Comparative
    analysis of recent fertility trends in East Asia.  In
    International Population Conference, Vol. 3.  Liege:
    International Union for the Scientific Study of
    Population.
Chojnacka, H. (1976)  Nuptiality patterns in an agrarian
    society.  Population Studies 30:203-226.
Chojnacka, H. (1980)  Polygyny and the rate of population
    growth.  Population Studies 34:91-107.
Chowdhury, A. K. M. A., S. L. Huffman, and G. T. Curlin
    (1977)  Malnutrition, menarche, and marriage in rural
    Bangladesh.  Social Biology 24:316-325.
Coale, A. J., and R. Treadway (1979)  A Summary of
    Changing Fertility in the Provinces of Europe.  Paper
    prepared for the summary conference on European
    Fertility, Princeton, N.J.
Coale, A. J., and T. J. Trussell (1974)  Model fertility
    schedules:  Variations in the age structure of
    childbearing in human populations.  Population Index
    40:185-258.

Coale, A. J., and C. Y. Tye (1961) The significance of age-patterns of fertility in high fertility populations. Milbank Memorial Fund Quarterly 39:631-646.

Coale, A. J., B. Anderson, and E. Harm (1979a) Human Fertility in Russia Since the Nineteenth Century. Princeton, N.J.: Princeton University Press.

Coale, A. J., N. Goldman, and L.-J. Cho (1979b) Nuptiality and fertility in the Republic of Korea. Paper presented at the International Union for the Scientific Study of Population Seminar on Nuptiality and Fertility, Bruges.

Cochrane, S. L. (1979) Fertility and Education: What Do We Really Know? Baltimore, Md.: The Johns Hopkins University Press.

Connell, K. H. (1950) Population of Ireland, 1750-1845. Oxford, Eng.: Clarendon Press.

Cox, P. R. (1970) International variations in the relative ages of brides and grooms. Journal of Biosocial Science 2:111-121.

Crafts, N. F. R. (1978) Average age at first marriage for women in mid-nineteenth century England and Wales: A cross-sectional study. Population Studies 32:21-25.

Crafts, N. F. R., and N. J. Ireland (1976) A simulation of the impact of changes in age at marriage before and during the advent of industrialization in England. Population Studies 30:495-510.

Croll, E. (1981) The Politics of Marriage in Contemporary China. Cambridge, Eng.: Cambridge University Press.

Davis, K. (1963) The theory of change and response in modern demographic history. Population Index 29:345-366.

Davis, K., and J. Blake (1956) Social structure and fertility: An analytic framework. Economic Development and Cultural Change 4:211-235.

Davis, N. J., and L. L. Bumpass (1976) The continuation of education after marriage among women in the United States: 1970. Demography 13:161-174.

Day, L. H. (1979) Fertility and Wife's Age at Marriage: A Causal Framework. Unpublished paper. Australian National University, Canberra.

Demeny, P. (1968) Early fertility decline in Austria-Hungary: A lesson in demographic transition. Daedalus 97:502-522.

De Tray, D. N. (1977)  Age of marriage and fertility:  A policy review. The Pakistan Development Review 16:89-100.

Dixon, R. B. (1970)  The Social and Demographic Determinants of Marital Postponement and Celibacy:  A Comparative Study. Unpublished Ph.D. dissertation. University of California, Berkeley.

Dixon, R. B. (1971)  Explaining cross-cultural variations in age at marriage and proportions never marrying. Population Studies 25:215-234.

Dixon, R. B. (1977) Late Marriage, Non-Marriage, and Population Policy. Paper presented at the annual meeting of the Population Association of America, Atlanta.

Dixon, R. B. (1978)  Late marriage and non-marriage as demographic response:  Are they similar? Population Studies 32:449-466.

Douglas, W. A. (1971)  Rural exodus in two Spanish Basque villages:  A cultural explanation. American Anthropologist 73:1100-1114.

Drake, M. (1969a)  Age at marriage in the pre-industrial west.  Pp. 196-208 in F. Bechhofer, ed., Population Growth and the Brain Drain. Edinburgh:  Edinburgh University Press.

Drake, M. (1969b)  Population and Society in Norway, 1735-1865. Cambridge, Eng.:  Cambridge University Press.

D'Souza, S. (1979)  Nuptiality Patterns and Fertility Implications in South Asia.  Paper prepared for the International Union for the Scientific Study of Population Seminar on Nuptiality and Fertility, Bruges.

Durand, J. (1975)  The Labor Force in Economic Development. Princeton, N.J.:  Princeton University Press.

Durch, J. S. (1980)  Nuptiality Patterns in Developing Countries:  Implications for Fertility. Reports on the World Fertility Survey, No. 1.  Washington, D.C.: Population Reference Bureau.

Duza, B., and C. S. Baldwin (1977)  Nuptiality and Population Policy:  An Investigation in Tunisia, Sri Lanka, and Malaysia. New York:  Population Council.

Easterlin, R. A. (1971)  Population change and farm settlements in the northern United States. Journal of Economic History 36:45-75.

Easterlin, R. A. (1978)  The economics and sociology of fertility:  A synthesis.  In C. Tilly, ed., Historical Studies of Changing Fertility. Princeton, N.J.: Princeton University Press.

Elder, G. H., and R. C. Rockwell (1976)  Marital timing
in women's life patterns.  Journal of Family History
1:34-53.

Ermisch, J. S.  (1981)  Economic opportunities, marriage
squeezes and the propensity to marry:  An economic
analysis of period marriage rates in England and
Wales.  Population Studies 35:347-356.

Fernando, D. F. S.  (1975)  Changing nuptiality patterns
in Sri Lanka1901-1971.  Population Studies 29:179-190.

Flinn, M. W.  (1980)  The European Demographic System,
1500-1820.  Baltimore, Md.:  The Johns Hopkins
University Press.

Foster, B. L.  (1977)  Adaptation to changing economic
conditions in four Thai villages.  Pp. 113-129 in W.
Wood, ed., Cultural-Recognition Perspectives on
Southeast Asia.  Athens, Ohio:  Southeast Asia
Program, Ohio University Center for International
Studies.

Freedman, R.  (1979)  Theories of fertility decline:  A
reappraisal.  Pp. 63-79 in P. M. Hauser, ed., World
Population and Development.  Syracuse, N.Y.:  Syracuse
University Press.

Freedman, R., and J. Casterline (1979)  Nuptiality and
Fertility in Taiwan.  Paper presented at the
International Union for the Scientific Study of
Population Seminar on Nuptiality and Fertility, Bruges.

Freiden, A. N.  (1972)  A Model of Marriage and
Fertility.  Unpublished. Ph.D. dissertation.
University of Chicago.

Friedlander, D.  (1973)  Demographic patterns and
socioeconomic characteristics of the coal-mining
population in England and Wales in the nineteenth
century.  Economic Development and Cultural Change
22:39-51.

Gamble, S. D.  (1954)  Ting Hsien.  New York:  Institute
of Pacific Relations.

Gaskin, K.  (1978)  Age at first marriage in Europe before
1850:  A summary of family reconstitution data.
Journal of Family History 3:23-76.

Goldschmidt, W., and E. J. Kunkel (1971)  The structure
of the peasant family.  American Anthropologist
73:1058-1076.

Goode, W.  (1963)  World Revolution and Family Patterns.
Glencoe, Ill.:  The Free Press.

Goode, W. J., E. Hopkins, and H. M. McClure (1971)
Social Systems and Family Patterns:  A Propositional
Inventory.  Indianapolis, Ind.:  The Bobbs-Merrill
Company, Inc.

Goody, J. (1976)  Production and Reproduction.
Cambridge, Eng.: Cambridge University Press.

Gronau, R. (1970)  An Economic Approach to Marriage:  The
Intrafamily Allocation of Time.  Paper presented at
the Second World Congress of the Econometric Society,
Cambridge, England.

Grossbard, A. (1978)  Towards a marriage between
economics and anthropology and a general theory of
marriage.  American Economic Review 68:33-37.

Grossbard-Shectman, A. (1981)  A Market Theory of
Marriage and Spouse Selection.  Paper presented at the
annual meeting of the Population Association of
America, Washington, D.C.

Gutman, M. P., and R. Laboutte (1980)  Early Industrialization and Population Change:  Rethinking
Protoindustrialization and the Family.  Paper
presented at the annual meeting of the Population
Association of America, Denver, Colo.

Habakkuk, H. J. (1955)  Family structure and economic
change in nineteenth century Europe.  Journal of
Economic History 15:1-12.

Habakkuk, H. J. (1971)  Population Growth and Economic
Development Since 1750.  Leicester, Eng.:  Leicester
University Press.

Haines, M. R. (1977)  Fertility, marriage and occupation
in the Pennsylvania anthracite region, 1850-1880.
Journal of Family History 2:28-55.

Haines, M. R. (1979)  Fertility and Occupation:
Population Patterns in Industrialization.  New York:
Academic Press.

Hajnal, J. (1965)  European marriage patterns in
perspective.  Pp. 101-143 in D. V. Glass and D. E. C.
Eversley, eds., Population in History.  Chicago:
Aldine Publishing Co.

Hammel, E. A., and K. W. Wachter (1977)  Primonuptiality
and ultimonuptiality:  Their effects on stem-family-
household frequencies.  Pp. 113-134 in R. D. Lee, ed.,
Population Patterns in the Past.  New York:  Academic
Press.

Hanley, S. B. (1977)  The influence of economic and
social variables on marriage and fertility in
eighteenth and nineteenth century Japanese villages.
Pp. 165-200 in R. D. Lee et al., eds., Population
Patterns in the Past.  New York:  Academic Press.

Hayami, A. (1980)  Class differences in marriage and
fertility among Tokugawa villagers in Mino Province.
Keio Economic Studies 7:1-16.

Henriques, M. H. F. da T. (1979) Legal and Consensual
    Unions: Their Fertility Implications in Latin
    America. Paper presented at the International Union
    for the Scientific Study of Population Seminar on
    Nuptiality and Fertility, Bruges.
Henry, A., and P. T. Piotrow (1979) Age at marriage and
    fertility. Population Reports Series M, No. 4.
Henry, L. (1961) Some data on natural fertility.
    Eugenics Quarterly 8:81-91.
Henry, L. (1972) Nuptiality. Theoretical Population
    Biology 3:135-152.
Henry, L. (1975) A model for studying fluctuations in
    nuptiality after large fluctuations in the number of
    births. Population 30:759-780.
Herlihy, D. (1977) Deaths, marriages, births, and the
    Tuscan economy (ca. 1300-1550). In R. D. Lee et al.,
    eds., Population Patterns in the Past. New York:
    Academic Press.
Hermalin, A. I., and E. van de Walle (1977) The civil
    code and nuptiality: Empirical investigation of a
    hypothesis. Pp. 71-111 in R. D. Lee et al., eds.,
    Population Patterns in the Past. New York: Academic
    Press.
Hirsch, F. (1978) The commercialization effect: The
    sexual illustration. Pp. 95-101 in F. Hirsch, Social
    Limits to Growth. Cambridge, Mass: Harvard
    University Press.
Hirschman, C., and J. Matras (1971) A new look at the
    marriage market and nuptiality rates, 1915-1958.
    Demography 8:549-560.
Hogan, D. P. (1978a) The effects of demographic factors,
    family background, and early job achievement on age at
    marriage. Demography 15:161-175.
Hogan, D. P. (1978b) The variable order of events in the
    life course. American Sociological Review 43:573-586.
Holsinger, D. B., and J. D. Kasarda (1976) Education and
    human fertility: Sociological perspectives. In R.
    Ridker, ed., Population and Development: The Search
    for Selective Interventions. Baltimore, Md.: The
    Johns Hopkins University Press.
Hugo, G. J. (1978) Population Mobility in West Java.
    Yogyakarta: Gadjah Mada University Press.
Hull, T. H., and V. J. Hull (1977) The relations of
    economic class and fertility: An analysis of some
    Indonesian data. Population Studies 31:43-57.
International Center for Research on Women (ICRW)
    (1979a) Variations in Nuptiality Age: An Inquiry

into its Trends and Determinants. Washington, D.C.:
International Center for Research on Women.

International Center for Research on Women (ICRW)
(1979b) Women in Migration: A Third World Focus.
Washington, D.C.: International Center for Research
on Women.

Iszaevich, A. (1975) Emigrants, spinsters and priests:
The dynamics of demography in Spanish peasant
societies. Journal of Peasant Studies 2:292-312.

Jain, A. K. (1981) The effect of female education on
fertility: A simple explanation. Demography
18:577-595.

Kasarda, J. D. (1979) How female education reduces
fertility: Models and needed research. Midamerican
Review of Sociology 4:1-22.

Katz, J. S., and R. S. Katz (1978) Legislating social
change in a developing country: The new Indonesian
marriage law revisited. American Journal of
Comparative Law 26:309-320.

Keeley, M. C. (1977) The economics of family formation:
An investigation of the age at first marriage.
Economic Inquiry (April):238-250.

Keeley, M. C. (1979) An analysis of the age pattern of
first marriage. International Economic Review
20:527-544.

Kennedy, R. E., Jr. (1973) The Irish: Immigration,
Marriage, and Fertility. Berkeley, Calif.:
University of California Press.

Kiernan, K. E. (1977) Age at puberty in relation to age
at marriage and parenthood: A national longitudinal
study. Annals of Human Biology 4:301-308.

Knodel, J. (1967) Law, marriage and illegitimacy in
nineteenth century Germany. Population Studies
20:279-294.

Knodel, J. (1972) Malthus amiss: Marriage relations in
19th century Germany. Social Science 47:40-45.

Knodel, J. E. (1974) The Decline of Fertility in
Germany, 1871-1939. Princeton, N.J.: Princeton
University Press.

Knodel, J., and M. J. Maynes (1976) Urban and rural
marriage patterns in Imperial Germany. Journal of
Family History 1:129-168.

Kobayashi, K., and Y. Tsubouchi (1979) Fertility
Implications of Nuptiality Trends in Japan. Paper
presented at the International Union for the
Scientific Study of Population Seminar on Nuptiality
and Fertility, Bruges.

Krause, J. T. (1958)  Changes in English fertility and mortality, 1781–1850. Economical History Review 9:52–70.

Lasch, C. (1977)  Haven in a Heartless World. New York: Basic Books.

Laslett, P. (1977)  Characteristics of the Western family considered over time. Journal of Family History 2:89–116.

Lee, C.-F., and J. C. Chao (1973)  A Comparative Investigation of Asian Fertility Transition:  Varying Patterns of Nuptiality and Marital Fertility.  Paper distributed at the International Union for the Scientific Study of Population General Conference, Liege.

Lee, R. D., ed. (1977)  Introduction.  In Population Patterns in the Past. New York:  Academic Press.

Lee, R. D. (1978)  Models of preindustrial population dynamics with application to England.  Pp. 155–207 in C. Tilly, ed., Historical Studies of Changing Fertility. Princeton, N.J.:  Princeton University Press.

Leibenstein, H. (1981)  Economic decision theory and human fertility behavior:  A speculative essay. Population and Development Review 7:381–400.

Lesthaeghe, R. (1971)  Nuptiality and population growth. Population Studies 25:415–432.

Lesthaeghe, R. (1973)  The feasibility of controlling population growth through nuptiality and nuptiality policies.  In International Population Conference, Vol. 3.  Liege:  International Union for the Scientific Study of Population.

Lesthaeghe, R. (1977)  The Decline of Belgian Fertility, 1800–1970.  Princeton, N.J.:  Princeton University Press.

Lesthaeghe, R. (1980)  On the social control of human reproduction.  Population and Development Review 6:527–548.

Levine, D. (1977)  Family Formation in the Age of Nascent Capitalism. New York:  Academic Press.

Libbee, M. J., and D. E. Sopher (1975)  Marriage migration in rural India.  Pp. 347–359 in L. A. Koskinski and R. M. Prothero, eds., People on the Move. London:  Methuen and Co.

Lindenbaum, S. (1981)  Implications for women of changing marriage transactions in Bangladesh. Studies in Family Planning 12:394–401.

Livi-Bacci, M. (1971) A Century of Portuguese Fertility. Princeton, N.J.: Princeton University Press.

Livi-Bacci, M. (1977) A History of Italian Fertility During the Last Two Centuries. Princeton, N.J.: Princeton University Press.

Lowrie, S. H. (1965) Early marriage: Premarital pregnancy and associated factors. Journal of Marriage and the Family 27:48-56.

MacDonald, M. M., and R. R. Rindfuss (1980) Earnings, Relative Income and Family Formation, Part I: Marriage. CDE Working Paper No. 80-7. Center for Demography and Ecology, University of Wisconsin, Madison.

Manser, M., and M. Brown (1980) Marriage and household decision making: A bargaining analysis. International Economic Review 21:31-44.

Marini, M. M. (1978) The transition to adulthood: Sex differences in educational attainment and age at marriage. American Sociological Review 43:483-507.

Matras, J. (1965) The social strategy of family formation: Some variations in time and space. Demography 2:349-362.

Mauldin, P., and B. Berelson (1978) Conditions of fertility decline in developing countries, 1965-75. Studies in Family Planning 9:90-147.

McArthur, N. (1961) Marriage in the Central South Pacific. International Population Conference, Vol. 2. Liege: International Union for the Scientific Study of Population.

McDonald, P. F. (1981) On Measuring the Onset of Fertility Decline When Age at Marriage is Increasing. Unpublished seminar paper. Department of Demography, Australian National University.

McDonald, P. F., and Katso (1978) The new Indonesian marriage law: Some impressions from village level research. The American Journal of Comparative Law 26.

McDonald, P. F., L. T. Ruzicka, and J. C. Caldwell (1980) Interrelations between nuptiality and fertility: The evidence from the World Fertility Survey. Pp. 77-146 in World Fertility Survey Conference, London, Vol 2. London: World Fertility Survey.

McFarland, D. C. (1970) Effects of group size on the availability of marriage. Demography 7:411-415.

McFarland, D. C. (1972) Comparison of alternative marriage models. Pp. 89-106 in T. N. E. Grenville, ed., Population Dynamics. New York: Academic Press.

McFarland, D. C. (1975)  Models of marriage formation and fertility. Social Forces 54:66-83.

McKeown, T., R. G. Brown, and R. G. Record (1972)  An interpretation of the modern rise of population in Europe. Population Studies 26:345-382.

McNicoll, G. (1980)  Institutional Determinants of Fertility Change. Center for Policy Studies Working Papers No. 59. Population Council, New York.

Medick, H. (1976)  The proto-industrial family economy: The structure and function of household and family during the transition from peasant to industrial capitalism. Social History 3:291-315.

Mendels, F. F. (1968)  Industry and marriages before the Industrial Revolution. Pp 81-93 in P. Deprez, ed., Population and Economics. Winnipeg: University of Manitoba Press.

Mendels, F. F. (1978)  Notes on the age of maternity, population growth and family structure in the past. Journal of Family History 3:236-250.

Mertens, W. (1965)  A comparative study of world nuptiality patterns. Unpublished Ph.D. dissertation. University of Chicago.

Mitchell, R. E. (1971)  Changes in fertility rates and family size in response to changes in age at marriage, the trend from arranged marriages, and increasing urbanization. Population Studies 25:481-489.

Moch, L. P. (1981)  Marriage, migration and demographic structure. Journal of Family History 6:70-88.

Modell, J., F. Furstenberg, Jr., and T. Hershberg (1976) Social change and transitions to adulthood in historical perspective. Journal of Family History 1:7-32.

Modell, J., F. Furstenberg, Jr., and D. Strong (1978) The timing of marriage in the transition to adulthood: Continuity and change, 1860-1975. In J. Demos and S. S. Babcock, eds., Turning Points. Supplement to Volume 84, American Journal of Sociology. Chicago, Ill.

Moore, C. A., and L. J. Waite (1981)  Marital dissolution, early motherhood and early marriage. Social Forces 60:20-40.

Mosk, C. (1977)  Demographic transition in Japan. Journal of Economic History 37:655-674.

Mosk, C. (1980a)  The Origins of Fertility Transition in Rural Japan. Working Papers in Economics. Department of Economics, University of California, Berkeley.

Mosk, C. (1980b)  Rural urban fertility difference and the fertility transition. Population Studies 34:77-90.

Mosk, C. (1981a)  The evolution of the pre-modern demographic regime in Japan. Population Studies 35:28-52.

Mosk, C. (1981b)  Fertility and occupation:  Mining districts in prewar Japan. Social Science Study 5:293-315.

Nag, M. (1962)  Factors Affecting Human Fertility in Nonindustrial Societies:  A Cross-Cultural Study. Yale University Publications in Anthropology No. 66. Reprinted by Human Relations Area Files Press.

Najmi, N. A. K. (1980)  Sex Role Perceptions and Singlehood Predisposition:  A Social Psychological Analysis of Contemporary Marriage Plans in the U.S. Montreal:  McGill University.

Nerlove, M. (1974)  Household economy:  Toward a new theory of population and economic growth. Journal of Political Economy 82(Part 2):S200-S211.

Ogle, W. (1980)  On marriage rates and marrige ages, with special reference to the growth of population. Journal of the Royal Statistical Society 53:253-280.

Ohlin, G. (1961)  Mortality, marriage and growth in pre-industrial populations. Population Studies 14:190-197.

Otto, L. B. (1979)  Antecedents and consequences of marital timing.  Chap. 5 in W. R. Burr et al., eds., Contemporary Theories About the Family, Vol 1. Research-Based Theories.  New York:  The Free Press.

Outhwaite, R. D. (1973)  Age at marriage in England from the late seventeenth through the nineteenth century. Transactions of the Royal Historical Society 23:55-73.

Page, H. J. (1977)  Patterns underlying fertility schedules:  A decomposition by both age and marriage duration. Population Studies 31:85-106.

Parish, W. L., and M. K. Whyte (1978)  Village and Family in Contemporary China.  Chicago:  University of Chicago Press.

Peipmeir, K., and E. Hellyer (1977)  Minimum Age at Marriage:  20 Years of Legal Reform.  London: International Planned Parenthood Federation.

Potter, J. M. (1981)  Marriage, Family and Kinship in Rural Guangdong Province, People's Republic of China: Retrospect and Prospect.  Paper presented at the Modern China Seminar, Columbia University.

Presser, H. B. (1975)  Age differences between spouses: Trends, patterns and social implications. American Behavioral Scientist 19:190-205.

Preston, S. H., and A. T. Richards (1975)  The influence of women's work opportunities on marriage rates. Demography 12:209-222.

Prothero, E. T., and L. N. Diab (1968)  Birth order and age at marriage in the Arab Levant. Psychological Reports 23:1236-1238.

Razzell, P. E. (1965)  Population change in eighteenth-century England: A re-interpretation. Economic History Review 18:312-332.

Rindfuss, R. R., C. Hirschman, and A. Parnell (1981)  The Timing of Entry into Motherhood in Asia: A Comparative Perspective. Paper prepared for the International Union for the Scientific Study of Population General Conference, Manila.

Roberts, G. W. (1979)  Family Unions in the West Indies and Some of Their Implications. Paper presented at the International Union for the Scientific Study of Population Seminar on Nuptiality and Fertility, Bruges.

Ryder, N. B. (1960)  Nuptiality as a Variable in the Demographic Transition. Paper presented at the annual meeting of the American Sociological Association, New York.

Salaff, J. W. (1976)  The status of unmarried Hong Kong women and the social factors contributing to their delayed marriage. Population Studies 30:391-412.

Santos, F. P. (1975)  The economics of marital status. Pp. 244-263 in C. B. Lloyd, ed., Sex, Discrimination and the Division of Labor. New York: Columbia University Press.

Schultz, T. P. (1981)  Economics of Population. Reading, Mass.:Addison-Wesley Publishing Company.

Shorter, E. (1975)  The Making of the Modern Family. New York: Basic Books, Inc.

Sklar, J. L. (1974)  The role of marriage behavior in the demographic transition:  The case of Eastern Europe around 1800.  Population Studies 28:231-247.

Smith, D. P. (1980)  Age at first marriage. World Fertility Survey Comparative Studies: Cross National Summaries (London) No. 1:1-18.

Smith, D. S. (1977)  A homeostatic demographic regime: Pattern in west European family reconstitution studies.  Pp 19-51 in R. D. Lee et al., eds., Population Patterns in the Past. New York: Academic Press.

Smitn, P. C. (1980)  Asian marriage patterns in transition. Journal of Family History 5:58-96.

Smith, P. C. (1982) Contrasting marriage patterns and fertility in Southeast Asia: Indonesia and the Philippines. Pp. 363-393 in L. Ruzicka, ed., Nuptiality and Fertility. Liege: Ordina Editions.

Smith, P. C., and M. S. Karim (1980) Urbanization, Education, and Marriage Patterns: Four Cases from Asia. Paper No. 70. Honolulu: East-West Population Institute.

Smith, P. C., M. Shahidullah, and A. Alcantara (1982) Cohort Nuptiality in Asia and the Pacific: An Analysis of the World Fertility Surveys. Paper prepared for the annual meeting of the Population Association of America, San Diego, Calif.

Smith, R. M. (1981) Fertility, economy, and household formation in England over three centuries. Population and Development Review 7:595-622.

Smith, T. C. (1977) Nakahara: Family Farming and Population in a Japanese Village: 1717-1830. Stanford, Calif.: Stanford University Press.

Spreitzer, E., and L. F. Riley (1974) Factors associated with singlehood. Journal of Marriage and the Family 36:533-542.

Sundt, E. (1980) On Marriage in Norway. Cambridge, Eng.: Cambridge Unversity Press.

Tella, A. (1960) The economic cycle in marriges. National Industrial Conference Board Business Record 17:20-22.

Thadani, V. N. (1980) Property and Progeny: An Exploration of Intergenerational Relations. Center for Policy Studies Working Paper No. 62. Population Council, New York.

Tilly, C. (1978) The historical study of vital processes. In C. Tilly, ed., Historical Studies of Changing Fertility. Princeton, N.J.: Princeton University Press.

Tilly, L. A., and J. W. Scott (1978) Women, Work, and Family. New York: Holt, Rhinehart and Winston.

Timur, S. (1977) Demographic correlates of woman's education: Fertility, age at marriage and the family. Pp. 463-495 in International Population Conference, Mexico 1977, Vol. 3. Liege: International Union for the Scientific Study of Population.

Trussell, T. J., J. Menken, and A. J. Coale (1979) A General Model for Analyzing the Effects of Nuptiality on Fertility. Background paper for the International Union for the Scientific Study of Population Seminar on Nuptiality and Fertility, Bruges.

Udry, J. R., and R. L. Cliquet (1982)  A cross-cultural examination of the relationship between ages at menarche, marriage and first birth. Demography 19:53-63.

United Nations (1962)  Demographic Aspects of Manpower. Report 1, Sex and Age Patterns of Participation in Economic Activities. New York: United Nations.

United Nations (1973)  Urban-Rural Differences in the Marital Status Composition of the Population. ESA/P/WP.51. New York: United Nations.

United Nations (1976a)  Population Aspects of Manpower and Employment: A Regional Overview. Asian Population Studies Series No. 35. Bangkok: Economic and Social Commission for Asia and the Pacific.

United Nations (1976b)  Updated Study of Urban-Rural Differences in the Marital Status Composition of the Population. Population Division Working Paper No. 59. New York: United Nations.

United Nations (1980)  Patterns of Urban and Rural Population Growth. New York: United Nations.

van de Walle, E. (1968)  Marriage in African censuses and inquiries.  In W. Brass et al., eds., The Demography of Tropical Africa. Princeton, N.J.: Princeton University Press.

van de Walle, E. (1974)  Female Population of France in the Nineteenth Century: A Reconstruction of 83 Departments. Princeton, N.J.: Princeton University Press.

Voss, P. (1977)  Social Determinants of Age at First Marriage in the United States.  Paper presented at the annual meeting of the Population Association of America, St. Louis, Mo.

Waite, L. J., and G. D. Spitze (1981)  Young women's transition to marriage. Demography 18:681-694.

Walsh, B. M. (1970)  A study of Irish country marriage rates 1961-66. Population Studies 24:205-216.

Walsh, B. M. (1973)  Marital status and birth order in a sample of Dublin males. Journal of Biosocial Science 5:187-193.

Watkins, S. C. (1981)  Regional patterns of nuptiality in Europe, 1870-1960. Population Studies 35:199-215.

Weber, A. F. (1899)  The Growth of Cities in the Nineteenth Century: A Study in Statistics. New York: The Macmillan Company.

Weekes-Vagliani, W. (1979)  Women in Development: At the Right Time for the Right Reasons. Paris: Organisation for Economic Cooperation and Development.

Wessels, W. J. (1976)  The Theory of Search in
    Heterogenous Markets:  The Case of Marital Search.
    Unpublished Ph.D. dissertation.  University of Chicago.
White, L. K. (1981)  A note on racial differences in the
    effect of female economic opportunity on marriage
    rates.  Demography 18:349-354.
Whiting, J. W. M., V. Burbank, and M. Ratner (1982)  The
    Duration of Maidenhood Across Cultures.  Paper
    presented at the Social Science Research Council
    Conference on School-Age Pregnancies and Parenthood,
    Elkridge, Md.
Willis, R. J. (1981)  The Direction of Intergenerational
    Transfers and Demographic Transition:  The Caldwell
    Hypothesis Reexamined.  Paper prepared for the
    International Union for the Scientific Study of
    Population Seminar on Individual and Families and
    Income Distribution, Honolulu.
Wolf, A. P. (1974)  Marriage and adoption in Northern
    Thailand.  Pp. 128-160 in R. J. Smith, ed., Social
    Organization and the Applications of Anthropology.
    Ithaca, N.Y.:  Cornell Unversity Press.
Wolf, A. P. (1976)  Childhood association, sexual
    attraction, and fertility in Taiwan.  In E. W. P.
    Zubrow, ed., Demographic Anthropology.  Albuquerque,
    N.M.
Wolf, E. R. (1966)  Peasants.  Englewood Cliffs, N.J.:
    Prentice-Hall, Inc.
Wrigley, E. A. (n.d.)  Age at Marriage in Early Modern
    England.  Unpublished paper.
Wrigley, E. A. (1961)  Industrial Growth and Population
    Change: A Regional Study of the Coalfield Areas of
    North-West Europe in the Later Nineteenth Century.
    Cambridge, Eng.:  Cambridge University Press.
Wrigley, E. A. (1966)  Family limitation in pre-industrial
    England.  Economic History Review 18:82-109.
Wrigley, E. A. (1978)  Fertility strategy for the
    individual and the group.  In C. Tilly, ed.,
    Historical Studies of Changing Fertility.  Princeton,
    N.J.:  Princeton University Press.
Wrigley, E. A., and R. S. Schofield (1981)  The
    Population History of England 1541-1871:  A
    Reconstruction.  Cambridge, Mass.:  Harvard University
    Press.
Wunsch, G. (1979)  Effects of Changes in Nuptiality on
    Natality in Western Europe.  Paper presented at the
    International Union for the Scientific Study of
    Population Seminar on Nuptiality and Fertility, Bruges.

Wyon, J. B., and J. E. Gordon (1971)  The Khanna Study:
    Population Problems in the Rural Punjab.  Cambridge,
    Mass.:  Harvard University Press.
Yaukey, D. (1973)  Marriage Reduction and Fertility.
    Lexington, Mass.:  Lexington Books.

Chapter 14

# The Impact of Forms of Families and Sexual Unions and Dissolution of Unions on Fertility

THOMAS K. BURCH*

## INTRODUCTION

For an individual woman to achieve maximum fertility, the following conditions must be met:

1. She must be in good physical health; that is, she must be without disease or malnutrition that might cause sterility or subfecundity or lessen the survival chances of the fetus.
2. She must engage in regular sexual intercourse throughout the fecund period, starting early, but not so early as to endanger health through untimely pregnancy.
3. She must avoid long periods of sexual abstinence due to physical separation, taboos on intercourse during pregnancy and the postpartum or lactation period, and taboos based on religious or other considerations.
4. She must be able to change her reproductive partner or take supplementary partner(s) in case the male is or becomes sterile or impotent.

*In preparing this review paper, the author benefited greatly from research on demographic decision making supported by the Rockefeller Foundation (GA SS 7839), and on comparative household structure supported by the Social Sciences and Humanities Research Council of Canada (410-80-0717) and the National Institute for Child Health and Human Development (HD 15004-SSP). The revised version of the paper was prepared while the author was on sabbatical leave from Western Ontario at the Population Studies and Training Center, Brown University.

5.  She must be able to take another partner in the
    event of widowhood.

However, there is an important distinction between
maximum fertility (children ever born alive) and maximum
surviving children (Easterlin, 1978).  Good infant and
child nutrition, for example, may require a prolonged
period of lactation extending postpartum amenorrhea and
perhaps delaying the resumption of intercourse until
another conception is deemed acceptable.  The taking of
multiple or supplementary partners may lead to sterility
or subfecundity through the spread of venereal disease;
it may also weaken the sense of responsibility for childcare and so lessen the child's survival chances.  Thus
maximizing surviving children depends on optimum, not
necessarily maximum values for a number of independent
variables; the functions linking the number of surviving
children and these independent variables often are not
linear but concave downward.

In this context, marital and familial institutions,
particularly those supported by tradition, are perhaps
the primary mechanisms used by society to optimize the
number of surviving children.  Marriage legitimizes
cohabitation and regular sexual intercourse between two
or more adults to provide for socially approved reproduction, where the offspring enjoy full rights and privileges
in relation to their parents, the kinship group, and the
larger society.  Kinship and family institutions also
establish responsibilities for the child, such as labor,
payments in money or kind, care in sickness and old age,
marriage in accordance with the interests of the kinship
group, and further reproduction.  Much of the variation
in kinship systems can be understood according to the
distribution of these responsibilities and rights.  In
almost all human societies, marriage, sex, and reproduction have traditionally been closely knit.  The distinctive feature of modern reproduction is a weakening of
these links, through normative changes (e.g., acceptance
of sex outside of marriage or of childless marriage) and
through the spread of modern fertility control technology.

To study the effects of variations in marital and
familial institutions on fertility or surviving children,
it would be helpful to characterize heterosexual unions
according to a number of abstract dimensions:  age of
participants; age difference between participants;
exclusiveness, or whether either participant is expected
or allowed to have other sexual partners; permanence or

dissolubility; repeatability, or whether the surviving
partner of a broken union is expected or allowed to form
another; formality, or the degree to which the union is
recognized and controlled by society or the broader kinship group; reproductive orientation, or whether offspring are expected or allowed; and autonomy, or the
extent to which the partners are socially and economically
independent of larger social groups, especially extended
family households or kinship networks.  However, theory
and empirical research have not progressed sufficiently
to permit such a systematic treatment.  The present discussion therefore focuses on a number of concrete patterns
of behavior that are important in the developing world and
have been studied extensively in the empirical literature.
These include polygyny, in Africa and the Middle East;
consensual and visiting unions, especially in Latin
America and the Caribbean, but also in Tropical Africa;
marital dissolution and remarriage; and family type.[1]

## POLYGYNY AND FERTILITY

### Prevalence

Apart from anomalies such as the Mormons in the nineteenth-century United States, the institution of polygyny
(a man having two or more wives) is confined to Africa
and the Middle East.  (Polyandry, the custom of a woman
having two or more husbands, is so rare as to have little
demographic significance.)

   In his survey of preliterate societies, Murdock (1957)
found that approximately 75 percent allowed polygyny;
however, its extent within any given society was limited
by practical considerations, notably the more or less
equal numbers of men and women.  Chojnacka (1980) reports
a range from 37 percent of males with more than one wife
in Guinea, to an average of 20 percent in West Africa as
a whole, to around 3 percent in North African nations
such as Egypt, Libya, and Algeria.  In her own data from
five separate Yoruba communities in Nigeria, she found
polygyny among 20 to 50 percent of households or husbands,
with 50 to 72 percent of the women surveyed involved.[2]
In her samples, as is typical, a large majority of polygynous husbands have two wives, with only 25 percent having
three or more.  Polygyny clearly does not have a major
demographic impact on the developing world as a whole;
however, its extent in Tropical Africa is large enough to
make it potentially important in that region.

Determinants and Differentials

Polygyny as an institution can be explained by male
domination; by the desire for the sexual, reproductive,
and economic services of more than one wife; and by the
status and prestige associated with the practice.  A
number of specific determinants are frequently mentioned.

  1.  Economic advantages:  Chojnacka (1980:92) describes this as the "underlying major determinant."  Given
a high land-labor ratio, a negligible role for capital,
and near-zero population growth, "labor is the critical
factor"; where the family is the dominant social institution, the major way to secure additional labor is to
increase the size of one's family by marriage and
reproduction.  In his study of a largely pastoral society
in the Negev, Muhsam (1956:16) cites the common practice
of splitting one's flock for grazing, and the convenience
of having an extra wife to send off with part of the
flock.  He describes the higher total number of children
of the male in polygynous households as "the main raison
d'etre of polygamy."
  2.  Sexual advantages:  With two or more wives, the
male is less apt to find himself separated from a
potential partner or denied access because of illness,
pregnancy, or postpartum taboos (Chojnacka, 1980;
Radcliffe—Browne and Forde, 1960; Muhsam, 1956).
  3.  Female infertility:  Where a male wants many
children, especially sons, the wife's infertility or
subfecundity in a monogamous marriage would motivate the
husband to take another wife (Muhsam, 1956; Chojnacka,
1980).
  4.  The levirate (a custom requiring a man to marry
his brother's widow):  Muhsam (1956) describes the
"economic reason of the levirate" as one of the main
incentives for polygyny, noting that second wives are
frequently older than first ones, as would be expected
when a man marries his older brother's widow.  In Nigeria,
Chojnacka (1980) finds that wives are "inherited" by a
deceased man's brother or even his son.  In a male-
dominated society, the levirate provides economic support
and social standing for a woman who otherwise might have
no acceptable social role.
  5.  Status and prestige for the male:  Polygyny and
high social status are associated in a complex reciprocal
relationship.  Polygyny is commonly seen as prestigious,
but can also be a source of greater wealth (through labor

supply) and resultant status.  At the same time, the
taking of an additional wife assumes a degree of wealth,
and is often seen as the duty of wealthy men.

6.  Distorted sex ratio:  Other things being equal,
polygyny is more likely where there is a chronic shortage
of males due to warfare, export of slaves, or sex-
selective outmigration.  Also, the sex ratio of marriage-
eligibles is low where males marry women much younger
than themselves.

In contemporary developing nations, as might be
expected, polygyny, a practice frowned on in the West and
in Asia, is less acceptable to the more educated and less
traditional.  Chojnacka (1980:100) found the practice more
common among farmers, petty traders, and manual workers,
and less common among nonagricultural, nonmanual, and
professional workers; it was more common among traditional believers and Moslems, and less among Christians.
Chojnacka sees the practice declining over time as the
motives for it decline:  good agricultural land is
becoming scarcer; capital and technology are replacing
labor; population increases are providing more abundant
labor; consumption patterns and tastes are changing; and
wives and children are becoming more of an economic
disadvantage, especially in urban areas.


Fertility Impacts

The impacts of polygyny on fertility can be studied at
the macro or micro level; at the latter level, they can
be studied with regard to the male or the female.  Only
for the individual male can the impact be stated unambigu-
ously and without qualification:  polygynous males have
more children than monogamous ones.  This is not only the
clear result of polygyny, but, as was noted earlier, one
of its chief motives.  It is generally thought that women
in polygamous unions, by contrast, will have fewer children than women in monogamous unions, and thus that
societies with a large proportion of women in polygamous
unions will tend to have lower fertility.  However, these
conclusions are much less certain than those pertaining
to individual males.

Comparative data on the impacts of polygyny at the
macro level are virtually nonexistent.  Nag's study
(1962) is an exception, but it generally applies only to
preliterate societies contained in the Human Relations

Area File.  Nag found no support for the hypothesis that polygyny is associated with reduced societal fertility. From a broad comparative perspective, it can be noted that there is no special connection between widespread polygyny and either high or low fertility.  Societal fertility rates are as high in many Asian or Latin American nations, where polygyny is largely absent, as they are in African nations where it is commmon; similarly, among populations in Africa where polygyny is widespread, fertility is sometimes high, sometimes relatively low.

There are some data at the micro level on the fertility of women by type of union.  These data are relatively scarce; moreover, because the studies are not comparable in a number of ways, including sample composition, fertility measures, and control variables, they have yielded conflicting results.  Many find no consistent difference between women in polygynous and monogamous unions (Pool, 1968; Chojnacka, 1980; Olusanya, 1971).  However, the most common finding is that women in polygynous unions tend to have lower cumulative or current fertility than those in monogamous unions (see, e.g., van de Walle, 1968:230-231).  In a pioneering study of Bedouins in the Negev, Muhsam (1956) found 1076.6 living children aged 0 to 4 per 1,000 women in monogamous unions compared to 735.8 for those in polygynous unions; thus the latter had almost one-third fewer children.  This difference persisted when age was controlled, when the analysis was confined to mothers (that is, childless women were excluded), and when known response errors were taken into account.  Muhsam concludes that there is a real fertility difference ". . . if it is assumed that there is no difference in infant and child mortality" (p. 9).  Olusanya (1971:173) has questioned this last assumption, arguing that "the standard of childcare is generally superior in families where there is only one wife."  Chojnacka (1980) has presented survey data from Nigeria showing that levels of living tend to be lower and infant and child mortality higher in polygynous households.  However, relations among polygyny, levels of living and childcare, and mortality may not be the same in all cultural contexts.

Explanations of why polygynous wives might be expected to have lower fertility than monogamous wives focus on three variables:  (1) frequency of coitus, (2) duration of marriage, and (3) childlessness.

1.  Frequency of coitus might be lower for polygynous wives for four reasons:  (a) the inability of the male to

have frequent intercourse with all his wives; (b) favoritism on his part; (c) a greater willingness to observe taboos on intercourse during pregnancy, the postpartum period, and lactation; and (d) physical separation from one or more wives. Muhsam (1956) tends to discount the role of favoritism, at least in a Muslim context where fair treatment of all wives is religiously enjoined, but attributes an important causal role to a lower average frequency of coitus. Olusanya (1971) expresses doubts that male capacity would become an important limiting factor in female fertility so long as the number of wives did not exceed two or three. He also questions the relevance of this factor in a society where abstinence from intercourse is already so extensive due to taboos on sex during pregnancy and lactation--for periods of up to three or four years around the birth of a child. Pool (1968) suggests that any difficulties with frequency of sex experienced by a woman in a polygyamous union could easily be offset by extramarital liaisons.

2. A frequent explanation for the lower fertility of women in polygynous unions is that they spend a smaller proportion of their reproductive years in marriage. Specifically, it is often suggested that second or higher-order wives have shorter marriage durations and/or later ages at marriage (Muhsam, 1956; Smith and Kunz, 1976). However, the evidence presented for this view involves problems of interpretation that cause its rejection by other authors. Assuming that males marry their several wives over a period of years, it is clear that for a sample of males, duration of marriage at the time of the survey will be lower for higher-order wives; however, it is not at all clear that the durations of different-order and monogamous wives within the same age group vary significantly, unless women in polygynous unions marry appreciably later than those in monogamous unions. The evidence on the latter point is not conclusive. Smith and Kunz (1976) find that second and third wives marry about two years later than first wives, but fail to distinguish first and later marriages of the women involved. If second and later wives are widowed or divorced from earlier unions, they might well have a higher average age at second marriage, thus driving up the overall average of higher-order marriages. Chojnacka (1980:107, Table 12) finds no tendency for later first marriages among second or higher-order wives, and rejects the marriage duration argument, at least for Nigeria. Olusanya (1971:168) reports that, at the time of survey,

women in polygynous unions had longer durations since first marriage, having married earlier.

Other arguments suggest that polygyny would have the aggregate effect of increasing the proportion of women of reproductive age married at any given time. For one thing, polygyny can favor the remarriage of women whose previous union was dissolved by death or divorce. Chojnacka (1980:106) notes that ". . . remarriage follows after a very short interval," with wives in Yoruba society inherited by brothers or even sons, so that the proportion of women currently widowed or divorced is quite low in the early reproductive years.

Another, and perhaps more important, argument is that polygyny tends to lower the average age at marriage for all women, including those in monogamous unions (Chojnacka, 1980:103-104). The argument is that polygyny "generates a constant disequilibrium between the demand for and supply of girls of marriageable age" as older men compete with younger ones. One response to this equilibrium is for men to seek wives among still younger female cohorts. Smith and Kunz (1976:465) question the scarcity of females in the marriage market, so long as males tend to marry women younger than themselves and the population is growing rapidly with a sharply sloping age structure; however, their argument also suggests that females will tend to marry young, certainly in relation to males and probably absolutely. On the other hand, the argument that polygyny promotes a general pattern of early and universal marriage for women must remain only a plausible hypothesis, since the formal demography of the issue has not been worked out adequately (e.g., by modeling or simulation). There is also no direct empirical evidence, since the kind of survey data reviewed above cannot easily be used to test an essentially macrodemographic hypothesis. In addition, many of the demographic, social, and economic factors that might lead to polygyny are also associated with early and universal marriage, and the implicit multivariate model (with indirect and direct effects distinguished) has barely been hinted at in the literature, much less tested empirically.

3. Still another argument for the observed lower fertility of polygynous wives relates to a higher incidence of childlessness (although, as noted above, in studies where there is a differential in fertility, it often persists when childlessness is controlled--see Muhsam, 1956). Two motivational explanations are given: (a) that a man whose first wife turns out to be sterile or

subfecund will be motivated to take an additional wife or
wives, given his basic desire for numerous children; and
(b) that men will be willing to take sterile and subfecund
women as second or higher-order wives (quite possibly on
favorable terms) since they can still serve such other
functions as the provision of labor. Empirically, however, none of these explanations yields clear predictions
of the expected pattern of childlessness when wives are
classified by type of union or by order in polygynous
unions. In fact, the data are highly erratic. Muhsam
(1956:5-6), for example, emphasizing the first explanation above, finds that first wives in polygynous marriages have a higher incidence of childlessness than
women in monogamous marriages, but that the incidence is
even higher among second wives in polygynous marriages.
Smith and Kunz (1976:469) find the highest incidence
among third wives.

Olusanya (1971) suggests yet another possible link
between polygyny and infertility: that polygyny is
associated with a higher frequency of divorce, which in
turn leads to the spread of venereal infection and a high
incidence of secondary sterility. This mechanism is
hypothesized for both the individual and the societal
levels.[3]

In summary, a review of the literature shows no conclusive evidence that polygyny has a substantial effect
on fertility levels at the micro or macro level, one way
or the other. Nor are there compelling theoretical arguments why it should. Census and survey data frequently--
but far from uniformly--find women in polygynous unions
with lower cumulative fertility than those in monogamous
unions; however, this cross-sectional finding could also
reflect selection of women into unions by fecundity/
fertility status. Data on current age-specific fertility
are more consistent with the view that polygyny lowers
female fertility. However, studies of these issues have
seldom included full reproductive histories, so that fertility cannot be apportioned among the woman's reproductive years spent in each type of union. Moreover, these
studies have not included full multivariate analyses:
although it is known that polygyny varies according to
the social and economic characteristics of husbands and
wives, these have seldom been adequately controlled; thus
it is not known if observed fertility differentials by
type of union can be attributed directly to union type or
to other, related variables.

CONSENSUAL AND VISITING UNIONS

The demographic treatment of marital status has been firmly rooted in Western custom and law.  In censuses and surveys, the adult population is categorized according to clear legal criteria:  a person is <u>single</u> if never legally married; <u>married</u> if currently in a legal marriage and cohabiting with the spouse; <u>separated</u> if still legally married but not cohabiting; <u>divorced</u> if not legally remarried after the dissolution of a previous marriage by legal means; and <u>widowed</u> if not legally remarried after the dissolution of a previous marriage by death.  Whatever the merits of this system, it does not accord with the real-world complexity and fluidity of adult heterosexual relationships.  Its inadequacies are being recognized increasingly in developed nations as nonlegal cohabitation becomes commonplace; the problem has been apparent much longer in African and Latin American societies, where nonlegal, more or less stable cohabitation has been socially approved.  Studies of illegitimacy indicate the extent to which human reproduction is not confined to the legally married.  In the West, illegitimate fertility has typically been a small part of a society's overall fertility; in Africa, Latin America, and the Caribbean, by contrast, a large share of fertility occurs to couples in unions that are nonlegal, or at least not fully formalized.  Demographic studies of "union type and fertility" have tried to provide more adequate descriptions of these varying patterns of heterosexual unions, to investigate their implications for individual and aggregate fertility, and to identify the causal links involved.

     In relation to fertility, the primary distinction among heterosexual unions is the extent to which they expose the female to intercourse and thus to the risk of pregnancy.  Exposure to intercourse, however, is a continuous variable; thus rather than discrete types of union, it is necessary to identify a "gradient of situations, ranging from celibacy (in which there may be considerable promiscuity), through free union, consensual union, and customary marriage, to religious and civil marriage" (van de Walle, 1968:186).  In practice, the following categorization has become commonplace:

1.   Unions involving some element of duration and stability, social recognition, and cohabitation (or at least more or less continual exposure to

intercourse). This category may be further broken
down as follows:

    a.  legal marriage--a union formed as the result
       of a ceremony having full legal effect in
       civil law. In Africa, this includes both
       customary marriage (based on traditional
       ceremonies), and marriage based on civil or
       religious (e.g., Christian, Moslem) ceremonies.

    b.  consensual union (also de facto union; in
       French, union de fait)--a socially recognized
       stable union, but with little or no legal
       standing.[4]

2.  More casual unions of various types, characterized
    by the absence of continuous cohabitation; often
    temporary and unstable. Free union, visiting
    union, and keeper union are terms frequently
    encountered.

### Prevalence

The extent to which adults participate in various forms
of union differs across societies. Although precise
country comparisons are difficult because of noncompar-
ability in the typologies used, it is possible to
distinguish situations in which nonlegal cohabitation
involves a small minority, and those in which it is a
majority or modal pattern. In a series for the Congo
presented by van de Walle (1968:213, Table 2.12), for
example, only 8 percent of females in stable unions were
involved in consensual rather than legal unions, with the
maximum proportion (18.6 percent) at ages 15-19. For
Jamaica, by contrast, Denton (1979:296, Table 1) presents
roughly comparable data showing approximately 60 percent
of women in stable unions in the "common-law" as opposed
to "married" category, with the highest proportion (87
percent) at ages 15-19, and the lowest (31 percent) at
ages 40-44. Although such large differences in the
prevalence of nonlegal unions could have important
implications for aggregate fertility levels, no systematic cross-national research on the topic seems to
have been undertaken.

    Type of union is closely related to age. The
proportion in stable unions tends to rise steadily with
age, as does the proportion in legal marriages among
those in stable unions. In Jamaica, for example, the
proportion of women legally married rises from 1.2

percent at ages 15-19 to 44.5 percent at ages 40-44;
among women in stable unions, the proportion married
rises from 13 percent to 69 percent (Denton, 1979:296).
In van de Walle's (1968:213) series for the Congo, the
proportion in legal marriages among women in stable
unions rises from about 81 percent at ages 15-19 to 96
percent at ages 55 and over.

The common interpretation of these age patterns is that
consensual unions (as well as other forms of nonlegal
union) represent "a transitional stage in conjugal status"
(van de Walle, 1968:213).  Most men and women are seen as
moving toward formal and stable unions during their lifetimes, rather than opting permanently for other types.
Viewed in this light, marriage becomes a process rather
than a status (Page, 1975:47).   This fluidity among union
types, as will be seen below, considerably complicates
the analysis of their fertility implications.


### Fertility Impacts

At the descriptive level, there is general agreement in
the literature on the relationship between type of union
and fertility.  When women are classified according to
current union type, those in formal marriages have the
highest cumulative (children ever born) and current
(age-specific fertility rates) fertility, followed by
those in consensual unions and those in free unions, in
that order (Henriques, 1980).  Ebanks' (1973:53) data for
Jamaica are typical:  women in formal marriages have 5.5
children ever born, those in common-law unions have 4.6,
and those in visiting unions have 3.2.  For the Congo, van
de Walle (1968:229) shows age-specific fertility rates to
be 50 percent higher for women in formal marriages than
for those in consensual unions across all age groups.

There are exceptions to this generalization, however,
notably in fertility surveys of several Latin American
metropolitan areas (Miro, 1966) that show cumulative
fertility of women in consensual unions as high as or
higher than that of legally married women.  In addition,
some investigators report differing patterns by age; for
example, Denton (1979:300) reports that, in Jamaica in
1960, married women had higher fertility than those in
consensual unions at all ages except the youngest (14-19).
Chi and Harris (1979), on the other hand, reporting on
survey data from four Colombian cities in 1971, find that
legal marriage is positively associated with current

fertility for zero-parity (and hence mostly young) women, but negatively associated for those of parities 1-3 and 4+.

Even thus qualified, however, the above generalization does not mean that union type determines fertility levels; the empirical evidence is also consistent with the proposition that conception or live birth helps determine union status. Existing studies cannot determine the direction of causation since they typically relate cumulative or current fertility (e.g., births within the twelve months preceding the survey) to union status at the time of the survey. The problem is aptly summarized by van de Walle (1968:230):

> The difference does not imply per se that formal marriage is more conducive to fertility than consensual union. There is normally an attrition of the numbers of women in consensual unions by the formalization of conjugal relations between a first conception and a first birth (or shortly thereafter). Indeed, the consensual union is frequently a transitional stage before marriage, and it is quite reasonable to assume that the transition may be speeded up by pregnancy or childbirth. Such change in conjugal status tends to raise the fertility rates for regular marriages and to lower those for consensual unions.

Resolving some of these complexities would require data on complete fertility and union histories; fertility at various periods of the woman's reproductive life could then be classified according to union type. This type of analysis was undertaken by Roberts and Braithwaite (1960), who related completed fertility to different patterns of unions. Their findings were a little more complex than those from the typical cross-sectional analysis, in that the relative fertility of women in legal and consensual unions varied according to the precise system of classification used (e.g., continuously in one type of union, in same type at beginning and end of reproductive period, etc.). Consistent with virtually all other studies, women involved in visiting unions had the lowest fertility.

The interpretation of the causal and selective mechanisms underlying the empirical results summarized above is complex, and probably must differ across the cultural areas in which informal unions are common. The statement from van de Walle quoted above, for example, is more pertinent to the traditional African situation, where an informal union is seen as a temporary step on the way to formal marriage, and where conception or birth may hasten that transition. In the Caribbean, by contrast, consensual unions frequently last longer, and visiting unions are more common throughout adult life, rather than being so concentrated in youth. In such a context, conception or birth often leads to the termination of a union instead of its strengthening or regularization. Blake (1961) and Nag (1971) report this phenomenon for Jamaica and Barbados, respectively, although Stycos and Back (1964) report opposite findings and conclude that fertility leads to greater stability in sexual unions.

As with polygyny, a more definitive interpretation of these relationships is hampered by the methodological problems of existing studies. The absence of longitudinal data has already been mentioned; also absent are adequate statistical controls for socioeconomic variables and explicit causal models. In the Caribbean and Latin America, for example, consensual and visiting unions are more common among the lower social strata; in some nations, such unions are more common among rural couples. Often it is not known whether the fertility observed by union type is due to the union type itself or to other socioeconomic variables. A particularly important contextual variable not included in the most commonly cited studies is the availability of modern fertility control methods. Until recently, in many of the societies at issue, the costs of avoiding pregnancy or a birth were quite high; thus women in casual unions may have been more willing to run the risk that a birth would lead to regularization. With modern contraceptives available, it should be less costly and therefore more rational to avoid pregnancy until there is greater promise of a stable union with the male involved.

The generally lower fertility of women in nonlegal unions is most commonly attributed to the instability of these unions, leading to extensive periods without exposure to intercourse. It is presumed further that women in visiting unions have less frequent coitus than those who cohabit. Moreover, both visiting and consensual unions are more apt to be dissolved than legal marriages, with reproduction time lost prior to the establishment of a new union. It has also been suggested that the instability of casual unions may result in a higher incidence of venereal disease, and thus of reduced fertility associated with secondary sterility (Nag, 1975:23).

Within the Easterlin (1978) framework, the lower fertility observed in visiting and consensual unions in the Caribbean can have a motivational explanation. In anticipating the consequences of pregnancy and birth, a woman may foresee a more stable sexual union with her mate, possibly even legal marriage. Failing that, however, she might foresee the costs and burdens of childcare falling primarily on herself alone, and thus try to avoid pregnancy or birth. This is consistent with Roberts' (1955) suggestion that induced abortion may be a relevant causal factor in the lower fertility rates observed.[5]

## MARITAL DISSOLUTION, REMARRIAGE, AND FERTILITY

If conceptualizing and measuring the frequency of various types of sexual unions are difficult cross-culturally and historically, they are doubly so for divorce and other, less formal kinds of union dissolutions. Not only do customs, laws, and statistical practices differ just as widely, but with union dissolutions there is the added complication of social disapproval and stigma. In many cultures, the parties to a divorce are motivated to deny the fact, or to call it by another name, making empirical data especially difficult to gather.

### Prevalence

Despite these data problems, it is possible to make some broad statements about the quantitative importance of divorce in the developing world. An old but authoritative study by Goode (1963) indicates the basic national or regional patterns.

In Islamic Arab societies, divorce (especially at the male's initiative) is allowed and carries relatively little stigma. As with polygyny, however, few men have been able to afford divorce, since it usually requires the return of a portion of the dowry. Still, the rate of divorce per 1,000 marriages has typically been much higher than that of the West. In Algeria, for example, the rate in 1905 was 410 divorces per 1,000 marriages, compared to 259 per 1,000 for the United States in 1960, and less than 200 per 1,000 for most other developed, Western societies (Goode, 1963:Tables 11-15). On the other hand, the trend in twentieth-century Islamic societies, contrary to that in the West, has been downward; in Algeria, for example, the rate had dropped to 35 per 1,000 by 1950.

Sub-Saharan Africa has a variety of patterns, although modern statistical data are virtually nonexistent: divorce is fairly frequent in matrilineal societies, where children belong to the wife's lineage and the bride-price is low; it is much less frequent in patrilineal societies, where children belong to the male line and the bride-price is large. Trends in the face of modernization and other social changes differ depending on the starting point.

In India, divorce was not permitted to Orthodox Hindus, but was common among the lower socioeconomic strata. It was made legal in 1955, and has been growing in frequency.

In China and Japan, divorce was traditionally rather infrequent and carried a measure of social stigma. Rates were lower than in the West, although higher than generally assumed. For the male in China, according to Goode, the alternative to divorce was concubinage, a system he terms "quasi-polygynous" marriage. In Japan, divorce rates were higher than in China despite apparently similar cultural views, but have tended to decline during much of this century.

Even this cursory review of selected evidence makes an important demographic point: unlike many demographic variables, rates of divorce and other forms of union dissolution are not consistently high or low in traditional Third World cultures; thus trends may be upward or downward, depending on the particular context. Patterns of dissolution may therefore have helped raise or lower birth rates in traditional cultures, and changes in these patterns may either accelerate or slow the fertility decline.


## Fertility Impacts

Divorce and other forms of union dissolution are generally thought to lower a woman's fertility (Lauriat, 1969; Cohen and Sweet, 1974; Nag, 1980; Reyna, 1975); however, much of the best evidence for this observation relates to developed rather than developing countries. Moreover, union dissolution patterns for a population with high and relatively uncontrolled fertility may differ from those for populations with low and controlled fertility (Downing and Yaukey, 1979). Nevertheless, it may be generally observed that union dissolution leads to periods of little or no sexual activity, and therefore to reduced risk of pregnancy (Downing and Yaukey, 1979).

Where venereal diseases are endemic, secondary sterility associated with a larger number of different sexual partners may also be a factor. Reyna (1975), for example, reports for a sample from Chad that the percent sterile increases from 17.4 percent for women with no divorces to 83.3 percent for those with three or more (although there is no control for age).

Of course, there is again a problem with direction of causation in such data. Where fertility is highly valued by the male or by society generally, female sterility has often been grounds for divorce. In addition, the dissolution of a union in any society is presumably simpler if there are no children (questions of inheritance, custody, and so forth do not arise), or a small number. Sterility or low fertility can thus be a causal factor in divorce.

The fertility effects of union dissolution clearly depend on the frequency and speed of the formation of new unions. Where new unions are discouraged or forbidden (e.g., the prohibition on widow remarriage in India), widowhood or divorce will have a strong negative impact on fertility; in other contexts, there will be little or no impact. For example, in some Caribbean and Latin American studies, there is a positive relationship between fertility and the number of unions a woman has experienced. Ebanks et al. (1974) report 2.6 live births for women who have had only one union, 3.2 births for those with two, 3.8 for those with three, and 4.7 for those with four or more; the general relationship persists when age is controlled (see also Chen et al., 1974). The explanation given is that women will want to have a minimal number of children by each successive mate (Downing and Yaukey, 1979; Blake, 1955; Stycos and Back, 1964; Ebanks et al., 1974; Chen et al., 1974). However, these studies do not show that the dissolution of the union as such causes higher fertility. Downing and Yaukey (1979) suggest that socioeconomic status may be a primary determinant, since lower class women typically have both higher fertility and higher rates of marital dissolution. In addition, a woman's fertility may affect her need and motivation to seek new partners and remarry. These analytic complexities are addressed and partially solved in a recent study by Koo and Suchindran (1980), who report an interaction effect of age at divorce on the remarriage prospects of women with children; however, similar analyses for developing countries do not exist.

## FAMILY TYPE AND FERTILITY

It is widely assumed that high fertility is closely associated with and indeed partly caused by certain family types, specifically "corporate kinship groups" (such as clans or lineages) or "extended families." The former include a large number of people who are or consider themselves to be descendants of a common ancestor; who acknowledge a common leader; and who act as a unit for a variety of social, political, and economic purposes. Such a group is typically comprised of residentially separate families. An extended (or "joint" or "group") family is usually defined to include a central person (commonly a male patriarch), along with his wife, his unmarried daughters, his sons and their wives and children, and other relatives, all of whom live together in the same household or in close proximity, and share the daily round of life and a common domestic economy. The term is also used more loosely to refer to any unified group of close kin more complex than the nuclear family (or husband, wife, and their children).

The thesis that such family systems promote high fertility was first developed at length by Lorimer (1954) and by Davis (1955; see also Davis and Blake, 1956). It has drawn recent interest because the variable "family nucleation" plays a central role in Caldwell's (1976, 1978) theoretical statements about the causes of high fertility and fertility decline processes. Despite a fairly large body of literature, however, both the theoretical treatment and empirical support of this thesis remain inadequate. The subsections below review the related literature:  the early theoretical work of Lorimer and Davis, the empirical testing of the thesis, and the more recent theoretical studies.[6]


### Early Theoretical Work

In his monograph <u>Culture and Human Fertility</u> (1954) Lorimer emphasized the role of the family/kinship system (as well as of religious values) in promoting high fertility in premodern societies. This emphasis was in keeping with his assignment in writing the monograph, which was to review the role of cultural factors, and does not imply that family or religion were considered the most important variables. Lorimer's study identifies two family systems that tend to promote high fertility:

(1) corporate kinship groups such as clans or lineages, especially in tribal societies that have not yet adopted settled agriculture but have been relatively successful in competing for resources; and (2) extended family systems of settled agrarian societies, especially in Asia. He sees the high-fertility effect of the former as stronger than that of the latter. In both cases, such an effect is likely, but not inevitable; the family system can also lead to fertility restriction.

Although Lorimer does not discuss mechanisms of influence in detail, he suggests that the family system provides "motivation and support" for high fertility, including social support (approval, encouragement) and economic support (childcare services, food, housing, employment). He also stresses the role of what he terms ego-group identification: the welfare of the individual (or reproducing couple) is so closely indentified with that of the kinship or family group that (in microeconomic terms) calculating individual and group utility would yield the same fertility choices. In demographic terms, the high fertility effect of family and kinship systems operates both on marriage patterns (promoting early and near-universal marriage) and on marital fertility.

In sharp contrast with such family systems are those emphasizing the individual reproducing couple and their responsibility for their own offspring, that is, systems dominated by the nuclear family. Lorimer associates this form primarily with Western Europe as far back as the Middle Ages, but quotes with approval Irene Taeuber's (1958) similar characterization of the Japanese.

Davis' (1955) classic treatment of this thesis is narrower in scope: it focuses only on contemporary underdeveloped societies that have reached the developmental stage of settled agriculture; preliterate, tribal societies, discussed at length by Lorimer, are glossed over. However, Davis is more explicit about the mechanisms by which the family system promotes high fertility. He defines families according to the degree of "subordination and incorporation of the nuclear family by wider kinship groups" (p. 34). Such subordination is greater among agrarian societies, and often takes the form of shared residence; even when the nuclear family lives separately, however, it tends to be close to and dominated by elder relatives. Such a family system, according to Davis, favors high fertility for a number of reasons: the economic costs and inconveniences of childrearing are

more shared; men can marry earlier because the burden on
the individual of supporting a wife is not so great; the
emphasis on family solidarity encourages marriage, as
well as early childbearing by the wife to improve her
status among the husband's kin; and men are more likely
to demand offspring, partly for similar reasons of family
status, and partly to ensure old age security.

Empirical Testing of the Thesis

The early work of Lorimer and of Davis understandably
lacked a number of theoretical specifications required
for rigorous empirical testing. There is some haziness
about (a) the level of aggregation to which their propositions apply; (b) key concepts; (c) the respective roles
of marriage variables and marital fertility; and (d)
causal mechanisms. Nevertheless, early empirical studies
used census or survey data collected for other purposes
to compare the cumulative fertility of women living in
extended and nuclear households. The results more often
than not failed to confirm the Lorimer-Davis thesis: in
many cases, women in nuclear families exhibited higher
fertility. In retrospect, most of these studies were not
methodologically appropriate for testing the thesis,
although they contributed greatly to its further clarification.[7] They were limited in three primary ways:

1. The time referent of the key variables was inappropriate: cumulative fertility, which occurred over the
woman's entire reproductive span up to the date of the
census or survey, was related to current family or residential status. Thus a woman who had spent her early
childbearing years, perhaps most of them, in an extended
family would be classified as "nuclear" if that were her
status at the time. The relationship between current
residence and cumulative fertility could therefore as
easily reflect the influence of fertility on residential/
family status as the other way around, as pointed out by
Rele (1963).
2. The family classification was based on the
criterion of joint residence within the same household as
defined for census or survey purposes, rather than on the
broader concepts of "ego-family identification" or
"nuclear family subordination and incorporation" used in
the original statements of the thesis. Thus a couple
living separately only a few yards from parents or

in-laws on whom they might be almost totally dependent
could be classified as a nuclear family.
   3. Analyses often did not introduce adequate controls
for other variables that might account for observed
relationships between family type and fertility, such as
socioeconomic status, education, modernity, attitudes
toward fertility, and availability of relatives. Explanations assuming causal influence from fertility to
family type or from a third variable to both fertility
and family type were not ruled out.

   Later empirical studies have tried to address some of
these methodological problems. Liu (1967), for example,
relating recent fertility (children under 5 years) to
women's current residence, found a fairly consistent
positive relationship between living in a stem or joint
household and fertility, especially in cities; the relationship with cumulative fertility was virtually nonexistent. Vlassoff and Vlassoff (1981) present Indian survey
data to show that, when age and life-cycle stage are taken
into account, relationships between family type and both
actual and expected fertility tend to disappear. Bebarta
(1977) introduced considerations of past as well as current family/household residence; he tended to find, if
anything, a negative relationship between fertility and
extended family residence.
   The best study of these issues is reported in a recent
paper by Freedman (1981). Although the analysis is in a
preliminary stage, the data avoid most of the problems
mentioned above. A probability sample was taken of 3,816
households in Taiwan containing a married woman 18-39
years of age. Questions were asked on the following:
current residence, that is, all the persons with whom the
respondent shares a housing unit and/or with whom the
respondent takes meals; past residence, back to the time
immediately after marriage; availability of kin, that is,
whether husband's parents and married brothers are alive
and how far away they live; financial contributions from
respondent/husband to kin or the reverse; visiting
patterns with kin; and expectations of assistance from
married sons. The resulting data provide some support
for the classic thesis on family type and fertility.
Women who have always lived in a nuclear family/household
show the lowest actual fertility (3.3 live births) and
preferred fertility (2.9 children); they also show the
highest percentage preferring fewer than three children
(28 percent), and having begun contraception for spacing

(38 percent). Past and present involvement in extended households, by contrast, is associated with higher fertility. Those currently in a joint-stem household (i.e., with husband's parents and married brothers) show the highest actual and preferred fertility (3.9 and 3.2, respectively); they also show a low (although not the lowest) percentage preferring fewer than three children or having begun contraception for spacing purposes (Freedman, 1981:Table 16).

Freedman also presents data showing that expectations about the functioning of kinship systems in later life may be as important as past or present residential and kinship involvements in determining fertility. Those respondents who thought it very important to have a male heir and those who expected to get financial aid from and co-reside with married sons later in life had the highest actual and preferred fertility (3.8 and 4.0 actual and 3.2 and 3.3 preferred, respectively). The lowest fertility was found among those who did not think a male heir important (3.3 actual and 2.7 preferred) and who did not expect to receive residential or financial assistance from their married sons (3.2 actual and 2.6 preferred).

The implications of these findings for the Lorimer-Davis thesis must await further analysis. Once again, the direction of causation is not entirely clear. For instance, it is possible that respondents with more children (and therefore more sons on average) naturally tend to place more importance on male heirs, and to have greater expectations of support from married sons. It is also interesting to note that none of the fertility differences reviewed above are massive, the largest being 0.8 live births; they do not suggest a powerful influence of family type or kinship expectations on fertility, and could disappear with the introduction of control variables. Finally, there may be some doubt about extrapolating the Taiwanese findings to societies with different cultural traditions or at much lower levels of development. For the moment, however, Freedman has presented the most convincing data thus far for a structural and attitudinal link running causally from family/kinship system to fertility.


## Some Recent Theoretical Developments

The widespread adoption of a microeconomic perspective on fertility behavior has paradoxically highlighted the importance of family structure, a variable traditionally neglected by economists. The family is seen as providing mechanisms for distributing income, wealth, and labor, as well as the costs of childrearing, among kin (see, e.g., Ben-Porath, 1980; Cain, 1977).

The most central role accorded family variables is in the recent theoretical writings of Caldwell (e.g., 1976, 1978, 1981, in these volumes), who argues that family nucleation is a key event in demographic transitions. The flow of wealth, which previously has gone from the younger generation to the older (thereby making high fertility economically rational) shifts direction. Young people begin to dissociate themselves from the traditional kinship system and its associated norms, to focus on themselves and their own nuclear families. The net flow of wealth is now from the older to the younger generation, making high fertility economically nonrational.

Caldwell's argument represents a fairly marked change in the classic thesis linking family structure and fertility. In contrast with Lorimer and with Davis, he sees the structure of the residential family group as almost completely irrelevant (determined largely by the ease of constructing separate housing); what matters for fertility is the kin network, and the economic exchanges that proceed irrespective of residence. Moreover, in contrast with Lorimer at least, Caldwell posits an economically rational and self-centered actor. If there is any "ego-group identification," it runs the opposite way from that described by Lorimer: what is good for the patriarch is defined as good for the group. Finally, Caldwell sees high fertility as motivated by the desire for eventual wealth flows from offspring in one's middle and later years; Lorimer and Davis emphasize the desire for the adult status and prestige within the family that go with marriage and parenthood. Similarly, Caldwell places no emphasis on the interim costs of childbearing and rearing; the reduction of these costs by the wider kinship group looms large in the Lorimer and Davis analyses.

Further empirical research is clearly needed. This research might focus on the following central questions:

1. Do certain family/kinship forms yield peculiarly favorable "economics of childbearing," either by reducing or spreading the costs of childbearing, or by yielding valuable economic benefits from children in the form of labor, income, anticipated old age security, and so forth? Recent work by Cain (1977), McNicoll (1980), and

White (1981), among others, represents a start in this direction.

2.  If the first question is answered in the affirmative, does this indicate a conscious choice by the individual, or conformity to a social and cultural system?   This is part of the broader question of the adequacy of traditional microeconomic explanations of demographic behavior.

A final specific theoretical result bearing on the question deserves mention, viz., that provided by Goodman et al. (1974), who demonstrate analytically the strong effect of fertility level on the average number of close kin a person has.  If one can accept as a general hypothesis that sheer number of close relatives may be an important determinant of the importance of kin-based institutions (both for society as a whole and for individuals), then many of the empirical results and theoretical ideas reviewed above have to be reexamined with an eye to the possibility that causation runs from fertility to family/kinship/household structure as well as or instead of the other way around.


PROPOSITIONS

The following propositions summarize the major points made in the foregoing discussion.

1.  Polygyny may have little effect on societal or female fertility, or may lower it slightly because of a lower frequency of intercourse for some women or sterility associated with marital instability and disease.  The number of surviving children in polygynous unions may be lower to the extent that the levels of childcare are poorer.

2.  Participation in free or consensual unions probably lowers a woman's fertility compared to what it would be in a more formal marriage.  Much of this effect is due to the greater instability of such unions and the consequent loss of reproductive time.

3.  Divorce and other forms of dissolution of heterosexual unions generally lower fertility, although there may be some exceptions when the rapid formation of new unions is common.

4.  Systems of extended family/kinship relations probably tend to raise fertility and surviving children, if only because they facilitate early marriage and repro-

duction and spread the costs and responsibilities of childbearing.

5. In general, the empirical evidence for these propositions is inadequate. Although detailed longitudinal data are required for proper empirical testing, most of the available data are cross-sectional. Direction of causality is always an issue, and other variables that could be determinants are not controlled or inserted into appropriate multivariate causal models.

In general, there is no particular reason to assume that the effects of particular marriage and family forms on fertility would be massive. Reproduction is only one of several ends served by marriage and family institutions, and these institutions are themselves powerfully shaped by ecological, economic, demographic, and sociocultural factors. The fundamental determinants of fertility in the less developed nations may after all be nonfamilial.

## NOTES

1. Particularly valuable reviews of many of the topics covered here are provided by Nag (1975) and by van de Walle (1968).

2. It is customary to report the extent of polygyny as the percent of men with more than one wife, although the proportion of women in polygynous unions is the more relevant statistic for assessing aggregate fertility effects.

3. Other a priori arguments on the effects of polygyny on fertility are encountered. Olusanya (1971) suggests that co-wives in polygynous marriages may compete for the husband's favor by trying to supply him with many children, especially sons, thus tending to drive up the fertility of polygynous women. Chojnacka (1980), on the other hand, suggests that, in contemporary developing nations where polygyny is giving way in the face of modernization and Westernization, monogamous women may try to make up for the potential offspring lost to the husband who refrains from taking additional wives.

4. The term "common-law" union or marriage is ambiguous, and often avoided: in some legal jurisdictions, a common-law union is in fact a legal marriage; in everyday speech, however, the phrase often is used to refer to consensual unions or even more casual relationships.

5. In the aggregate, a pattern of widespread casual unions like those in the Caribbean tradition probably has favored high fertility in the past, and has militated against fertility reduction because the lines of responsibility for both fertility control and the care of offspring are uncertain, diffused, and fluid. Where it is not clear that the reproducing woman or couple will bear the costs of children, the motivation to control fertility (as defined in Easterlin's model) is proportionately reduced.
6. Relevant review articles are by Burch and Gendell (1970), Nag (1975), and Caldwell et al. (1980).
7. For a review of several earlier studies and their methodological inadequacies, see Burch and Gendell (1970).

## BIBLIOGRAPHY

Bebarta, P. C. (1977) Family Type and Fertility in India. North Quincy, Mass.: Cristopher Publishing.

Ben-Porath, Y. (1980) The F-connection: Families, friends, and firms and the organization of exchange. Population and Development Review 6:1-30.

Blake, J. (1955) Family instability and reproductive behavior in Jamaica. Pp. 24-41 in Current Research in Human Fertility. New York: Milbank Memorial Fund.

Blake, J. (1961) Family Structure in Jamaica. New York: The Free Press.

Burch, T., and M. Gendell (1970) Extended family structure and fertility: Some conceptual and methodological issues. Journal of Marriage and the Family 32:227-236.

Cain, M. (1977) The economic activities of children in a village in Bangladesh. Population and Development Review 3:201-227.

Caldwell, J. C. (1976) Toward a restatement of demographic transition theory. Population and Development Review 2:321-366.

Caldwell, J. C. (1978) A theory of fertility: From high plateau to destabilization. Population and Development Review 4:553-578.

Caldwell, J. C. (1980) Mass education as a determinant of the timing of fertility decline. Population and Development Review 6:225-255.

Caldwell, J. C. (1981) The mechanisms of demographic change in historical perspective. Population Studies 35:1-27.

Caldwell, J. C., G. Immerwahr, and L. T. Ruzicka (1980) Family structure and fertility. Unpublished manuscript. World Fertility Survey, International Statistical Institute, London.

Chen, K., S. M. Wishik, and S. Scrimshaw (1974) The effects of unstable sexual unions on fertility in Guayaquil, Ecuador. Social Biology 21:352-359.

Chi, P. S. K., and R. J. Harris (1979) An integrated model of fertility: A multivariate analysis of fertility differentials in Colombia. Canadian Studies in Population 6:111-125.

Chojnacka, H. (1980) Polygyny and the rate of population growth. Population Studies 34:91-107.

Cohen, S. B., and J. A. Sweet (1974) The impact of marital disruption and remarriage on fertility. Journal of Marriage and the Family 36:87-96.

Davis, K. (1955) Institutional patterns favoring high fertility in underdeveloped areas. Eugenics Quarterly 2:33-39.

Davis, K., and J. Blake (1956) Social structure and fertility: An analytic framework. Economic Development and Cultural Change 4:211-235.

Denton, E. H. (1979) Economic determinants of fertility in Jamaica. Population Studies 33:295-305.

Downing, D., and D. Yaukey (1979) The effects of marital dissolution and remarriage on fertility in urban Latin America. Population Studies 33:537-547.

Easterlin, R. A. (1978) The economics and sociology of fertility: Asynthesis. Pp. 57-133 in C. Tilly, ed., Historical Studies of Changing Fertility. Princeton, N.J.: Princeton University Press.

Ebanks, G. E. (1973) Fertility, union status, and partners. International Journal of Sociology of the Family 3:48-60.

Ebanks, G. E., P. M. George, and C. E. Nobbe (1974) Fertility and number of partnerships in Barbados. Population Studies 28:449-461.

Freedman, R. (1981) Trends in Household Composition and Extended Kinship in Taiwan and Relation to Reproduction: 1973-1980. Paper prepared for International Union for the Scientific Study of Population Seminar on Family Types and Fertility in Less-Developed Countries, Sao Paulo, Brazil.

Goode, W. J. (1963) World Revolution and Family Patterns. New York: The Free Press.

Goodman, L. A., N. Keyfitz, and T. W. Pullum (1974) Family formation and the frequency of various kinship

relationships. Theoretical Population Biology
5:1-27. (See also 8:376-381.)

Henriques, M. H. F. T. (1980) Unioes legais e
consensuais: Incidenciae fecundidade na America
Latina. FIBGE, Rio de Janeiro. Boletin Demografico
10(3).

Koo, H. P., and C. M. Suchindran (1980) Effects of
children on women's remarriage prospects. Journal of
Family Issues 1:497-515.

Lauriat, P. (1969) The effect of marital dissolution on
fertility. Journal of Marriage and the Family
31:484-493.

Lesthaeghe, R. (1980) On the social control of human
reproduction. Population and Development Review
6:527-548.

Liu, P. K. C. (1967) Differential fertility in Taiwan.
Pp. 363-370 inContributed Papers, Sydney Conference.
Liege: International Union for the Scientific Study
of Population.

Lorimer, F. (1954) Culture and Human Fertility. Paris:
UNESCO.

McNicoll, G. (1980) Institutional determinants of
fertility change. Population and Development Review
6:441-462.

Miro, C. A. (1966) Some misconceptions disproved: A
programme of comparative fertility surveys in Latin
America. Pp. 615-634 in B. Berelson et al., Family
Planning and Population Programs. Chicago:
University of Chicago Press.

Muhsam, H. V. (1956) The fertility of polygamous
marriages. Population Studies 10:3-16.

Murdock, G. P. (1957) World ethnographic sample.
American Anthropologist 59:664-687.

Nag, M. (1962) Factors Affecting Human Fertility in
Non-Industrial Societies: A Cross-Cultural Study.
New Haven, Conn.: Yale University.

Nag, M. (1971) The influence of conjugal behavior,
migration and contraception on natality. Pp. 105-123
in S. Polgar, ed., Culture and Population: A
Collection of Current Studies. Cambridge, Mass.:
Schenkman.

Nag, M. (1975) Marriage and kinship in relation to human
fertility. Pp. 11-54 in M. Nag, ed., Population and
Social Organization. The Hague: Mouton.

Nag, M. (1980) How modernization can also increase
fertility. Current Anthropology 21:571-587.

Olusanya, P. O. (1971) The problem of multiple causation in population analysis, with particular reference to the polygamy-fertility hypothesis. The Sociological Review 19:165-178.

Page, H. J. (1975) Fertility levels, patterns and trends. Pp. 29-57 in J. C. Caldwell, ed., Population Growth and Socio-Economic Change in West Africa. New York: Columbia University Press.

Pool, D. I. (1968) Conjugal patterns in Ghana. Canadian Review of Sociology and Anthropology 5:241-253.

Radcliffe-Browne, A. R., and D. Forde (1960) African Systems of Kinship and Marriage. London: Oxford University Press.

Rele, J. R. (1963) Fertility differentials in India: Evidence from a rural background. Milbank Memorial Fund Quarterly 41:183-199.

Reyna, S. P. (1975) Age differential, marital instability, and venereal disease: Factors affecting fertility among the Northwest Barma. Pp. 55-73 in M. Nag, ed., Population and Social Organization. The Hague: Mouton.

Roberts, G. W. (1955) Some aspects of mating and fertility in the West Indies. Population Studies 8:199-227.

Roberts, G. W., and W. L. Braithwaite (1960) Fertility differentials by family type in Trinidad. Annals of the New York Academy of Sciences 84:963-980.

Smith, J. E., and P. R. Kunz (1976) Polygyny and fertility in nineteenth century America. Population Studies 30:465-480.

Stycos, J. M., and K. W. Back (1964) The Control of Human Fertility in Jamaica. Ithaca, N.Y.: Cornell University Press.

Taeuber, I. B. (1958) The Population of Japan. Princeton, N.J.: Princeton University Press.

van de Walle, E. (1968) Marriage in African censuses and inquiries. In W. Brass et al., eds., The Demography of Tropical Africa. Princeton, N.J.: copyright 1968 by Princeton University Press.

Vlassoff, C., and M. Vlassoff (1981) Family Type and Fertility in Rural India: A Critical Analysis. Paper presented at the Canadian Population Society Annual Meeting, Halifax, Nova Scotia.

White, B. (1981) Child labor and population growth: Some studies from rural Asia. Workshop on Child

Labor.   Institute of Development Studies and the
   Anti-Slavery Society, Sussex University.
Willis, R. J. (1980)  The old-age security hypothesis and
   population growth.   Pp. 43-69 in T. K. Burch, ed.,
   Demographic Behavior:   Interdisciplinary Perspectives
   on Decision-Making.   Boulder, Colo.:  Westview Press.

Part IV
# SOCIAL INSTITUTIONS AND FERTILITY CHANGE

# Chapter 15

# Modernization and Fertility: A Critical Essay

RICHARD A. EASTERLIN*

The most challenging problem today in the social study of
human fertility is the causes of the shift from high to
low fertility during the process of modernization. Most
of the preceding papers focus on the state of knowledge
about only one of the main determinants of fertility--
supply, demand, or regulation costs. The purpose of the
present paper is to clarify the conceptual links between
modernization and fertility as suggested by the overall
theoretical framework of these volumes, and to note some
thoretical and empirical implications of the approach.
This is, therefore, a conceptual essay rather than a
state-of-the-art survey. The central point made is that
supply, demand, and regulation costs can be thought of as
a new set of "intervening variables" through which
modernization influences fertility, and that this perspective offers a number of benefits. First, the
transition from high to low fertility has taken place
under a wide variety of socioeconomic, institutional, and
cultural conditions (Knodel and van de Walle, 1979), and
the use of these intervening variables provides possible
explanations for that diversity. These variables also
indicate important gaps in empirical knowledge and thus
new research needs. In addition, they provide a way of
comparing and testing different theories about the
effects of modernization on fertility.

Although this paper is based on a particular view of
the mechanisms through which modernization operates, it
is not commited to any one of these mechanisms or any
specific set of modernization influences; rather, the

*The author wishes to acknowledge the excellent
assistance of Nancy Zurich, and helpful comments by
Eileen M. Crimmins and the reviewers.

framework presented here encompasses existing theories of
the effect of modernization on fertility to facilitate
their empirical testing and evaluation. The first section
below discusses briefly the meaning of modernization and
associated changes in fertility behavior; the second
focuses on the conceptual links between modernization and
fertility; and the third presents some theoretical and
empirical implications of the analysis.

## THE NATURE OF MODERNIZATION AND ASSOCIATED CHANGES IN FERTILITY BEHAVIOR

### Modernization

Modernization may be defined as a transformation in economic, social, and political organization and in human
personality observed in a growing number of nations since
the mid-eighteenth century (Coleman, 1968; Easterlin,
1968; Kuznets, 1966; Lerner, 1968; United Nations, 1970).
On the economic side, this transformation involves a
sustained rise in real output per capita. It encompasses
wide-ranging changes in techniques of producing, trans-
porting, and distributing goods; in the scale and
organization of productive activities; and in types of
outputs and inputs. It embraces major shifts in the
industrial, occupational, and spatial distribution of
productive resources and in the degree of exchange and
monetization of the economy. On the social and demographic side, modernization involves significant
alterations in fertility, mortality, and migration; in
place of residence; in family size and structure; in the
educational system; and in public health services. Its
influence extends into the areas of income distribution,
class structure, government organization, and political
structure. For the human personality, modernization means
an increased openness to new experience, increased independence from parental authority, belief in the efficacy
of science, and greater ambition for oneself and one's
children (Inkeles, 1969).

The international spread of modernization has so far
been limited, although few parts of the world have
remained untouched. The pattern of its diffusion in time
and space cannot be established with quantitative precision, but the picture in broad outline is as follows.
Elements of the transformation were increasingly apparent
in parts of northwestern Europe in the seventeenth and

eighteenth centuries.  In the course of the nineteenth
century, as the process made increasing progress in these
areas of origin, it gradually diffused southward and
eastward thoughout Europe.  By the end of the century,
its beginnings could be identified in easternmost Europe,
including Russia, and also in Japan.  A somewhat similar
development was taking place concurrently in overseas
areas settled by Europeans, mirroring to some extent the
diffusion pattern within Europe.  The process was first
apparent in areas initially settled chiefly by migrants
from northwestern Europe--the United States in the first
part of the nineteenth century, followed by Canada,
Australia, and New Zealand.  Subsequently, it could be
discerned in parts of Latin America, where migration from
southern and eastern Europe was especially important.  In
the twentieth century, and increasingly since World War
II, its early signs have become more widely apparent in
parts of Asia and, to a lesser extent, Africa.


## Fertility Behavior

The principal changes in reproductive behavior associated
with the process of modernization relate to nuptuality,
fertility, and fertility control.  Since the concern here
is with the reproductive behavior of the family or similar
conjugal unit, the present discussion is confined to married women, and thus to marital fertility and fertility
control.
   The most widely recognized change in reproductive
behavior associated with modernization is the shift from
high to low fertility.  This shift, together with a similar (and usually prior) decrease in mortality levels, is
termed "the demographic transition."  For the crude birth
rate, this means a shift from magnitudes often of 40 or
more per thousand to under 20.  This fertility decline
has been chiefly accomplished by conscious family-size
limitation on the part of individual couples.  In the
last few decades, this development has been formalized
conceptually as a shift from a "natural-fertility regime"
to one of deliberate fertility control.  There are two
types of evidence for this shift:  survey data in which
households report explicitly on their knowledge and use
of fertility control, and analyses of census or other
data on observed age-specific fertility rates, using a
technique developed by Coale and Trussell (1974) based on
Henry's work.  Although these data sets embody somewhat

different concepts of natural fertility, both yield
similar results (Easterlin et al., 1980:104-110; Knodel
and van de Walle, 1979:223; Robinson, 1981).

The combined process of fertility decline and this
shift to deliberate fertility control is hereafter called
the "fertility transition." Although this transition has
accompanied the process of modernization in all societies,
capitalist and communist alike, the specific links between
the two are not clear. As noted above, the transition
has occurred under a wide variety of conditions. Also,
in comparison with the time required for modernization of
a country, the fertility transition is usually comparatively rapid (Knodel and van de Walle, 1979:235-236).

CONCEPTUAL LINKS BETWEEN MODERNIZATION
AND FERTILITY BEHAVIOR

In seeking to identify specific links between the
processes of modernization and fertility transition just
described, a frequent approach is to regress fertility
(as measured, say, by children ever born) on measures
that reflect various aspects of social, economic, and
political modernization, along with other possible determinants such as cultural conditions (see, e.g., Richards,
in these volumes). The recent development of the "intermediate variables" approach (Davis and Blake, 1956;
Bongaarts, 1978) has introduced an intervening stage into
this analysis: fertility is now seen as being directly
influenced by a set of "proximate determinants"; modernization, in turn, operates only indirectly on fertility
through these determinants (see Bongaarts, 1978:106).

Panels I and II of Figure 1 present these two
approaches schematically. The approach adopted in the
present discussion can be thought of as a further evolution. It singles out one subset of the proximate
determinants--that relating to deliberate fertility
control. It then inserts still another set of what will
hereafter be called "intervening variables"--supply,
demand, and regulation costs--between deliberate control
and modernization (see Panel III, which is a very abbreviated version of Figure 1 in Chapter 1). As applied to
the fertility transition, this appoach thus sees the
various modernization variables as directly influencing
supply, demand, and regulation costs. These three
factors, in turn, shape the trends in use of deliberate
control. Finally, the latter, in conjunction with the

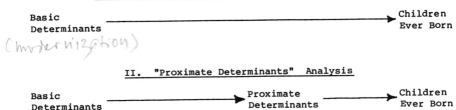

I. Multivariate Regression on Basic Determinants

Basic
Determinants ——————————————————————→ Children
Ever Born

(modernization)

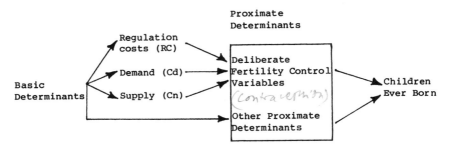

II. "Proximate Determinants" Analysis

Basic                    Proximate                Children
Determinants ——————→ Determinants ——————→ Ever Born

III. Approach of "Synthesis" Framework

Proximate
Determinants

Regulation
costs (RC)

Deliberate
Fertility Control
Demand (Cd) —→ Variables
(contraception)

Basic
Determinants        Supply (Cn) —→

Children
Ever Born

Other Proximate
Determinants

FIGURE 1  Modernization and Fertility:   Evolving
Approaches

Note:  The basic determinants comprise modernization
variables (education, urbanization, etc.), cultural
factors (ethnicity, religion, etc.), and other
determinants.

other proximate determinants, determine observed fertility.  The other proximate determinants—postpartum
infecundability, waiting time to conception, and so
on—are, of course, also affected by modernization; the
justification for focusing primarily on deliberate
control is that changes in this variable have been the
source of the observed fertility decline.
    The present approach can thus be thought of as a
continuation of the theoretical trend started by proximate
determinants analysis, designed to establish new links
between modernization and fertility.  Like that earlier
approach, it draws considerably on extant data in its
empirical implementation, especially in this case on data

from family planning knowledge, attitude, and practice
(KAP) surveys.  Also, as in the case of proximate determinants analysis, its justification is the promise of
useful insights and guidance for further empirical study,
rather than final, definitive answers on basic causali-
ties.  To illustrate the approach more fully, the next
section singles out a few aspects of modernization and
traces their possible impact on fertility via supply,
demand, and regulation costs.  The analysis proceeds in
two stages:  first, from the modernization factors to
supply, demand, and regulation costs; second, from the
latter to deliberate fertility control and fertility
decline.

Links from Modernization to Potential Supply,
Demand, and Regulation Costs

Four widely recognized, empirically identifiable aspects
of modernization are selected here for purposes of
illustration:

1.  innovations in public health and medical care,
2.  innovations in formal schooling,
3.  urbanization, and
4.  the introduction of new goods.

As is clear from the earlier discussion, these aspects
are far from exhaustive.  There are many other obvious
candidates for inclusion, such as per capita income
growth, female employment in the modern sector, mass media
developments, modernization of government administration,
and the introduction of private or public family planning
programs.  Moreover, none of these aspects adequately cap-
tures what some might consider more fundamental aspects
of modernization, such as subtle changes in human attitudes and personality.  However, the logic of the relationships will remain the same regardless of the measures
used.
    Table 1 presents a summary view of the channels through
which conscious family-size limitation may be influenced
by each of the four selected aspects of modernization.
In the table, the modernization variables are listed on
the left hand side, and the intervening variables immediately relevant to deliberate fertility control--demand,
supply, and regulation costs--run across the top as column
headings.  An entry in a cell indicates that the item on

TABLE 1 Direction of Effect of Various Aspects of Modernization on Indicated Determinants of Deliberate Fertility Control

| | Factors Through Which Fertility Control is Influenced | | | | | | |
| | Demand (Cd) | | | Supply (Cn) | | Regulation Costs (RC) | |
| Aspect of Modernization | Tastes | Income[a] | Prices | Natural fertility | Survival prospects | Subjective costs | Market costs |
|---|---|---|---|---|---|---|---|
| Better public health and medical care | | | | + | + | | |
| Growth in formal education | − | | − | + | + | | − |
| Urbanization | − | | − | | | − | − |
| New consumer goods | − | | | | | | |
| New fertility control methods | | | | | | − | − |

[a]See text for treatment of this factor.

the left influences the intervening variable at the top
in the direction shown. For example, the negative sign
at the bottom of the first column indicates that, other
things being equal, the introduction of new consumer
goods during modernization tends to reduce the strength
of preferences for children relative to goods, and thus
the demand for children. It should be noted that the
effects shown in Table 1 are illustrative; no attempt is
made to be exhaustive. A brief sketch of the reasoning
underlying the specific cell entries is given below; more
comprehensive discussion of the points made here can be
found in the preceding papers in these volumes.


Public Health and Medical Care

Improved public health and medical care affects the
family's reproductive situation by tending to increase
potential supply in two principal ways. First, they may
increase the natural fertility of women within marriage,
though there are conflicting views on this (on the pro
side, see Bourgeois-Pichat, 1967a, and Poston and Trent,
1984; on the con side, see Gray, in these volumes).
Second, even if natural fertility remains unchanged,
infants are more likely to survive to adulthood, and
potential supply is correspondingly increased. These
relationships are indicated in Table 1 by the positive
signs in the top row.
    Better public health and medical care may also raise
per capita income since a healthier, more energetic population is likely to be more productive (Malenbaum, 1970);
increased per capita income, in turn, may have effects on
demand and potential supply beyond those of better health
mentioned above. However, to simplify the table, only
those effects directly attributable to public health and
medical care improvements are shown, not those that might
be induced indirectly through the effect of better health
on per capita income. The same treatment has been followed in Table 1 with regard to the other aspects of
modernization, each of which may raise per capita income
in addition to influencing the adoption of deliberate
control directly.


Education and the Mass Media

One of the most pervasive influences on fertility control
behavior is the growth of formal education (Cochrane,

1979; in these volumes). As shown in Table 1, education operates on all three of the intervening variables--demand, potential supply, and regulation costs.

The impact on potential supply is much like that of public health and medical care improvements. Formal education improves health conditions by diffusing improved knowledge about personal hygiene, food care, environmental dangers, and so on. It may also break down traditional beliefs and customs and thus undermine such cultural practices as an intercourse taboo or prolonged lactation that have had the latent function of limiting reproduction. In these ways, it tends to enhance potential supply by raising natural fertility and/or increasing the survival prospects of babies; hence the positive signs in the second row.

Education also tends to lower the costs of fertility regulation, as shown by the negative signs in the second row under regulation costs. It may provide information not formerly available on various means of fertility control, reducing time costs. It may also alter cultural norms opposed to the use of fertility control and thus lower subjective costs, challenging traditional beliefs and encouraging a problem-solving approach to life.

Finally, formal education tends to reduce the demand for children by shifting tastes in a way unfavorable to children and decreasing the price of goods relative to children (see Lindert, in these volumes). With regard to the relative price of children (row 2, column 3), if better education improves the income-earning possibilities of women, then the opportunity cost of the mother's childrearing time is increased. Although this cost may be somehow offset, for example, through the help of other family members or domestic workers, there is still probably some net positive effect on the cost of children and thus a tendency toward a reduction in demand. In addition, compulsory education may increase the relative cost of children by reducing the possible contribution of child labor to family income. Tastes for children, or the intensity of the desire for children relative to goods (row 2, column 1), are affected negatively by education because children, and the life style associated with them, are essentially an "old" good, whereas education presents images of new life styles that compete with children. Also, education may lead to higher standards of childcare, creating greater emphasis on quality rather than quantity of children. In these ways, education increases the subjective attractiveness of expenditures

that compete with having more children, and thus tends to
lower demand.


Urbanization

The process of modernization requires a population density
in urban areas that is accomplished in part by a vast
increase in rural-urban migration. Urbanization in turn
decreases the demand for children by reducing tastes for
children and lowering the price of goods relative to them
(row 3, columns 1 and 3). The mechanism of the effect
via tastes is like that for education--the promotion of
antinatal life styles. With regard to costs, the relative
price of children of a given "quality" is usually higher
in urban than in rural areas (Lindert, 1980; in these
volumes; Cochrane, in these volumes). A variety of
factors are responsible for this. The price of food is
higher in urban than in rural areas; moreover, farm children take less time away from a mother's paid work and
contribute more time toward family work than do urban
children. Thus, the effect of urbanization is to place
the population in an environment where goods become
relatively less expensive than children, and, other
things being equal, correspondingly more attractive.

With regard to potential supply, urbanization probably
had a significant negative influence in the past, tending
to lower the survival prospects of children since concentration in densely populated areas increased exposure to
disease. However, this effect is less applicable today
given the more modern public health and medical conditions
of urban areas in many of the less developed nations; for
this reason, no entry appears in the table linking urbanization to potential supply. Another mechanism through
which urbanization might influence potential supply is by
reducing lactation.

Finally, urbanization tends to reduce both the subjective and market costs of fertility regulation, via mechanisms much like those for formal education (row 3,
columns 6 and 7). In higher-density urban situations,
access to fertility control knowledge is likely to be
greater, and market costs consequently reduced. Subjective costs are also likely to be lower because of the
tendency of the urban environment to break down traditional attitudes, including the reluctance to try new
ways of doing things.

## New Goods

Another facet of modernization is the continuing introduction of new goods (Rosovsky and Ohkawa, 1961). Within
the present framework, this tends to lower the demand for
children by shifting tastes in a way adverse to children,
as shown by the negative sign in row 4, column 1. The
enjoyment of new goods tends to require life styles that
do not center on children, since new goods are typically
substitutes for, rather than complements to, children
(see Potter, in these volumes). At any given level of
income, households tend to shift expenditure toward new
purposes and away from old goods, with the latter including having and raising children.

Among the new goods associated with modernization are
some that relate specifically to fertility control.
Historical examples are the modern condom and improved
methods of induced abortion; more recent examples are the
oral contraceptive pill and the IUD. Such developments
typically reduce the costs of fertility regulation by
expanding alternatives. They may also lower the subjective drawbacks of fertility regulation by providing less
objectionable options; for example, an advantage claimed
for both the pill and the IUD compared with most other
methods is that they separate the contraceptive act from
that of intercourse. Allowance for the effects of new
methods of fertility control is made in Table 1 by the
negative signs in columns 6 and 7 of the bottom row.

## Links from Potential Supply, Demand, and
## Regulation Costs to Fertility Control and Fertility

The preceding section suggests some specific ways that
several aspects of modernization affect the demand for
children, potential supply, and costs of fertility regulation. This section extends that analysis by indicating
how the latter three factors may in turn shape the trend
in use of deliberate fertility control as modernization
progresses. As in the foregoing section, the discussion
is hypothetical, for lack of the requisite empirical
studies.

Assume, to start with, that in a premodern society the
typical couple cannot produce as many children as they
want, that is, that demand exceeds supply. This might be
because of an agricultural environment that generates a
high demand for children, adverse mortality conditions

and extended lactation practices that make for a low supply, or a combination of the two. Under these circumstances, a couple would have as many children as possible; that is, natural fertility would prevail.

Though the analysis of the preceding section is confined to only a few aspects of modernization, it suggests that modernization tends on balance to lower the demand for children, raise potential supply, and reduce regulation costs, a pattern that is consistent with the general trend of the more detailed papers elsewhere in these volumes (see, for example, the summary essays by Lee and Bulatao, Bongaarts and Menken, and Hermalin). A couple tends to be pushed from an initial excess demand situation into one of excess supply; that is, in the absence of deliberate attempts to limit family size, the typical couple will have more children than are wanted. The prospect of unwanted children provides a motivation for family-size limitation, say, via contraception; however, such action is costly, both psychologically and economically, and the disadvantage of unwanted children must be weighed against these costs. Early in the modernization process, the excess of supply over demand and, consequently, the motivation for fertility regulation are likely to be low, while regulation costs are likely to be high. As a result, the typical couple is likely to forego deliberate family-size limitation, and natural fertility will continue to prevail. Because modernization may be raising natural fertility, an increase in fertility may consequently be observed during this early phase of modernization (Nag, 1980). However, as modernization progresses and the excess of supply over demand grows, the prospective number of unwanted children increases, generating a corresponding growth in the motivation to limit family size. Moreover, regulation costs and thus the obstacles to family-size limitation are declining. At some point, the balance between the motivation for and cost of regulation tips in favor of the former, and deliberate actions to limit family size are taken. At this point, actual family size starts to fall below potential supply, though it still exceeds demand. As modernization continues, motivation rises farther, and regulation costs fall still more—perhaps approximating a "perfect contraceptive society" (Bumpass and Westoff, 1970); a point is eventually reached at which actual family size corresponds to demand.

The above analysis is represented schematically in Figure 2. For simplicity of exposition, modernization is

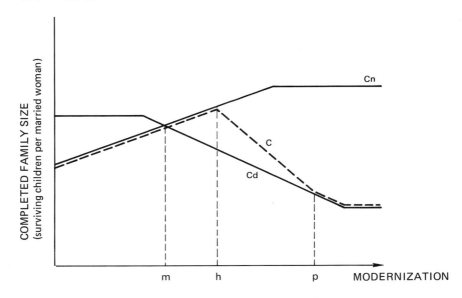

FIGURE 2   Hypothetical Trends in Supply (Cn), Demand
(Cd), and Actual Family Size (C) Associated with
Modernization

represented as a one-dimensional process, corresponding
to a rightward movement along the horizontal axis.
Supply and demand, measured according to surviving
children per married woman, are shown on the vertical
axis.   Initially, demand (Cd) exceeds supply (Cn), and
actual family size (C) corresponds to supply.   As
modernization occurs, an excess supply condition emerges
(point m), generating a motivation for fertility control.
Initially, this motivation is low and does not offset
regulation costs sufficiently to result in deliberate
family-size limitation; hence actual family size continues to correspond to supply.   However, as modernization progresses, with motivation growing and regulation
costs falling, at some point deliberate restriction sets
in (point h).   Eventually, family size falls to a level
corresponding to demand (point p).
    The precise nature of the trends in demand, supply,
and regulation costs is, of course, a matter for empirical
inquiry.   For example, the transition as depicted here
starts from a premodern situation in which supply is less
than demand and a motivation for regulating family size

is therefore absent. However, there is nothing in the framework that requires this view. The premodern situation might be one in which motivation exists, but the practice of fertility control is absent because regulation costs are very high (that is, the premodern position would be between points m and h in Figure 2). Clearly, the true nature of the premodern situation is an empirical issue.

Point h might be thought of as the dividing line or "threshold" (Kirk, 1971; United Nations, 1965) between two modes of fertility regulation. To the left of point h, fertility is "regulated" by a variety of social and biological mechanisms working though natural fertility (see LeVine and Scrimshaw, in these volumes; Bourgeois-Pichat, 1967b). The modernization process, which shifts the typical household to a position to the right of point h, creates a fundamental change in the circumstances of family reproduction, moving parents from a situation where childbearing is a matter "taken for granted" to one that poses difficult problems of individual choice regarding the limitation of family size. To the left of point h, although there is a demand for children, parents may be quite imprecise about the number desired (stating, e.g., it is "up to God"); the usual demand mechanisms emphasized in the economic theory of fertility do not influence observed fertility, though fertility may be affected by economic variables via natural-fertility mechanisms. The explanation of fertility in such a situation calls for inquiry into the determinants of natural fertility. To the right of point h, the household decision-making approach of economics comes more into its own.

Of course, such sweeping distinctions are never fully satisfactory. Social sanctions are operative in both premodern and modern circumstances, while the idea that there is no individual choice whatsoever in a premodern society is too strong. Moreover, no society shifts en masse at a single point of time from "social" to "individual" control situations, as suggested in this highly simplified sketch. Rather, at any given time, individual couples are distributed about the mean with regard both to motivation and regulation costs, and the modernization process pushes some couples across the threshold earlier than others; indeed, even under premodern conditions there may be some couples actually practicing deliberate family-size limitation. Hence, at the societal level, there may be no "threshold" clearly identifiable in time; however, if there are rapid and sizable changes in supply, demand,

or regulation costs that occur in common among many
families (see, e.g., Retherford and Palmore, in these
volumes, on diffusion processes; Retherford, 1980), a
societal threshold may be observable.


SOME THEORETICAL AND EMPIRICAL IMPLICATIONS

Introducing supply, demand, and regulation costs as
intervening variables between modernization and deliberate fertility control helps clarify a number of theories
and empirical findings on the relationship between modernization and the fertility transition; as has already
been seen, it also suggests new empirical research needs.
This section first analyzes certain empirical findings
and then examines some theoretical views.


Empirical Findings

Variability in the Time Series Relationship Between
Modernization and Fertility

As noted earlier, perhaps the most striking finding about
the fertility transition in Europe is that "it occurred
under remarkably diverse socioeconomic and demographic
conditions," in particular, that "there was no clear
threshold of social and economic development required for
the fertility transition to begin (Knodel and van de
Walle, 1979:220, 225). This diversity can be readily
understood in light of the present analysis. Assume that
two countries have identical trends in potential supply
(reflecting, say, identical improvements in infant and
child mortality as public health programs are introduced);
different levels of demand due to differing child cost
environments; and, for simplicity, zero regulation costs.
Graphically, this situation may be depicted as in Figure
3 (the superscripts refer to countries A and B, respectively, and the passage of time is represented by movement
from left to right).
    Note that, despite identical trends in mortality and
hence in potential supply, the onset of fertility decline
occurs earlier in Country A. This is because of its lower
level of demand at each point in time, which, coupled
with growing supply, results in earlier motivation for
fertility control. Similarly, even if the trends in
demand and supply were identical in the two countries,

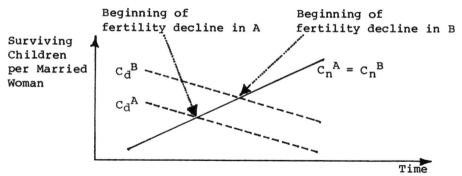

FIGURE 3   Hypothetical Trends in Supply (Cn) and Demand
(Cd) in Two Countries and the Timing of Fertility Decline

but regulation costs were different, there would be a
difference in the onset of fertility decline.

Knodel and van de Walle (1979:235) also make the point
that cultural setting "influenced the onset and spread of
fertility decline independently of socioeconomic conditions". To see why this might be true, one need merely
assume that the differing levels of demand in the preceding diagram reflect differences in cultural conditions
operating through tastes--perhaps because of differences
in son preference or the status of women. As a result of
these cultural differences, the same socioeconomic trend
(declining mortality) would be accompanied by a difference in the timing of the onset of fertility decline.
Clearly, cultural conditions could also operate via potential supply (e.g., by influencing lactation practices) or
regulation costs (e.g., through attitudes toward the
acceptability of induced abortion).

These illustrations show that the effect of any given
modernization factor, such as public health, varies
depending on the initial conditions of (and, implicitly,
changes in) other modernizing and cultural variables; thus
no one aspect of modernization, nor any selected set of
modernization variables, need exhibit an invariant pattern
in relation to observed fertility and the adoption of
fertility control. Indeed, it is surprising that mortality and fertility change were ever closely enough related
in historical experience to suggest the well-known model
of the demographic transition. Although in all countries
that have modernized or are modernizing there are a number
of similar changes in social, economic, and political
conditions, the relative timing of these changes has by

no means been uniform. Moreover, economic changes, such
as shifts in industrial structure, are often protracted,
whereas social changes, such as those in public health or
compulsory elementary education, may be more temporally
concentrated.  In addition, in today's developing countries, advances in public health and compulsory education
often occur at an earlier time relative to economic
modernization than was true of the now-developed countries; in these countries, new modernizing influences are
also at work, such as mass media in the form of radios,
television, and movies, new modes of fertility regulation
such as the pill and the IUD, and government population
programs that are sometimes highly coercive in nature.
Cultural conditions also vary widely, both within and
between the more and less developed blocs.  Hence it
should not be expected that the ways in which various
modernizing and cultural influences come together to
shape the fertility transition will be identical from one
place to another.  However, the present effort to identify
how these influences shape supply, demand, and regulation
costs, and thus the adoption of fertility control during
modernization, as well as how they affect the noncontrol
proximate determinants, should help to explain differences
among countries in the timing and pace of the fertility
transition more coherently.


The Trend in Fertility Differentials
by Socioeconomic Status (SES)

The present approach also has implications for findings
on trends in fertility differentials during modernization.
Cross-sectional empirical studies linking fertility to a
given modernization variable often yield mixed results,
even after a variety of controls have been introduced.
For example, the review of evidence by Mueller and Short
(in these volumes) finds that fertility is related to
income positively in rural and negatively in urban areas.
Cochrane (in these volumes) reports a frequent finding of
a positive relationship between fertility and education
over part of the educational range in low-income countries and, consistent with this, that the "cross-section
effect on fertility is more negative at later than at
earlier points of time."  Such results should not be
surprising since there is reason to expect that the cross-
section pattern of fertility differentials by socioeconomic status may change during modernization.  As is

evident from Table 1, any given modernization factor may
influence fertility through more than one intervening
variable, and the net effect on fertility may differ
according to which intervening variables dominate.
Therefore, the observed relationship between fertility
and a given modernization variable may vary in time and
space if the dominant intervening variables change. In
particular, if the prevailing variables yield a natural-
fertility regime at one time and a situation of partially
or wholly deliberately controlled fertility at another, a
change in the nature of the observed relationship is
quite possible.

As an illustration, consider the relation of fertility
to education. Suppose that, at a given time within a
country, potential supply (Cn) varies positively with
education (say, because of higher natural fertility among
the more educated due to shorter lactation), while demand
(Cd) varies negatively, reflecting the antinatal effect
of education via the taste and cost mechanisms described
earlier. Suppose further that the cross-sectional
schedules relating supply and demand to education are
positioned as shown in panels a and b of Figure 4 in two
succesive periods. Figure 4a is the premodern case, and
Figure 4b the early modern one. In Figure 4a, neither
those at low nor at high education levels can have as
many children as they would like (supply, Cn, is less
than demand, Cd); hence, those at both levels have as
many as they can. In this situation, one would expect
observed fertility to vary positively with education, as
a result of the lactation mechanism just mentioned. In
Figure 4b, the early modern case, the supply schedule is
shifted upward and the demand schedule downward at all
levels of education, as modernization exerts its expected
effects. As a result, there is a motivation to control
fertility among those of higher education. Assuming that
no obstacle arises from regulation costs, natural fertility will prevail among less-educated parents and
controlled fertility among more-educated parents. In
this situation, fertility differentials by education
might shift from a positive to a negative slope, as
antinatal taste and cost mechanisms working through
demand and lower regulation costs come to prevail at
higher educational levels.

This example suggests that, for developing countries,
estimates of the elasticity of fertility with regard to a
given modernization variable such as education based on
cross-sectional data may yield results differing in

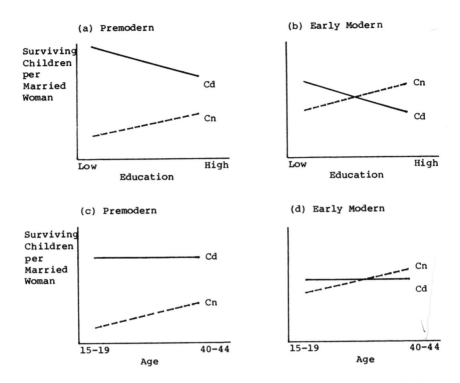

FIGURE 4   Hypothetical Relationship Between Supply (Cn) and Demand (Cd) and Education and Age in Premodern and Early Modern Settings

magnitude and/or sign, depending on the mechanisms governing the determination of fertility. It also implies that time series observations on national averages of, say, education and fertility in a given country will not necessarily show the same relationship in different phases of modernization. If, for example, potential supply were rising over time as a result of decreased lactation associated with growing education, but remained below demand so that natural fertility conditions persisted, then education and observed fertility would be positively associated in time; in some later period, education and fertility might be negatively associated in time as deliberate control came increasingly to prevail.

The Trend in Fertility Differentials by Age

Several studies reported on by Knodel (in these volumes)
show a "tilt" in the age-specific marital fertility
schedule with the onset of modernization--an increase at
younger and a decrease at older ages.  Knodel links this
development to the effect of natural fertility at younger
ages and of deliberate family-size limitation at older
ages.  Reference to the intervening variables suggested
by the present analysis indicates the underlying
mechanisms involved.

As sume that for any given couple, potential supply
varies with duration of marriage--the longer the marriage, the greater the potential supply; for simplicity,
also assume that demand and regulation costs are independent of duration of marriage.  If duration of marriage
and age are positively correlated, the hypothetical
cross-sectional patterns of supply and demand by age in
successive periods shown in panels c and d of Figure 4
will obtain.  Figure 4c is a hypothetical sketch of how
demand (Cd) and supply (Cn) might vary as the typical
woman in a premodern society goes through her reproductive
career.  As shown, even by the end of her reproductive
career, the typical woman has fewer surviving children
than are desired.  If for simplicity of exposition one
disregards variations around the mean at each age, no
motivation for or adoption of fertility control exists at
any reproductive age.  This means that, in such a society,
the observed age-specific marital fertility schedule and
a natural fertility schedule would correspond.

Figure 4d is a hypothetical sketch of the same two
curves later in the process of modernization; it assumes
that the supply curve shifts upward and the demand curve
downward, in keeping with the effects of modernization
discussed earlier.  As a result of this, a motivation to
control fertility emerges at the later reproductive ages,
and, assuming no obstacle from regulation costs, deliberate family-size limitation occurs.  With regard to the
schedule of age-specific marital fertility, this implies
that the _trend_ in age-specific marital fertility rates at
the younger reproductive ages between situations 4c and
4d will reflect developments in natural fertility alone,
and hence will be upward; however, the trend at older
ages will be influenced, in addition, by a shift from
uncontrolled to controlled fertility, and hence may be
downward.  The overall result may be a tilt in the marital
fertility schedule like that observed.  Also, as Knodel

points out, the net balance of these contrasting fertility changes at younger and older ages may yield a stable
or even upward movement in the total fertility rate at an
early stage in the shift to deliberate fertility control.

## Theories of the Fertility Transition

Although the present approach views modernization as
influencing fertility through the intervening variables
of supply, demand, and regulation costs, it does not
adopt a particular theory of the dominant mechanisms at
work. However, by providing a framework that encompasses
different views, it facilitates their comparison and
empirical testing. To illustrate this, the following
discussion touches briefly on several theories.

To start with, there are those whose theories either
explicitly or implicitly stress influences working through
the demand for children. Lindert (in these volumes; see
also Schultz, 1976) provides an excellent and succinct
statement:

> In all countries and all eras, fertility follows
> changes in the demand for children, driven by
> considerations of both economics and taste. Fertility
> fails to fall in the early phases of most countries'
> development, and falls thereafter, for a straight-
> forward reason: the relative costliness of extra
> children fails to rise until a fairly advanced stage
> in development. . . . It appears, therefore, that the
> fertility transition parallels the long-term pattern
> of child costs and benefits.

Caldwell's "wealth flows" theory (see Caldwell, in these
volumes) also stresses factors working wholly through the
demand for children, though the underlying mechanisms
shaping demand differ in important respects from
Lindert's.

In contrast, other analysts focus on supply. Consider,
for example, Carlsson's (1966) well-known article on the
historical experience of Sweden, "The Decline of Fertility: Innovation or Adjustment Process?" In the terminology of the present analysis, the adjustment process
Carlsson has in mind is the response that occurs when
rising supply due to declining infant and child mortality
pushes households across (or further to the right of) the
fertility control threshold (point h in Figure 2). He

contrasts this with an explanation of the fertility
decline according to "innovation," for example, in methods
of fertility regulation that would, in the present terminology, reduce regulation costs.  Carlsson argues that
the Swedish evidence favors an interpretation of that
country's fertility decline as an adjustment to increasing
supply caused by lower infant and child mortality, rather
than a response to an innovation that lowers costs of
regulation.

Still other scholars place primary emphasis on regulation costs. Knodel and van de Walle (1979), for example,
argue that the motivation for fertility control (an excess
supply situation) already existed in many parts of Europe
prior to the fertility transition:  "[T]here was latent
motivation for reduced fertility among substantial portions of the population before fertility began to fall,"
and "births were frequently unwanted, especially among
women . . ." (pp. 226, 227). As regards the availability
of or access to fertilty control, they argue that "family
limitation was not widely available or acceptable . . .
[and] its use . . . [was] extremely limited because it
was either unknown or objectionable" (p. 231).  They
therefore identify a decline in regulation costs as the
key development behind the fertility transition:

> [W]e believe that what is understood by the "cost of
> fertility regulation," a term that covers a variety of
> factors including sheer familiarity with the concept
> and means of family limitation, is an extremely
> important component of an explanation of the secular
> fertility decline, as it occurred in Europe. . . (p.
> 239).

Others propose some combination of the intervening
variables stressed here.  Freedman (1975), for example,
places particular emphasis on two sets of social norms--
those about family size and those about each of the
"intermediate variables" of the Davis-Blake (1956)
framework.  The former would work through the demand for
children. As for the latter, norms regarding those
intermediate variables that are under voluntary control
relate to regulation costs; others relate to supply.  As
another example, Potter's discussion (in these volumes)
of institutional influences primarily stresses those
shaping the demand for children, either through cost or
taste factors.  However, in considering institutional
influences on social values relating to appropriate

fertility behavior, such as religious opposition to birth control, he also touches on influences of regulation costs.

Clearly, resolution of these differing views would be helped by empirical studies of the trends in supply, demand, and regulation costs. Time series and cross-sectional data for different countries could be mobilized to answer questions such as the following (Crimmins et al., 1983; Easterlin and Crimmins, 1982): Is the prevalence of natural fertility in premodern societies due to an inability on the part of the typical household to have as many children as are wanted, and therefore to an absence of motivation for fertility control (i.e., is demand [Cd] greater than supply [Cn])? Or does the motivation for fertility control exist (demand is less than supply), but regulation costs (RC) are perceived to be so high that fertility control is not adopted? As modernization occurs and growth in deliberate fertility control eventually sets in, what is the proximate source of this increase in fertility control--increasing motivation (an excess of supply over demand), declining regulation costs, or both? If it is increasing motivation, to what extent is this due to a growth in supply (Cn) rather than a reduction in demand (Cd)? If supply grows, what is the relative role in this growth of changes in natural fertility compared with infant and child survival? The answers to these questions would help sort out the relative roles of supply, demand, and regulation costs at different stages of the fertility transition. This would help assess the relative plausibility of different theories of the moving forces behind the transition, and identify which lines of further research are likely to be most fruitful.

## BIBLIOGRAPHY

Bongaarts, J. (1978) A framework for analyzing the proximate determinants of fertility. Population and Development Review 4:105-132.

Bourgeois-Pichat, J. (1967a) Relation between foetal-infant mortality and fertility. Pp. 68-72 in Proceedings of the World Population Conference, 1965, Vol. 2. New York: United Nations.

Bourgeois-Pichat, J. (1967b) Social and biological determinants of human fertility in non-industrial societies. In Proceedings of the American Philosophical Society 3:160-163.

Bumpass, L., and C. F. Westoff (1970) The perfect
contraceptive population. Science 169:1177-1182.

Carlsson, G. (1966) The decline of fertility:
Innovation or adjustment process? Population Studies
20:149-174.

Coale, A. J., and T. J. Trussell (1974) Model fertility
schedules: Variations in the age structure of
childbearing in human populations. Population Index
40:185-258.

Cochrane, S. H. (1979) Fertility and Education: What Do
We Really Know? World Bank Staff Occasional Papers
No. 26. Baltimore, Md.: The Johns Hopkins University
Press.

Coleman, J. S. (1968) Modernization: Political
aspects. Pp. 395-402 in International Encyclopedia of
the Social Sciences. New York: Macmillian.

Crimmins, E. M., R. A. Easterlin, S. J. Jejeebhoy, and K.
Srinivasan (1983) New perspectives on the demographic
transition: A theoretical and empirical analysis of
an Indian state, 1951-1975. Economic Development and
Cultural Change, forthcoming.

Davis, K., and J. Blake (1956) Social structure and
fertility: An analytical framework. Economic
Development and Cultural Change 4:211-235.

Easterlin, R. A. (1968) Economic growth: An overview.
Pp. 395-408 in International Encyclopedia of the
Social Sciences. New York: Macmillan.

Easterlin, R. A., and E. M. Crimmins (1982) An
Exploratory Study of the 'Synthesis Framework' of
Fertility Determination with World Fertility Survey
Data. WFS Scientific Reports, No. 40. London: World
Fertility Survey..

Easterlin, R. A., R. A. Pollak, and M. L. Wachter (1980)
Toward a more general economic model of fertility
determination: Endogenous preferences and natural
fertility. Pp. 81-135 in R. A. Easterlin, ed.,
Population and Economic Change in Developing
Countries. Chicago: Chicago University Press.

Freedman, R. (1975) The Sociology of Human Fertility.
New York: John Wiley.

Inkeles, A. (1969) Making men modern: On the causes and
consequences of individual change in six developing
countries. American Journal of Sociology 75:208-225.

Kirk, D. (1971) A new demographic transition. Pp.
123-147 in Rapid Population Growth. Baltimore, Md.:
The Johns Hopkins University Press.

Knodel, J., and E. van de Walle (1979)  Lessons from the past:  Policyimplications of historical fertility studies.  Population and Development Review 5:217-245.

Kuznets, S. (1966)  Modern Economic Growth:  Rate, Structure and Spread.  New Haven, Conn.:  Yale University Press.

Lerner, D. (1968)  Modernization:  Social aspects.  Pp. 386-395 in International Encyclopedia of the Social Sciences.  New York:  Macmillan.

Lindert, P. H. (1980)  Child costs and economic development.  Pp. 5-69 in R. A. Easterlin, ed., Population and Economic Change in Developing Countries.  Chicago:  University of Chicago Press.

Malenbaum, W. (1970)  Health and productivity in poor areas.  Pp. 31-54 in H. E. Klarman, ed., Empirical Studies in Health Economics.  Baltimore, Md.:  The Johns Hopkins University Press.

Nag, M. (1980)  How modernization can also increase fertility.  Current Anthropology 21:27-36.

Poston, D. L., and K. Trent (1984)  Modernization and childlessness in the developing world.  Comparative Social Research 7, forthcoming.

Retherford, R. D. (1980)  Modeling Sudden and Rapid Fertility Decline.  Working Paper No. 1.  East-West Population Institute, Honolulu.

Robinson, W. C. (1981)  Demand Versus Supply Factors in the Fertility Transition.  Unpublished paper. Pennsylvania State University, University Park, Pa.

Rosovsky, H., and K. Ohkawa (1961)  The indigenous components in the modern Japanese economy.  Economic Development and Cultural Change 9:476-501.

Schultz, T. P. (1976)  Determinants of fertility:  A micro-economic model of choice.  Pp. 89-124 in A. J. Coale, ed., Economic Factors in Population Growth. New York:  Halsted Press.

United Nations Department of Economic and Social Affairs (1965)  Population Bulletin of the United Nations, No. 7.  New York:  United Nations.

United Nations, Research Institute for Social Development (1970)  Contents and Measurement of Socio-Economic Development:  An Empirical Inquiry, Report No. 70.10. Geneva:  United Nations.

# Chapter 16
# Effects of Education and Urbanization on Fertility

SUSAN H. COCHRANE *

The purpose of this paper is to document the effects of education and residence on fertility. The effect of education has been much more carefully documented (Cochrane, 1979) than that of residence; however, both raise similar methodological issues.

First, neither education nor residence can affect fertility directly in the same way as age at marriage, lactation, and contraceptive use, but must operate through such variables. Although these intervening channels are not the focus of this paper, they must be recognized if the "true" effects of education and residence are to be assessed. If all these channels were included in the analysis, the measured effect of education would be reduced to zero.

In addition to these problems of causal modeling, there is a second problem--linearity. If the relationship between two variables is linear, one can aggregate with impunity. Unfortunately, the evidence indicates that the relationship between education and fertility is nonlinear, and is in fact not even monotonic. In a previous literature review, uniformly inverse relationships were found in only 49 percent of the cross-tabular studies; significant negative coefficients were found in only 31 percent of the regression studies in which income and wealth were controlled along with age and residence (Cochrane, 1979). In most cases, if the relationship was not monotonically

---

*This paper was supported in part by the Population and Human Resources Division of the World Bank. The views and interpretations, however, are those of the author and should not be attributed to the World Bank, to its affiliated organizations, or to any individual active in their behalf.

587

inverse, fertility first rose with education and then
fell. In these cases, peak fertility was generally found
at lower primary education. The new data reviewed in
this paper confirm the existence of two different
patterns--the inverse pattern and an inverted "U."
Similarly, it is unlikely that the relationship between
residence and fertility is linear, although this has not
been documented. Therefore, studies should probably be
restricted to the individual rather than the aggregate
level.

The methodological issues involved in assessing the
effects of education and residence on fertility are
discussed in detail below. Following this discussion is
a summary review of the literature on these effects.

## MEASURING THE EFFECTS OF EDUCATION AND RESIDENCE ON FERTILITY:  METHODOLOGICAL ISSUES

### Measuring Education's Effect

To measure the effect of education on fertility, one must
first eliminate spurious correlations between education
and other fertility determinants, most obviously age and
residence. In developed countries, younger women are
generally more educated than older women, and of course
age is highly correlated with number of children ever
born. Therefore, if age is not controlled, the effect of
education on fertility will be overestimated. Likewise,
education tends to be higher in urban than in rural areas,
and fertility is generally higher in rural than urban
areas. Thus if residence has effects other than those
through education and if it is not controlled, education's
effect will be overestimated. Beyond these generalizations, however, there is not even agreement on how to control appropriately for residence or exposure to childbearing. Moreover, although other background variables such
as caste probably determine both education and fertility
and therefore need to be controlled, these factors vary
among countries so that generalizations cannot can be
made.

There is also considerable disagreement about which
effect of education one wishes to estimate, depending on
the objective of the research. This paper focuses on the
total effect of education. As noted above, education acts
through many other variables, such as age at marriage,
lactation, and contraceptive use. If these intervening

TABLE 1 Education--the Intervening Variables Through Which It Affects Fertility, and the Biases Introduced by Including these Variables with Education in Regression Models

| Intervening Variable (IV) | Effect of Education on IV | Effect of IV on Fertility | Bias in Estimating Education's Effect if Controlling for IV Without Adding Indirect Effects |
|---|---|---|---|
| **Supply of Births** | | | |
| Age of marriage | + | − | + |
| Breastfeeding | − | − | − |
| Abstinence (noncontraceptive) | − | − | − |
| **Demand for Children** | | | |
| Income[a] | + | ? | ? |
| Wealth | + | ? | ? |
| Female wage | + | − | + |
| Mass media | + | − | + |
| Female labor participation[a] | + | ? | ? |
| Child labor participation[a] | − | + | + |
| Child schooling[a] | + | − | + |
| Child survival[a] | + | − | + |
| Perceived cost of children | + | − | + |
| Perceived benefits of children | − | + | + |
| Migration[b] | + | − | + |
| **Fertility Regulation** | | | |
| Contraceptive use | + | − | + |
| Knowledge of birth control | + | − | + |
| Access to birth control | + | − | + |

[a] Variables affected by as well as affecting fertility. Income is included in the list since it depends on labor participation, which in turn is affected by fertility; income is also affected by education independently of labor participation as a result of assortive mating.

[b] Education may affect migration, but migration's effect on fertility is uncertain. Most of its effect is probably captured by residence.

variables (IV) are included in the analysis, then education's total effect on fertility will be biased. Therefore, education's effect on fertility through these variables must be added to its "direct" effect. Table 1 lists a number of these variables; the effect of education on each; the effect of the IV on fertility; and the resultant bias in estimating education's total effect if the IV is controlled but the effect of education on that IV is not added.[1] These variables have been arranged under the three broad determinants of fertility: the supply of children, the demand for children, and fertility regulation.

In most cases (14 of 15), the inclusion of an intervening variable will bias the education variable positively (i.e., toward zero if the effect is negative). On
the other hand, while the direction of the bias can be
determined in most instances, the magnitude can not,
since it depends on how strong an effect education has on
the intervening variable. For example, if mass media
exposure includes mainly written communication, education
will have a strong effect on exposure; inclusion of
exposure in the analysis will then lead to a serious
underestimate of education's effect (assuming that mass
media exposure has a strong effect on fertility). On the
other hand, if mass media exposure represents primarily
radio, the bias resulting from inclusion of this variable
will be less serious.

These points can be illustrated by Mason and Palan's
(1980) Malaysian study. Starting with the basic controls
of age and marital duration,[2] they estimate the coefficient of education for six racial-residence groups and
then successively show the effect on these estimates of
the following variables: occupation prior to marriage,
residence when growing up, husband's education, a sanitary
and amenities scale, family income, and the minimum
education for sons. When these variables are added,
significant inverse (linear or nonlinear) relationships
are eliminated in four out of five groups; in the fifth
group--rural Malays--for whom the positive effects of
education were initially strongest, the negative effect
of education is increased. (In the sixth group, the
coefficient was not significant initially.) The neutral-
izing effect of the variables differs from group to
group. This variation among groups in the channels
through which education operates makes it impossible to
formulate a priori statements about the size of the biases
introduced (or eliminated) by introducing variables.[3]

The indirect effects of education can be easily
adjusted for if sufficient information is available and
causation is unidirectional. However, if causation runs
in two directions, it is much more difficult both conceptually and empirically to determine the effect of education on fertility. Two kinds of problems may arise here.
First, education and some other variable may be simultaneously determined. The most important example is the
education of husband and wife. Assortive mating will
result in more educated women being married to more
educated men. To the extent that the husband's education
also affects fertility, it would be a mistake to attribute

all of education's effect to either the wife or the husband. If the wife's education is used alone, its effect will be biased away from zero; if both the husband's and the wife's education are included, then the effect of each education measure will be biased toward zero. Although there is no clear-cut solution[4] to this problem, it helps to be aware of the upper and lower limits on "education's" effect (see Hermalin and Mason, 1980).

A second kind of problem arises if fertility, rather than education, is jointly determined with some other variable. For example, if fertility and female labor participation are interdependent, then the inclusion of the latter causes the coefficients of other explanatory variables such as education to be biased. Since the importance of this bias is a matter of degree, there is considerable disagreement over which variables should be treated as simultaneous with fertility.[5]

In Table 1, those variables most commonly considered to be simultaneous with respect to fertility have been marked. There are no variables on this list which might be considered to have feedback effects on education, primarily because these variables are measured in adulthood, generally long after education has already been completed. The one important exception might be age at marriage if there is overlap between marriage ages and levels of education.

To summarize, residence and age are necessary controls if one is to avoid overestimating the negative effect of education.[6] Inclusion of other variables determined by education may bias the effect of education (usually toward zero). Inclusion of husband's and wife's education together will reduce the measured effect of each individual measure, while exclusion will lead to an overestimate (unless they differ in the sign of their effect); the "proper" specification will depend on the use to be made of the model. Finally, inclusion of simultaneous variables will cause biases of unknown direction and magnitude.

## Measuring Residence's Effect

The effect of education on fertility cannot be studied separately from that of residence. The reason for this is that many of the factors affecting individual decision making are determined at least in part by the community

of residence. These factors include presence in the
community of contraceptive services; schooling opportunities and health facilities; economic opportunities and
costs, such as the demand for labor of men, women, and
children; the costs of food and housing; and the less
easily defined factors of social milieu, climate, and
exposure to disease. All of these factors vary between
urban and rural areas. Ideally, one would control for
these factors individually; however, sufficient data are
rarely available. Therefore, residence is used as a
control to approximate these factors. This is at best a
very gross control, especially if a dichotomous variable
is used for residence.

The effect of residence on fertility operates through
all these intervening factors. As in the case of education, if these factors are included with residence in a
model of fertility determination, a bias will be introduced in estimating residence's effect. Table 2 shows
the direction of such biases. It should be recognized
that because the intervening community variables (ICV)
will in turn affect intervening family variables (IFV),
the inclusion of the latter will affect estimates of the
effect of residence. One major advantage of ICVs over
IFVs in an analysis is that, unlike the ICVs, the IFVs
may be simultaneously determined with family fertility.
Thus although both introduce biases, the ICVs are
exogenous to the family, and the biases are of known
direction.


Interactions, Nonlinearities, and Measurement Problems

To this point, residence and education have been discussed
separately. However, it is important to recognize that
interactions may exist. These interactions can arise
from (1) the effects of one variable on the other; (2)
the fact that education operates differently in various
environments; and (3) a combination of nonlinear effects
and different levels of education in different areas.

The first of these possibilities depends on whether
place of birth or place of current residence is used as
the residence variable. In the former case, the places
of birth, childhood, and adolescence can affect educational opportunities and thus determine educational
achievement; thus the total effect of place of birth on
fertility would have to include its effect through
educational achievement. If current residence is used,
education may affect residence through migration; thus

TABLE 2 Urbanization--the Intervening Variables Through
Which It Affects Fertility, and the Biases Introduced by
Including these Variables with Urbanization in Regression
Models

| Intervening Variable | Effect of Urbanization on ICV or IFV | Effect of ICV or IFV on Fertility | Bias in Estimating Residence's Effect if Controlling for ICV or IFV Without Adding Indirect Effects |
|---|---|---|---|
| **Intervening Community Variables (ICV)** | | | |
| Presence of family planning facilities | + | − | + |
| Presence of schools | + | − | + |
| Presence of health facilities | + | − | + |
| Demand for labor of | | | |
| Men | + | + | − |
| Women | + | − | + |
| Children | − | + | + |
| Housing costs | + | − | + |
| Food costs | + | − | + |
| Sociocultural milieu | + | − | + |
| Disease exposure | ? | − | ? |
| **Intervening Family Variables (IFV)** | | | |
| Income[a] | + | ? | ? |
| Female wage | + | − | + |
| Mass media | + | − | + |
| Knowledge of birth control | + | − | + |
| Access to birth control | + | − | + |
| Female labor participation[a] | + | ? | ? |
| Child labor participation[a] | − | + | + |
| Child schooling[a] | + | − | + |
| Child survival[a] | + | − | + |
| Cost of children | + | − | + |
| Benefits of children | − | + | + |
| Modernism | + | − | + |

[a]Endogenous variable.

education's effect would have to include its effect
through migration. (Migration is included in Table 1.
However, there is little evidence on whether migration
per se or residence before and after migration affects
fertility, although those who migrate from rural to urban
areas generally have lower fertility.)

The second of these possible interactions, the fact
that education operates differently in urban and rural
areas, has frequently been discussed, but with little
certainty. One possible interaction is through labor
markets. Increased education opens modern-sector
employment opportunities for women in urban areas; it
does not generally have this effect in rural areas. Of
course, migration would allow rural women to avail themselves of urban opportunities, but at higher cost than
that incurred by urban women.

Although such behavioral interactions between education
and residence are not precisely defined, a statistical
interaction clearly exists. The evidence that urban areas
have a different educational distribution from rural areas
is very convincing. In addition, it is fairly clear that
education's effect on fertility is nonlinear in some environments. Therefore, if linear estimates of education's
effect are made, that effect will appear different in
urban and rural areas; if the correct nonlinear specification is used and no other interactions exist, that effect
will not differ between urban and rural areas.

In addition to these considerations of interaction and
nonlinearity, there are problems of measurement. Both
education and residence can be measured as either dichotomous or continuous variables. It is much more common,
however, to use an urban/rural dichotomy for residence
than to use a literate/nonliterate dichotomy for education. Therefore, the measurement of education is usually
more detailed than that of residence. This point will be
raised in the following review of the literature on the
effects of education and residence on fertility.

## LITERATURE REVIEW

As noted earlier, only studies having a direct or indirect
age control will be included in the present review. This
review is also limited to studies having a minimum sample
size or degrees of freedom of over 150 in the relevant
age-residence group. Moreover, because of the nonlinearities noted above, studies based on regional aggregates
of data will not be included. Finally, if the same
methodology were used in all studies, the results would
be easy to summarize; however, studies differ substantially in how they analyze fertility determinants.
Therefore, this review will be restricted to studies in
which the dependent variable is a measure of completed
fertility, either children ever born or the total
fertility rate, and in which age or marital duration is
implicitly or explicitly used as a control.

The subsections below first review a study that uses a
common methodology to estimate the effects of education
and residence on fertility for several countries. This
study, prepared by Rodriguez and Cleland for the 1980
World Fertility Survey (WFS) Conference in London,
addresses the separate effects of education and residence,
as well as their interaction. Next, two other types of

studies of education's effect on fertility are examined:
Hermalin and Mason's meta analysis, and a number of multivariate studies within countries. Finally, two important
considerations in studying the effects of education and
residence on fertility are examined: the issue of the
stability of educational differentials over time, and
evidence on urban-rural differences in fertility.

## Comparative Analysis of WFS Data

The Rodriguez and Cleland paper (1980) is a comprehensive
report on the effects of education, residence and a number
of other explanatory variables on fertility for 22 countries in which WFS surveys have been conducted. This
paper is extremely useful in illustrating the points discussed above, as well as in quantifying the relationships
between education and residence and fertility.

Rodriguez and Cleland use regression analysis both to
create their primary dependent variable--marital
fertility--and to estimate the effects of education and
residence on fertility. The dependent variable is
constructed by estimating the effect of marital duration
and duration squared on fertility in the last 5 years
(weighted by exposure), and then predicting total
fertility over 25 years of marriage using the estimated
effects of duration. Thus the dependent variable, an
approximation of completed fertility based on recent
fertility, resembles the total fertility rate in its
characteristics.[7]

### Education

Rodriguez and Cleland estimate the effects of education
and other variables on fertility using dummy variables
and regression. Average marital fertility can be determined for every category of education (see Table 3).
Other variables can also be introduced, and average
marital fertility determined controlling for these
factors.

Table 3 shows the relationship between fertility and
the education of the wife (or woman) and that of the
husband. In Panel A, fertility is estimated, using total
fertility rates, for all women in the household; in Panel
B, only ever-married women are included, and fertility is
estimated at marital durations of 25 years. Before

TABLE 3   Effect of Education on Predicted Completed Fertility

| | Panel A. Total Fertility Rate (all women) | | | | Panel B. Adjusted for Marital Duration (ever-married women) | | | | | | | |
| | Woman's Education | | | | Wife's Education | | | | Husband's Education | | | |
| Country | No School | Lower Primary | Upper Primary | Secondary | No School | Lower Primary | Upper Primary | Secondary | No School | Lower Primary | Upper Primary | Secondary |
|---|---|---|---|---|---|---|---|---|---|---|---|---|
| Bangladesh | 6.2 | 6.5 | 6.9 | 5.0 | 6.2 | 6.6 | 7.1 | 6.1 | 6.0 | 6.9 | 6.6 | 6.8 |
| Fiji | -- | -- | -- | -- | 4.8 | 5.2 | 4.8 | 4.1 | 4.9 | 5.3 | 4.7 | 4.3 |
| Indonesia | -- | -- | -- | -- | 4.9 | 5.5 | 5.6 | 5.4 | 4.5 | 5.4 | 5.3 | 5.7 |
| Korea | 5.8 | 5.2 | 4.5 | 3.3 | 6.2 | 6.0 | 5.0 | 4.0 | 6.1 | 6.1 | 5.5 | 4.5 |
| Malaysia | 5.2 | 5.1 | 4.6 | 3.2 | 6.3 | 6.0 | 5.4 | 4.6 | 5.9 | 6.3 | 5.8 | 5.1 |
| Nepal | -- | -- | -- | -- | 6.1 | 6.5 | 6.1 | 2.8 | 6.1 | 5.4 | 6.2 | 5.4 |
| Pakistan | 6.6 | (5.9) | (5.7) | 3.6 | 7.0 | 6.7 | 7.1 | 5.8 | 7.0 | 6.6 | 7.3 | 6.8 |
| Philippines | 5.2 | 6.9 | 6.0 | 3.8 | 6.4 | 7.1 | 6.6 | 5.3 | 6.5 | 7.2 | 6.6 | 5.5 |
| Sri Lanka | -- | -- | -- | -- | 5.3 | 5.1 | 5.3 | 4.8 | 5.4 | 5.3 | 5.2 | 5.0 |
| Thailand | -- | -- | -- | -- | 5.5 | 5.7 | 5.3 | 3.6 | 5.1 | 6.8 | 5.5 | 4.0 |
| Colombia | 6.4 | 5.5 | 3.5 | 2.5 | 6.7 | 5.9 | 4.1 | 3.3 | 6.7 | 6.1 | 4.3 | 3.3 |
| Costa Rica | (4.9) | 4.5 | 3.3 | 2.7 | 5.2 | 4.5 | 3.4 | 3.3 | 4.7 | 4.5 | 3.6 | 3.3 |
| Dominican Republic | (6.6) | 6.4 | 4.1 | (2.3) | 6.9 | 6.7 | 4.9 | 3.7 | 6.6 | 7.1 | 5.1 | 3.5 |
| Guyana | -- | 5.4 | 5.3 | 4.0 | 6.0 | 5.1 | 4.8 | 4.4 | 4.6 | 5.3 | 5.0 | 3.9 |
| Jamaica | -- | 5.4 | 5.1 | 3.2 | 6.6 | 5.3 | 5.0 | 3.4 | 6.0 | 5.4 | 4.9 | 3.4 |
| Mexico | 7.6 | 6.6 | 4.7 | 3.3 | 7.4 | 7.2 | 5.5 | 4.6 | 7.6 | 7.2 | 5.9 | 4.7 |
| Panama | -- | 6.1 | 4.3 | 2.9 | 6.7 | 6.2 | 4.5 | 3.6 | 6.6 | 6.2 | 4.5 | 3.7 |
| Peru | 7.0 | 6.4 | 3.7 | 3.4 | 7.7 | 6.9 | 5.4 | 4.5 | 7.2 | 7.4 | 6.3 | 5.1 |
| Jordan | 9.2 | 6.8 | 5.4 | (3.6) | 9.3 | 7.7 | 6.7 | 5.6 | 9.3 | 9.1 | 7.9 | 6.8 |
| Kenya | 8.4 | 8.9 | 8.0 | 5.5 | 7.4 | 8.1 | 7.7 | 7.8 | 7.2 | 8.2 | 7.9 | 7.8 |
| Average of all available countries | 6.6 | 6.1 | 5.0 | 3.5 | 6.4 | 6.2 | 5.5 | 4.5 | 6.2 | 6.4 | 5.7 | 4.9 |
| Average for countries with data in Panel A only | 6.6 | 6.1 | 5.0 | 3.5 | 6.8 | 6.4 | 5.6 | 4.7 | 6.5 | 6.6 | 5.8 | 5.0 |

Note:  Dash indicates not available or n less than 250; parentheses denote n less than 500.

Source:  Rodriguez and Cleland (1980:Tables 4, 7, A-2).

reviewing the data in Panel B, it is important to determine if restricting the sample to ever-married women
causes any bias.  If education has an effect on age at
marriage, as many studies have shown, then this restriction, used in most fertility surveys, will result in an
underestimation of the effect of education on fertility.
Panel A offers some guidance in making this determination
because it includes education and total fertility data
for married and unmarried women combined.  On average,
the difference between the effects of education shown for
all women and only married women are substantial (compare
Panel A with the effects of wife's education in Panel
B).  Over the entire education range, the difference in
fertility is 3.1 when all women are included, but only
2.1 if only married women are included.[8]  Thus, a
priori, surveys of married women will tend to underestimate the effect of education on fertility substantially, depending on the importance of education in
determining age at marriage.  This point needs to be
considered in reviewing any comparative analysis of data
drawn from surveys of ever-married women.

These data for ever-married women show that the relationship between education and fertility is monotonically
inverse for women in Latin America; outside Latin America,
female education is monotonically related to fertility
only in Jordan, Korea, and Malaysia.  (Sri Lanka is a
marginal case.)  For males, the relationship is monotonic
only in five of the eight Latin American countries,
Jordan, and Sri Lanka.

This irregular relationship between female education
and fertility outside Latin America is not inconsistent
with the pattern found in Cochrane (1979).  The nonlinearities differ according to the education level at which
the highest fertility is observed, the regularity of the
increases and decreases in fertility on either side of
the peak, and the magnitude of the differences in fertility among those with no education and those with maximum
education.  In Sri Lanka and Pakistan, the overall pattern
is irregular, showing two peaks; in the other countries,
only one peak is evident, and the fertility differences
between the extreme education categories are typically at
least one-half a child.  Although these irregularities
defy simple description, they are sufficiently persistent
and based on adequately large samples that they cannot be
dismissed as mere flukes.

In an attempt to determine if such nonlinearities are
regionally determined or a function of development, some

additional analysis was done for this paper: literacy, urbanization, caloric intake, income, and total fertility rates were compared for countries with and without monotonic fertility-education relationships. Simple comparisons show that only for per capita income is there a clear separation between the two groups of countries: all countries with 1978 per capita income at or below $510 have a pattern of increased fertility with education prior to a decline; all countries with an income of $740 or above have monotonic inverse relationships.

However, income is not the only important variable for some very low-income countries, such as Sri Lanka, that have small increases in fertility, or for richer low-income countries, like the Philippines, that have large increases in fertility before a decline is observed. A test of the relative importance of variables in explaining the shape of the education-fertility relationship is shown in Table 4. The differences in fertility between particular levels of education were regressed on per capita income, the total fertility rate, urbanization (proportion urban), the literacy rate, and per capita calories. Urbanization is the most consistent variable explaining the differences in fertility between education groups. For the first four steps of education given in Table 4, the greater the degree of urbanization, the more likely it is that fertility will fall with each increment in education, and the larger these decreases will be. GNP behaves similarly for the differences between no schooling and upper primary, and between lower primary and upper primary. Caloric intake is also significant at these steps in education. Rather surprisingly, neither aggregate education (literacy) nor total fertility rate is significant in explaining the changes in fertility between particular levels of education. This suggests an important interaction between poverty (GNP and caloric intake) and urbanization and the effect of education on fertility. It is interesting to note that, for husband's education, urbanization and GNP have the same relationship as for wife's education; however, caloric intake, literacy, and total fertility rate have perverse signs. Of these, caloric intake is the most interesting in that it is significant in three equations.

In Cochrane (1979), it was shown that female education was much more likely than male education to be inversely related to fertility. This is confirmed in the WFS data by the unweighted average fertility for males and females in each education group. These average values, given at

TABLE 4  Relationship Between Fertility at Different Education Levels and Aggregate Characteristics

| | $F_{LP}-F_{NO}$ | $F_{UP}-F_{NO}$ | $F_S-F_{NO}$ | $F_{UP}-F_{LP}$ | $F_S-F_{LP}$ | $F_S-F_{UP}$ |
|---|---|---|---|---|---|---|
| **Wife's Education** | | | | | | |
| GNP | -- | -.002 (3.99) | -- | -.001 (2.60) | -- | -- |
| TFR | -- | -- | -- | -- | -- | -- |
| Urbanization | -.020 (1.98) | -.044 (5.53) | -.047 (2.31) | -.025 (2.95) | -- | -- |
| Literacy | -- | -- | -- | -- | -- | -- |
| Daily calories | -- | -.002 (2.83) | -- | -.002 (2.34) | -- | -- |
| Constant | -.0495 | -3.43 | -6.82 | -2.94 | -- | -- |
| $R^2$ | .39 | .88 | .38 | .67 | -- | -- |
| d.f. | 12 | 12 | 12 | 12 | -- | -- |
| **Husband's Education** | | | | | | |
| GNP | -- | -.001 (2.92) | -- | -.001 (3.24) | -- | -- |
| TFR | -- | .254 (2.03) | -- | -- | -- | -- |
| Urbanization | -.023 (2.39) | -.043 (5.57) | -.054 (3.77) | -.020 (2.95) | -.031 (2.35) | -- |
| Literary | .022 (2.25) | .017 (2.08) | -- | -- | -- | -- |
| Daily Calories | -- | .002 (2.90) | -- | .003 (4.63) | .003 (2.77) | -- |
| Constant | .555 | -4.49 | -4.62 | -4.99 | -- | -- |
| $R^2$ | .38 | .83 | .71 | .77 | .66 | -- |
| d.f. | 13 | 12 | 12 | 12 | 12 | -- |

Note:  The dependent variable is the difference in fertility between education groups:  those with lower primary school and no education ($F_{LP}-F_{NO}$), upper primary and no education ($F_{UP}-F_{NO}$), etc.  Only significant coefficients are shown; t values are in parentheses.

Source:  Regressions based on data in Table 3 and World Bank (1980).

the bottom of Table 3, show that there is a difference of
1.9 children over the education spectrum from no education
to secondary schooling for females, and a difference of
only 1.3 for males. In addition, males with some education have higher fertility on average than those with no
schooling--6.4 versus 6.2 (these values are reversed for
females). In considering the extent to which these differences accurately reflect the effect of education,
several adjustments need to be considered. Adjustments
for residence and for spouse's characteristics are
addressed by Rodriguez and Cleland, and are discussed in
the subsections below.


Residence

Table 5 summarizes Rodriguez and Cleland's urban-rural
fertility estimates. The difference between urban and
rural areas is greater for the data on all women (1.6
children) than for those on married women only (1.2).
This is similar to the finding for education. However,
the residential differential using either group of women
is smaller than the educational differential, perhaps
because residence is measured dichotomously, whereas
education is classified into four groups.
     A particularly interesting finding is that urban
fertility is always lower than rural fertility when all
women are included, but not when only married women are
sampled. In Bangladesh, Indonesia, and Pakistan, the
marital fertility of urban women is higher than that of
rural women. In Indonesia and Pakistan, this difference
is large, one-half a child. This implies that, particularly in these two countries, age at marriage is very
important in explaining residential differentials.
     Multivariate comparisons of urban-rural differences in
fertility, similar to those in Table 4 and using the same
variables, show that only the degree of urbanization is
significant. The higher the level of urbanization in a
country, the greater the difference between rural and
urban fertility. Findley and Orr (1978) also found the
percentage of the population urban significant in
explaining urban-rural differentials in fertility.[9]
These findings suggest that in countries with greater
degrees of urbanization, those classified as urban are
more likely to be from large cities where fertility is in
fact lower than in rural areas.

TABLE 5   Effect of Residence on Predicted Completed
Fertility

| Country | Total Fertility (all women) | | Marital Duration Adjusted (ever-married women) | |
|---|---|---|---|---|
| | Rural | Urban | Rural | Urban |
| Bangladesh | 6.2 | 6.0 | 6.3 | 6.5 |
| Fiji | 4.6 | 3.6 | 5.2 | 4.3 |
| Indonesia | 4.8 | 4.6 | 5.1 | 5.6 |
| Korea | 5.1 | 3.7 | 5.9 | 4.5 |
| Malaysia | -- | -- | 6.1 | 5.5 |
| Nepal | 6.2 | -- | -- | -- |
| Pakistan | 6.4 | 6.2 | 6.8 | 7.3 |
| Philippines | 6.0 | 3.9 | 6.8 | 5.4 |
| Sri Lanka | 3.8 | 3.2 | 5.3 | 4.8 |
| Thailand | 4.9 | 2.9 | 5.5 | 4.3 |
| Colombia | 6.6 | 3.5 | 7.2 | 4.2 |
| Costa Rica | 4.7 | 2.9 | 4.8 | 3.3 |
| Dominican Republic | 7.1 | 4.1 | 7.6 | 5.0 |
| Guyana | 5.1 | 4.3 | 5.1 | 4.1 |
| Jamaica | 5.3 | 3.9 | 5.4 | 4.1 |
| Mexico | 7.3 | 4.8 | 7.7 | 5.7 |
| Panama | 5.7 | 3.3 | 5.9 | 3.9 |
| Peru | 7.0 | 4.6 | 7.6 | 5.8 |
| Jordan | 9.8 | 7.1 | 9.7 | 8.5 |
| Kenya | 8.4 | 6.1 | 8.0 | 6.5 |
| Total | 6.0 | 4.4 | 6.4 | 5.2 |

Note:  Dash indicates not available.

Source:  Rodriguez and Cleland (1980).

## Interaction of Residence and Education

The question of interaction between residence and
education was also addressed by Rodriguez and Cleland.
Although they found that such interactions were not
statistically significant in most instances, their test
of interaction was not symmetrical for husband's and
wife's education.

Husband's education was adjusted for residence by the
inclusion in the regression of a dummy variable for
residence.  In many cases, there was no perceptible
difference in education's effect before and after this
adjustment.  In those cases where the interaction term

was significant, the residential adjustment reduced the impact of husband's education in all cases except Kenya, where education's effect became more positive, and in Guyana, where there was no change. Overall, the average (unweighted differential) before adjustment was -1.9; after adjustment the average was -0.85.

On the other hand, wife's education was adjusted not only for residence, but also for husband's characteristics (education, occupation, and work status).[10] These adjustments reduced female education's average effect from -1.9 to -0.955, making it less negative in most cases, although in one case (Indonesia), it made that effect negative rather than positive. Adjustment for residence seems desirable to estimate the "true effect" of education; however, adjustment for husband's work status and occupation is not desirable since these are at least partially the effect of the wife's education through assortive mating.

Residence's effect was also measured by Rodriguez and Cleland, adjusting for all other variables (husband's education, occupation, and work status, and wife's education and work status). Again, such adjustments generally reduced the effect of residence from an average of -1.2 to -0.66.

The effects of these various adjustments are summarized in Table 6. After controlling for other variables (some of which are endogenous to education, residence, or both), the effect of female education is still to reduce fertility by almost one child; the effect of male education is one-third as large; and the effect of urban residence is about two-thirds of a child. Although these figures support a strong negative effect of female education, this effect is not linear, as was noted above. After all other variables have been controlled, the difference in fertility for married women is only a tenth of a child between no and some primary education, and the negative effect increases thereafter. In contrast, the fertility of husbands with some primary education is one-third of a child larger than that of husbands with no education after controlling for all other factors, including residence, wife's education, and work status. Thus adjustment for other variables does not eliminate the nonlinear relationship between education and fertility.

TABLE 6  Differences in Predicted Completed Fertility Between Specific Education-Residence Groups

| | Wife's Education | | | Husband's Education | | | Residence |
|---|---|---|---|---|---|---|---|
| | $F_{LP}-F_{NO}$ | $F_{UP}-F_{NO}$ | $F_{S}-F_{NO}$ | $F_{LP}-F_{NO}$ | $F_{UP}-F_{NO}$ | $F_{S}-F_{NO}$ | $F_{U}-F_{R}$ |
| All women | -0.5 | -1.6 | -3.1 | -- | -- | -- | -1.6 |
| Married women | -0.2 | -0.9 | -1.9 | 0.0 | -0.5 | -1.3 | -1.2 |
| Controlling for residence | -- | -- | -- | 0.6 | -0.3 | -0.9 | -- |
| Plus husband's characteristics | -0.9 | -0.4 | -1.0 | -- | -- | -- | -- |
| Plus all other variables | -0.1 | -0.4 | -0.9 | 0.3 | 0.0 | -0.3 | -0.7 |

Source:  Summarized from Rodriguez and Cleland (1980) using unweighted averaging of results.

Other Studies of Education's Relationship to Fertility

Meta Analysis

Another study using WFS data from several countries was done by Hermalin and Mason (1980). This paper, which addressed strategies for comparative analysis of WFS data, used an approach falling between micro and macro analysis. Instead of using individual or countrywide data to estimate regressions between education and fertility, it used as the dependent variable the average fertility of women of various education and marital duration groups from WFS tabulations. The independent variables were education and marital duration, and their values were estimated by the approximate midpoints for each group.

Using these data points from WFS tabulations in each of 10 countries, Hermalin and Mason fitted a nonlinear model to the data. The model used was $\ln (P + .5) = a + bE + c \ln D$, where $P$ is parity, $D$ is duration, and $E$ is education.[11] This formulation implies that the higher the level of education, the stronger its effect. In all cases except Nepal, the coefficients for education were negative, although they varied in size from $-0.0077$ in Sri Lanka to $-0.04085$ in Panama and $+0.02531$ in Nepal. These variations in the effect of education were then studied at the national level to determine what macro characteristics affect the relationship between education and fertility.

The analysis most relevant to this review is that which relates the effect of education on fertility in a country, $B_1$, to that country's level of development and to characteristics of the education system. Generally, the more "modern" the country, the more negative was education's effect. Five correlations were significant at the 5 percent level for a two-tailed test: (1) 1957/58 per capita expenditures on education, in U.S. dollars; (2) percentage rural; (3) females in teacher training as a percentage of all students in teacher training, secondary and higher, 1960; (4) percentage of economically active females aged 14 to 65 in occupations other than agriculture in the early 1960s; and (5) females as a percentage of total school enrollment at first, second, and third levels. The most interesting finding is the robustness of the effect of the percentage rural:

We would conclude on the basis of the analysis thus far that the effect of education on fertility is weaker in more rural settings.  Whether this is due to the content of education or to the opportunity of individuals to use education remains to be studied and the general hypothesis needs to be further tested with more observations (Hermalin and Mason, 1980:116).

The summary of Hermalin and Mason's work presented here is very abbreviated.  However, it does illustrate the pattern of nonlinearity in the education-fertility relationship, as well as the interaction of education and residence.

## Multivariate Studies Within Countries

A great number of multivariate studies of fertility determinants have been done on micro data within countries. For this reason, the present discussion must be selective. For comparability, only studies using children ever born as the dependent variable and a sample size of over 150 will be included.  Estimates of both linear and nonlinear relationships between education and fertility will be examined.

The Appendix Table summarizes the results of 30 multivariate studies of the effect of education on fertility. These studies vary substantially in their methodology. However, in all cases but five, both husband's and wife's education are included, and most use linear estimation of the relationship between education and fertility.  Of these, 19 include husband's education.  In six cases, the relationship is negative and significant, whereas in two cases it is positive and significant; in the rest it is insignificant.  The two perverse cases are for a group of urban men in Brazil in 1960 and for 717 heads of household in Sierra Leone in 1966-67.

For women's education, 13 of the 26 estimates are negative and significant, and two cases are positive and significant.  The two atypical cases are the rural Laguna survey, in which a matching analysis of the same data revealed a negative significant value, and a rural Bangladesh sample of 265 women in 1968-69.  In the latter case, the positive relationship would be reduced from +0.13 to +0.03 if the effect of female education on child mortality and of child mortality on fertility were considered in the ordinary least squares estimates; it would

TABLE 7   Significance of Linear Estimates of the Effect of
Education on Fertility, by Methodology Used

Panel A.   Results by Sample Size

| | Sample Size | | | | | |
| | Under 300 | | 300-1,000 | | Over 1,000 | | |
| Statistical Significance | Male | Female | Male | Female | Male | Female | Total |
|---|---|---|---|---|---|---|---|
| Negative significant | 0 | 2 | 0 | 5 | 6 | 9 | 22 |
| Not significant | 5 | 5 | 6 | 2 | 5 | 7 | 30 |
| Positive significant | 1 | 2 | 0 | 1 | 1 | 0 | 5 |
| Percent negative significant | 0 | 29 | 0 | 63 | 50 | 56 | 39 |

Panel B.   Results by Inclusion of Age at Marriage in Regression

| | Age at Marriage Included | | | Age at Marriage not Included | | |
| Statistical Significance | Male | Female | Total | Male | Female | Total |
|---|---|---|---|---|---|---|
| Negative significant | 6 | 11 | 17 | 0 | 6 | 6 |
| Not significant | 9 | 10 | 19 | 7 | 4 | 11 |
| Positive significant | 1 | 1 | 2 | 1 | 1 | 2 |
| Percent negative significant | 38 | 50 | 45 | 0 | 55 | 32 |

be reduced from +0.42 to +0.26 if the mortality effect
were adjusted for in the two-stage least squares
estimates.[12]

These linear estimates can also be used for other
analyses. For example, Table 7 (Panel A) shows a very
clear relationship between sample size and significance:
for small samples (under 300) only 13 percent of the
results are negative and significant; for samples 300 to
1,000, 36 percent; and for samples over 1,000, 54 percent.

Another conclusion to be drawn relates to the effect
of controlling for age at marriage.[13]  Table 7 (Panel
B) shows that, if age at marriage is included, 45 percent

of the cases are inverse for males and females; if age at marriage is not included, none of the male and 55 percent of the female results are negative and significant. Thus inclusion of age at marriage has a different effect on the sign and significance for males and females.

To summarize, with the best methodology and the largest sample sizes, most studies show inverse results. However, even with the best methodology, the proportion of inverse results does not rise above 60 percent. This confirms what was suggested earlier: in an important number of cases, education is not monotonically, much less linearly, related to fertility.

In 11 studies, the authors explore the nonlinearity in the relationship between education and fertility. Anderson (1979) uses a semilog specification, four authors use a quadratic term, and six authors use dummy variables for various levels of education. To briefly summarize these results, Anderson's formulation showed that the negative impact of female but not male education increased as education rose. Studies using a quadratic specification find that fertility first increases with education and then decreases. The level of education with maximum fertility (obtained by solving for the maximum point on the quadratic curve) varies from 2.8 years in the Philippines to 10 in Sierra Leone. In studies using dummy variables for the different levels of education, the patterns observed vary among age groups and regions within countries. In general, the impact on fertility is more negative at higher education levels. In some cases, no level of female education has a significantly negative impact (women over 45 in Korea, landless households in India, urban households in Kenya, rural households in Egypt); in one case, education has a significantly positive effect (male primary education in rural Egypt). Part of this uneven pattern of significance may be due to small sample sizes in particular age and education groups.

It is not easy to get an overall picture of the education-fertility relationship from these studies. Averaging the coefficients is inappropriate because of the nonlinearity of the relationship. In addition, given the variety of methodologies used, most estimates are "biased" in one direction or another from some ideal effect. To explore the true relationship further in a multivariate context would require some explicit causal modeling of the channels through which education acts. Mason and Palan (1980) have done this for Malaysia, and Smock (1980:87) for Kenya. Both studies show that, as

more channels are included, the direct effect of education
diminishes to zero; however, neither goes through the
final step of adding up the effect of education through
various channels.

Several papers have carried out rather complete path
analyses of fertility. Loebner and Driver (1973) have
done such a study with data from Central India. In this
study, although neither husband's nor wife's education
was directly related to children ever born, both affect
fertility indirectly. Husband's education operates
through occupation (0.267), husband's income (0.275),
wife's age at marriage (0.130), family structure (0.131),
and absence of husband and wife (-0.12 and 0.08). Among
these, only age at marriage affects fertility (0.052);
therefore, husband's education has a small indirect positive path of 0.130 x 0.052 = 0.0068. The path between
wife's education and fertility is more tortuous: direct
through age at marriage 0.191 x 0.052 = 0.0099, and more
indirect through marriage duration 0.191 x -0.272 x 1.032
x 0.721 = -0.0387. Thus the net effect of female education through these indirect paths is -0.0288.

Another study traces the effects of education on
current fertility (rather than children ever born) for a
sample of Colombian women (Chi and Harris, 1979). The
analysis is done separately for women of zero parity,
parities one to three, and parities of four or more. The
direct effects of education are not significant for those
of zero parity, -0.109 for those of parities one to three,
and -0.099 for those of higher parities; the indirect
effects are +0.025, -0.001, and -0.062 for the three
groups. Thus the total effects are +0.025, -0.110, and
-0.161, respectively. The principle channels through
which education acts indirectly are spouses' discussion
about family size; contraceptive attitudes, knowledge,
and use; and infant mortality experiences. This study
illustrates the shift in education's effects as family
size increases, as well as the importance of indirect
effects.


## Other Considerations

### Stability of Educational Differentials Over Time

It is important to determine the stability of educational
differentials in fertility across time. Unfortunately,
in very few countries is this possible. Many censuses do

not report fertility differentials by education controlling for age; even more rarely are there two such censuses
for one country.  Since most WFS data are standardized by
marital duration rather than age, the educational differentials cannot be directly compared with census data.

Three countries do provide data of this kind:  the
Philippines, 1968 and 1973; Jordan, 1972 and 1976; and
Egypt, 1960 and 1976.  The results of these comparisons
are given in Table 8, showing that education has a more
negative effect on fertility at the later point in all
three cases.  Although this is a very small amount of
evidence, it does seem to be confirmed by much more
tenuous comparisons of census (age) data with duration
data from comparable WFS surveys.[14]  Comparisons of
CELADE data with WFS data for urban areas (or specifically
for city or metropolitan areas where available) also
confirm this pattern if women 25-44 are compared with
women of all marital durations in the WFS.  Any attempt
at a finer breakdown (women 35-44 and durations 10-19 and
20-29), yields confirmation for the longer durations
only.[15]

Although these data are suggestive, retabulation of
WFS data by age would considerably increase our ability
to make these comparisons across time.  This would permit
testing of the hypothesis that education's impact increases over time until fertility is relatively low, at
which point the absolute but not the relative differentials decrease.


Other Evidence on Urban-Rural Differences in Fertility

A number of country-specific studies specifically address
or indirectly control for residence in the analysis of
fertility.  In addition to these studies and the WFS data
used by Rodriguez and Cleland, there have been a number
of other fairly comprehensive studies of urban and rural
differences in fertility.

Kuznets (1974) reviewed data on urban-rural variations
in fertility for the late 1950s and early 1960s, and
Findley and Orr (1978) reviewed data from the period
around 1970.  These two studies use different methodologies, though they do share two similarities:  (1) they
examine the fertility of all, not just married, women;
and (2) they introduce no controls except for age.
Although differences in methodology prevent close comparison, these studies agree on some points that give
considerable insight into urban-rural variations.

TABLE 8   Relationship Between Education and Fertility at
Two Points in Time:   The Philippines, Egypt, and Jordan

Panel A.   Philippines, Children Ever Born to Women 40-44 (ESCAP, 1978)

| Education | CEB 1968 | Percentage Difference from CEB of Uneducated | CEB 1973 | Percentage Difference from CEB of Uneducated |
|-----------|----------|----------------------------------------------|----------|----------------------------------------------|
| No school | 6.11 |        | 6.85 |        |
| 1-4 years | 6.49 | +6.0   | 7.04 | +2.8   |
| 5-7 years | 6.77 | +10.8  | 6.75 | -1.5   |
| High school | 5.93 | -2.9 | 6.09 | -11.1  |
| College | 4.27 | -30.1   | 4.57 | -33.0  |

Panel B.   Egypt, Standardized Average Parity (World Bank, 1981)

| Education | Parity 1960 | Percentage Difference from Parity of Uneducated | Parity 1976 | Percentage Difference from Parity of Uneducated |
|-----------|-------------|-------------------------------------------------|-------------|-------------------------------------------------|
| Illiterate | 4.21 |       | 4.21 |        |
| Read and write | 4.53 | +7.6 | 4.37 | +4.2 |
| Elementary | 4.26 | +1.2 | 3.66 | -13.1 |
| Secondary | 3.59 | -14.7 | 2.80 | -33.5 |

Panel C.   Jordan, Children Ever Born Among Women Married over 20 Years
(Rizk, 1977; Jordan WFS, 1979)

| Education | CEB 1972 | Percentage Difference from CEB of Uneducated | CEB 1976 | Percentage Difference from CEB of Uneducated |
|-----------|----------|----------------------------------------------|----------|----------------------------------------------|
| Illiterate | 8.79 |       | 9.00 |        |
| Primary and secondary | 7.86 | -10.6 | 7.23 | -19.7 |
| Secondary+ | 4.70 | -46.5 | 4.50 | -50.0 |

Findley and Orr found that the average total fertility rate was 4.95 for urban areas and 6.35 for rural areas, yielding a difference of 1.4 and a ratio of 1.28. This absolute difference falls between the two estimates found using data from Rodriguez and Cleland,[16] but the ratio of fertility rates indicates much larger differences than those found by Kuznets. Kuznets found a ratio of 1.09 for developing countries as a whole, this ratio varying from 1.03 for sub-Saharan Africa to 1.12 for Asia and 1.15 for Latin America. At least some of the contrast with Findley and Orr is due to differences in methodology. Kuznets used children under 5 per 1,000 women of reproductive age as his measure of fertility. Using this measure, differences between urban and rural areas would result from differences not only in fertility, but also in age structure and child mortality, although it is possible that these latter two factors cancel each other out somewhat. To the extent that Kuznets' results are accurate for the period around 1960, it is also quite possible that urban and rural differences in fertility widened over the decade. Further support for a widening gap is found in the fact that, in Western Europe, residential differences widened during the period of fertility decline and then began to narrow in the post-World War II period (United Nations, 1973:97).

Additional findings of interest from these two studies concern regional differences. Findley and Orr found that the larger the city, the lower the level of fertility in Asia and Latin America; however, this relationship did not hold for Africa. Kuznets found greater urban-rural differences in Latin America than elsewhere in the developing world, whereas in Africa urban fertility was in some cases higher than rural. This pattern can be checked against the Findley and Orr data from the 1970s, showing that African differentials (1.29-1.39) are midway between those of Latin America (1.56-1.43) and Asia (1.20-1.12). This change in pattern may arise from differences in measurement, actual changes in differentials, or the effect of selecting particular countries for study. Unfortunately, the latter point can not be checked on a country-by-country basis since Kuznets did not report country-specific data. These varying results may also arise not from regional factors per se, but from differences in the degree or pattern of urbanization in different regions. Thus one must interpret these regional patterns cautiously.

Relatively little insight into the effect of urbanization on fertility is gained from the multiple regression studies reviewed above (see the Appendix Table) since they were not designed for that purpose. Only 11 of the 26 studies include residence or a proxy in their analysis.[17] In these studies, significant negative effects of urbanization are shown in five cases and positive significant effects in one; the rest are insignificant. Given the relatively small number of cases, it is impossible to derive patterns of significance and nonsignificance from these data.

On the other hand, three multivariate studies yield some insight into the channels through which residence operates. A study of Costa Rica by Michielutte et al. (1975) shows that adding other variables (education, income, age at first conception, and church attendance) significantly reduces the effect of residence. Of these variables, the addition of income has the greatest effect on the association, reducing the correlation coefficient from $-0.32$ to $-0.24$; no other variable had an effect even a third this size. Ketkar's (1979) study also shows that fairly large urban-rural differentials in fertility (0.85) are reduced to statistical insignificance when income, education, infant mortality, size of extended family, religion, and occupation are added to a regression. The Loebner and Driver (1973) path analysis of fertility in India examines residence as well as education and shows no direct effect of residence. Although residence affects husband's income, family structure, and education, its only indirect effects on fertility are those through education, which is itself an indirect effect. Residence's effect is thus much smaller than education's. It is somewhat surprising that residence does not have an effect more directly through age at marriage; however, for this particular sample, no significant effect of this kind exists. On the other hand, this sample is perhaps atypical in that even the zero-order correlations between residence and children ever born are very small (0.039).

There are other studies giving some fragmentary evidence on the channels through which urbanization may operate. However, it seems more efficient to examine broader issues in addressing the effects of changing socioeconomic circumstances on fertility. The propositions below summarize these issues.

PROPOSITIONS

## Education and Fertility

1. The effects of education on fertility vary according to whether male or female education is considered and whether all or only married women are included, and with the degree of urbanization.

2. A major effect of education on fertility is through age at marriage; thus the observed negative effect of education on fertility is smaller in samples including only ever-married women than in those including both married and unmarried women.

3. Monotonic inverse relationships between education and fertility are much less likely to be observed in countries having low levels of urbanization, per capita income, and daily caloric intake. Of these three factors, urbanization appears to be the most important. This may explain the stronger observed negative relationship between education and fertility in Latin American than in Asia.

4. Female education is more often inversely related to fertility than is male education: the negative effect across the total range of female education is about three times greater than that of male education after adjusting for many other factors, including spouse's education, occupation, and residence. Male education at low levels is more likely to be positively related to fertility than is female education; however, this may well reflect a positive income effect of education since income is more closely related to male than to female education.

5. In multiple regression studies, the observed magnitude of the relationship between education and fertility is highly dependent on whether or not the regression equation includes variables through which education operates. Although several recent studies have illustrated this by including these variables, the relative importance of the different channels is still unclear and probably varies among countries.

6. The cross-section effect of education on fertility is more negative at later than at earlier points in time, at least until fertility levels become very low. This topic needs more research, which would be facilitated by a simple retabulation of WFS data in more comparable form to those of earlier surveys and censuses. In addition to comparing differentials at various points in time, research should attempt to determine what aggregate factors,

such as development or income growth, affect the changes in differentials over time.

7.  Reanalysis of the Value of Children data could provide insight into the extent to which education's effect operates through differential values.

## Residence and Fertility

8.  Differences in fertility between urban and rural areas are smaller than those between the least and most educated; however, this may result from the dichotomous classification of residence and may thus be an artifact.

9.  The greater the degree of urbanization in a country, the greater the urban-rural differences in fertility. This may arise in part from measurement problems since, as urbanization increases, those classified as urban generally come from larger cities.

10.  The mechanisms through which residence operates are less clear than those through which education operates.  The former are more difficult to identify because of the need to separate out factors specific to location (place factors), as well as those specific to individuals and themselves correlated with place factors.  The WFS analysis of such community variables as access to markets and average education levels offers some hope of eventually disentangling these channels; reanalysis of Value of Children data could also provide insight into the extent to which residence operates through the perceived costs and benefits of children.

### NOTES

1.  For example, if education affects age at marriage, then the inclusion of age at marriage (M) in a regression between age-controlled fertility (F) and education (E) will have the following bias. Let $F = a + bE + cM$ and $M = d + eE$. The effect of education on fertility cannot be measured by b alone, but must be measured by $b + ec$. If c is negative and e is positive, then the coefficient of b will be biased upward. This explains the plus in column 3 of Table 1.

2.  Including age and marital duration is equivalent to including age at marriage; this will cause a positive bias in the education coefficient.

3.  It is interesting to note that in no case was husband's education the most important variable in reducing the negative effect of wife's education, and that, for rural Malays, controlling for husband's education had the most important impact on increasing the negative effect of wife's education.
4.  Studies using the total education of husband and wife introduce other problems--such as nonlinearities and the differential effects of husband's and wife's education.
5.  Two solutions to the problem of variables determined simultaneously with fertility are two-stage least squares and reduced-form equations.
6.  Other background variables, such as religion, caste, and parental status and education, cause less well-defined problems because the direction of bias depends on the effect of the background variable on education and fertility.
7.  Therefore, in countries where the timing of fertility is undergoing significant change, these variables will be an inaccurrate reflection of completed fertility.
8.  The value obtained for countries in which both estimates are available is 2.1; for all countries, the average difference is 1.9 for married women.
9.  Rather surprisingly, Findley and Orr also found that the percentage of the population in small cities (under 20,000) was significantly related to larger urban-rural differentials.
10. Rodriguez and Cleland give no explanation for the asymmetrical treatment of male and female education in this respect.
11. This description glosses over very detailed, careful discussions of the measurement of the variables and the choice of model specification.
12. If income or wealth is controlled, female education is significantly inverse to fertility in 46 percent of the cases, and male education in 29 percent. If there is no control for income or wealth, female education is inversely related 58 percent of the time and male education 20 percent. If wealth, income, or husband's education is controlled, wife's education is inversely related in 49 percent of the cases.
13. If age and marital duration are both in the equation, this is equivalent to including age at marriage.

APPENDIX TABLE   Multivariate Studies of Education and Children Ever Born in Developing Countries, by Region

| Region and Study | Sample: Location, Year, Size | Estimation Technique | Education Measure | Education's Effect and Significance (t values in parentheses) [elasticities in brackets] | Other Variables Included (sign if significant) | Comments |
|---|---|---|---|---|---|---|
| **LATIN AMERICA** | | | | | | |
| Iutaka et al., 1971 | Brazil (1959-60) 1,280 urban males | OLS | Husband's levels | .077 (2.46) | Age +, age at marriage -, city size +, migratory status +, color -, social status +, father-in-law's status +, father's status. | Major bias due to inclusion of age at marriage and social status. |
| Kogut, 1974 | Brazil (1960 census) 2,083 NE 3,287 S 2,872 E | OLS | Years | HE              WE<br>-.088 (2.93)   -.035 (0.87)<br>-.065 (5.66)   -.030 (1.84)<br>-.059 (3.85)   -.058 (2.68) | Age -, marital duration +, income (varying sign), type of marriage consensual - (NE and S), rural +, suburban. | Major bias due to marital duration, which affects the coefficient of wife's education more than husband's.[a] |
| Davidson, 1973 | Mexico Mexico City (1963-64) 269 women 35-39 | Step-wise | Wife's years | -.096 (0.80) | Age at marriage -, desired number of children +. | Age at marriage causes education to be underestimated, as does desired size. Author recognizes former effect in text. |
|  | Venezuela Caracas (1963-64) 192 women 35-39 | Step-wise | Wife's years | -.101 (0.76) | Age at marriage -, desired number of children +, wife's work status, husband's occupation. |  |
| Michielutte et al., 1975 | Costa Rica (n.d.) 292 women 35-49 (clinic and control) | OLS | Wife's years | -.38[b] | Residence -, income, church attendance -, age at first conception -. | Bias probably introduced by age at first contraceptive use; also perhaps by sample design. |

616

| Study | Method | Variable | HE | WE | Effects | Notes |
|---|---|---|---|---|---|---|
| Stycos, 1980 | Costa Rica (1978) 966 women over 35 | OLS | Wife's years | -.16[b] | | Years married +, mass information -, modern psychology. | Since mass information depends on education, education is underestimated. Adjustment not possible with given data. |
| | Sterilized<br>No (550)<br>Yes (267) | | | HE<br>-.05<br>.00 | WE<br>-.05<br>-.17[b] | Years since union +, consumer durables -, siblings +, urban church attendance +, work history, parent's education, current work. | No residence control. |
| Anderson, 1979 | Guatemala (1974-75) 657 households | OLS (in CEB) | Years | HE<br>-.008 (1.00)<br>[-.021] | WE<br>-.029 (3.22)<br>[-.054] | Wealth, location, wife's age +. | Does not include imputed wage for husband.[c] |

EAST ASIA

| Study | Method | Variable | HE | WE | Effects | Notes |
|---|---|---|---|---|---|---|
| Kiranandana, 1977 | Thailand (1969-70) 1,546 women 478 rural 1,068 urban | OLS | Levels | HE<br>-.155 (4.05)<br>-.097 (0.95)<br>-.162 (4.09) | WE<br>-.059 (1.31)<br>.049 (0.43)<br>-.073 (1.70) | Age +, marital duration +, ideal family size +, contraceptive use +, proportion dying +, proportion male +, (urban) -.[d] | If husband's education is deleted, wife's is negative and highly significant. |
| Lee et al., 1978 | Korea (1971) 2,334 women 35-49 | OLS | Age 35-39<br>0<br>7-9<br>10-12<br>12+ | HE<br>0.29(2.17)<br>-0.08(0.66)<br>-0.22(1.79)<br>-0.26(1.47) | WE<br>0.23(2.27)<br>-0.52(3.58)<br>-0.64(3.17)<br>-0.45(0.88) | Mortality +, mortality squared -, surviving sons -, wife urban -, modern objects owned, family structure, children in agriculture, children in nonagriculture +, regional mortality, children enrolled, children under 6 +, regional unemployment, demand for female labor, husband's unemployment. | Education underestimated due to the inclusion of mortality, child enrollment, and employment. |
| | | | Age 40-44<br>0<br>7-9<br>10-12<br>12+ | 0.01(0.07)<br>-0.20(1.10)<br>-0.17(0.77)<br>-0.18(0.56) | 0.39(2.51)<br>0.08(0.28)<br>-1.07(3.00)<br>-0.95(1.41) | | |
| | | | Age 45-49<br>0<br>7-9<br>10-12<br>12+ | -0.36(1.59)<br>-1.15(3.87)<br>-0.31(0.79)<br>-0.96(1.99) | 0.20(0.84)<br>0.05(0.10)<br>-0.24(0.45)<br>-0.85(0.69) | | |

| Region and Study | Sample: Location Year, Size | Estimation Technique | Education Measure | Education's Effect and Significance (t values in parentheses) [elasticities in brackets] | Other Variables Included (sign if significant) | Comments |
|---|---|---|---|---|---|---|
| Mason and Palan, 1980 | Malaysia (1974) 6,147 | OLS | Years, Race: Malay, Chinese, Other, Malay | Urban: $E$ .095, -.117b, -.180b, $E^2$ -.015b; Rural: $E$ .127, -.096b, .034, $E^2$ -.016b | Age, marital duration. | Biased due to marital duration, but see text for expanded discussion. |
| Chernichovsky and Meesook, 1980 | Indonesia (1976) 60,000 households | OLS | Wife: Elementary, Jr. Hi. Voc., Jr. Hi. Gen., Sr. Hi. Voc., Sr. Hi. + | Java-Bali: -.076(1.79) [-2.0], .023(0.16), -.133(1.38), -.479(3.61), -.960(7.92); Outer Islands: .083(1.75) [1.9], .061(0.44), -.313(3.42), -.663(4.70), -.888(6.72) | Age +, age at marriage -, marital status -, religion, work in home +, work outside +, modern durables -, household expenditure +, expenditure squared -, knows contraception +, rural - (Java-Bali). | Education's effect probably biased positively by age at marriage, but knows contraception has a perverse sign, as does work outside the home. Thus overall direction of bias is unclear. |
| Encarnacion, 1974 | Philippines (1968 NDS) 3,629 women under 50 | OLS | Wife's years | $WE$ = .214(3.05)e, $WE^2$ = -.040(3.56) | Age at marriage -, duration (nonlinear), family income (nonlinear) +/-. | Biased due to inclusion of age at marriage. |
| Rosenzweig, 1978 | Philippines (1968 NDS) 1,830 women 35-49 | OLS | Years | $HE$ = .022(0.65), $WE$ = -.091(3.51) | Age of husband +, age of wife +, child wage +, regional infant mortality +, religion, contraceptive knowledge, predicted husband's wage, farm. | Husband's education may be biased slightly due to predicted wage; wife's education may be biased due to contraceptive knowledge. |
| Banskota and Evenson, in press | Philippines Laguna (1977) 320 rural households | OLS | Years | $HE$ = -.049(1.43), $WE$ = .172(3.31) | Infant deaths +, 1963 husband's wage, predicted wife's wage -, predicted child wage +, full income, land, home technology -, year married -, father's farm background +, mother's farm background, mother's nonfarm. | Compare results with next study. This specification has far more variables endogenous with respect to education so results are more biased. |

| Study | Sample | Method | Education measure | Coefficients | Other variables | Comments |
|---|---|---|---|---|---|---|
| Navera, 1978 (in Evenson et al., 1979) | Philippines Laguna (1977) 320 rural households | OLS | Years | HE = -.131(1.58)<br>WE = -.182(2.07) | Wife's age at marriage, duration of marriage +, household income, wealth. | Wife's education underestimated due to age at marriage and duration. |

## SOUTH ASIA

| Study | Sample | Method | Education measure | Coefficients | Other variables | Comments |
|---|---|---|---|---|---|---|
| Chernichovsky, forthcoming | India (1968-69) 213 rural households (one village) | OLS | Husband's years<br>Wife's literacy | HE = .058(0.85)<br>WE = .341(0.952) | Log mother's age +, age at marriage -, agricultural income +, unskilled income +, skilled income -. | Wife's education biased positively by age at marriage; husband's education biased downward due to effect of his education on income. |
| Sarma, 1977 | India (1970-71) 1,111 landed households 505 landless | OLS | Wife<br>Some primary<br>Above primary<br>Matriculated<br>Husband<br>Primary or above | Landed<br>-.247(0.89) [-.0029]<br>-.599(1.66) [-.0040]<br>-1.44 (2.57) [-.0039]<br>.95 (6.90) [.1401]<br><br>Landless<br>-.165(0.48) [-.0038]<br>-.431(0.82) [-.0036]<br>-.464(0.72) [-.0026]<br>1.19 (5.36) [.1726] | Age of wife +/0, child death rate +/+, value of livestock, cultivated area +, intensive development program, health center in village +/+, school in village, factory in village, household electricity -/0, distance to town 0/-, value of farm instruments | Careful effort to exclude endogenous variables. However, if education affects landownership, some selectivity bias may exist. |
| Chaudhury, 1977 | Bangladesh Dacca (n.d.) 1,130 women | OLS | Years<br>1-5<br>6-9<br>Secondary<br>BA<br>MA | HE<br>-1.03 (2.60)<br>-0.64 (1.22)<br>-0.548(1.00)<br>-0.446(0.78)<br>-0.39 (0.67)<br><br>WE<br>-0.675(2.05)<br>-0.953(3.32)<br>-1.25 (5.04)<br>-1.50 (5.56)<br>-1.83 (6.67) | Duration of marriage, age at marriage, labor force status, income, exposure to mass media.f | Husband's, wife's education entered separately. Underestimates wife's education due to inclusion of age at marriage. |
| Khan, 1979 | Bangladesh (1968-69) 265 rural women 35-49 who want no more children | OLS | Years | HE = -.06 (1.00)<br>WE = .13 (2.17) | (Dead children) +/+, (montly income) +/+, (wife worked), land owned -/0, income adequacy -/-, age of wife, aware of family planning, nuclear family, age of wife at marriage 0/+, education of children +/0.d | See comments on next study. |

619

APPENDIX TABLE (continued)

| Region and Study | Sample: Location, Year, Size | Esti-mation Tech-nique | Education Measure | Education's Effect and Significance (t values in parentheses) [elasticities in brackets] | Other Variables Included (sign if significant) | Comments |
|---|---|---|---|---|---|---|
| Khan and Sirageldin, 1979 | Pakistan (1968-69) 269 women 35-49 who want no more children | TSLS | Husband's years Wife's literacy | HE = .04(0.10)<br>WE = -.48(0.68) | (Number of dead children) -, (income), (wife worked) -, urban +, nuclear +, land owned -, house owned +, wife's age +, age at marriage -, know of family planning -, income adequacy -, education of children -.d | Wife's education underestimated due to other variables. Also possible bias due to selection of those who want no more children. See text. |
| De Tray, 1979 | Pakistan (1968-69) 861 women 35-49 | OLS | Years | HE = .38(2.00)<br>HE² = -.09(2.10)<br>WE = -.33(3.30) | Electricity +, house type +, rural, wife born urban, current age +, mortality +. | Only child mortality is likely to bias results. |
| Afzal et al., 1976 | Pakistan Lahore (1973) 674 women | OLS | Levels | HE = -.037 (0.87)<br>WE = -.234 (3.68) | Mortality rate, age of mother, marital duration +. | Age and marital duration are implicit control for age at marriage and bias may exist. |
| Sathar, 1979 | Pakistan (1975) 4,949 women 15-49 | OLS | Years<br>Total<br>Urban<br>Rural | HE_____ WE<br>-.017(2.10)  -.058(3.85)<br>-.022(1.83)  -.052(2.83)<br>-.012(0.99)  -.070(2.07) | Age +, age squared -, age at marriage -, mortality +, use of contraception +. | Wife's education probably underesti-mated due to age at marriage, mortality, and use of contraception. |
| MIDDLE EAST |  |  |  |  |  |  |
| Zurayk, 1977 | Lebanon (1976) 16 villages 1,050 women 15-44 | OLS | Levels | HE = -.08(1.82)<br>WE = -.06(2.73) | Duration of marriage +, number of child deaths +, religion -. | Education's effect probably underesti-mated due to mortality. |
| Kelley et al., 1980 | Egypt (n.d.) 3,812 rural households | OLS | Wife<br>Some primary (19%)<br>Primary + ( 4%)<br>Husband<br>Some primary (23%)<br>Comp. primary (6%) | .05(0.71)<br>.02(0.15)<br><br>.16(2.48)<br>.15(1.35) | Wife's age +, age squared -, age at marriage -, electricity +, child death +, personal assets, real assets +. | Age at first marriage and child deaths cause educa-tion coefficient to be biased. |

| Snyder, 1974 | Sierra Leone (1966-68) 228 women 35-49 | OLS | Levels | HE = .21(3.71) WE = -.19(2.17) HE = .19(1.56) WE = -.19(1.40) | Wife's working age, child survival -, age +. Wife's wage if working, labor participation, survival of children -, age, age squared -, child education. | Probable bias upward by child survival. |
|---|---|---|---|---|---|---|
| Ketkar, 1978  1979 | Sierra Leone (1966-68) 1,999 women | OLS | Years | HE = .016(1.11) WE = -.011(0.61) $WE_2$ = .06 (1.03) $WE^2$ = -.006(1.17) | Wife's age +, number of adult females +, community infant mortality +, religion, residence, occupation, migration. | Careful use of reduced form. |
| Knowles and Anker, 1975 | Kenya (1974) 1,073 women | OLS | Years | WE = .0256(0.697) | Years married +, urban -, nonfarm employment +, breastfeeding, household income, land owned +, other wife, community family planning. | None of the independent variables that are dependent on education are significant. |
| Kelley et al., 1980 | Kenya (n.d.) 401 urban nuclear households | OLS | Husband Comp. primary Secondary Wife Comp. primary Secondary | -0.32(-0.67) -2.82( 1.83)  -0.29 (0.70) -3.88(2.72) | Child death +, income +, age +. | Probable bias due to child deaths, but female education is not significant in child death equation. |

|  | NE | S | E |
|---|---|---|---|
| Husband's | .144 | .214 | .244 |
| Wife's | .325 | .322 | .305 |

[a]Age at marriage is highly dependent on education, but more dependent on wife's education. The coefficients of husband's and wife's education on age at marriage in each region are shown below:

All values are highly significant, but adjustment of education coefficients is not possible given the specification.

[b]t values not reported, but result is significant at 5 percent level.

[c]This is the third specification. With an imputed wage added, husband's education has a positive coefficient and is marginally significant if the imputed wage is a reservation wage. In another paper, the author also used an imputed wage for the wife. In that case, wife's education had a value of -0.956, but a t value of only 1.55 (Anderson, 1978:146).

[d]Variables in parentheses are endogenous.

[e]This is not the regression equation focused on by Encarnacion. His focus was on a more complex equation (p. 125) which uses a threshold treatment. That treatment confirms the above: at low levels of education, there is a positive effect of education; at high levels, there is a negative effect. The threshold value is 2.75 years.

[f]Significance not reported for any of these variables.

14.     The approximate comparisons are as follows:   for
        Kenya, women 45-49 in 1962 and over 45 in 1977-78;
        for Indonesia, women 45-49 in 1971 and marital
        duration over 20 in 1976; and for Malaysia, women
        35-44 in 1966-67 and duration over 20 in 1974.
15.     This is not surprising since in most cases, the
        negative impact of education increases over the
        life cycle.
16.     For all women, the average difference was 1.6 and
        for ever-married women 1.2.
17.     Many control for residence by having samples
        restricted to urban or rural areas.

## BIBLIOGRAPHY

Afzal, M., Z. Khan, and N. A. Chaudhry (1976)  Age at
    marriage, fertility and infant-child mortality in a
    Lahore suburb.  Part I, Pakistan Development Review
    15(1):90-109.  Part II, Pakistan Development Review
    15(2):195-210.

Aghajanian, A. (1979)  The relationship of income and
    consumption of modern goods to fertility:  A study of
    working class families in Iran.  Journal of Biosocial
    Science 11:219-226.

Anderson, K. H. (1978)  The Effect of Child Mortality on
    the Quantity and Quality of Children in Guatemala.
    Unpublished Ph.D dissertation.  North Carolina State
    University, Raleigh, N.C.

Anderson, K. H. (1979)  Determination of Fertility, Child
    Quality, and Child Survival in Guatemala.  Economic
    Growth Center Discussion Paper No. 332.  Yale
    University, New Haven, Conn.

Banskota, K., and R. E. Evenson (in press)  Fertility,
    schooling and home technology in rural Philippines
    households.  Philippine Economic Journal.

Bulatao, R. A. (1975)  The Value of Children:
    Philippines, Vol. 2.  Honolulu:  East-West Population
    Institute.

Buripakdi, C. (1977)  The Value of Children:  Thailand,
    Vol. 4.  Honolulu:  East-West Population Institute.

CELADE and CFSC (1972)  Fertility and Family Planning in
    Metropolitan Latin American.  Community and Family
    Study Center, University of Chicago.

Chaudhury, R. H. (1977)  Education and fertility in
    Bangladesh.  Bangladesh Development Studies 5:81-110.

Chernichovsky, D. (forthcoming)  Fertility behavior in developing economies:  An investment approach.  In J. L. Simon and P. Lindert, eds., Research in Population Economics.  Greenwich, Conn.:  JAI Press.

Chernichovsky, D., and O. A. Meesook (1980)  Regional Aspects of Family Planning and Fertility Behavior in Indonesia.  World Bank Mimeo.  World Bank, Washington, D.C.

Chi, P. S. K., and R. J. Harris (1979)  An integrated model of fertility:  A multivariate analysis of fertility differentials in Colombia.  Canadian Studies in Population 6:111-125.

Cochrane, S. H. (1979) Fertility and Education:  What do we Really Know?  Baltimore, Md.:  The Johns Hopkins University Press.

Davidson, M. (1973)  A comparative study of fertility in Mexico City and Caracas.  Social Biology 20:460-472.

De Tray, D. (1979)  The demand for children in a "natural fertility" population.  Pakistan Development Review 18:55-67.

Encarnacion, J., Jr. (1974)  Fertility and labor force participation:  Philippines 1968.  Philippine Review of Business and Economics 11:113-144.

ESCAP (Economic and Social Commission for Asia and the Pacific) (1978)  Population of the Philippines.  ESCAP Country Monograph Series No. 5.  Bangkok:  United Nations.

Evenson, R. E., B. M. Popkin, and E. King-Quizon (1979) Nutrition, Work, and Demographic Behavior in Rural Philippine Households:  A Synopsis of Several Laguna Household Studies.  Economic Growth Center Discussion Paper No. 308.  Yale University.

Findley, S. E., and A. C. Orr (1978)  Patterns of Urban-Rural Fertility Differentials in Developing Countries:  A Suggested Framework.  Washington, D.C.: Office of Urban Development, Development Support Bureau, Agency for International Development.

Goldberg, D. (1976)  Residential location and fertility. In R. G. Ridker, ed., Population and Development. Baltimore, Md.:  The Johns Hopkins University Press.

Hermalin, A. I., and W. M. Mason (1980)  A strategy for the comparative analysis of WFS data, with illustrative examples.  In The United Nations Programme for Comparative Analysis of World Fertility Survey Data.  New York:  United Nations Fund for Population Activities.

Hull, T. H., and V. J. Hull (1977)   The relation of
    economic class and fertility:   An analysis of some
    Indonesian data.   Population Studies 31:43-57.
Indonesia, Central Bureau of Statistics (1978a)
    Indonesia Fertility Survey 1976.   Principal Report,
    Vol. I.   Jakarta:   Central Bureau of Statistics.
Indonesia, Central Bureau of Statistics (1978b)
    Indonesia Fertility Survey 1976.   Principal Report:
    Statistical Tables, Vol. II.   Jakarta: Central Bureau
    of Statistics.
Iutaka, S., E. W. Bock, and W. G. Varnes (1971)   Factors
    affecting fertility of natives and migrants in urban
    Brazil.   Population Studies 25:55-62.
Jordan, World Fertility Survey (1979)   Jordan Fertility
    Survey, 1976 Principal Report, Vol. I.   Amman:
    Department of Statistics.
Kelley, A. C. (1980)   Interactions of economic and
    demographic household behavior.   Pp. 403-470 in R. A.
    Easterlin, ed., Population and Economic Change in
    Developing Countries.   Chicago: University of Chicago
    Press.
Kelley, A. C., A. M. Khalifa, and M. N. El-Khorazaty
    (1980)   Demographic Change and Development in Rural
    Egypt.   Paper presented at the Institute of
    Statistical Studies Seminar on the Demographic
    Situation in Egypt, Cairo.
Kenya (1966)   Kenya Population Census, 1962.   African
    Population, Vol. III.   Nairobi:   Statistics Division,
    Ministry of Economic Planning and Development.
Ketkar, S. L. (1978)   Female education and fertility:
    Some evidence from Sierra Leone.   Journal of
    Developing Areas 13:23-33.
Ketkar, S. L. (1979)   Determinants of fertility in a
    developing society:   The case of Sierra Leone.
    Population Studies 33:479-488.
Khan, M. A. (1979)   Relevance of human capital theory to
    fertility research:   Comparative findings for
    Bangladesh and Pakistan.   Research in Human Capital
    and Development 1:3-43.
Khan, M. A., and I. Sirageldin (1979)   Education, income,
    and fertility in Pakistan.   Economic Development and
    Cultural Change 27:519-547.
Kiranandana, T. (1977)   An Economic Analysis of Fertility
    Determination Among Rural and Urban Thai Women.
    Institute of Population Studies Paper No. 20.
    Bangkok:   Chulalongkorn University.

Knowles, J. C., and R. Anker (1975)  Economic
    Determinants of Demographic Behavior in Kenya.
    Population Employment Working Paper No. 28.
    International Labour Organization, Geneva.
Kogut, E. L. (1974)  The Economic Analysis of Fertility:
    A Study for Brazil. Population and Employment Working
    Paper No. 7. International Labour Organization,
    Geneva.
Kuznets, S. (1974)  Rural-urban differences in fertility:
    An international comparison.  Proceedings of the
    American Philosophical Society 118:1-29.
Lee, B. S., R. E. Paddock, and B. F. Jones (1978)
    Development of an Econometric Fertility Model for Less
    Developed Countries:  The New Home Economics Approach
    to Female Status and Age at Marriage and Fertility.
    First Draft.  Interim Report prepared for the Office
    of Population Policy Development Division, Department
    of State, Agency for International Development.
Loebner, H., and E. D. Driver (1973)  Differential
    fertility in central India:  A path analysis.
    Demography 10:329-350.
Malaysia, World Fertility Survey (1977)  Malaysian
    Fertility and Family Survey--1974. First Country
    Report.  Kuala Lumpur:  Department of Statistics.
Mason, K. O., and V. T. Palan (1980)  Female Education,
    Fertility and Family Planning Behavior in Peninsular
    Malaysia.  Unpublished manuscript.  University of
    Michigan, Ann Arbor, Mich.
Michielutte, R., C. A. Haney, C. M. Cochrane, and C. E.
    Vincent (1975)  Residence and fertility in Costa
    Rica.  Rural Sociology 40:319-331.
Navera, E. (1978)  Home Investment in Children in Rural
    Philippines.  Paper presented at the International
    Center for Research on Women Workshop, "Women in
    Poverty, What Do We Know?", Elkridge, Md.
Rizk, H. (1977)  Trends in fertility and family planning
    in Jordan.  Studies in Family Planning 8:91-99.
Rodriguez, G., and J. Cleland (1980)  Socio-Economic
    Determinants of Marital Fertility in Twenty
    Countries:  A Multivariate Analysis.  World Fertility
    Survey Conference, Substantive Findings Session No. 5,
    London.
Rosenzweig, M. R. (1978)  The value of children's time,
    family size and non-household child activities in a
    developing country:  Evidence from household data.
    Pp. 331-347 in J. L. Simon, ed., Research in
    Population Economics, Vol. 1.  Greenwich, Conn.:  JAI
    Press.

Sarma, M. T. R. (1977)  The Economic Value of Children in Rural India. Economic Growth Center Discussion Paper No. 272. Yale University, New Haven, Conn.

Sathar, Z. A. (1979)  Rural-urban fertility differentials: 1975. Pakistan Development Review 18:231-251.

Smock, A. C. (1980)  The Relationship Between Education and Fertility in Kenya. Nairobi:  Central Bureau of Statistics, Ministry of Economic Planning and Development.

Snyder, D. W. (1974)  Economic determinants of family size in West Africa. Demography 11:613-627.

Stycos, J. M. (1980)  Education, Modernity, and Fertility in Costa Rica. Unpublished manuscript. International Population Program, Department of Sociology and Center for International Studies, Cornell University, Ithica, N.Y.

Thailand, World Fertility Survey (1977)  The Survey of Fertility in Thailand:  Country Report, Vol. II, Report No. 1. Institute of Population Studies. Bangkok:  Chulalongkorn University.

United Nations (1973)  The Determinants and Consequences of Population Trends, Vol. I. Department of Economic and Social Affairs. Population Studies, No. 50.  New York:  United Nations.

UN/WHO Advisory Mission (1969)  Pakistan:  Report on the family planning program. Studies in Family Planning 40.

U.S. Agency for International Development (1978) Patterns of Urban-Rural Fertility Differentials in Developing Countries:  A Suggested Framework. Washington, D.C.:  Office of Urban Development, Development Support Bureau, Agency for International Development.

World Bank (1980)  World Development Report, 1980. Washington, D.C.:  World Bank.

World Bank (1981)  Some Issues in Population and Human Resource Development in Egypt. World Bank Mimeo. Population and Human Resources Division, Development Economics Department, World Bank, Washington, D.C.

Wu, T.-S. (1977)  The Value of Children:  Taiwan, Vol. 5. Honolulu:  East-West Population Institute.

Zurayk, H. C. (1977)  The effect of education of women and urbanization on actual and desired fertility and on fertility control in Lebanon. Population Bulletin of the United Nations Economic Commision for Western Asia 13:32-41.

# Chapter 17
# Effects of Societal and Community Institutions on Fertility

JOSEPH E. POTTER*

## INTRODUCTION

In studies of the determinants of fertility, much more attention has traditionally been given to the characteristics of individuals, households, and families than to the characteristics of the environments in which they are found. This review attempts to delineate some of the questions that arise when the emphasis is reversed, and attention is focused on social and economic contexts and the institutions of which they are comprised. Such a perspective brings to the fore a vast and diverse subject matter with only a slight correspondence to identifiable niches in the literature on fertility, on the demographic transition, or even on population and development. The institutions in question range from such concrete entities as schools, churches, and local welfare systems to less tangible aspects of economic, social, and administrative organization. Their existence may be rooted in the local community, or stem from the national capital city; their influence on behavior is apt to work through a loose

*The author exploited the goodwill, time and patience of more colleagues than he would care to admit in the course of the preparation of this review. Particularly generous and helpful were Geoffrey McNicoll, Norman Ryder, Brigida Garcia, Ron Lesthaeghe, and Raul Urzua. The participants in a seminar at El Colegio de Mexico and in the Seventh Meeting of the Working Group on Processes of Population Reproduction provided critical comments on the first draft of the manuscript, as did reviewers of these volumes. Hilda Nava de Coletta provided dedicated secretarial assistance from start to finish.

articulation that comprehends large portions of the more familiar socioeconomic determinants of fertility.

The discussion that follows is organized according to three distinct primary routes by which alterations in an institutional setting can be seen to elicit corresponding shifts in fertility:

1.  by changing the economic costs and benefits of children;
2.  by changing internalized values concerning the family, marriage and fertility; and
3.  by changing the social and administrative pressures bearing on the reproductive behavior of individuals and couples.

The approach is a crude one.  The primary concern is with the objective reality of the incentives created by institutional arrangements and the messages transmitted by institutions and their agents.  The complexities of decision making and behavioral response are beyond the scope of this review, as are important issues regarding the sources and functions of institutions.

In the discussion, considerable place will be given to illustrative examples of the sorts of questions that can and should be addressed by research on the institutional determinants of fertility.  Given the limited amount of work that has been done on most of these, and the sorts of data that available studies have been able to marshal, only occasionally will it be possible to respond to the editors' injunction to indicate conclusions that can be safely drawn from the evidence.  This might not have been the case if mainstream research on fertility in the past two decades--whether focused on the historical populations of Western Europe or contemporary societies of the South-- had not been so singlemindedly preoccupied with the analysis of data collected from censuses and individual or household surveys.  To make further progress in understanding the effects of societal and community institutions, a major effort will be required to collect the appropriate data; a recommendation along these lines is offered in the concluding section of the paper.

## INSTITUTIONAL INFLUENCES ON THE ECONOMIC COSTS AND BENEFITS OF CHILDREN

Although it is altogether reasonable to suppose that institutions and institutional change play an important

role in shaping the economics of fertility, the subject
is inevitably complex and open to a wide variety of interpretations. The approach taken here is to consider the
problem by separating the economic value of children into
several components. On the benefit side, there is a distinction between the everyday labor that children contribute (both as children and as adults) towards production
and household maintenance, and the value of children as
sources of risk insurance and old age support. Costs of
children, the third component, are seen as the opportunity
costs attached to time spent by parents or others in
childrearing and direct costs arising from expenditures
on food, clothing, shelter, and education. Component by
component, an attempt is made to delineate some of the
more frequently mentioned ways in which institutional
factors and arrangements influence the economic value of
children, and what changes may be expected to take place
in the course of development.[1]

## The Labor Value of Children

The belief that the labor contributions of children are
both needed and desired in pretransition settings is
shared by almost everyone who has written on the economics
of fertility. However, what determines differentials in
the labor value of children between different contexts,
and what determines change over time, are not so well
established. The discussion below focuses on influences
that derive from the social organization of production.

### Familial or Household Production

In conditions characterized by relatively primitive technology, there is apt to be ample scope for the productive
employment of child and family labor when production takes
place within the household, or on land or in enterprises
controlled by networks of relatives. This is a familiar
and almost tautological thesis, but it is one that has
important implications for the economics of fertility.
In the past, familial or household production characterized a very large proportion of all economic activity
in the Western world, and it probably still characterizes
a substantial proportion of economic activity in the
contemporary countries of the South.

A wide variety of institutional arrangements for economic production fall into the loosely defined category
of familial or household production.  In agriculture,
smallholders, sharecroppers, tenant farmers, squatters,
and those who farm communal or lineage lands would all
qualify, with (temporary) wage labor providing the major
exception.  Elsewhere, one would think first of artisans
and those engaged in cottage industry, but family-owned
and (at least to some extent) family-operated enterprises
clearly extend into industry, commerce, and various kinds
of services.

Recognizing that definitional issues command a lot of
attention in this realm, it may be worth noting that most
delimitations of the "peasant economy" or "domestic mode
of production" would constitute a distinct subset of the
activities and arrangements listed in the preceding para-
graph.  Thadani (1980:19), for example, recently characterized the salient features of peasant social organization as "the dependence of the household on family labor,
production largely for self consumption, for use rather
than for exchange, and the combination of production,
consumption, and reproduction within the household."  In
contrast, the present discussion will not exclude from
consideration units that market a significant fraction of
the goods they produce:  peasant societies often have
numerous forms of highly institutionalized exchange, and
production for markets has been common in villages where
modern or capitalist relations of production have made
few inroads.

The peasant or household economy is generally seen as
fundamentally different from the capitalist or commercial
economy.  Some of these distinctions are relevant to the
way child labor and, thereby, fertility are evaluated by
parents (and other relatives).  First, household production units do not maximize profits.  Since labor is provided by the family, and family income is not divisible
into wages and rents, the eventual tradeoff that determines the intensity of the use of the factors of production at the disposition of the household is between the
"disutility" of additional work and the utility of
additional consumption.  Apart from differences in
preferences, just how intensely factors will be used
depends, of course, on the amounts of land, labor, and
capital available to the household; the number of consumers it must support; and the amount of surplus that is
extracted from the household by way of taxes, payments in
kind to a landlord, or the like.  It may also be said of

the peasant economy that "assymetrical relationships to
other segments in both rural and urban society" (Thadani,
1980:19) will ensure unfavorable terms of trade for peasant products in the overall or local market; thus peasants
will tend to reduce the purchase of inputs and means of
production to the lowest possible level, and take maximum
advantage of their (abundant) labor resources (Schejtman,
1980:124).

Most economic and anthropological work on the peasant
economy has emphasized the removal of surplus production
by the politically powerful; whatever coercion and
exploitation may exist in the internal relations of
production of the peasant family has received relatively
little attention. It is this apparent vacuum that provided Caldwell with the opportunity to make a host of
far-reaching generalizations about the control of familial
labor and consumption in peasant households. Caldwell's
(1978:560) thesis is that, in the "familial mode of production," the powerful or the decision makers (usually
elder males) use their authority to secure a host of
advantages:

> They include consumption: the kind and amount of food
> eaten, precedence in feeding, the clothing customarily
> worn, use of house space and facilities, and access to
> transport. They include power and access to services:
> who can tell whom to do what; the right to be pampered
> and have the little services performed that make life
> graceful; the guarantee of support in argument, danger,
> or a bid for social or political power, and the right
> to make unchallenged decisions. They include labor:
> the amount of work done, the kind of work done, the
> right to control one's own working time, and access to
> leisure or to activities (such as bargaining) that
> give real pleasure.

If Caldwell is right, the economic calculus of peasant
production units begins to look like that of a miniature
capitalist firm, and is by no means as "antisurplus" as
has often been maintained.

A final aspect of the logic of the peasant economy has
to do with its reproduction. The length of time that
children will work for their parents is influenced by the
requirements for establishing a new productive unit
(household). When the nuclear family is an independent
unit of production and the inheritance of land is a
critical factor, parents may benefit directly from their

children's labor for their entire lives.  In the geronto-
cratically controlled kinship groups prevalent in African
societies, since the lineage elders retain their prerogatives until death, a similar result may obtain, but without the nuptiality check implicit in the previous case
(Lesthaeghe, 1980).  In the case of the protoindustrial
households of historical Europe, however, the requirements
for forming a new productive unit were slight, and children tended to leave the household at a relatively early
age.  "Employment in proto-industry provided the means to
a livelihood not contingent upon customary practices of
retirement and inheritance" (Thadani, 1980:45); thus the
period during which parents could benefit from the labor
contributions of their children was cut short.  Considering the range of land tenancy arrangements to be found in
developing countries, the variations here would seem to
be endless.

In synthesis, the expected economic value of the labor
contributions of a child in a peasant economy will vary
with the economic and demographic circumstances of the
particular household or family, and with the characteristics of the relations of production in the setting
under consideration.  The implications of this conclusion
for fertility, however, are not as straightforward.

At one extreme is Caldwell (1978:554), who writes that
"as long as the internal relations of the familial mode
of production remain intact, marital fertility will not
be restricted for the purposes of limiting family size."
His basis for this statement seems to be a belief that,
as long as children can be exploited, there is no danger
of their consumption requirements exceeding their marginal
productivity.  In short, children are either exploitable
and economically worthwhile, or they are not; if they are,
it makes economic sense to have as many as possible.
Needless to say, this sort of theorizing raises the
hackles of those who are convinced of "the intrinsically
'antisurplus', 'non-maximizing' basis of household enterprise" (Thadani, 1980:20).

The notion that child labor represents an argument for
limitless high fertility in the domestic mode of production has recently been challenged.  Both Thadani (1980)
and Smith (1981) have made use of the example of a
sizeable proportion of peasant households in historical
England sending their adolescent children away to work as
agrarian servants in the households of others, who for
the most part were not their kin.  The apparent motivation
was to restore balance between the consumption require-

ments of the household and its productive capacity, rather than to secure additional income by way of obliging the children to return their earnings to their parents (Smith, 1981:605).[2]  Cain (1981a:7) has made a similar point about the market for servants in the rural societies of South Asia.  In particular, he has emphasized that "one can purchase labor, including child labor, for practically any service or activity," and that this alternative is often an inexpensive way to meet seasonable labor demands.

## Modern Organizational Forms

Although the number of children that provides a peasant household with an optimal balance between its productive capacity and its consumption requirements may vary between contexts, it seems clear that household or familial production generally offers greater opportunities for parents to benefit from the labor of their children than do other forms of production.

The polar opposite of familial or household production would seem to be "modern" organizational forms in which the means of production are owned and controlled either by private entrepreneurs or by the state, and labor is supplied by individuals in exchange for monetary compensation.  The characteristic of these forms of production which most decreases opportunities for the productive employment of children is the fundamental separation between family and economy that they entail:  labor contracts are with individuals rather than families; moreover, the place of work is no longer the place of residence, so that there is a differentiation between childcare and the supervision of child labor.  Of course, in reality, the purely institutional effects of new forms on child labor will be complemented by the effects of the shifts in technology, mechanization, specialization, and required skill levels that are associated, in the first place, with the shift in organizational forms.[3]

On the other hand, although one can be reasonably sure that the labor contributions of children will be considerably diminished when virtually all production is organized along moderns lines of one type or another, and although this is in effect what eventually came to pass in the now developed countries of the North, it is by no means certain that the changes in the relations of production that are currently taking place in many countries of the South have similar implications.  For one thing, as Caldwell (1978:568) has pointed out, "the transformation from familial to capitalist production is a process rather than a sudden change. What is formed first and is sustained for long periods of time is a two-tiered system in which the two forms of economies coexist." With respect to the historical experience of Western Europe, he goes on to note that "at the early stages only the husband participated in the capitalist mode of production; services within the house were provided on a subsistence basis by a familial mode of production not very different from that found in the peasant household." This sketch bears an obvious similarity to descriptions of what is taking place today in many countries of the South, especially where wage labor is combined with subsistence farming on "private plots" of one sort or another.

Moreover, not all of the changes in the relations of production taking place in the Southern countries involve an increase in wage labor. McNicoll (1978a:137) has written that "forced occupational diversification out of agriculture into micro-scale trading, fodder or fire-wood gathering, and the like, creates a self-employed class without capital--in status even below the proletariat--competing both within itself and with increasingly favored townbased enterprise." In both rural and urban settings, a wide range of intermediate or peripheral organizational forms have emerged that are neither classic cases of familial production nor reasonable facsimiles of modern capitalist or socialist modes of production. Although the economic activities of children in such settings have not been thoroughly studied, there is evidence, at least for Latin America, that children make significant contributions to the family economy of the marginal self-employed (e.g., Garcia et al., 1982).

Despite the fact that the changes in the relations of production taking place in the South are complex and unstudied, there are important cases to be found where these changes are having a significant impact on opportunities for exploiting child labor. This discussion concludes with two agricultural examples where major changes in the social organization of production seem to be having just such an impact.

Over the past two decades, the structure of Brazil's agricultural economy changed dramatically as the country became one of the world's greatest agricultural exporters. This metamorphosis--achieved at the cost of increased resource concentration, shortfalls in domestic food

supply, and ecological deterioration--led to new patterns
in the organization of agricultural work and a dramatic
increase in temporary wage labor, known commonly as "boia
fria" (Saint, 1981).

In Brazil, the system replaced by a capitalist agriculture based on mechanization, modern inputs, and temporary wage labor was that of fazendas, large landholdings
cultivated by resident tenant farmers under arrangements
that permitted landowners full access to family labor,
and provided tenants (parceiros and moradores) with income
from the commercial harvest that varied directly with the
number of workers in the family.  Presumably, larger
families also had the advantage of economies of scale in
domestic food production and suffered no disadvantage in
terms of housing, which did not represent a financial
cost (Carvalho et al., 1981; Paiva, 1982).

Somewhat surprisingly, there is some debate about
whether the advent of boia fria has led to more or less
exploitation of child labor than existed on traditional
fazendas.  The idea that child labor has increased may
stem from a misguided tendency to compare the Brazilian
example of proletarianization to that which took place in
historical Europe with the development of protoindustry.
It may also be inspired by census and survey data showing
increased participation of children in the agricultural
labor force (Saint, 1981); however, this probably just
reflects the fact that children who work for wages are
more likely to appear in such statistics than those who
participate in family production.  In fact, it seems
probable that the boia fria has led to a rather drastic
reduction in opportunities for child labor for several
reasons:  the labor contracts are made on a short-term,
individual rather than a long-term, collective basis; the
distance between place of work and place of residence has
greatly increased; and greater speed and skill are
demanded of workers.  This shift in labor relations has
been identified as one of the important determinants of
the rapid fertility decline now taking place among the
poorer segments of the Brazilian rural population
(Carvalho et al., 1981; Paiva, 1982).

Another example of a diminished role for child labor
is provided by a study of village and family life in
contemporary Kwangtung province recently conducted by
Parish and Whyte (1978).  In the years following their
military triumph, the Chinese Communists carried out land
reform, the collectivization of agriculture, and then the
formation of people's communes.  The economic and politi-

cal organizations that emerged are radically different
from the systems that existed prior to 1949.  The new
organizational unit is the production team, a group of
about 20 to 40 households that corresponds in most cases
to a village.  Landholdings are of two types:  the bulk
of the best land is collectively held and controlled by
the production team, and the rest is allocated as private
plots to individual households.  Individuals are given
points for work in the collective fields; these amount to
income credits that are eventually paid in cash if a
positive balance remains after deductions for payments in
kind (grain allowances) and cash advances.  Although
points are awarded on an individual basis, accounting is
by household, and it is usually the household head who
receives the lump sum payment at the end of the year.
One of the most important changes in the lives of children
has been the advent of compulsory primary education.  As
Parish and Whyte (1978:228) point out, "the major economic
consequence of children attending school is not the cost
of tuition but the lost labor the children could provide."
Even so, children provide a considerable amount of labor
to the household:  before they begin to attend school by
aiding with childcare and other duties, while attending
school by dedicating their spare time to household chores
and/or work on the private plot, and after completing
school by contributing work points earned in regular
fulltime labor in the collective fields.

Although the structure of production in Kwangtung
province clearly includes both traditional and modern
elements, there are some parallels with the Brazilian
case.  There is at least limited separation between place
of work and place of residence; moreover, since both
parents are apt to be actively engaged in field work for
the production team, the possibilities for supervising
the work of children in domestic endeavors are greatly
limited.  Perhaps the other major change is in the length
of time that a son or daughter will remain economically
active in the parents' household.  In the pre-1949 scheme,
a son labored on the family farm after marrying and until
it became his through inheritance or the father's retirement; similarly, after marriage, a daughter worked for
her mother-in-law in the household of her husband's
family.  As Parish and Whyte (1978:133) note, "land
reform and collectivization have curtailed the economic
authority of the father and his power and desire to keep
sons together under his rule."  Finally, it may be
speculated that specialization and increased skill levels

not only made possible the impressive
yields documented by the authors, but
opportunities for the productive empl‹
at least on collective lands.

## Children as a Source of Risk and Old Age Support

The value of children to their parents
economic support in old age is a famil
fertility theory (e.g., Caldwell, in these volumes);
somewhat less familiar is the value of children as a
source of insurance against various risks.  In both
cases, children are a source of income when the regular
earnings of the parent(s) are reduced or eliminated.  The
drop in income with old age is foreseeable, although
there may be considerable uncertainty about the timing
and duration of the required support; risk insurance
relates to any unforeseeable drop in income that might
result from, say, a natural disaster like a drought, from
an illness, or from the closing of a factory.
    The value of children as a source of economic security
clearly depends on what alternative forms of insurance
are available, as well as on the gravity of the risks
parents face.  In the course of development, there are
likely to be important changes in both of these variables,
with institutional factors playing a major role.  For
example, the development of capital markets would have a
clear effect on the value of children as a source of both
old age support and insurance against natural disasters.[4]
Given efficient credit institutions, parents are able to
accumulate financial assets through savings and interest
during good (productive) years, and to borrow at similar
rates of interest or draw down savings during bad years
(in their retirement).  Institutional change can also
directly affect the risks to which families are exposed.
For example, development of effective law enforcement and
adjudication within an effective system of economic
administration would help to protect against the violation
of property rights, the risk of depredation, and the
threat of physical violence.[5]
    In a recent paper, Cain (1981b) analyzed the insurance
value of children in four poor agricultural villages in
South Asia, three in India, and one, Char Gopalpur, in
Bangladesh.  One of his principal conclusions is that
children, particularly adult males, are a vital source of

risk insu
no such
analy
to

...ance in Char Gopalpur, but they have little or
...value in the Indian villages. According to Cain's
...sis, this difference can be attributed almost totally
...institutional factors.

To begin with, two critical aspects of the Bangladesh
social setting make Char Gopalpur a much higher-risk environment than the Indian villages. First, Char Gopalpur's
system of patriarchy and division of labor by sex effectively excludes women from most wage employment and from
cultivation of their own land; thus the consequences of
the illness or death of the principal male provider are
greatly intensified. Second, because there is no credible
system of justice and law enforcement in rural Bangladesh,
there is more lawlessness and a greater likelihood of
property loss through either outright expropriation or
fraud.

The second important difference between the Indian and
Bangladesh villages is that the former offer several possible sources of risk insurance, whereas in Char Gopalpur
parents apparently have almost no alternative to children
(especially adult male children) as a means of reducing
economic vulnerability in times of stress. The Indian
villages have well-functioning credit cooperatives, and
villagers have been able to obtain public relief employment in periods of prolonged drought. In Char Gopalpur,
the major way of adjusting to severe economic stress due
to either bad weather or widowhood is the sale of land.
Cain argues that this can only be interpreted as the
worst outcome next to loss of life. As the last step in
his analysis, he observes that fertility is now low and
declining in the Indian states of Maharashtra and Andhra
Pradesh. He notes that Bangladesh, in contrast, "has one
of the highest and most unyielding fertility rates in all
of South Asia" (Cain, 1981b:467).

In contrast to the Cain study, two examples may be
cited in which a relationship between fertility decline
and the availability of alternate, institutional forms of
security was not observed. First, the Parish and Whyte
(1978) Kwangtung study provides a vivid example of planned
institutional change producing, albeit somewhat inadver-
tently, a major decline in fertility; however, this
institutional change did not result in a significant
curtailment of the role of children as providers of old
age support. Parish and Whyte state categorically: "For
the vast majority of old people in rural Kwangtung,
support is the obligation of the family, not of the
collective or the state" (p. 76). The responsiblity lies

almost entirely with sons, and may or may not involve
living in a stem family arrangement with the aged
parents. The authors also note that the relationship
between sons and economically dependent parents who have
retired from field labor is, in most cases, seen as
mutually beneficial, since older relatives can assist in
childcare, domestic chores, private-plot work, and other
activities. This is in marked contrast to many higher-
income developing countries such as Singapore, where most
parents do not expect to rely on their children for old
age support, but rather on their personal savings (Fawcett
and Khoo, 1980:569). In this respect, there is also a
big difference between Kwangtung and Char Gopalpur. In
China, all is not lost for parents with no surviving sons
since they are eligible for "five guarantee support" in
their old age. This is seen not as a substitute for
family support, but as something to fall back on together
with private endeavors such as raising chickens and
tending a private plot. The communist revolution in
China has produced some institutions that have done away
with many of the traditional dangers to family incomes,
and others that constitute effective insurance mechanisms.
However, in an environment that is still very poor and
harsh, many risks remain, and children in Kwangtung
continue to help out their parents, for example, when
they have run short of grain or become ill or lame. Thus
although the Chinese revolution clearly reduced the
"indispensability" of children as a source of risk insurance and old age support, it did so without losing the
benefits of the traditional system and without going to
the expense of replacing it.

Another somewhat anomalous illustration of institutional influence on the value of children as sources of
risk insurance and old age support is offered by Smith's
(1981) study of historical England. Smith argues that
the welfare institutions operating from the late six-
teenth through the first half of the nineteenth century
did much to make children redundant as a means of dealing
with "nuclear family hardship." Furthermore, in marked
contrast to contemporary China, a large proportion of the
poor seem to have spent their old age as dependents of
the parish whether they had adult children or not. The
striking fact about this case, however, is that marital
fertility remained high in England until the late nineteenth century. The onset of controlled marital fertility came much later than in other European societies
where the role of children as a source of economic
security was presumably greater.

## Costs of Children

Before evaluating how institutions may influence the economic costs of children, it is important to define what is meant by costs. First of all, in the framework of this paper, benefits and costs are considered separately; no attempt is made to balance the two in some net measure. Second, following the logic of the microeconomists, the concern here is with price influences rather than with changes in the amount of time and resources parents invest in their children as a result of changes in their tastes or incomes. This distinction is important in that it excludes from the present discussion "Caldwell effects," whereby parents gradually decide to grant their children a larger share of family consumption as a result of changes in the cultural environment.

Although the composition of child costs will vary greatly from setting to setting, it will usually include a mix of the following:

   a.  food and other material goods such as clothing, shelter, and toys;
   b.  services--principally formal education and health; and
   c.  time, such as that spent on general childcare (including breastfeeding) and at-home training and instruction.

### Food Costs

Among the material inputs to childrearing, food seems to merit special attention. Household budget studies in many parts of the world have confirmed the "food intensity" of children (Lindert, 1980:29), and in very poor settings the cost of food may dominate that of all other inputs together. It is therefore at least possible that institutional arrangements affecting the cost of food could in turn affect fertility.

An interesting attempt to develop and explore this hypothesis in the context of the Brazilian Northeast has recently been made by Almeida (n.d.). Her analysis focuses on the cost of two alternative "investments in the future"--land, on the one hand, and children, on the other--and on how the relative prices of these two assets depend upon the terms under which a family has obtained access to the means of production. There are four predominant land-tenure arrangements in this part of Brazil, and over 60 percent of agricultural laborers are either posseiros (squatters), minifundistas (small landowners), parceiros (sharetenants), or moradores (sharecroppers). The data used for the study were collected in several municipios of a hot, semi-arid region called the sertao, where cotton and cattle are the main cash-earning economic activities, and in a township characterized by heavier rainfall, shallow topsoil, and slash-and-burn agriculture in the state of Maranhao. Farming is a very risky proposition throughout these areas, with droughts a perennial threat in the sertao, and with soil erosion and the onrush of weeds making it imperative to change locations frequently in the pre-Amazonic Maranhao region.

In the event of a bad year, tenant farmers, squatters, and small landowners employ quite different strategies. Almeida's argument takes special account of the credit systems operating in the region. Tenants on large farms may obtain food on credit throughout the course of the year, and repay their debts in kind at harvest time. Small landowners and squatters, on the other hand, have only local usurers to finance their consumption. Thus the interest cost of food is considerably lower for tenants than for other agricultural laborers. Almeida goes on to argue that tenants are also at an advantage in the subsistence production of beans and corn since landlords provide them with an elastic supply of land that increases with household size; thus they never encounter the diminishing returns that small landowners and squatters must contend with as their families grow. Tenants, however, are not in a good position to acquire their own land. The cost of land is money, and tenants have no special advantage in acquiring financial credit. Indeed, their lack of any collateral places them at a disadvantage with respect to those who already own some land. These considerations lead Almeida to predict that sharetenants would want and have more children than other rural residents in the study areas.

The empirical analysis supports this prediction, and also indicates that tenants are somewhat less conscious of the cost of children than are small landholders or squatters. Since the available data are from a pilot survey of a small population, these conclusions are only tentative. However, perhaps the most attractive contribution of the study is its careful delineation of one of the ways the Brazilian sharetenancy system promotes high fertility. With respect to landlord-tenant relations,

Almeida's argument clearly complements the child-labor
thesis discussed above.


## Education and Health Services

Demographic considerations may play a limited or negligible role in discussions of the important issues of
equity, efficiency, and administrative feasibility involved in providing basic services such as education or
health care.  However, by way of the fees that they do or
do not charge for their services, schools, hospitals, and
health clinics may have an important impact on the cost
of children.  When demographic incentives are purposely
built into a price structure, as for example in the case
of delivery fees in Singapore, a certain amount of
research attention is likely to focus on the fertility
impacts of those incentives (e.g., Fawcett and Khoo,
1980).  Less attention, however, has been given to the
finding that "some important (but unknown) proportion of
the cost of rural schools is borne by the parents of
students" in contemporary China (Parish and Whyte,
1978:80).  Indeed, in most of the voluminous literature
on the links between education and fertility, there is
very little to be found on the elementary question of
what schooling costs parents (e.g., Cochrane, 1979).


## Time Costs

A consistent finding of time-use surveys the world over
is that "the mother's childcare time far outweighs that
of the father and accounts for most of the total care
time, regardless of socioeconomic class or nation of
residence" (Lindert, 1980:38).  Since the opportunity
cost of a mother's time depends on the economic activities
that she would be able to engage in were she not rearing
children, it seems likely that patriarchy--defined as a
set of social relations with a material base that enables
men to dominate women--suppresses the cost of children in
societies such as Bangladesh.  Here again Cain's work on
Char Gopalpur is particularly illuminating.  There he and
his colleagues find that the "same patriarchal structures
that force (women) into relative seclusion in the household compound also deny them access to most forms of
market work" (1979:411).  Although Cain is careful to
point out that the pronounced labor market segregation

found in this setting is "not simply a neutral accommodation of women's childrearing role," it seems clear that the opportunity costs of childcare would rise considerably if this segregation were removed (see Standing, in these volumes).

In addition to discrimination against women in various forms, other institutional developments that might have an important influence on the opportunity costs of children are those that affect the sharing of childcare in large family-based groupings or the availability of domestic help (Oppong, in these volumes).

## INSTITUTIONAL INFLUENCES ON FERTILITY-RELATED VALUES

Beliefs, attitudes, and motivations are prominent among the recognized determinants of fertility (see Mason, in these volumes; Fawcett, in these volumes). They clearly affect the way people react to changes in institutional settings such as those discussed above and are sometimes said to have an important independent influence on fertility.

Many survey questionnaires have been designed to collect information on fertility-related values. The crude attempts of the first KAP surveys have recently given way to more sophisticated efforts such as the Value of Children surveys. In these analyses, much attention has been focused on the associations between particular value orientations and such variables as educational achievement, urbanization, and industrial employment. Although the reasons for such associations are not always made explicit, the rationale often has to do with the influence of the individual's institutional context. This is, to be sure, a very indirect way of testing hypotheses about the influence of certain institutions on fertility-related values; a more direct approach would involve studying the institutions and their agents to find out what sort of messages they actually transmit.

Of course, there is debate over the sorts of ideological influences that are eventually related to fertility. Attention is restricted here to influences related to two areas of clear importance: family life and appropriate reproductive behavior. The discussion examines the role of institutions as agents of ideological change in each of these areas, albeit in a highly simplified manner. The focus is on the content of the images or messages transmitted, with no attempt made to

explore how these are incorporated into norms or decision-
making processes.  Similarly, the difficult background
questions of how different institutions relate to each
other and why they "say" what they do are largely ignored.


## Images of Family Life

Caldwell takes values very seriously, and has not limited
his attention to survey data.  In advancing the thesis
that mass education has done a great deal to destroy
traditional family morality, and thereby to generate new
patterns of fertility behavior, he has focused his
analysis directly on the institution of education itself.
The framework of family morality that he believes is
under attack is one "which enjoins children to work hard,
demand little, and respect the authority of the old.
Under this system, the patriarch, as head of the family,
exercises authority.  Children are employed from an early
age and are valued as an addition to the work force"
(Caldwell, 1980:226).  As long as domestic production of
goods and services remains important, this system makes
high fertility beneficial to parents.
    Caldwell is quick to recognize two economic mechanisms
through which education has an impact on fertility--by
reducing "the child's potential for work inside and
outside the home" (p. 227), and by increasing the cost of
children.  However, he rests the bulk of his case on
three ideological effects.  First, schooling creates
dependency:  it is responsible for the social construction
of children as dependents, where they were previously
regarded primarily as producers.  Second, "schooling
speeds up cultural change and creates new cultures" (p.
228); these cultures, oriented towards a capitalist
economy, are in conflict with the morality of the domestic
mode of production.  Third, the school is the major
instrument "for propagating the values . . . of the
Western middle class" (p. 228).  Caldwell also identifies
a particularly devastating idea conveyed by national
education systems:  the ethic that one has to do things
for the good of the country rather than for the good of
one's father or parents.
    In his analysis, Caldwell focuses on school books,
curricula, and the impressions of teachers and school
administrators.  He notes that there are exceptions to
the general rule, such as Catholic schools that "taught
and implied the need for more traditional (and more

authoritarian) family relationships" (p. 234); however, he does not take up the question of why these schools teach a different family morality.[6]

Parish and Whyte's (1978) Kwangtung study can be used to "test" several of Caldwell's hypotheses. Most of the prerequisites for a powerful "Caldwell effect" would seem to be present. First, there was an impressive increase in school enrollment: before 1949, a minority of rural males and a few rural females received schooling; currently, almost all youths of both sexes receive some education. Moreover, in China, schools are considered a major source of moral and ideological training, and official Chinese policy on intrafamily relations would seem to be very much at odds with the traditional family morality that prevailed before the communists came to power: there is an emphasis on more egalitarian marital relationships, and parents are expected to encourage children's awareness of their extrafamilial obligations. However, education in Kwangtung province does not seem to have produced the dramatic conflict between the generations that Caldwell posits. Parents do not view their children's schooling as a threat, and new ideas can apparently be accepted without a weakening of family ties and roles.

On the other hand, the educational system seems to have adapted in important ways to the local environment; moreover, "school authorities take pains not only to avoid conflict with familial authority but to stress values that parents strongly approve of: hard work, discipline, harmonious relationships with others, and helpfulness around the home" (Parish and Whyte, 1978:232). On the other hand, those changes in intrafamily relations that have occurred seem to accord well with the new institutional realities. For example, new wives, who now have the opportunity and obligation to earn income laboring on the team's fields, no longer serve their mothers-in-law like domestic slaves until they demonstrate their son-bearing abilities. Sons may be somewhat less fearful of their fathers than in earlier times, but no longer will they spend an important fraction of their adulthood working on the family farm under their father's supervision.

A reasonable conclusion might be that, although family life has undergone some change in Kwangtung, the introduction of mass education has been in relative harmony with that change. It does not seem to have had the destructive impact on family morality that Caldwell posits.

## Appropriate Reproductive Behavior

While entities such as schools, enterprises, and the
media may promote or propagate a wide variety of values
that affect fertility indirectly, a smaller number of
institutions are likely to attempt to influence the way
people think about fertility itself. Organized religion
is clearly one of these. In numerous studies of historical Europe, it is argued that the Church has had an
important influence on the timing and speed of the
fertility transition. In a paper reviewing the results
of the European Fertility Project, Coale (1973) identifies
the moral acceptability of birth control as one of the
three conditions necessary for a major fall in marital
fertility. In a similar vein, Lesthaeghe (1980:537)
assigns an important role to secularization and to changes
such as those that took place in England, where "the
Churches gradually accommodated to the altered facts of
life without a strong fundamentalist revival, thereby
allowing fertility to fall more closely in line with what
one might expect on the basis of formal economic
reasoning."

Organized religion is undoubtedly an important arbiter
with respect to the moral acceptability of birth control
in many societies of the contemporary South. Yet perhaps
just as frequently, its competence in this realm is being
eroded by the increased importance of the medical community. A recent investigation in Brazil provides interesting evidence about the changing prominence of different
institutions in propagating and sustaining values regarding appropriate reproductive behavior. This is a valuable
case for present purposes since it is not complicated by
the influence of a national family planning program.

The Brazilian National Survey of Human Reproduction
(PNRH), unlike most fertility surveys, was focused on
only nine municipalities.[7] In each of these, a study
of different aspects of the community was undertaken
before a representative sample of households was drawn
and their members interviewed. The community studies
included a component that, by way of extended structured
interviews with agents and clients of a variety of institutions, attempted to determine whether organizations
such as churches, private businesses, the media, schools,
and the medical community were attempting to influence
reproductive behavior. A few generalizations that seem
to apply to most of the municipalities can be summarized
here.

In a country where, at least nominally, most of the population is Catholic, the Church could be expected to have an important influence on attitudes toward fertility limitation and modern contraception. That, however, does not seem to be the case in these communities in contemporary Brazil. In addition to the apparent atrophy of the Church itself, there is no uniformity of opinion among priests, and there are indications that attitudes are rapidly changing to a "hands-off" approach to the question of birth control. A common stance is that of "responsible parenthood": each case is taken individually, and couples should try to find the proper balance between economic pressures and their obligation to reproduce. The question of birth control methods, more often than not, is recognized as a problem outside the province of the priest; Lamounier (1981:19) interprets the trend as a gradual transfer of responsibility for the matter to the broader medical community.

On the other hand, medical institutions and doctors in particular were found by the PNRH researchers to be eager and willing to provide both counseling and services with respect to fertility limitation. In fact, given that Brazil has no official policy to curb population growth and devotes few resources to government health programs, medical institutions in that country seem to do a remarkably effective job of legitimizing modern contraceptive methods and promoting their widespread use.

## INSTITUTIONAL PREREQUISITES FOR THE
## SOCIAL REGULATION OF FERTILITY

The previous two sections have focused on how institutions can have a more or less direct impact on reproductive behavior, either by contributing to the incentive structures faced by individuals and families, or by influencing the normative values of a community and its members. This section turns to a slightly different set of issues related to the social control of fertility. Here a distinction is drawn betwen local efforts to either restrict or increase natural population growth, and fertility policies designed and implemented at the national level. With respect to the former, the question asked is what sort of insitutional arrangements are likely to foster social regulation of fertility at the community level. With respect to national policies, the focus is on institutional prerequisites for effective implementation.

## Local Fertility Policies

In all but the most primitive or otherwise exceptional circumstances, it can be taken for granted that fertility has social consequences. That is, the reproductive behavior of individuals in one way or another affects the welfare of other people. To the extent that the overall fertility level of the population residing within a geographically bounded local community affects the collective welfare of the members of that community, or at least the welfare of established interest groups within the community, there is good reason for establishing some sort of "social regulation" of the phenomenon.

McNicoll (1975) has argued forcefully that conscious community-level regulation of fertility is important both in explaining historical experience and in designing effective population policies in the countries of the South. He has been particularly concerned with identifying the characteristics of local organizational forms that are likely to elicit social incentives and sanctions that encourage demographic restraint. He suggests that, in addition to having a legitimate internal administrative structure or some less formal means of influencing its members, a community is likely to be successful in this regard if it is small, closed, and autonomous, and if its members can at least partially identify their own interests with those of other members. The advantage of smallness is that it permits face-to-face contact—a frequently mentioned requirement for effective social control. Communities able to regulate in-migration can benefit from restrained fertility without fear that their success will be offset by an influx of new entrants; similarly, a community that can transfer its unemployment problems to other parts of the society through out-migration will have little incentive to "invest" in local fertility control. A village's self-regulating capacity is likely to be enhanced if its authority is not crippled by "alliances such as large kin groups that extend over village boundaries and compete with village economic functions" or by "government apparatuses that extend down to the village (and interfere) with intra-village relations." Finally, the felt need for cooperative effort in addressing mutual problems is likely to be greatest where "all member households have a stake in the village economy" (p. 16).

McNicoll's policy orientation directs his attention away from communities in which economic advantage and

political authority have been concentrated among a few
members, and local efforts to regulate fertility have
been decidedly pronatalist. The list of prerequisites
for the emergence of social control along these lines is
notably shorter. Again, however, an open population
severely limits the incentive to invest in reproductive
policy of any kind.

Several of the papers cited earlier in this discussion
make some reference to social controls operating at the
local level for the benefit of the ruling group.
Lesthaeghe notes (1980:530) that "appropriation of
resources takes place . . . at very early stages of
social organization. Such an appropriation leads
inevitably to inequality with respect to access to
resources, and its maintenance (both as a short-term and
a long-term goal) implies the imposition of restraints
and the emergence of social controls". Caldwell
(1978:568) includes this resounding statement: "It is
not the factories and the steel mills that count in the
reduction of fertility; it is the replacement of a system
in which material advantage accruing from production and
production flows to people who can control or influence
reproduction by a system in which those with economic
power either gain no advantage from reproduction or
cannot control it." Indeed, the African lineages that
Lesthaeghe refers to and the haciendas described by
Almeida could both be taken as cases of community level
fertility control.[8]

The problem of demonstrating a link between particular
characteristics of local-level organization and the
emergence of social regulation of fertility clearly does
not lend itself to easy empirical tests. As McNicoll
(1980:449) himself admits, "persuasive post hoc theorizing is essentially the present state of the art." As
examples of communities in which social or administrative
pressures have been mobilized to advance the collective
demographic interest, he has taken up the cases of
Tokugawa Japan (1975), China in the 1950s (1975), contemporary Kwangtung province (1980; based on Parish and
Whyte, 1978), and Bali since the late 1960s (1980). He
also presents Bangladesh as a case where dysfunctional
social organization has prevented the emergence of
community interest in fertility (1980; based on Arthur
and McNicoll, 1978).

The late fertility transition in historical England,
because of the controversy it has stirred, may serve as a
useful basis for further speculation about organizational

forms and community-level regulation of fertility.  Several elements of the English institutional setting are critical to the interpretation offered here.  Foremost is the presence of very marked class differentiations: there was a readily identifiable elite in this society that retained economic and political power as well as social status.  Next are the institutions highlighted in Smith's (1981) analysis.  The first of these is agrarian service, whereby "so many young people in this society spent many years between the onset of sexual maturity and marriage residing and working in households of others who for the most part were not their kin" (p. 603).  The second is parish relief, which served as "a system of social welfare to buttress households and individuals whose self-sufficiency was frequently impaired," and which "required a local revenue-gathering and re-distributional system of considerable sophistication" (p. 608).  A third development highlighted by Smith is the growing importance of markets, wage labor, and the monetization of exchange.  A prominent feature of the English institutional setting hardly mentioned by Smith is the strict administrative control exercised over such matters as the enforcement of labor, the prohibition of vagrancy, and restrictions on the physical mobility of labor.  A last feature, emphasized by Lesthaeghe (1980) if not by Smith, is the existence of a strong, unified church.

The primary unit of social, economic, and political activity was the parish or village.  This unit was small, territorially bounded, and closed to migration.  Within it, economic, administrative, and moral authority was concentrated in the hands of a well-defined few.  Moreover, English village society exhibited a remarkable amount of organizational coherence, with a notable absence of conflicting or overlapping alliances or interest groups.  Indeed, it seems likely that agrarian service and parish relief did quite a bit to preempt the emergence of kin-based alliances that might compete or interfere with the established village power structure.  The institution of service certainly weakened ties between parents and their children, while the ready availability of community support for the casualties of "nuclear family hardship" such as widows, the disabled, and the aged meant that there was no need for kin groups to serve as a welfare agency in this society.

Parish relief and the system of taxes and transfer payments it entailed also seem to have created important

incentives with regard to marital fertility: if this
institution downgraded the need for children as a source
of risk insurance and old age support, it also did much
to reduce the cost of childbearing. Smith (1981:608)
notes that "it is frequently possible to observe persons
excused from rate payments while they contended with the
presence of a youthful and expensive family on fixed
household resources only to contribute more heavily as
their children left home," and that "those with few
family dependents who were economically active gave to
those with costly dependents or those who were economically inactive." The effect was clearly to take the
weight off the nuclear family and to spread the cost of
fertility over the wider community, thus removing or at
least diminishing economic incentives for couples to
control marital fertility.

The institutions of English village society also seem
to have fit together in a remarkable way that yielded
late (if variable) age at marriage—what Lesthaeghe (1980)
refers to as the nuptiality valve. Age at marriage, on
average if not for individuals, was effectively controlled
by two rules. The first was the rule that "after marriage a couple was in charge of their own household"
(Smith, 1981, drawing on a forthcoming paper by Hajnal);
that is, the newly formed nuclear household was economically independent of the families of both the wife and
the husband. The second rule, really a supplement to the
first, concerned the minimum economic standard that a new
family was supposed to meet by having acquired a certain
amount of capital (physical or human), and/or a suitable
"economic niche."

Controls of these sorts were certainly convenient for
the rate payer in a parish. Most immediately, through
the influence of nuptiality on the level and age pattern
of fertility, they limited the number of child dependence
allowances. Equally important, if less direct, was the
effect that such controls had in limiting the number of
paupers that might burden the parish. Of course, both
effects were entirely dependent on the ability of the
parish to restrict in-migration. As Smith emphasizes,
this household formation regime also meshed well with the
institution of agrarian service. So, too, it was part of
a social system that gave little place to the extended
family, both with respect to residence and to household
economy. In this characterization, English village
society is seen as coherent, tightly controlled, paternal-
istic, and thus moderately cohesive. It was exploitative

in that the bulk of economic and human resources were appropriated by a small elite; however, appropriation was limited by a quid pro quo that guaranteed all members of the parish a certain minimum economic standard. Social and economic mobility, like physical mobility, were greatly restricted.

The transition from this demographic regime to one of controlled marital fertility would seem to hinge on the breakdown of one or more components of the system. Indeed, by the end of the eighteenth century, many of these components were clearly facing some rather momentous forces for change. Prominent among these were economic factors such as the expansion of markets, urbanization, and factory-based industrialization. The complex of changes known as the industrial revolution, in which England was clearly a pioneer, seemed to demand social changes that would convert the system just described into one much better attuned to the needs of a fast-growing industrial economy. Not by any means the least of the changes "required" was an increase in the physical mobility of labor.

It may well be that it is on this front that one may find important clues to why the demographic transition occurred later in England than one would have expected on the basis of aggregate economic indicators alone. For a series of idiosyncratic cultural and political reasons, many of which undoubtedly had to do with the "cohesive- ness" of the old system, English society put off these social changes until well past the time that they occurred in other European societies less advanced along the path of industrialization. The Speenhamland system, in effect from 1795 to 1834, which prevented the mobilization of labor and promoted new heights in paternalism, may have been the most overt example of the phenomenon referred to (Polanyi, 1944).

In this view, the sine qua non for the transition to controlled marital fertility was the elimination or replacement of locally financed welfare systems, combined with the removal of restrictions on the physical mobility of the population. When this happened, the family rapidly came to bear a much larger share of the costs of fertil- ity, and the village elites no longer had much incentive to invest in local population policies. Moreover, the wide range of risks and opportunities to which the bulk of the population was rather suddenly exposed greatly increased the incentive to invest in the education of one's children. In short, the "new household economics of fertility," which had little place in the old system, had a prominent place in the new one.

The interpretation advanced here may be clarified by comparison with the views of Lesthaeghe and Smith. Lesthaeghe's (1980) study of England is largely confined to the transitional stage. In accordance with the "secularization hypothesis," he suggests that the belated adaptation of an unchallenged moral or ethical code delayed marital fertility decline in the face of rapid changes in the "formal aspects of household economics" (p. 537). The present interpretation also stresses the parson's influence on sexual behavior in the village; however, that influence is seen as part of the efforts of an elite to regulate the demography of the local population, and the formal aspects of household economics are seen as being more responsive to the incentives built into the parish rates than to changes in the level of aggregate (economywide) economic indicators. In Smith's (1981:618) view, in England "the family, demographic, economic, and political systems were linked in a culturally determined moral economy"; however, he strongly objects to the notion that the control system was "imposed by the social and economic elite who have appropriated resources and are intent upon maintaining the prevailing social structure" (p. 616). He bases his objection on two arguments. The first is that "it was in a practical sense not easy for the social and economic elites to control the reproductive activities of those in lower status groups" (p. 615). The second is that the relationship between changes in real income and fertility was not instantaneous enough to suggest that either parental or social elite controls were functioning very well. Since the control exerted was not so much a matter of directly intervening in individual decisions as of setting up a system with the appropriate incentives, the first argument seems somewhat shortsighted; the second seems to be based on the dubious proposition that the welfare of the village elite was directly related to the real wage.

It seems quite clear that, in a small, closed population with a well-defined power structure, the elite is likely to be concerned with the rate and pattern of household formation, and with growth or shrinkage in the amount of labor at its disposal. A great deal of attention has been focused on the operation of preventive checks in such societies; at least recently, however, much less attention has been given to the ways elites may

have sought to ensure that fertility never fell to a
level that would endanger an adequate future supply of
labor.  Another broad but tentative conclusion might be
that, in village societies of the type posited here for
England, theoretical approaches to the analysis of
fertility that place great weight on the family and on
intrafamilial relations have only limited applicability.
In such contexts, class rather than family relations are
what are of central importance to social organization.
This is not to say that many of the propositions advanced
by Caldwell have no relevance to England; however, they
should be recast in terms of wealth flows between classes
rather than between generations, in a system where those
with social and economic power are the elite of the
village rather than patriarchs standing at the head of
lineages, extended families, or other kin-based
associations.


## National Population Policies

One way to carry out a national population policy is to
alter local environments to ensure that their incentive
structures are consistent with the desired fertility
outcome; most of the discussion to this point has potential applications in this regard.  In practice, however,
national policies are not usually so broad in their
scope; generally, they are confined to programmatic
attempts to increase the availability of contraceptive
services, and to convince people that low fertility is in
their own, as well as the nation's, best interest.  Sometimes, governments may complement such efforts with
administrative pressure or the establishment of outright
sanctions for those unwilling to cooperate.

Given their mixed success in the past, it is worth
asking whether there are certain institutional prerequisites for effective family planning policies of this
sort, or how they are limited by various existing institutional arrangements.  Two issues may be raised in this
regard.  First is the existence of local interest groups
that are unresponsive or, worse, outwardly hostile to the
government policy, whether because they have conflicting
demographic interests or because they have their own,
nondemographic uses for the family planning resources
available.  A second issue concerns the sort of "presence"
the central government is able to muster at the local
level.  The government's local agents or representatives

might not be responsible in any real sense to higher
levels of administration; they might be controlled by
local interest groups, or they might simply be their own
men--caciques bent on using public office for private
gain.  In addition, there are issues related to the
resources at the government's disposal--financial constraints and the range and quality of the services
provided.

As an example of these issues, Arthur and McNicoll
(1978) argue convincingly that the institutional prerequisites (among other sorts of necessary prior conditions) for an effective government-sponsored family
planning program are lacking in Bangladesh.  There, they
note, "the various colonial regimes did not leave behind
a strong system of local government capable of responding
to national goals and providing a firm institutional
setting for rural change" (p. 43); this condition has
persisted to the present.  The local system is dominated
by the rural elite, whose interests take precedence over
national concerns.

In contrast, McNicoll's (1980) sketch of the local
administrative system on the Indonesian island of Bali
indicates a much greater responsiveness of local
authorities to initiatives of the central government.
According to McNicoll, in the aftermath of the 1965
attempted coup in Indonesia, the local administrative
system was greatly strengthened; moreover, its interests
were in harmony with those of the prevailing social and
political structures.  This harmony was in turn favorable
to implementation of the national government's fertility
control policies, with local authorities given responsibility for meeting target numbers of birth control
acceptors, and these targets being compatible with local
social interests.

Another example of a context where government initiatives are not undercut by factional interests is provided
by Fawcett and Khoo's (1980) recent description of public
administration in Singapore.  Here, a strong, wide-ranging
national population policy is administered by a bureau-
cracy having two essential qualities.  First, it is both
powerful and efficient, and perceived as such by the
public.  Second, it is subject to political direction,
particularly the dominance of Prime Minister Lee Kuan Yew
and his People's Action Party.

CONCLUSIONS AND RECOMMENDATIONS

The preceding discussion has necessarily been limited in scope. In particular, institutional influences on the process of household formation were mentioned only in passing, and virtually no attention was given to the effect of institutional and cultural environments on decision-making processes, an area in which McNicoll (1980) has suggested that there is fruitful work to be done.

A more fundamental limitation, however, may arise from what might be called the "partial derivative" approach taken here, which effectively divides the problem into many small parts whose relationships may not be specified. This strategy precludes consideration of important "second-order" or "feedback" effects, such as those that demographic change may have on institutional developments. More important, perhaps, it means omitting discussion of what sorts of institutional change are likely to take place in combination, and what their net effect on fertility is likely to be, an issue that may well be at the heart of many Latin American discussions of the relations between development style and population change.

The avoidance of this and other difficult questions about the forms and dynamics of institutional change may, however, generate some useful insight: just as it is now possible to analyze the influence of the various so-called intermediate fertility variables in "determining" a particular level or trend in fertility without addressing fundamental ideological assumptions about how the world works, it may soon be possible to analyze the fertility-related incentive structures embedded in particular institutional settings in an ideologically neutral manner. The earlier discussion of temporary wage labor in Brazil may illustrate this point. Similar transformations in agricultural labor markets are apparently taking place in a number of countries of the South. There is wide variation in the causes and consequences of this phenomenon being suggested in the literature--from the human capital type of interpretation of the Philippine experience in a recent paper by Roumasset and Smith (1981) to a neo-Marxist interpretation of the boia fria (Gomes da Silva, 1975). Ideology will form an important component of such discussions for a long time. Meanwhile, however, although the forces generating a shift from traditional production relations to temporary wage labor may be difficult to assess empirically, it may be relatively simple to determine whether that shift decreases the opportunity (if not the need) for families to exploit child labor--regardless of whether the new system is viewed as fair and efficient, or exploitative and wasteful.

Finally, a number of thoughtful recommendations have been made for additional work on the institutional determinants of fertility (see, e.g., McNicoll, 1978, 1980); certainly, work could be undertaken on virtually all of the topics that have been addressed in the preceding pages. This being the case, rather than set forth yet another research agenda, it might be more profitable to take the present opportunity to address the strategic question of how to proceed with research in this area.

Much of the research that has been reviewed is of relatively little use when it comes to drawing conclusions about why fertility is behaving the way it is in a particular country. At one extreme are the highly empirical micro or village-level investigations; although these have yielded a wealth of interesting and empirically verified hypotheses, their results can only be taken as suggestive of what might be happening beyond the particular area considered. At the other extreme are the wide-ranging and qualitative arguments about the effects of particular institutions. These studies make skillful use of a kaleidoscope of evidence, often drawn from various parts of the world, but once again there is nothing much that can be said about what happens in a particular country.

If work done by people such as Caldwell and Cain has produced a wealth of interesting hypotheses but few if any nationally representative results, almost the opposite can be said about the mainstream efforts to discover the causal factors underlying fertility change on the basis of data collected in the World Fertility Survey. This is not the place to engage in a thorough critique of this much-debated research instrument; the point is simply that the WFS made only a very limited attempt in its community survey to collect data on the institutional environment surrounding the household. Indeed, it may well be true that "the community factors most pertinent to the explanation of demographic behavior cannot, by their very nature, be measured in one-visit surveys, in which the content of the instrument must necessarily be restricted to a set of straightforward factual items" (Casterline, 1981:2).

There would seem, however, to be a way out of this dilemma. The use of heavily clustered samples in future surveys would permit a two-pronged investigative effort;

collecting detailed community-level data on social and economic organization on the one hand, and individual and family-level data on fertility, economic activity, and the like, on the other. The object would still be to collect nationally representative data, but the tradeoff between sampling efficiency and the collection of satisfactory data on local institutional environments would be heavily weighted towards the latter. An example of this type of investigation is the Brazilian National Survey of Human Reproduction referred to above.

There is, of course, no readily available prescription for drawing a sample and designing research instruments for this kind of a survey, and a large amount of conceptual and experimental effort would be required of any such attempt to break away from the traditional mold. With regard to sample design, there would be important questions about the number, size, and character of the "communities" to be included as primary sampling units; indeed, there would even be the important question of whether the primary sampling units should be defined geographically or according to some other criteria. In any event, the selection of a stratification scheme would raise major theoretical as well as statistical problems.[9]

The design of research instruments for such investigations would be a major challenge. Still lacking, as McNicoll (1980:459) has pointed out, are "well designed empirical measures of the forms and dynamics of fertility-relevant institutions." What is more, the field work involved in this sort of research would make much greater demands on the talented social scientists available in a country than does the normal one-visit fertility survey. However, these difficulties should not be exaggerated. In-depth interviews with both the agents and clients of, say, local government, the church, the school system, the health system, and private enterprise can, as the Brazilian PNRH has shown, reveal much about the ideological influences exercised by such institutions. An examination of institutional products, such as curricula for educational programs, can contribute additional information. Although incentive structures may be more difficult to document, Cain's work on villages in India and Bangladesh, Parish and Whyte's study of Kwangtung Province, and Almeida's analysis of the Brazilian Northeast provide examples of successful empirical attempts to trace the influence of the social relations of production on the economics of reproduction. Of crucial importance is a direct attempt to determine the rules and procedures that govern the operation of, say, markets for temporary agricultural labor, haciendas, factories, and credit institutions, as well as to form a picture of how such institutions work from the information gathered on individual behavior.

In conclusion, an institutional approach to the analysis of fertility determinants holds considerable promise for the future. Such a focus may well enable researchers to overcome two of the major stumbling blocks they face: the much-discussed divorce between micro and macro levels of analysis, and the less frequently mentioned but equally fundamental contradiction between the Malthusian and transitional perspectives on historical demographic experience.

Arguably, the former problem results from the disparate findings generated by two parallel and somewhat misguided research traditions: the first was comprised of correlation and regression analyses in which individual fertility was arrayed against one or more explanatory variables such as household income, women's labor force participation, and education; the second consisted of attempts to estimate the relationship between national or state-level indicators of fertility and aggregate socioeconomic variables associated with modernization and economic development. Missing was an intermediate level of analysis--"empirical investigation of how social, economic, political, administrative, and cultural structures create fertility incentives or disincentives and otherwise impinge on reproductive behavior" (Population Council, 1981:315). It seems likely that research concentrating on local institutional settings would supply much of the "mediation" needed between global and individual levels of analysis, whatever the theoretical framework adopted by the analyst.

The second stumbling block arises from the positive association hypothesized by demographic transition theory between declining fertility and mortality--and, eventually, decelerating natural increase--and economic growth. In the Malthusian perspective, over the long run, population growth and economic expansion generally accompany each other. "Likewise, economic decline and demographic contraction tend to occur together. In the short run, fertility and nuptiality tend to respond positively, mortality to respond negatively, to upswings in economic well-being" (Tilly, 1978:24). This contradiction, however, is readily explained within the framework of local-level population policies. The

Malthusian relationships held as long as territorially based systems of social control were working effectively. With the onset of industrialization and the expansion of markets, along with rapid economic growth, the control systems broke down. The result was a radical change in the environment in which individual couples found themselves, and fertility was among those behaviors affected by the new structure of opportunities and obligations. Again, the institutional approach provides a useful research frame.

## NOTES

1. It is important to emphasize that this evaluation is not tied to a particular view of how the economic value of children eventually influences reproductive behavior. How economic considerations are evaluated in parental decisions about an additional child or in the formation of social norms about fertility-related behavior are questions addressed elsewhere (Hollerbach, in these volumes).

2. It should be observed, though, that Smith does not provide empirical support for his belief that servants did not send an appreciable portion of their earnings back to the household of origin. If they did, the institution of agrarian service could be seen as having constituted an important prop for high fertility in this setting, permitting poorer households to export their surplus family labor "to the farms of the more comfortably situated members of the agrarian populace" (p. 605) in exchange for either remittances or guarantees of support in times of crisis.

3. The belief that wage labor in urban-industrial settings is associated with fewer expected returns from child labor was at least partly responsible for the inclusion of variables such as the "proportion of the labor employed in agriculture" in a variety of macro-level multivariate analyses of the relations between modernization and fertility (Richards, in these volumes). A recent empirical study that sought to explicitly test the influence of a "familial, labor intensive mode of production" on the speed of the fertility transition in the subdivisions of various European countries at (about) the turn of the last century has been circulated in draft form by Lesthaeghe and Wilson (forthcoming). The proxy used depended on

the country under consideration; in the cases of
Belgium, Switzerland, and Germany it was the proportion
of the economically active population in agriculture
or cottage industry rather than in agriculture alone.
While the mode-of-production variable accounted for a
large proportion of the variance in the dependent
variable, here, as in previous studies, the results
lend themselves to a variety of interpretations besides
those based on the declining role of child labor.

4. On the other hand, Ben-Porath (1980:18) has reasoned
   that "the initial entry into a turbulent labor market
   is associated with increased risks:    parents may gamble
   and reduce risks by pooling the fortunes of several
   children.   The simultaneous entry into the market of
   several relatives may have the advantage of information
   and connections that strengthen rather than weaken
   family ties."   Much the same idea was expressed by
   Caldwell (1976:340) when he wrote that a large family
   "forms an excellent springboard to success for young
   aspirants in the modern sector of the economy."
   Lastly, in a similar vein, Ben-Porath (1980:18) makes
   reference to the complementarities that are likely to
   exist between the family and the emerging capital
   market.

5. In a recent paper, Caldwell (1981) pointed out that
   violence is an important fact of life in many parts of
   the South and that large family size is an essential
   defense against this threat.  Ben-Porath (1980:12)
   makes essentially the same point when he notes that
   "family relationships also play an important part in
   the struggle over the establishment of property rights
   and their physical protection, as is evident in any
   frontier movie."

6. Lesthaeghe (1980:536) appears to have a very clear
   idea of the church's self-interest in teaching a
   stricter family morality.

7. The results of the first phase of the analysis of the
   PNRH were published in individual monographs on the
   respective study areas, two of which included both a
   rural and an urban municipality.  A general description
   of the objectives and content of the survey is available in a paper by Berquo (1978).  Very recently, a
   comparative study of the role of institutions in
   influencing reproductive behavior was published by
   Loyola and Quinteiro (1982); their volume contains a
   good summary of the findings related to institutions
   that appear in the previous seven volumes.

8. Note that both are, at least partially, closed populations. Only women have the possibility of leaving the lineage (by marriage outside of it, which may be infrequent), and only those tenants who have avoided falling into debt with the landlord may leave the hacienda.

9. Perhaps this difficulty should not be exaggerated, however, since the great structural heterogeneity found in most societies of the South may guarantee that the sorts of geographically defined communities to be included in a sample would be relatively insensitive to the theoretical framework underlying the stratification scheme. In the Brazilian PNRH, for instance, mode of production was chosen as the principal basis for stratifying the sample of nine communities, but a quite similar set of communities might well have been drawn if the basis had been some index of modernization.

## BIBLIOGRAPHY

Almeida, A. L. O. de (n.d.)   Share Tenancy and Family Size in the Brazilian Northeast.   Instituto de Planeamiento Economico e Social, Rio de Janeiro.

Arthur, W. B., and G. McNicoll (1978)   An analytical survey of population and development in Bangladesh. Population and Development Review 4:23-80.

Ben-Porath, Y. (1980)   The F-connection: Families, friends, and firms and the organization of exchange. Population and Development Review 6:1-30.

Berquo, E. (1978)   A pesquisa nacional sobre reproducao humana.   In San Jose Dos Campos, Estado de Caso: Dinamica Poblacional, Transformacoes Socio-economicas, Atuacao das Instituicoes, Vol 1. Sao Paulo:   CEBRAP.

Cain, M. (1981a)   Extended Kin, Patriarchy, and Fertility.   Paper presented to the Seminar on Family Types and Fertility in Less Developed Countries, Sao Paulo, Brazil.

Cain, M. (1981b)   Risk and insurance:   Perspectives on fertility and agrarian change in India and Bangladesh.   Population and Development Review 7:435-474.

Cain, M., S. R. Rokeya, and S. Nahar (1979)   Class, patriarchy, and women's work in Bangladesh. Population and Development Review 5:405-438.

Caldwell, J. C. (1976)  Toward a restatement of demographic transition theory. Population and Development Review 2:321-366.

Caldwell, J. C. (1978)  A theory of fertility:  From high plateau to destabilization. Population and Development Review 4:553-577.

Caldwell, J. C. (1980)  Mass education as a determinant of the timing of fertility decline. Population and Development Review 6:225-255.

Caldwell, J. C. (1981)  The mechanisms of demographic change in historical perspective. Population Studies 35:5-27.

Carvalho, J. A. M. de, P. de T. A. Paiva, and D. R. Sawyer (1981)  The Recent Sharp Decline in Fertility in Brazil:  Economic Boom, Social Inequality, and Baby Bust. Working Paper No. 8.  Population Council, Mexico.

Casterline, J. (1981)  Community Effects on Individual Demographic Behavior:  Multilevel Analysis of WFS Data.  Paper presented to the International Union for the Scientific Study of Population International Population Conference, Manila.

Coale, A. J. (1973)  The demographic transition reconsidered.  Pp. 53-71 in International Population Conference, Liege, 1973, Vol. 1.  Leige:  International Union for the Scientific Study of Population.

Cochrane, S. H. (1979)  Education and Fertility:  What Do We Know?  Baltimore, Md.:  The Johns Hopkins University Press.

Fawcett, J. T., and S.-E. Khoo (1980)  Singapore:  Rapid fertility transition in a compact society. Population and Development Review 6:549-579.

Freedman, R. (1979)  Theories of fertility decline:  A reappraisal.  In P. M. Hauser, ed., World Population and Development.  Syracuse, N.Y.:  Syracuse University Press.

Garcia, B., H. Munoz, and O. de Oliveira (1982)  Hogares y Trabajadores en la Ciudad de Mexico.  Mexico City:  El Colegio de Mexico.

Gomes da Silva (1975)  O boia fria:  Contradicao de una agricultura em tentativa de desenvolvimiento. Reforma Agraria 5:2-44.

Lamounier, B. (1981)  Instituicoes e Comportamento Reprodutivo:  O Caso de Recife.  Mimeo.  Sao Paulo, CEBRAP

Lesthaeghe, R. (1980)  On the social control of human reproduction. Population and Development Review 6:527-548.

Lesthaeghe, R., and C. Wilson (forthcoming)  Modes of production, secularization, and the pace of fertility decline in Western Europe, 1870-1930.  In S. Watkins, ed. Proceedings of a Conference on the European Fertility Project.  Princeton, N.J.:  Princeton University Press.

Lindert, P. H. (1980)  Child costs and economic development.  In R. A. Easterlin, ed., Population and Economic Change in Developing Countries.  Chicago: University of Chicago Press.

Loyola, M. A., and M. de Conceicao Quinteiro (1982) Instituicoes e Reproducao, Vol. 8.  Sao Paulo:  CEBRAP.

McNicoll, G. (1975)  Community level population policy: An exploration.  Population and Development Review 1:1-21.

McNicoll, G. (1978a)  The demography of post-peasant society.  In Economic and Demographic Change.  Issues for the 1980s:  Proceedings of the Conference, Vol. 2.  Liege:  International Union for the Scientific Study of Population.

McNicoll, G. (1978b)  On fertility policy research. Population and Development Review 4:681-693.

McNicoll, G. (1980)  Institutional determinants of fertility change.  Population and Development Review 6:441-462.

Paiva, P. de T. A. (1982)  O Proceso de Proletarizacao como Fator de Destabilizacao dos Niveis de Fecundidade no Brasil.  Paper presented to the Seventh Meeting of the Working Group on Human Reproduction, Commission on Population and Economic Development, CLACSO, Cuernavaca, Morelos, Mexico.

Parish, W. L., and M. K. Whyte (1978)  Village and Family in Contemporary China.  Chicago:  University of Chicago Press.

Polanyi, K. (1944)  The Great Transformation.  Boston: Beacon Press.

Population Council (1981)  Research on the determinants of fertility:  A note on priorities.  Population and Development Review 7:311-324.

Roumasset, J. R., and J. Smith (1981)  Population, technological change, and the evolution of labor markets.  Population and Development Review 7:401-419.

Saint, W. S. (1981)  The wages of modernization:  A review of the literature on temporary labor arrangements in Brazilian agriculture.  Latin American Research Review 16:91-110.

Schejtman, A. (1980)  The peasant economy:  Internal
    logic, articulation and persistence.  CEPAL Review
    11:115-134.
Smith, R. M. (1981)  Fertility, economy, and household
    formation in England over three centuries.  Population
    and Development Review 7:595-622.
Thadani, V. N. (1980)  Property and progeny:  An
    exploration of intergenerational relations.  Center
    for Policy Studies Working Paper No. 62.  Population
    Council, New York.
Tilly, C. (1978)  The historical study of vital
    processes.  Pp. 3-56 in C. Tilly, ed., Historical
    Studies of Changing Fertility.  Princeton, N.J.:
    Princeton University Press.

# Chapter 18

# Effects of Culture on Fertility: Anthropological Contributions*

ROBERT A. LEVINE and SUSAN C. M. SCRIMSHAW

The value of anthropological research for understanding human population patterns in general and those of the developing world in particular has been recognized for some time, though its relevant findings and perspectives are not always considered in demographic theory and policy analysis. There is a growing literature of population anthropology containing empirical evidence and theoretical formulations bearing on the determinants of fertility. That literature has been reviewed by Barlett (1980), Nag (1973, 1980), Oppong (in these volumes), Nardi (1981), and Weiss (1976). Although an exhaustive review of this literature is not possible within the confines of the present paper, its major concepts can be outlined. In addition to briefly describing the major anthropological approaches to understanding fertility-related behavior, the discussion will focus on areas in which the anthropological contribution seems most relevant to these volumes, particularly in complementing the work of the other population sciences.

This chapter reflects, without attempting to report, the proceedings of a February 1981 Workshop on the Anthropology of Human Fertility at the National Academy of Sciences.[1] It begins by reviewing the concept of culture and its application to fertility, in particular the critical perspective it provides on some current demographic concepts, such as natural fertility. It then

---

*Editors' note: Unlike the other papers in this report, this paper does not confine itself to particular fertility determinants but discusses in broad terms the contributions of one discipline, illustrating in its approach the anthropological preference for dealing with specific elements in their social and cultural context.

briefly reviews anthropological areas of research related
to fertility. Next, it discusses the important issue of
research methodology, and how the anthropological method
complements demographic approaches. Finally, a brief
summary of research needs in the area of culture and
fertility is presented.


CULTURE AND FERTILITY

This is an area in which the anthropological contribution
to the understanding of fertility determinants should be
strongest and most integrated with demographic research.
A good deal has been written about culture and fertility,
both in general and for specific populations, and there
have been efforts to incorporate cultural factors into
demographic theory and research. Problems remain, however, particularly conceptual ones. The discussion below
attempts to clarify those that seem to pose the greatest
obstacles to productive research.

The first of these problems concerns the concept of
culture itself. When demographers and economists write
about cultural factors in the determination of fertility
in the developing countries, they tend to treat those
factors as discrete rules or beliefs: "irrational" norms,
tastes, and taboos on the one hand, and "rational" perceptions of local cost-benefit contingencies on the other.
Anthropologists, however, tend (particularly in recent
years) to see culture as an organized system of shared
meanings, often more pervasive than explicit, a set of
basic assumptions and images that generates rules and
beliefs, but is not reducible to them. In the influential
formulation of Geertz (1973), culture refers to "models
of" and "models for" reality--organized images and conceptions that reflect environmental contingencies and guide
social behavior, respectively. A cultural model thus
includes both existential and normative aspects (implications of what is and what ought to be) combined in a
single symbolic code that is not merely shared by a community, but taken for granted as a matter of "common
sense."

The rules generated from such a model presume as the
context for their application the validity of certain
beliefs about reality; those beliefs are in turn shaped
by the normative or moral standards of the model. This
unreflective fusion of fact and value, rejected by Western
positivism, is nevertheless the basis of folk cultures,

as well as religious doctrines and political ideologies. The most important research implication is that no rule or belief can be interpreted out of the context that gives it meaning, and that is uncovered by ethnographic work. Geertz (1973) has argued this view of culture in terms derived from epistemology, aesthetics, and social theory, and has published superior examples of cultural interpretation. In so doing, he has become the spokesman for anthropologists in the field who have found that observed rules and beliefs derive their meaning from tacit assumptions retrievable through ethnographic work. While not all social anthropologists hold this view, it prevails among those who put the concept of culture at the center of anthropological research.

Culture is also seen by anthropologists as having facilitated humanity's adaptation in the Darwinian sense: it has helped us to increase our reproductive success and to compete in a wide variety of environments. Obviously, a key feature of this adaptation is the ability to communicate and to pass information from one generation to the next; however, the content of that communication is also seen as having adaptive value. Cultures evolve in response to specific environmental pressures; thus, behaviors that affect birth, death, and disease rates reflect adaptive responses to the environment (Alland, 1970:203). Because culture evolves over a long time, many of the behaviors that affect fertility and mortality rates are not necessarily perceived as doing so directly. They are, however, supported by other aspects of the culture, as noted above.

The implications of this are that human populations have always regulated fertility and mortality to some degree. Many anthropologists believe this regulation has been greater than frequently acknowledged by demographers, and that there has been a good deal of variation in the amount and type of fertility regulation from one society to the next (Polgar, 1972:203-211). Polgar, Hassan (1973), and Cowgill (1975), among others, have demonstrated that both fertility and mortality have been controlled since before the existence of written records. As Polgar points out, this has implications for the interpretation of fertility-related behavior. It is one thing to posit that women have as many children as possible, unaware that mortality is dropping and they will now have more living children; it is another to see them making a careful adjustment between fertility and mortality, disrupted by external forces (such as public

health measures that reduce disease rates).  The latter
model implies an underlying purpose to the behavior, and
social systems that support it.  To ignore this is to
misunderstand both the behavior and its place in the
culture.  White (1981:6) puts it as follows:

> Population growth, then, must be seen as a positive
> rather than a passive response of the society (or more
> precisely, of the class) concerned.  The question
> whether changes in a population are due primarily to
> reductions in mortality or to increased fertility is
> not the basic question.  The matter at issue is not
> how, but why a population . . . allows itself to
> depart from the state of demographic equilibrium in
> which fertility and mortality vary inversely in the
> short term.

Applying this perspective to the determinants of
fertility implies that there are cultural models for
reproduction; these models reflect the shared beliefs and
expectations of a population about the reproductive
process in general and its own fertility-mortality
situation in particular, and prescribe and proscribe
certain reproductive behaviors.  The meanings of
conception, pregnancy, birth, lactation, infant care,
infant mortality, and lifetime fertility for a population
are constituted by their place in the model.  The fertility pattern that characterizes a population in
demographic terms--e.g., its crude birth rate, age-
specific fertility rates, and total fertility rate--has a
cultural rationale based on certain assumptions, some
"rational" (reflecting the actual environment) and others
"irrational" (reflecting normative traditions), but all
accepted by the population to be principles of common
sense.  This cultural rationale for a fertility pattern,
though often unstated, is accessible through ethnographic
study.  Because it provides the best indication of why
the pattern is being maintained, descriptions of this
rationale, and of the cultural models of reproduction and
parenting from which it is derived, are highly relevant
to the design of programs seeking to change fertility
levels.
   The cultural approach to fertility can be illustrated
by discussion of the conceptual problem of natural fertility, a concept well known to demographers but not to
anthropologists.  Knodel (in these volumes) provides a
lucid introduction to this concept.  A society is char-

acterized by natural fertility if its reproducing women make no deliberate effort to stop bearing children. There can be much variation in fertility among natural-fertility populations, based on factors such as length of the birth interval, age at marriage, and health factors affecting fecundity, but not on deliberate termination of childbearing.

From the viewpoint of anthropology, the term "natural" is misleading since it suggests something genetically determined, as in "nature vs. nurture"; precultural, as in Levi-Strauss' "nature vs. culture"; or free of technological intervention, as in "natural childbirth." Such connotations are not meant to be implied by the concept of natural fertility, which is straightforward and extremely useful within the context of historical and comparative demography. At the same time, it is likely to be of limited value for anthropological research on fertility, for reasons that illustrate the complementarity of the two disciplines in the population field. The concept of natural fertility combines historical and contemporary populations with high birth rates, and contrasts them with those (largely industrialized) populations which deliberately limit their fertility. One advantage of this division is that it permits operationalization of demographic transition theory, with standard census categories as the basis of quantitative and revealing differences between stages (pretransition, transitional, and posttransition). For example, the Coale-Trussell (1974) index of family limitation, m, is based on the fact that widespread birth limitation affects age-specific fertility rates (concentrating childbearing in a woman's young adult years). Thus societies with controlled fertility show concave curves of age-specific fertility, while those with natural fertility show convex curves—regardless of their total fertility rates. The effect of m in homogenizing natural-fertility societies according to the shape of their age curves is considered an advantage, the better to heighten contrasts with controlled-fertility societies and to detect the effects of parity-dependent limitation when it appears (Knodel, 1977; in these volumes). This accords with the aims of demographic research on fertility.

Anthropologists work largely with societies lacking (or which until recently lacked) parity-dependent birth limitation; their aims are to identify and analyze the social and cultural aspects of reproduction that have significant fertility outcomes in those societies. To

categorize societies according to what they lack (as the
distinction between natural and controlled fertility
does) is of limited value in understanding how they
operate the way they do. Natural-fertility societies
vary widely in their total fertility rates because of
variations in the proximate and indirect determinants of
fertility that are the primary objects of anthropological
investigation. African societies, for example, differ in
fertility rates as a result of diverse periods of abstinence in their childspacing systems (Page and Lesthaeghe,
1981), as well as the varying prevalence of diseases
causing infertility, to mention just two of the factors
involved. The anthropologist focuses on these differences not only to explain fertility variations among
populations at a given point in time, but also to help
forecast the direction of change when the social and
cultural supports for a particular fertility level are
altered by changing conditions of health, infant care,
marriage, and sexual conduct. Some anthropologists
believe that the concept of natural fertility obscures
these differences, and that it creates a category which
may well prove to be as variable internally as the stages
of the demographic transition are from each other. Future
research may help decide these issues. There can be no
doubt, however, that anthropological research can make
major contributions by continuing to emphasize the diversity within natural-fertility patterns.

The study of culture also involves the study of when,
how, and why cultures change. As advocates of modern
contraception have discovered, people do not always welcome a new technology enthusiastically. Arensberg and
Niehoff (1971) comment that, in the past, cultural change
took a long time, and the persistence of obsolete behaviors or other aspects of culture was less significant.
Today, because change is more rapid, there is a greater
need to understand how the process of change affects
behaviors related to fertility and mortality. Changes
that led to the increased population growth rates of the
twentieth century provide a dramatic example.

In most cases, forces of cultural conservatism, competition between groups, and diffusion from other cultures
operate simultaneously. Cultural change often begins at
the individual level, although individuals function within
society. When contemplating a change, people weigh their
wants and needs against the prevailing norms, beliefs,
and customs in the society (Goodenough, 1963). Each
person perceives the need for action according to his or

her own precepts; for example, if a woman expects half her children to die, she may not view another pregnancy in a negative way.  Goodenough suggests that cultural change depends on people's ability to organize new experience and relate it to conditions they cannot handle within their own cultural context.  They may revert to former habits if the new ones do not produce the desired results.  This happens frequently with contraceptive technology, particularly when undesirable side effects are attributed to a given method, or when pregnancy occurs after either method or user failure.  People also tend to adapt one form of behavior to another purpose if it seems feasible, or even to rearrange or substitute behaviors. Thus anthropologists suggest that new contraceptive methods that resemble existing ones or accepted medications are most likely to be adopted.

Both in understanding the cultural context of fertility and in examining the process of cultural change, anthropologists can make important contributions to demographic transition theory.  For example, Nag (1980) has shown that earlier and simpler views of the fertility transition must be modified in the face of growing evidence that "modernizing influences" increase fertility in natural-fertility societies, at least temporarily, mainly through social changes that reduce age at marriage and decrease the interval between births.  This finding, like the description of childspacing patterns as fertility determinants (Page and Lesthaeghe, 1981), illustrates one contribution of anthropological research:  the identification of apparently culture-specific, short-term patterns that in fact have widespread and substantial effects on fertility and its direction of change.

Anthropologists can also contribute to an understanding of the relationship between mating patterns and fertility. In most of the demographic literature, people are treated as married or unmarried, with the implicit assumption that children are desired by married and not by unmarried couples.  There has also been the assumption that marital unions are more stable than nonmarital ones (Stycos, 1963:226).  These assumptions have led to endless difficulty in the interpretation of fertility behavior. In fact, what in U.S. society is called marriage might better be called a formalized union, that is, formalized by the social mechanisms appropriate for that culture; however, in many societies (for example, in most of Latin America), individuals can spend years in unions which are not formalized, but which function like marriage in every

other way. Because they look at the form and not the
function, demographers have trouble understanding why
unions they assume to be "unstable" produce as many
children as "marriages." To complicate matters further,
there are other union types, such as visiting relationships, which may be expected to produce children, as well
as multiple unions such as polygamy and polyandry.
Desires for children and fertility-related behavior (such
as frequency of intercourse) may vary from one union type
to another and from one spouse to another in a polygamous
union. In addition, individuals and couples can move
from one union type to another, presenting a dynamic
rather than a static pattern. This may necessitate
longitudinal studies, or at least longitudinal analyses.
Understanding the motivations and behaviors surrounding
union types can help explain variations in fertility and
mortality rates; however, as Nag (1975a:289) says,
"Demographers have concentrated on the end-products of
such interaction without relating those to family and
kin" (cf. Burch, in these volumes).

This contrast between the demographer's tendency to
concentrate on behavioral results and the anthropologist's concerns with intention, planning, volition, and
context indicates a number of specific potential anthropological contributions to the study of the intermediate
fertility variables (Davis and Blake, 1956) and in
particular the proximate variables (Bongaarts, 1978).
Newman (1981) has suggested an additional set of variables
which she calls context variables. These include ideological, interpersonal, contraceptive, and reproductive
variables; for example, under reproductive she includes
the wantedness or value of children. These variables are
seen as influencing the intermediate or the proximate
variables. Anthropologists can also contribute to the
understanding of all these variables because many are not
easily derived from survey material or secondary data
sources, but instead are amenable to ethnographic investigation. The discussion that follows focuses on the
major areas in which anthropological research can
contribute to the study of fertility.


MAJOR ANTHROPOLOGICAL AREAS OF FERTILITY RESEARCH

Anthropological work on the determinants of human fertility can be divided into two broad areas:  macro
(treating large populations such as societies and

TABLE 1   Anthropological Areas of Fertility Research:
Macro-Level

| Topic | References |
|---|---|
| 1. Population homeostasis | Alland, 1970; Abernethy, 1980; Swedlund, 1978; Polgar, 1973 |
| 2. Culture and reproductive success | Irons, 1979, 1980; Blurton-Jones and Sibley, 1978; Chagnon, 1979 |
| 3. Social structure and fertility | Harris, 1976; Yengoyan, 1972; Schneider, 1955; Wagley, 1952; Abernethy, 1979 |
| 4. Cultural evolution and population growth | Nag, 1973; Polgar, 1975; Bartlett, 1980; Netting, 1974; Dumond, 1965; Harner, 1970 |
| 5. Environment and reproduction | Baker, 1978; Clegg, 1978; McClung, 1969 |

communities) and micro (treating individuals and
families).  At each level, fertility behavior and its
determinants have been studied both in the past (including the archeological and paleontological records
predating written history) and in the present.  Major
topics of study at both levels are described in the
subsections below.  Each topic could easily be the subject of its own chapter; all that is possible here is to
provide a brief definition and example for each, with a
few sample references.

## Macro-Level Areas of Research

The major macro-level areas of anthropological fertility
research are listed in Table 1, and briefly described
below.

## Population Homeostasis

The concept of population homeostasis, based on Wynne-
Edwards' (1962) work, centers on the idea that population
size represents an adaptation to a specific environment,
including the way that environment is utilized (in
extracting food and other resources from it).  If an
environment and the way it is used remain the same, the
population also remains stable, and does not grow enough
to damage the environment to the point at which the
population's survival chances are threatened (usually
expressed in terms of food scarcity).  A key point in

this theory is that human populations have not simply
been victims of high mortality rates necessitating high
fertility rates, but have always regulated both fertility
and mortality to some degree (Alland, 1970; Abernethy,
1979; Swedlund, 1978; Polgar, 1971, 1972, 1973). As
Alland (1970:2) puts it, "beliefs and behaviors that
affect fertility, death, and disease rates are major
factors in the adaptations of human societies. Over
time, every society develops behavioral strategies which
maximize gains and minimize losses in its population size
relative to particular environments."


Culture and Reproductive Success

Culturally patterned behaviors will frequently ensure
maximum reproductive success in the form of genetic
representation in the next generation. For example,
Blurton-Jones and Sibly (1978) argue that Kung Bushman
birth spacing ensures the survival of more children to
adulthood than if birth intervals were shorter. Although
the cultural spacing norm of four to five years produces
fewer children, mortality rates are lower, guaranteeing
more and healthier representatives in the next generation.


Social Structure and Fertility

Although environment, particularly food resources, is a
major potential limiting factor, societies may find many
different ways to function effectively in the same environment. Thus, Australian aborigines and sheepherders
have very different cultures, but both function successfully in the same environment. Social structure, the way
a society is organized, produces behavioral norms that
influence fertility (among many other facets of life).
Sometimes these norms function to limit fertility more
than is absolutely necessary in the particular environment, but in ways consistent with harmonious social
organization. An example is two Amazon cultures studied
by Wagley (1969). Although the Tapirape had a social
structure that made forming new communities difficult or
impossible, the agricultural and hunting system could not
support villages larger than 200 people. The Tapirape
had a strict policy limiting families to three children,
and this was enforced through infanticide. In the same
environment, the Tenetehara had a social structure that

facilitated dividing villages to form new ones when the
original village became too large to be practical; there
were no limitations on family size (see also Potter, in
these volumes).

## Cultural Evolution in Relation to Population Growth

These discussions tend to center around the role of
population pressure (or its lack) in the development of
many cultural patterns, particularly agriculture and
social stratification (Barlett, 1980; Dumond, 1975;
Harner, 1970; Polgar, 1975). For example, there is much
discussion of whether population growth stimulated the
intensification of agriculture or whether new agricultural techniques permitted population growth. Much of
this debate is summarized by Netting (1974), who provides
evidence of increasing intensification of agriculture as
at least a concomitant of increased population density.

## Environment and Reproduction

Physical anthropologists have looked specifically at the
effects of various environments on the probability of
conception, the maintenance of gestation, and intrapartum
mortality. For example, much has been done on the effects
of high altitudes on reproduction (Baker, 1978; McClung,
1969). The evidence suggests that, despite compensations
such as larger placentas, more fetal wastage is experienced at high altitudes (10,000 feet and over), as is
higher perinatal mortality, in part due to lower birth
weights (McClung, 1969; Clegg, 1978).

## Micro-Level Areas of Research

The major micro-level areas of anthropological fertility
research are shown in Table 2, and briefly described in
the following subsections. Some of these areas, such as
the intermediate fertility variables described by Davis
and Blake (1956), have, of course, been discussed by
sociologists and others. Anthropologists have taken these
topics and explored them in depth, looking not only at
actual behaviors but also at etiology and causality and
at relationships between the behaviors.

TABLE 2   Anthropological Areas of Fertility Research:
Micro-Level

| Topic | References |
|-------|-----------|
| 1. Union formation and dissolution | Nag, 1980; Gulick and Gulick, 1975; Chen et al., 1974 |
| 2. Sexual intercourse within unions | Nag, 1967, 1968; Abernethy, 1979; Ford, 1964; Mead, 1949; Malinowski, 1929; Saucier, 1972 |
| 3. Contraceptive use: acceptability, method preferences, consistency of use | Hines, 1963; Polgar, 1971, 1972, 1973; Carr-Saunders, 1922; Polgar and Marshall, 1976; Scrimshaw, 1972, 1976, 1980a, 1980b; Shain, 1980; Marshall, 1977 |
| 4. Abortion | Ford, 1964; Schneider, 1955; Devereux, 1967 |
| 5. Infanticide | Dickeman, 1975, 1979; Wagley, 1952; Ford, 1964; Langer, 1974; Abernethy, 1979; Firth, 1961 |
| 6. Fertility decision making | Hull, 1982; Shedlin and Hollerbach, 1981; Scrimshaw, 1978 |
| 7. Family form and fertility | Lorimer, 1954; Nag, 1968; Sipes, 1974; Hammel, 1961, 1977 |
| 8. Women's activities and roles | Ford, 1964; LeVine, 1980; Oppong, 1981 |
| 9. Value of children | Nag et al., 1978; Cain, 1977; Yengoyan, 1974 |
| 10. Infant mortality and fertility | Scrimshaw, 1978; Harris, 1977; Lewis, 1963; Neel, 1970 |

## Union Formation and Dissolution

Mating patterns have been a classical area of anthropological study, so their analysis in relation to fertility
is no surprise.  Anthropologists have looked at age at
marriage and fertility (Gulick and Gulick, 1975b;
Scrimshaw, 1978a; Low, 1978); nonmarital fertility (Low,
1978); interruptions in unions and fertility (Chen et
al., 1974); and many similar behaviors.  Some of the most
detailed work in this area has been done by Nag (1968),
who first explored the Davis and Blake (1956) variables
from an anthropological perspective and found that their
assumptions about factors affecting fertility in nonindustrial societies needed revision.  For example, he found
that methods of fertility regulation in nonindustrial
societies were not determined solely by factors most
closely related to gestation and parturition (Nag,
1968:149).  In a more recent article on relationships
between modernization and fertility, Nag (1980:579) has
continued to explore areas such as the effect of improved

mortality rates on the duration of unions, and hence on fertility.


Sexual Intercourse Within Unions

This is a difficult area to research either qualitatively or quantitatively. Sexual behavior has been studied by many anthropologists, including Mead (1949), Malinowski (1929), Ford (1964) and Nag (1967, 1968). The qualitative, descriptive work is useful in that it gives some indication of attitudes towards intercourse and hints at frequency. For example, stories about the illnesses or disorders that can result when intercourse does not take place several times a week hint at cultural expectations of frequency. Women's accounts of fearing intercourse and their search for excuses to avoid it also allow the researcher to ask about actual frequency with some sense of the accuracy of the answer. In a society where intercourse is regarded as a very private matter and where there are few opportunities for privacy, frequency may be more limited than in contexts where those constraints do not exist. For example, Nag (1967:161-163) mentions lower frequency of intercourse for extended families than for nuclear families because of the lack of privacy in the former. Anthropological research can also help establish behavioral ideals, and the extent to which these are upheld or disregarded. For example, many cultures have ritual periods when intercourse is forbidden; these are frequently related to preparation for warfare or hunting (Ford, 1964:28-29), or to the postpartum period (Saucier, 1972; see also Nag, in these volumes).


Contraceptive Use

This area includes the concepts of method and program acceptability as well as contraceptive choice and consistency (Hermalin, in these volumes; Bogue, in these volumes). When family planning programs began to proliferate in the 1960s, the underlying assumption of some population activists and some demographers was that there was a large, eager population just waiting for the opportunity to use modern contraceptives. When programs did not have the success expected, anthropologists began pointing out that there might be instances where people wanted to prevent fertility, but where either the methods themselves or the programs delivering them were not culturally acceptable (Polgar, 1973; Polgar and Marshall, 1976; Newman, 1972; Shain, 1980; Scrimshaw, 1972, 1976, 1980a, 1980b).

Questions of both method and program acceptability have been addressed to some extent by fields other than anthropology. One of the important aspects of the anthropological treatment of these topics is the range and scope of factors considered. Acceptability of both methods and programs is looked at in light of such diverse factors as social structure, sexuality, male and female roles, women's modesty, family structure, marriage patterns, perceptions of blood and other body secretions, and so on. For example, see the collection of papers in Culture, Natality, and Family Planning (Marshall and Polgar, 1976). Because human behavior is not unilinear or unidimensional, such broadly based analyses of contraceptive behavior are likely to be extremely valuable.


Induced Abortion

This topic has been widely discussed in the anthropological literature (Ford, 1964; Schneider, 1955; Devereux, 1955). Much of the work has focused on the existence of induced abortion in a given society, on the techniques used, and on the way it is perceived within the culture. Some studies have examined its demographic impact (see, e.g., David, in these volumes; see also Schneider, 1955, for a discussion of its role in the depopulation of Yap).


Infanticide

This topic has also been frequently mentioned in the anthropological literature (Ford, 1964; Langer, 1974; Scrimshaw, in these volumes); analyses of infanticide in relation to fertility have been done by Wagley (1969), Dickeman (1975), Abernathy (1979), and Firth (1961). Infanticide and fertility have also been discussed in relation to East Indian social behavior, such as decisions to keep newborn females more frequently in the lower than the upper classes because of the tendency for women to marry "up" (Dickeman, 1979). Perhaps the most controversial discussion of infanticide was provided by

Divale and Harris (1976), who related the practice to
warfare, with war generating higher status for males and
thus creating an incentive for female infanticide; they
therefore suggested that war and female infanticide
together act as population-regulating mechanisms.   This
argument has been strongly criticized, particularly for
its lack of precise quantitative data (Lancaster and
Lancaster, 1978).


## Fertility Decision Making

This subject has been discussed at the levels of the
individual, the couple, and the family.   For example,
Shedlin and Hollerbach (1981) provide a classic anthro-
pologically oriented analysis in describing and docu-
menting the complex factors influencing fertility
decision making in a Mexican community.   Similarly,
Scrimshaw (1978b) discusses the changes in men's and
women's relative influence on the fertility decision-
making process as the woman passes through different
stages in her life cycle, stages which are both bio-
logically and culturally determined.   Many other examples
are provided by Hull (in these volumes) and Beckman (in
these volumes).


## Family Form and Fertility

Family form refers to distinctions such as nuclear versus
extended families, and can also be used to refer to
residence patterns, (matrilocal, patrilocal, neolocal).
For example, as noted above, there has been a great deal
of discussion on whether couples living in extended family
situations have fewer children because of a lack of privacy (Nag, 1967, 1974, 1980); alternatively, they may
have more children since there are more potential care-
takers around.   The consensus in the literature seems to
favor the former argument (Sipes, 1974).   Another series
of studies has looked at strong corporate descent groups
and found that they are not associated with high fertility
(Sipes, 1974; Nag, 1968; see also Burch, in these
volumes).

Women's Activities, Parental Roles, Childcare, and
Fertility

This area covers topics ranging from women's work and
lactation (Nerlove, 1974) to women's status and fertility
(see Oppong, in these volumes). For example, Newman
(1978) argues that children are so important to the
status of East Indian women that it is essential to
produce them as soon as possible after marriage. Women's
work and its relationship to fertility seems to be influenced by the availability of childcare (Nardi, 1981; see
also Standing, in these volumes). Research relating
women's schooling to fertility in developing countries
has been reviewed by LeVine (1980).


Value of Children

Along with psychologists and sociologists (Fawcett, in
these volumes), anthropologists have looked closely at
the value of children, taking advantage of participant
observation and time budget studies, observing as well as
interviewing. A series of studies under Nag's direction
showed that children in large families work more than
those in small families, so that large families may be
more productive (Nag et al., 1978; White, 1975). These
same studies and others (Cain, 1977; Marshall, 1972)
indicate that, in many societies, children are economically valuable at a relatively young age (but see
Lindert, in these volumes; Lee and Bulatao, in these
volumes). Caldwell has also shown that older children
continue to be valuable by contributing money to the
household, even from a distance (1974, 1977, in these
volumes). The question of the quality of children has
also been discussed by anthropologists who have suggested
that spacing may be a way of ensuring heathier, better-
educated children, considered more valuable than a larger
family of poor-quality children (Nag et al., 1978;
Scrimshaw and Pelto, 1979).


Relationships Between Infant Mortality and Fertility

Some anthropologists feel there is evidence that in some
societies and subcultures (particularly where there are
economic constraints), differential parental care (conscious or unconscious) results with children who are not

wanted: those that are too closely spaced, a sex considered less desirable (usually females), a high birth
order in a large family, the product of an illegitimate
union, or a child not wanted for some other reason
(Scrimshaw, 1978c; Harris, 1977; Lewis, 1963: Neel, 1970).
Thus high mortality can be a behavioral consequence of
high fertility, rather than the reverse; that is, people
who lose children to mortality may not necessarily rush
to replace them as had been thought (Taylor et al., 1976).
Anthropologists are continuing to study the specific
behavioral mechanisms through which differential care
might operate (Scrimshaw and Pelto, 1979). These include
infant and child feeding, response to illness (use of
medical services), accident prevention, and other physical
and emotional support.

## METHODS

The most distinctive feature of social anthropology is
ethnographic field work, its method of data collection in
contemporary populations (Pelto and Pelto, 1978; Johnson,
1978). Ethnography involves a single anthropologist (or
a couple) in direct and prolonged contact with individuals
of the population under study, using various techniques
and perspectives to record social behavior patterns in
their natural contexts--ecological, socioeconomic, linguistic, and cultural. Like natural historians of
Darwin's day and contemporary ethologists investigating
animal behavior, the ethnographer selects methods
appropriate to the particular setting, its patterns of
adaptation, and its peculiar opportunities for and
constraints on observation. The ethnographer collects
both quantitative and qualitative data, interprets them
in context, and synthesizes them in a detailed published
description made available to the scientific community
and the general public. The use of specific bodies of
data to test hypotheses and evaluate policy follows this
contextual study.

This approach is clearly limited for examining large-
scale problems of population change. However, it serves
as a unique complement to the macro-level methods of
demography. In fact, ethnographic data are strongest
just where standard demographic data are weakest.

First, ethnography can provide contextual knowledge.
Unlike the analyst of national censuses or large-scale
surveys, the ethnographer is personally involved in both

the collection and analysis phases of research and, having lived in the communities studied, knows the local scene and many of the individuals in it. Conducting a small-scale survey, he or she is able to examine each interview in the light of other information already collected on the same respondent individuals and families, checking for errors and discrepancies while there is still a chance to correct them. This cross-checking of data sources guarantees the validity of the data to a degree not possible in large-scale surveys. Contextual knowledge also facilitates valid interpretation, particularly for anomalous and deviant findings, since the ethnographer has, in his reservoir of local information, an empirical basis for explanation that is independent of any particular survey. The ethnographer is also in a position to assess the relative plausibility of alternative explanations, such as whether results reflect errors of reporting or demographic realities with vernacular meanings. In an example noted by Page and Lesthaeghe (1981), demographers examining African birth histories believed they had no grounds for deciding whether long birth intervals represented a real social constraint on fertility or defective sampling or reporting. The anthropologists who reported such data, however, knew from their ethnographic research on African families that these intervals were due not to methodological errors, but to institutionalized postpartum abstinence, a cultural pattern of great normative significance in some African communities that has important consequences for total fertility. The anthropological interpretation was confirmed by subsequent demographic research (Caldwell and Caldwell, 1977; Page and Lesthaeghe, 1981), thus demonstrating the value of contextual knowledge to the scientific understanding of fertility.

Another area where the anthropological method is particularly effective is in measuring proscribed behavior. Since such behavior is often related to reproduction, this has important implications for demographers. Depending on the culture, behaviors such as induced abortion, infanticide, contraceptive use, and forbidden sexual intercourse may all be concealed to some extent. Anthropologists can obtain data on these behaviors through repeated, subtle conversations, through observation, through the flexibility of changes in approaches to a topic, and through the increased trust that comes from time spent in a community. For example, each of several women interviewed during the first two months of field work in Barbados claimed to have had a single father for all her children; later, one by one, they "confessed" that their children had "several fathers," and then provided accurate union and fertility histories (Scrimshaw, 1969).

Population researchers have had a great deal of difficulty in addressing the related questions of achieved behavior versus intentions and real versus ideal behavior, questions that are important in understanding fertility and family planning.  Here, the strength of the anthropological method lies in its combination of questions, conversation, and observation over time in the field.  A woman who states she will seek contraception can be observed to see if she actually does, and what obstacles she encounters along the way.  A woman who categorically states she is against induced abortion and later asks the researcher to loan her money so she can get one is demonstrating the discrepancy between real and ideal behavior. Typically, the anthropologist accumulates cases like these, and uses them as a basis for estimating the frequency of such occurrences.  Often, a few case histories can reveal problems which survey researchers had not suspected were present, thus allowing appropriate questions to be incorporated into surveys.

The ethnographic method is particularly important for population studies in developing countries that lack birth and death registration, where national census interviews are used to estimate ages and proportions of children who have died.  Although government census bureaus have become more sophisticated in constructing local event calendars for age determination, and demographers have devised methods of estimating ages and other vital statistics from censuses known to be based on approximations, community census surveys conducted by anthropologists can make unique contributions.  In some cases, they provide census material in which ages have been carefully ascertained, taking much more time and effort than a government enumerator could afford, and including exact birth dates for children born during the field research period.  An increasing number of anthropologists have worked in the same communities over 20 years or more, collecting data indicative of demographic trends and dynamics in a small population.  There is reason to believe that much more information of this kind has been collected on peoples throughout the developing world than has been published to date; were these data to be made available to the demographic research community, research on fertility change would probably benefit substantially.

Ethnographic work is thus stronger in validity and in the extent to which one is actually measuring what one is attempting to measure; however, survey work is stronger in its reliability and replicablity (Pelto and Pelto, 1978). Because of this complementarity, researchers are increasingly attempting to combine the two. Ideally, this combination should consist of ethnographic work applied to the survey design, and then some in-depth work with a small, randomly selected subsample of the survey population. The presurvey ethnographic work provides the research investigation with the contextual richness described above, and guides the framing of the questions themselves. For example, when this combination of methods was applied in Ecuador in the early 1970s, barriers to contraceptive use such as fears of specific methods and of family planning clinics, as well as problems with access to the clinics, emerged from conversations between the ethnographer and women in the community. Related questions were then built into the survey which confirmed the existence of these problems in the larger population and established their magnitude. At the same time, a question on whether or not women knew how to "avoid children," which had successfully elicited information about contraception from Puerto Rican women in New York, was interpreted in Ecuador as meaning knowledge about abortion. The wording had to be changed to "avoid becoming pregnant." Even working in the same language, it was necessary to make such changes from one country to another (Scrimshaw, 1974).

Ethnographic work done concurrently with a survey can be used to establish greater depth on a subsample, thus enhancing the interpretation of survey results. For example, in one study of seasonal migration in Guatemala, the researcher migrated with a subsample from one of the communities studied. She rode the trucks from the highlands to the coast, ate and slept under the same conditions as the migrants, and picked up a great deal of detail on their feelings about migration, their reasons for it, and their methods of coping with it (Hurtado, 1980).

Finally, surveys and ethnographies can be combined in the data analysis and writing phase. In Ecuador, 65 families studied ethnographically were interviewed as a special subsample of the survey, so that the researcher had both kinds of data for them. It was gratifying that

the fertility histories were identical, down to admitted
induced abortions, since the ethnographic work had led to
the development of detailed probes and questions for each
topic. Other items, however, were less accurate. A
question about sanitary facilities was designed as both
an economic and a health measure. Unfortunately, people
surveyed (2,200 families throughout the city) often
insisted they had facilities which the ethnographer knew
did not exist in their areas. The information on family
income was not consistent with ethnographic records;
however, other culturally appropriate measures of socioeconomic status, developed during the ethnographic phase,
appeared to place each family accurately (Scrimshaw,
1974).

The ethnographic data often also served to reveal the
meaning behind the statistics. For example, women's
determination to obtain contraception despite their husbands' objections could be illustrated by their stories
of how they tried to do so. In another example, detailed
analysis of fertility histories revealed that the second
of two closely spaced infants was more likely to die than
its older sibling, a reverse of the usual mortality pattern. The survey data yielded no clue as to the reason
for this (Wolfers and Scrimshaw, 1975); however, the
reason was painfully clear from the ethnographic observations of differential treatment of siblings, with the
older likely to receive more food and medical attention
than the younger (Scrimshaw, 1978c). Without the data
from both methods, the two halves of this puzzle could
not have been put together.

Although it will not always be possible to conduct such
combined field research, demographers can make greater use
of existing ethnographic research and of ethnographers in
areas where survey research or other data analysis will
be conducted. Moreover, ethnographic work and ethnographers can be used in the design of data collection and
analysis and in the interpretation of results.


CONCLUSIONS


Anthropologists and demographers have examined many of
the same problems, although often in different populations and from different perspectives. However, the
mutual influence that might have been expected has been
relatively slight, in part because of a lack of awareness
by investigators of relevant research outside their own

disciplines. The contributions that anthropology and its unique methods can made to the scientific understanding of fertility and its determinants in developing countries will be realized only when more anthropologists read the population literature, address their research and writings to issues in population studies, and include demographic methods in their research. Conversely, more demographers, especially those working in developing countries, need to be aware of the anthropological evidence. More specifically, the advantages of ethnographic inquiry should be combined with quantitative research, as separate stages of a single project and through the intensive study of subsamples from survey populations.

Anthropological research, as reviewed in this chapter, has made some contributions to the understanding of fertility determinants, but these could be substantially enhanced by field studies focused on such topics as factors affecting fertility decline, particularly in some of the larger national populations; factors affecting contraceptive acceptability; and changes in the value of children with migration from rural to urban areas. Whatever the location and problem focus of their studies, however, anthropologists should continue to do what they do best: provide holistic and accurate pictures of communities and the cultures, behaviors, relationships, and motivations of people within those communities, in this case with respect to fertility and fertility change. To be fully effective at this, anthropologists must learn enough of the problems, language, and culture of demography to put their research into terms comprehensible to other disciplines within the population field.

## NOTE

1. Participants at the workshop were John W. Adams, J. Lawrence Angel, Mead T. Cain, John C. Caldwell, Mary Elmendorf, B. M. Gray, John Gulick, Eugene A. Hammel, Nancy Howell, William Jansen, Alice Bee Kasakoff, Robert A. LeVine, Richard Lieban, Moni Nag, Robert M. Netting, Lucile F. Newman, Priscilla Reining, Susan C. M. Scrimshaw, Michele Shedlin, Mayling Simpson-Hebert, Richard G. Sipes, Benjamin White, and Aram Yengoyan, in addition to members and staff of the Panel on Fertility Determinants: Rodolfo A. Bulatao, Ronald Freedman, Paula E. Hollerbach, Robert J. Lapham, W. Parker Mauldin, Toni Richards, and Carol Bradford

Ward. Many of the anthropologists prepared short papers for the workshop, which are reflected to some extent in this chapter. In particular, the chapter draws on the extensive bibliographic work and discussion paper prepared for the workshop by Reining (1981).

BIBLIOGRAPHY

Abernathy, V. (1979) Population Pressure and Cultural Adjustment. New York: Human Sciences Press.

Alland, A. (1970) Adaptation in Cultural Evolution: An Approach to Medical Anthropology. New York: Columbia University Press.

Arensberg, A., and A. Niehoff (1971) Introducing Social Change: A Manual for Community Development. Chicago: Aldine-Atherton.

Baker, P. T. (1978) The Biology of High Altitude Peoples. London: Cambridge University Press.

Baker, P. T., and J. S. Dutt (1972) Demographic variables as measures of biological adaptation: A case study of high altitude populations. In G. H. Harrison and A. J. Boyce, eds., The Structure of Human Populations. Oxford, Eng.: Clarendon Press.

Barlett, P. F. (1980) The anthropological approach to fertility decision-making. In T. K. Burch, ed., Demographic Behavior: Interdisciplinary Perspectives on Decision-Making. Boulder, Colo.: Westview Press.

Blurton-Jones, N. B., and R. M. Sibly (1978) Testing adaptiveness of culturally determined behavior: Do Bushmen women maximize reproductive success by spacing births widely and foraging seldom? In N. B. Blurton-Jones and V. Reynolds, eds., Human Behavior and Adaptation. Symposium Number 18 of the Society of the Study of Human Biology. London: Taylor-Francis.

Bongaarts, J. (1978) A framework for analyzing the proximate determinants of fertility. Population and Development Review 3:63-102.

Cain, M. T. (1977) The economic activities of children in a village in Bangladesh. Population and Development Review 3:201-228.

Caldwell, J. C. (1974) The Study of Fertility and Fertility Change in Tropical Africa. WFS Occasional Papers, No. 7. London: World Fertility Survey.

Caldwell, J. C. (1977) The economic rationality of high fertility: An investigation illustrated with Nigerian survey data. Population Studies 31:5-27.

Caldwell, J. C., and P. Caldwell (1977)  The role of marital sexual abstinence in determining fertility:  A study of the Yoruba in Nigeria.  Population Studies 31:193-217.

Carr-Saunders, A. M. (1922)  The Population Problem. Oxford, Eng.:  Clarendon Press.

Chagnon, N. A. (1979)  Kin selection and conflict:  An analysis of a Yanomano ax fight.  In N. A. Chagnon and W. Irons, eds., Evolutionary Biology and Human Social Behavior:  An Anthropological Perspective.  North Scituate, Mass.:  Duxbury Press.

Chen, K. H., S. Wishik, and S. Scrimshaw (1974)  The effects of unstable sexual unions on fertility in Guayaquil, Ecuador.  Human Biology 21:353-359.

Clegg, E. J. (1978)  Fertility and early growth.  In P. Baker, ed., The Biology of High Altitude Peoples. London:  Cambridge University Press.

Coale, A. J., and T. J. Trussell (1974)  Model fertility schedules:  Variations in the age structure of childbearing in human populations.  Population Index 40:185-258.

Cowgill, G. (1975)  On causes and consequences of ancient and modern population changes.  American Anthropologist 77:505-525.

Davis, K., and J. Blake (1956)  Social structure and fertility:  An analytical framework.  Economic Development and Cultural Change 4:211-235.

Devereux, G. (1955)  A Study of Abortion in Primitive Societies.  New York:  Julian Press.

Dickeman, M. (1975)  Demographic consequences of infanticide in Man.  Annual Review of Ecology and Systematics 6:100-137.

Dickeman, M. (1979)  Female infanticide, reproductive strategies and social stratification:  A preliminary model.  In N. A. Chagnon and W. Irons, eds., Evolutionary Biology and Human Social Behavior:  An Anthropological Perspective.  North Scituate, Mass.: Duxbury Press.

Divale, W., and M. Harris (1976)  Population, warfare and the male supremist complexes.  American Anthropologist 78:521-538.

Dumond, D. E. (1975)  The limitation of human population: A natural history.  Science 187:713-721.

Firth, R. (1957)  We, The Tikopia.  London:  Allen and Unwin.

Firth, R. (1961)  Elements of Social Organization, 3rd ed.  Boston:  Beacon Press.

Ford, C. S. (1964) A Comparative Study of Human Reproduction. New Haven, Conn.: Human Relations Area Files Press.

Geertz, C. (1973) The Interpretation of Cultures. New York: The Free Press.

Goodenough, W. (1963) Cooperation in Change. New York: Russell Sage.

Gulick, J., and M. E. Gulick (1975a) Final Considerations About Their Children Among Parents in the Iranian City of Isfahan. Paper presented at the annual meeting of the American Association for the Advancement of Science, New York.

Gulick, J., and M. E. Gulick (1975b) Migrant and native married women in the Iranian city of Isfahan. Anthropological Quarterly.

Hackenberg, R. A. (1974) Genealogical method in social anthropology: The foundations of structural demography. In J. Honigman, ed., Handbook of Social and Cultural Anthropology. New York: Rand McNally.

Hammel, E. A. (1961) The family cycle in a coastal Peruvian slum and village. American Anthropologist 63:989-1005.

Hammel, E. A., and D. W. Wachter (1977) Primonuptuality and ultimonuptuality: Their effects on stem-family-non-household frequencies. In R. D. Lee, ed., Population Patterns in the Past. New York: Academic Press.

Harner, M. J. (1970) Population factors and the social evolution of agriculturalists. Southwestern Journal of Anthropology 26:67-86.

Harris, M. (1977) Cannibals and Kings: The Origins of Cultures. New York: Random House.

Hassan, F. A. (1973) On the mechanisms of population growth in the neolithic. Current Anthropology 14:535-542.

Himes, N. E. (1963) Medical History of Contraception. New York: Gamut Press.

Hurtado, E. (1980) Personal communication.

Irons, W. (1979) Culture and biological success. In N. A. Chagnon, and W. Irons, eds., Evolutionary Biology and Human Social Behavior: An Anthropological Perspective. North Scituate, Mass.: Duxbury Press.

Irons, W. (1980) Is Yomut social behavior adaptive? In G. W. Barlow, and J. Silverberg, eds., Sociobiology: Beyond Nature? American Association for the Advancement of Science Selected Symposium 35. Boulder, Colo.: Westview Press.

Johnson, A. W. (1978)  Quantification in Cultural Anthropology: An Introduction to Research Design. Stanford, Calif.: Stanford University Press.

Kaplan, B. A. (1976)  Anthropological Studies of Human Fertility. Detroit, Mich.: Wayne State University Press.

Katz, S. H. (1972)  Biological factors in population control. In B. Spooner, ed., Population Growth: Anthropological Implications. Cambridge, Mass.: MIT Press.

Knodel, J. (1977)  Breastfeeding and population growth. Science 198:111–115.

Kunstadter, P. (1971)  Natality, mortality and migration of upland and lowland populations in northwestern Thailand. In S. Polgar, ed., Culture and Population: A Collection of Current Studies. Cambridge, Mass.: Schenkenmapp.

Kunstadter, P., R. Buhler, F. Stephan, and C. F. Westoff (1963)  Demographic variability and preferential marriage patterns. American Journal of Physical Anthropology 21:511–519.

Lancaster, C., and J. Lancaster (1978)  On the male supremist complex: A reply to Divale and Harris. American Anthropologist 80:115–117.

Langer, W. (1974)  Infanticide: A historical survey. History of Childhood Quarterly 1:353–365.

LeVine, R. (1980)  Influences of women's schooling on maternal behavior in the Third World. Comparative Education Review 24:S78–S104.

Lewis, O. (1963)  Life in a Mexican Village. Pregnancy and Birth. Urbana, Ill.: University of Illinois Press.

Lorimer, F. et al. (1954)  Culture and Human Fertility. Paris: UNESCO.

Low, S. (1978)  Family formation in Costa Rica. In W. B. Miller and L. F. Newman, eds., The First Child and Family Formation. Chapel Hill, N.C.: Carolina Population Center.

Malinowski, B. (1929)  The Sexual Life of Savages. New York: Harcourt, Brace and World.

Marshall, J. F. (1972)  Culture and Contraception: Response Determinants to a Family Planning Program in a North Indian Village. Unpublished Ph.D. dissertation. Department of Anthropology, University of Hawaii, Honolulu.

Marshall, J. F. (1977)  Acceptability of fertility regulating methods: Designing technology to fit people. Preventative Medicine 6:65–73.

Marshall, J. F., and S. Polgar, eds. (1976) Culture,
    Natality, and Family Planning. Chapel Hill, N.C.:
    University of North Carolina.
McClung, J. (1969) Effects of High Altitude on Human
    Birth. Cambridge, Mass.: Harvard University Press.
Mead, M. (1949) Male and Female: A Study of the Sexes
    in a Changing World. New York: William Morrow and
    Company.
Nag, M. (1967) Family type and fertility. Pp. 160-163
    in Proceedings of the World Population Conference,
    Vol. 2. New York: United Nations.
Nag, M. (1968) Facts Affecting Human Fertility in
    Non-Industrial Societies: A Cross Cultural Study.
    New Haven, Conn.: Human Relations Area Files.
Nag, M. (1973) Cultural factors affecting family
    planning. Journal of Family Welfare (India) 19:3-7.
Nag, M. (1974) Socio-cultural patterns, family cycle,
    and fertility. Pp. 289-312 in The Population Debate:
    Dimensions and Perspectives, World Population
    Conference 3, Bucharest, Vol. 2. New York: United
    Nations.
Nag, M. (1975a) Population anthropologists at work.
    Current Anthropology 16:264-266.
Nag, M. (1975b) Population and Social Organization. The
    Hague: Mouton.
Nag, M. (1980) How modernization can also increase
    fertility. Current Anthropology 21:571-587.
Nag, M., B. N. F. White, and R. C. Peet (1978) An
    anthropological approach to the study of the economic
    value of children in Java and Nepal. Current
    Anthropology 19:293-306.
Nardi, B. A. (1981) Modes of explanation in
    anthropological population theory: Biological
    determinism vs. self-regulation in studies of
    population growth in Third World countries. American
    Anthropologist 83:28-56.
Neel, J. V. (1970) Lessons from a 'primitive' people.
    Science 170:815-822.
Nerlove, S. B. (1974) Women's workload and infant
    feeding practices: A relationship with demographic
    implications. Ethnology 13:207-214.
Netting, R. M. (1974) Agrarian ecology. Annual Review
    of Anthropology 3:21-56.
Newman, L. F. (1970) Cultural factors in family
    planning. Annals of the New York Academy of Sciences
    175:833-846.
Newman, L. F. (1972) Birth Control: An Anthropological
    View. Reading, Mass.: Addison-Wesley.

Newman, L. F. (1978)  Symbolism and status change:
Fertility and the first child in India and the United
States.  In W. B. Miller and L. F. Newman, eds., The
First Child and Family Formation.  Chapel Hill, N.C.:
Carolina Population Center.

Newman, L. F. (1981)  Anthropological Contributions to
Fertility Research.  Paper presented at the annual
meeting of the American Anthropological Association,
Los Angeles, Calif.

Page, H. T., and R. Lesthaeghe, eds. (1981)  Childspacing
in Tropical Africa:  Tradition and Change.  New York:
Academic Press.

Pelto, P. J., and G. H. Pelto (1978)  Anthropological
Research:  The Structure of Inquiry.  New York:
Cambridge University Press.

Polgar, S., ed. (1971)  Culture and Population:  A
Collection of Current Studies.  Carolina Population
Center Monograph No. 9.  Chapel Hill, N.C.:
University of North Carolina.

Polgar, S. (1972)  Population history and population
policies from an anthropological perspective.  Current
Anthropology 13:203-211.

Polgar, S. (1973)  Modernization, Population and the
Family:  Cultural and Historical Perspectives.  Paper
for the World Population Conference Symposium on
Population and the Family, UNESCO, Honolulu, Hawaii.

Polgar, S. (1975)  Population, Ecology and Social
Evolution.  The Hague:  Mouton.

Polgar, S., and J. F. Marshall (1976)  The search for
culturally acceptable fertility regulating methods.
In J. F. Marshall and S. Polgar, eds., Culture,
Natality, and Family Planning.  Chapel Hill, N.C.:
University of North Carolina.

Reining, P., ed. (1977)  Village Women:  Their Changing
Lives and Fertility.  Studies in Kenya, Mexico, and
the Philippines.  Publication No. 77-6.  Washington,
D.C.:  American Association for the Advancement of
Science.

Reining, P. (1981)  Anthropology of Fertility.  Paper
prepared for the Workshop on the Anthropology of Human
Fertility, Washington, D.C.

Saucier, J. F. (1972)  Correlates of the long postpartum
taboo:  A cross-cultural study.  Current Anthropology
13:238-249.

Schneider, D. M. (1955)  Abortion and depopulation on a
Pacific island.  In B. Paul, ed., Health, Culture and
Community.  New York:  Russell Sage.

Scrimshaw, S. C. M. (1969)  A Critique of the
   Anthropological Method as an Instrument for Research
   on Human Reproduction:  A Case Study in Barbados.
   Unpublished Ph.D. dissertation.  Columbia University,
   New York.
Scrimshaw, S. C. M. (1972)  Anthropology and Population
   Research:  Application in Family Planning Programs.
   Evaluation Manual.  New York:  International Institute
   for the Study of Human Reproduction.
Scrimshaw, S. C. M. (1974)  Culture, Environment, and
   Family Size:  A Study of Urban In-Migrants in
   Guayaquil, Ecuador.  Ph.D. Dissertation.  Columbia
   University, New York.
Scrimshaw, S. C. M. (1976)  Women's modesty:  One barrier
   to the use of family planning clinics.  In J. Marshall
   and S. Polgar, eds., Culture, Natality and Family
   Planning.  Chapel Hill, N.C.:  University of North
   Carolina.
Scrimshaw, S. C. M. (1978a)  Family formation and first
   birth in Ecuador.  In W. B. Miller and L. F. Newman,
   eds., The First Child and Family Formation.  Chapel
   Hill, N.C.:  University of North Carolina.
Scrimshaw, S. C. M. (1978b)  Stages in women's lives and
   fertility decision-making in Latin America.  Medical
   Anthropology 2:41-58.
Scrimshaw, S. C. M. (1978c)  Infant mortality and
   behavior in the regulation of family size.  Population
   and Development Review 4:383-403.
Scrimshaw, S. C. M. (1980a)  Cultural factors affecting
   the acceptability of vaginal contraceptives.  In G. I.
   Zatuchni, A. J. Sobrero, J. J. Speidel, and J. J.
   Sciarra, eds., New Developments in Vaginal
   Contraception.  New York:  Harper and Row.
Scrimshaw, S. C. M. (1980b)  Acceptability of new
   contraceptive technology.  In G. I. Zatuchni, M. H.
   Labbock, and J. J. Sciarra, eds., Research Frontiers
   in Fertility Regulation.  New York:  Harper and Row.
Scrimshaw, S. C. M., and G. H. Pelto (1979)  The impact
   of nutrition and health programs on family size and
   structure.  Pp. 183-217 in R. Klein, M. S. Read, H.
   Riecken, A. Pradilla, and C. Daza, eds., The Practice
   of Impact Evaluation.  New York:  Plenum Press.
Shain, R. M. (1980)  Acceptability of contraceptive
   methods and services:  A cross-cultural perspective.
   In R. M. Shain and C. J. Pauerstein, eds., Fertility
   Control:  Biological and Behavioral Aspects.
   Hagerstown, Md.:  Harper and Row.

Shedlin, M. G., and P. E. Hollerbach (1981)  Modern and traditional fertility regulation in a Mexican community:  The process of decision-making.  Studies in Family Planning 12:278-296.

Sipes, R. (1974)  A Hologeistic Investigation of the Influence of Three Sociocultural Factors on Population Growth Rates.  Unpublished Ph.D. dissertation.  SUNY, Buffalo.

Stycos, J. M. (1963)  Culture and differential fertility of Peru.  Population Studies 16:257-270.

Swedlund, A. C. (1978)  Historical demography as population ecology.  Annual Review of Anthropology 7:137-173.

Taylor, C. E., J. S. Newman, and N. U. Kelley (1976)  The child survival hypothesis.  Population Studies 30:263-278.

Wagley, C. (1969)  Cultural influences on population:  A comparison of two Tupi tribes.  In A. P. Vayda, ed., Environment and Cultural Behavior.  New York:  The Natural History Press.

Weiss, K. M. (1976)  Demographic theory and anthropological inference.  Pp. 351-381 in B. J. Siegel, A. R. Beals, and S. Tyler, eds., Annual Review of Anthropology, Vol. 5.  Palo Alto, Calif.:  Annual Reviews.

White, B. (1975)  The economic importance of children in a Javanese village.  In M. Nag, ed., Population and Social Organization.  The Hague:  Mouton.

White, B. (1981)  Statement Prepared for the Workshop on the Anthropology of Human Fertility.  Committee on Population and Demography, National Research Council, Washington, D.C.

Wolfers, D., and S. C. M. Scrimshaw (1975)  Child survival and intervals between pregnancies in Guayaquil, Ecuador.  Population Studies 29:479-496.

Wynne-Edwards, V. C. (1962)  Animal Dispersion in Relation to Social Behavior.  Edinburgh:  Oliver and Boyd.

Yengoyan, A. A. (1972)  Biological and demographic factors in Aboriginal Australian socio-economic organization.  Oceana 43:88.

Yengoyan, A. A. (1974)  Demographic and economic aspects of poverty in the rural Philippines.  Comparative Studies in Society and History 16:58-72.

# Chapter 19

# Statistical Studies of Aggregate Fertility Change:
# Time Series of Cross Sections

TONI RICHARDS

## INTRODUCTION

The statistical analysis of the determinants of fertility change in developing countries is a difficult problem. The long time series needed to disentangle trend, cycle, and short-run fluctuations are simply not available. At best, we have replicated short time series for some set of cross-sectional units or time series of cross sections. The cross-sectional units are geographically defined and may be countries (cross-national analysis) or areal units within a country (within-country analysis). The time period for which data are available is typically short. The analysis of time series of cross sections presents special interrelated theoretical and statistical problems. Most theoretical work has assumed what will be called "structural stability"; that is, most work has assumed that the same process that accounts for cross-sectional variability can account for changes over time. Thus, if some association between variables is observed in the cross section, structural stability would suggest that a change in one variable will produce a change in the other over time. Empirically, this turns out to be unjustified. (This is not a new point. It has been made repeatedly by other authors, for example, Hermalin [1978] and Schultz [1973]). The reasons for this are relatively straight-forward. Much of the research has concerned the impact of modernization on fertility decline. In the rather short periods for which data are available, these vari-ables tend to change rather slowly. However, cross-sectional differentials, either between countries or between regions within countries, tend to be rather large; these cross-sectional differentials can be thought of as the result of some long historical process. It is unlikely that the same model that accounts for changes in fertility over the period of observation will also account for differentials arising from long-term historical evolution. Indeed, it seems plausible that any model used to account for fertility change over some period must somehow take into account (condition on) the history of the areas that form the basis of the analysis. This makes assessing the impact of modernization on fertility decline somewhat delicate. This point will be reiterated below when statistical models appropriate to the analysis of time series of cross sections are considered.

The present paper reviews a sampling of recent work that analyzes fertility change in developing countries using time series of cross sections as data sets. These include both studies of a single country, such as Schultz's (1973) Taiwan study, and cross-national studies, such as Gregory and Campbell's (1976), that include a longitudinal component. The work of both sociologists and economists is represented. All of the studies are based on aggregate data, and all include at least some time series information for repeated cross-sectional units. The discussion has five parts. First is a brief examination of theoretical models; this is necessitated by the controversy over the relevance of socioeconomic factors as explanations of fertility change (see, e.g., van de Walle and Knodel, 1980; Freedman, 1979), as well as by the variety of approaches used by the authors reviewed. Next is a section on methodology. This is followed by a discussion of the empirical literature in two parts: within-country and cross-national studies. Finally, some suggestions for further research are offered, followed by a number of propositions summarizing and assessing the evidence discussed in the paper.


### THEORETICAL ASPECTS

Arguments concerning the effects of socioeconomic development on fertility decline seem to have fallen out of favor as explanations of the demographic transition in Europe. However, measures of socioeconomic development, along with mortality, are the principal independent variables used to predict fertility change in the studies reviewed for this paper.[1] Another common variable is information on contraception or family planning programs. When the research is carried out by sociologists, the arguments are based on the "theory of the demographic transition." This view has been summarized in a critical essay by Freedman (1979:2):

> Briefly, changes in macro-developmental variables-- urbanization, industrialization, literacy, and the like--resulted in a shift from major dependence on relatively self-contained local institutions to dependence on larger social, economic, and political units.  Such a shift implies a change in the division of labor from one in which the family and local community are central to a larger complex [to one] in which the family gave up many functions to larger, specialized institutions.  The satisfactions derived from children and family are both economic and noneconomic; and for both, new nonfamilial institutions were of growing importance.  Greater literacy and the development of effective communication and transportation networks were essential to all these changes.
>
> As units of interdependence expanded and took over familial functions, the benefits and satisfactions derived from numerous children lessened.  The costs of children increased, partly because they interfered with new nonfamilial activities and partly because improving standards of living, the increased education, and the opportunities in the new expanded system of interaction led to rising aspirations.  Parents wanted more for themselves and their children.  Under the new conditions, many satisfactions, such as those derived from the achievements of their children, were more likely to be derived from investing in fewer rather than more children.
>
> In this classical model, primary emphasis was on the changes in the objective structural developmental levels as primary in fertility decline.  The new aspirations, the changes in the functions of the family, and the new perceptions of the costs and benefits of children were seen as the necessary and almost incidental consequences of the developmental changes which lead to the demand for fewer children.

Recently, transition theory has been criticized for being too automatic, for paying too little attention to the mechanisms through which modernization leads to fertility decline, and for being empirically inaccurate. In the same article, Freedman points out that there are cases where less advanced areas began their decline before more advanced ones and that culturally similar

areas tend to have similar fertility regardless of their
level of development. He suggests that some subset of
changes in life conditions along with access to new ideas
may be sufficient for fertility decline; he emphasizes
the importance of legitimation of family limitation, and
the importance of the availability of contraceptive
methods. In many ways, this is a restatement of Coale's
preconditions for fertility decline, with a much-
diminished emphasis on economic aspects (Coale, 1973).
In a somewhat similar vein, van de Walle and Knodel
(1980) have also criticized transition theory. They
argue that a "new mentality" is required for the onset of
fertility decline (p. 35). The support for their argument
is largely the same as Freedman's. Given the concentration in time of fertility decline in historical Europe
and the diversity of socioeconomic conditions then
existing, van de Walle and Knodel argue that "differences
in the start and speed of fertility decline seem to have
been determined more by cultural setting than by socioeconomic conditions" (p. 21). Pointing to the relative
invariance of the mean age at last birth (p. 11), they
emphasize the absence of target family size in pretransition populations. They conclude that a new mentality was
required for fertility decline, and that this predisposition is governed by cultural factors (p. 34).

Criticism of transition theory is not new. Earlier
criticism emphasized its lack of precision. In 1975,
Teitlebaum remarked: "The theory of the demographic
transition is essentially a plausible description of
complex social and economic phenomena which took place in
19th century Europe. It is notably lacking in such components of theories as a specifiable and measurable
mechanism of 'causation' and a definite time scale." The
new criticisms both deny the theory's empirical accuracy
for Europe and seek new culturally based mechanisms to
account for fertility decline. The question that must be
raised is whether, in light of these criticisms, it still
makes sense to include measures of modernization among
the independent variables used to account for fertility
change in developing countries, and how well such models
are likely to perform. The principal issue is what can
be reasonably expected from statistical models of fertility decline.

It will be argued here that some of the results cited
by van de Walle and Knodel and by Freedman as evidence
for the relative unimportance of modernization for fertility decline may have been far too strict a test of the

theory. Critics of transition theory have regarded the onset of family limitation as a decisive break with the past. In empirical analysis, they have examined the date when fertility declined 10 percent or more, never to return to its previous levels. On this basis, they have noted that regions with far different levels of modernization tend to have similar dates of fertility decline and that those regions with similar dates of decline tend to cluster geographically and culturally. On this basis, they have concluded that economic modernization is relatively unimportant for fertility decline and that cultural and linguistic factors that facilitate the communication of new ideas are more important. However, this analysis may be too strong a test for what seems to be a relatively weak hypothesis. What the test amounts to is predicting the turning point in fertility from the level of modernization. This is a difficult task. If the level of fertility at any given point in time is regarded as the outcome of some long historical process (Hermalin, 1975), it seems unreasonable to expect to predict the turning point in such a series from a single factor, without more knowledge of the process. It is like trying to draw inferences about a moving picture from a single still frame. A perhaps less restrictive test is to ask whether, in some set of regions over some time period, an increase in modernization is associated with a decline in fertility, once one has somehow accounted for the history of the process. A variety of statistical models are available for such analyses; the present discussion will emphasize selecting a model that makes sense theoretically, at the same time pointing out how different statistical models make different assumptions about the dynamics of fertility and its responsiveness to change.

The arguments just described have been primarily among sociologists; the hypotheses involved properly concern aggregate behavior. However, the causal mechanisms are sometimes ambiguous. In contrast, the work of economists examined next proceeds from an explicit model of decision making developed at the household level,[2] so that the causal mechanisms are clearly stated. However, aggregation from the household to the population level is somewhat vague. The model of decision making assumes some desired family size or target number of surviving children, and proceeds from the theory of consumer choice. Schultz (1973) summarizes it as follows: "The object is to specify a relation between the birth rate parents want and the price, income, and information

constraints that are not themselves determined simultaneously with or subsequently by, the objective number of
births." The result is a single reduced-form derived
demand equation for (surviving) children.[3] The price
and income effects arising from some structural change
are traced through the model of the demand for children,
with a goal of predicting at least the sign on the
elasticities.[4] Even so, considerable indeterminancy
can result. This is exacerbated when the households are
aggregated and when indicators must be used instead of
prices and income. This work of economists differs
substantially from that of the sociologists who have
criticized transition theory; it resembles more the older
view in which the demographic transition is seen not as a
drastic change in the decision-making process, but as the
result of a change in opportunities and constraints
resulting from structural economic change.

## A NOTE ON DATA AND METHODS

All of the data sets in the studies considered here are
time series of cross sections. The estimation procedures
rely on the general linear model. These data sets pose
specific methodological problems that must be handled
carefully. First, the cross-national data sets raise
questions of comparability both cross-sectionally and
over time. Such problems are less severe for the within-
country studies. Cavanaugh (1979), for example, questions
the quality of international fertility data, given the
variability of estimates from different sources, and
suggests that it may be impossible to draw conclusions
from such dubious data. However, examination of the data
he presents indicates that the problems may be less
serious than originally suggested. Although the level of
fertility in any particular country at any particular
time may not be precisely known, the overall pattern is
quite consistent among the various sources, and the
conclusions to be drawn from regression estimates are
likely to be largely the same since the coefficient
estimates depend not on the level but on the pattern.[5]
The discussion below will describe some of the sources of
bias that can be controlled through suitable estimation
procedures. A more serious problem is the cavalier
treatment of missing data and sampling problems in
cross-national studies.[6]

The present discussion will focus only on the most basic issues involved in analyzing time series of cross sections, and will describe only some of the simpler statistical models. In recent years, there has been an explosion of new models and new estimation techniques, many of which have been collected in the Annales de l'INSEE, 1978. However, although these new models are substantially more sophisticated than the simpler ones described here, the basic principles remain the same. Moreover, the available empirical research relies on the simpler models; the more sophisticated models appear not to have been applied to demographic problems.

A time series of cross section data set can be thought of as an analysis of covariance design with a two-way layout (with or without interactions): the cross-sectional units--regions or countries in this case--form one classification; the time observations--years--form the second classification.[7] As with any analysis of variance problem of this sort, for each classification, the total sum of squares can be decomposed into two orthogonal components--the within and the between sums of squares--and independent parameter estimates can be computed from each sum of squares.[8] Clearly, the results can be quite different depending on which component of the variance is analyzed. This independence of the within and the between sum of squares estimates is fundamental to the remainder of this discussion.

In addition to analysis of variance issues, time series of cross sections raise some of the same questions as standard time series, without having the necessary observations to resolve them. Relevant here are the consequences of focusing on one classification rather than another--regions or countries versus time periods-- and what is represented by each component of the variance. The theoretical and statistical problems are further compounded by some of the characteristics of the data sets analyzed. This will be discussed below, following a review of some of the more formal aspects of the problem. Recall that the basis of the analysis of variance and of covariance is the decomposition of the total sum of squares into between- and within-category variation. The analysis of the between sum of squares is based on the category means; the analysis of the within sum of squares is based on deviations from those means. First consider the country or region classification. Do the country or region means, computed over time, reflect persisting characteristics resulting from the unique historical experience of the region or country that either cannot be explained by variables typically available or are not of interest? Or do they represent long-term trends that it is essential to understand? Does the within-country or within-region over time variance (the deviations from the country or region means) represent only short-run fluctuations, or can inferences about trends be drawn from this component? Now consider the time period classification. It can be argued that, under conditions of structural stability, where coefficients do not change with time or with different levels of development (no interactions), estimates based on within-cross-section variance represent the long term by averaging effects for several time periods (see Chenery and Syrkin, 1977). Unfortunately, hypotheses about stability of coefficients are rarely verified, and, when verification is attempted, seem unfounded.[9]

In addition to these theoretical questions, the data sets themselves have certain characteristics that complicate the issues. The period of analysis tends to be relatively short, and the variables in question tend to change slowly; as a consequence, the data sets tend to have considerably more cross-sectional than temporal variation. In the context of the analysis of variance just discussed, this means that the total sum of squares is dominated by the region or country means, where these are computed over time. It is the contention here that these region or country means are correctly viewed as the result of a long-term historical process about which relatively little is known. It seems unlikely that, in the context of the demographic transition, the assumption of structural stability will be met, that is, that the pretransition and posttransition processes that describe the time path of fertility will be the same. Thus the between-region variability must be treated with special care, since the regional means are presumably the result both of pretransition differentials and of the process of transition, and special modeling is required. Examination of the within-region variability eliminates this long-run variability from the analysis, making it possible to ask about relationships among the variables within regions over time, and in a limited sense takes into account (conditions on) the longer-term process. Because variability between and within regions may arise from different processes, and because the estimates are statistically independent, analyses based on one component or the other may give different results. It is therefore

important that researchers carefully consider which
portion of the variance they wish to analyze and which is
more relevant to the hypotheses of interest. In this
context, the choice of statistical model is far from
arbitrary.

The paucity of time series observations not only makes
it difficult to distinguish long-run from short-run
variability; it also creates problems in cases where the
response of the dependent variable depends not on the
value of the independent variable at some specified time
point, either present or past, but on a set of current
and lagged values of the independent variables, that is,
where a distributed lag is required. Usually, only contemporaneous values or a single lag is available; thus
the estimated coefficient may be biased due to the omitted
lags, and the dynamics of the relationship obscured.[10]

On the positive side, the analysis of covariance framework does make it possible to eliminate some of the
effects of certain systematic errors in the data. This
may be particularly valuable for cross-national studies
that are plagued by data problems. Removing the regional
or country means and analyzing the within-country
variance simultaneously removes any consistent country-
or region-specific biases from the data. Similarly,
removing time-period means and analyzing within-cross-
section variance removes any consistent bias that affects
all countries from a particular period. In this way, the
country or region means (calculated over time) capture
the biases of particular countries; likewise, the cross-
sectional means (calculated over countries) capture the
global time trend in such biases as it affects all
countries in a given period. This is yet another reason
why the between sum of squares must be handled with
particular care.


EMPIRICAL STUDIES

Within-country Studies

Only three studies are examined in this section. This is
due in part to the difficulty of obtaining repeated time
series observations for a reasonably fine areal partition
of a country. Two of the studies examined are Schultz's
(1973) Taiwan study and Nerlove and Schultz's (1970)
Puerto Rico study (also see Schultz, 1969); the other is
Hermalin's (1978) Taiwan study. The first two studies

have similarly structured data sets, and use the same
methodology and the same theoretical framework of household decision making; Hermalin analyzes largely the same
data set as Schultz, although the approach is somewhat
different. From the point of view of statistical
analysis, as well as from a substantive point of view,
these three studies are some of the best work on fertility change, providing a model for future research.

Nerlove and Schultz's (1970) Puerto Rico study examines
five aspects of the demographic system: family size,
female labor force participation, marriage patterns,
personal income, and rural-urban migration. Data were
recorded for 75 municipios (regions) for the period
1950-60, with the bulk of information on population
characteristics coming from the two censuses (1950 and
1960), supplemented by vital registration data (births
and deaths) for the intercensal years. Fertility equation
estimates are based on 11 annual observations. Values of
the relevant independent variables, taken from the census,
are interpolated for the intercensal years.[11] The other
equations are estimated only for the census years.

The results for the fertility equation are summarized
here. The dependent variable is the crude birth rate.
The independent variables include measures of income,
education of children, education of adults, female labor
force participation, consensual and legal unions, age
composition,[12] and mortality. Three sets of estimates
for the births equation are presented: (1) based on the
pooled sample of time series of cross sections (total sum
of squares); (2) based on deviations from the regional
means, where the means are computed over time (within-
region temporal variation); and (3) error components
estimates that weight the within and between sum of
squares by the inverse of the error variance. As with
the other studies reviewed, there is considerably more
variability between the municipios than there is change
over the period of study. Thus the results for the pooled
model tend to be heavily dominated by cross-sectional
variability. This problem is exacerbated by the use of
interpolated values for the independent variables.
Nerlove and Schultz present both ordinary least squares
(OLS) and instrumental variables (IV) estimates;[13] they
do not present estimates based primarily on cross-
sectional variation, nor do they test the hypothesis that
the coefficients are constant over time (interaction
model).

The results of these estimation procedures are quite
erratic and are correspondingly difficult to interpret
and summarize.  Aside from expected differences between
estimates relying on the total sum of squares—which
tends to be dominated by cross-sectional variation—and
those based on temporal variation,[14] the IV and the OLS
estimates based on the same component of variance often
differ substantially.[15]  The authors give most weight
to the IV estimates based on an error components model.
In addition, they find that the age-composition variable
tends to reflect persisting characteristics of municipios.
For example, a young age structure is the result of persisting high fertility, and, for this reason alone, the
age composition variable tends to be highly correlated
with the level of fertility in the estimates based on the
total sum of squares (pooled).  The variable does not
perform much better in the deviations model, and the
coefficient is consistently much smaller than would
theoretically be expected.  An increase in legal unions
is associated with a somewhat higher birth rate, with the
effect somewhat larger for legal than for consensual
unions.  Female labor force participation is negatively
related to the birth rate if one considers only temporal
variability, but positively related to the birth rate in
the pooled model.  This suggests that, although regions
with high fertility have a high rate of female labor
force participation for reasons that are unaccounted for
by the model, within regions over time, female labor
force participation may be associated with fertility
decline.  The OLS estimate for the income coefficient is
negative, but the effect is positive or zero in the case
of the IV estimates.  Nerlove and Schultz conclude that
this evidence suggests children are not a superior good.
Although increased education among parents is associated
with lower fertility, increased education for children,
which would be expected to increase the cost of children,
has only a small effect on the birth rate.  Nerlove and
Schultz suggest that this weak result may be due to their
failure to take into account the supply of schools.
Mortality, lagged three or four years, is positively
associated with fertility.

Schultz's (1973) Taiwan study focuses exclusively on
fertility.  Data cover a period of six years for 361
administrative units.  A reduced-form demand equation for
the number of births is estimated.  The independent
variables that predict the demand for births are child
mortality (returns to investments in children), proportion

of males in agriculture (relative prices), male educational attainment (income effects), female educational attainment (price effects),[16] and two measures of family planning activity information (p. 243). All variables are lagged three years, except the family planning variables, which are lagged two years. These discrete lags were chosen after examination of more complex distributed lags. The estimation procedure is similar to that of Nerlove and Schultz (1970), but includes a better sampling of estimates based on cross-sectional variability. Since the dependent variables are age-specific fertility rates, it is possible to graphically trace the pattern of coefficients across various age groups, although Schultz does not fully exploit this opportunity. Because this is an exemplary piece of work that demonstrates some of the advantages and problems of time-series cross-section analysis, some of Schultz's estimated coefficients are shown graphically in Figures 1 and 2.

Figure 1 shows the estimated coefficients for child mortality. Age groups are arrayed along the horizontal axis, with the values of the estimated coefficients on the vertical axis. The lower panel shows estimates based on two cross sections (1965 and 1969) and for the pooled sample based on all six cross sections; the upper panel shows estimates based on pooled, deviations and error components estimates, and estimates based on first-differenced data. Comparison of the lower and upper panels shows how estimates based on the pooled sample are dominated by cross-sectional variability, and how estimates based on the cross section can differ substantially from those based on temporal change. First consider the effects of infant and child mortality on fertility. On theoretical grounds, older women should be more likely than younger ones to try to replace children who die. Thus larger coefficients should be expected in the older than in the younger age groups, tapering off for the oldest age groups as fewer and fewer women are fecund. Estimates based on the within-region temporal variation shown in the upper panel (the broken lines) display a cohesive age pattern in which the expected greater propensity of older women to replace children who have died is clearly evident.[17] In contrast, estimates based on the pooled data set (the solid line in both the top and bottom panels) deviate considerably from this pattern for the two youngest age groups. The lower panel allows a comparison of these results: the estimates for

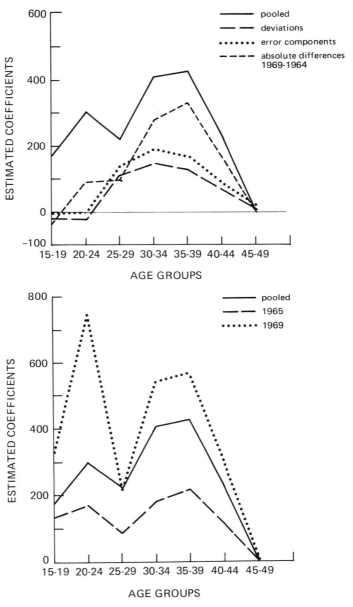

FIGURE 1   Estimated Coefficients for Child Mortality in Regressions for Age-Specific Fertility, Taiwan

Source:   Schultz (1973).

the pooled model fall between those for the two cross sections, and it is apparent that the large coefficients for the two youngest age groups are the result of cross-sectional variability rather than temporal change. Schultz (1973:253) suggests that this result is due to long-run differences between regions in the proportion married among teenagers. Thus persisting regional characteristics that may not be of theoretical interest can dominate estimates based on pooled time series of cross sections if care is not taken in the choice of estimation procedure.

Estimates of the effect of the proportion of males in agriculture, given in Figure 2, show a similar disparity. From the cross-sectional evidence, one would infer that there is higher fertility in agricultural areas. However, the coefficients based on temporal variability behave erratically and are not statistically significant. Thus it cannot be inferred that decreases in the proportion employed in agriculture are associated with lower fertility.

In contrast, male education shows no consistent, theoretically explicable impact on fertility in the cross section, but has a clear and consistent impact when temporal variability is considered. Results for female education are similarly well behaved when temporal variation is considered. Likewise, the impact of family planning workers is clear within regions over time, but not in the cross section. These results demonstrate, at least to some extent, the contention here that, although socioeconomic characteristics may not account for the onset of fertility decline, they can sometimes help explain temporal change in fertility.

Hermalin (1978) analyzes nearly the same data set as Schultz (1973). However, Hermalin's approach is theoretically and methodologically different: while Schultz's work focuses primarily on economic change, Hermalin pays special attention to family planning programs and to the spatial and temporal pattern of fertility decline. In particular, he notes that those areas which decline later tend to decline more rapidly, and that decline begins first in the cities, then in the rural areas. Thus there is more rapid fertility decline in urban areas in the first part of the period of analysis (1961–65) and more rapid decline in rural areas in the second part (1965–72). His strategy for handling this problem is rather different from that used by Schultz or Nerlove and Schultz and implies a different view of the process of fertility

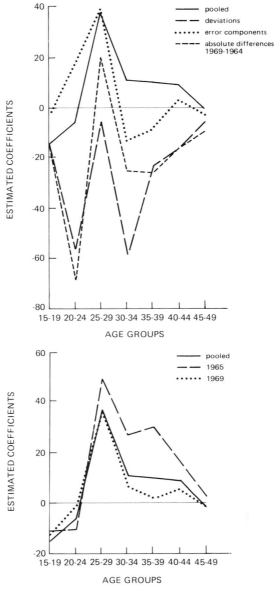

FIGURE 2   Estimated Coefficients for Agricultural
Composition in Regressions for Age-Specific Fertility,
Taiwan

Source:   Schultz (1973)

decline. Hermalin analyzes three dependent variables:
the total fertility rate in 1966, the slope of fertility
decline 1961-65, and the slope 1965-72. The analysis of
the first of these is a straightforward cross-sectional
analysis. The analysis of the slopes is more complex:
for each region in each subperiod, Hermalin regresses the
annual total fertility rate on time; the estimated slope
of this regression or the estimated average annual rate
of change in fertility for each of the regions is the
dependent variable.[18] The independent variables in all
three cases are the levels of child mortality, education
of adults, school attendance, percent of the male labor
force engaged in agriculture, population density, and
distance to the nearest city. The levels of these variables are measured near the midpoint of the first subperiod used in the analysis, and are used for both
subperiods. Hermalin also examines a first difference
model. However, results for this estimation procedure
rely on only two time points, and the estimated coefficients vary considerably depending on the choice of year
for the endpoints (1965-70 versus 1965-72). This indicates the danger of analyzing only two time periods and
the need for sampling as many time points as possible.

Before turning to the empirical results, let us
consider the substantive implications of this model. As
specified, it states that the level of a set of independent variables, all measuring socioeconomic conditions
(roughly for the years around 1963-64), is related first
to the level of fertility two or three years later (1966),
second to between-region differences in the rate of fertility decline for a time period (1961-65) straddling the
date at which the independent variables are measured, and
third to between-region differences in the rate of fertility decline for a time period (1965-72) following the
date at which the independent variables are measured.
Although the independent variables may change rather
slowly over the period in question, it is not clear that
their value at the midpoint of some interval should be
expected to predict between-region differences in the
rate of fertility decline, or how differences in the
performance of the statistical model for the three
dependent variables should be interpreted since quite
different conceptual models of the dynamics of fertility
change are implicit in each case. In particular, it
seems inappropriate to compare the two estimates where
the slope of fertility is the dependent variable: in one
case, the independent variables are measured at the

midpoint of the interval; in the other, they are measured
before the start of the interval. Because rather different results are obtained from the three sets of estimates,
it is unclear which set of findings to report. Not all
variables will change at the same rate for all regions;
thus researchers should take special care that the leads
and lags defining the dynamics of fertility decline are
the same when they wish to compare results across
subperiods.

Hermalin's results for the family planning variables
are largely cross-sectional. These results suggest that
areas that are more modern and those with a high cumulative acceptance rate for contraceptives tend to have
lower fertility. A recursive structural equations model
shows that more modern areas tend to have lower proportions married in the younger age groups, and that the
most important determinant of contraceptive acceptance is
fieldworker input. Elsewhere in the paper, Hermalin
demonstrates the importance of the intermediate variables
such as breastfeeding and nonprogram contraception in
accounting for differences between areas in fertility
levels. He also examines a model in which both the
independent and the dependent variables are differenced.
These results most closely approximate within-region
temporal change in terms of the portion of the variance
analyzed. When only temporal change is considered,
increases in worker input are associated with fertility
decline, but increases in the acceptance rate for contraceptives are not, and increasing modernization has no
statistically significant impact on fertility decline.
Increased proportions married in the age group 20–24 and
higher rates of child mortality are both associated with
higher fertility.


Cross-national Studies

The number of cross-national studies of fertility determinants that include a temporal dimension is somewhat
larger than the number of within-country studies.
Although the variables included in these studies often
overlap, each study tends to focus on a different aspect
or determinant of fertility decline, and the same variable is often interpreted differently. These differences
in theoretical approach and substantive focus make a
cohesive summary difficult.

Gregory and Campbell's (1976) study is based on a theoretical framework similar to that of Schultz (1973) and Nerlove and Schultz (1970), reviewed above. Data are based on 18 Latin American countries for two time points, 1950 and 1960. Since Gregory and Campbell have only two time series observations, there is no decomposition into cross-sectional and temporal variation.[19] Instead, there is a careful examination of multiplicative interactions among the variables. The dependent variable is the crude birth rate; the independent variables are per capita income, the infant mortality rate, percent urban, the female labor force participation rate, and per capita energy consumption. The percent urban is used as a proxy for attitudinal changes. Other variables measure income and child costs (p. 162). In addition, interactions of percent urban with the other independent variables are also examined.[20] The authors present both ordinary least squares (OLS) estimates and two stage least squares (2SLS) estimates where per capita income is endogenous.

From a theoretical point of view, Gregory and Campbell (1976:61) claim to be estimating a demand equation for births, with the insertion of percent urban regarded as an integration of economic and sociological theory. The interaction model looks at income and substitution effects on fertility, net of the level of modernization. The measures are not pure, since urbanization also modifies the costs of children. Even if Gregory and Campbell's arguments about attitude change are not compelling to sociologists, or if the integration of economic and sociological theory is not satisfactory, they are to be commended for testing a substantively interesting set of interactions. Such an examination can indicate important nonlinearities and may lead to new theoretical developments.

Their most interesting substantive findings in fact come from the examination of "modernization turning points," the values of the percent urban at which the elasticities of fertility with respect to other variables change sign.[21] For example, the elasticity of fertility with respect to per capita income changes from positive to negative when the percent urban reaches 69 percent, reflecting a lessening of the income effect at higher levels of modernization. This sort of empirical result may help resolve some of the indeterminacies in the theory of household choice, since it allows researchers to trace the points at which substitution effects replace income effects. However, it is difficult to tell just how much

weight to give estimates of turning points when the
estimation procedures fail to take into account the
structure of the data. Gregory and Campbell simply pool
the data from the two cross sections without explicitly
considering time series aspects. As was suggested above,
such estimates are likely to be dominated by cross-
sectional variability. An examination of differences
between 1950 and 1960 would have focused on temporal
variability and provided an interesting comparison. In
any case, two points is a very small sample from a time
series. Moreover, because all estimates refer to contemporaneous association of variables, the results may be
contaminated with considerable long-run variability,
unexplained characteristics of countries, and misspecifi-
cation of the lag structure. For example, the authors
find that infant mortality is positively associated with
fertility until the population is about 80 percent urban,
at which point the coefficient changes sign. They attribute this to replacement effects dominating cost over most
of the course of modernization. However, this change may
just as well reflect changes in the cause structure of
mortality and the proxy effect of morbidity on fertility
that may accompany urbanization. In any case, it seems
reasonable that Gregory and Campbell's results cannot be
given any time series interpretation.

An alternative investigation of economic modernization
can be found in Chenery and Syrkin (1977), who study
patterns of development, with extensive exploration of
national income accounts. Although fertility is not a
central focus of this study, some of the information from
their typology of development might usefully be included
in studies of fertility. Data are based on 100 countries,
for 20 years, with some estimates based on subsets of
countries and many on a single cross section for 1965.
Unfortunately, the study is not clear as to what data are
available for particular years and countries and how
missing data are handled. Typically, pooled estimates
pay attention to the classification by year only; Chenery
and Syrkin argue that the estimated average cross-
sectional coefficients are representative of the long
run. However, since there are no tests for interactions,
this hypothesis is not verified. There is some analysis
of within-country variability, which the authors claim
represents short-run relationships.

Ten development processes are defined based on national
income accounts. The independent variables in each case
are income level (an overall index of development) and

population (a measure of market size). The model assumes
uniformity in the development process; that is, a consistent pattern of change in resource allocation, factor
use, and other structural features (p. 17). Results are
broken into allocation and accumulation processes. The
goal of the analysis seems to be to determine the income
level at which visible shifts in production, trade,
resource use, and so on take place. Development is seen
as an S-shaped curve, involving a transition from one
relatively constant structure to another (p. 10).

Chenery and Syrkin find that theories of balanced
growth most aptly describe large countries where levels
of exports and imports are sufficient to offset the
implied relationship between domestic demand and domestic
supply of major commodities, and specialization is therefore not pronounced. In small countries, imports and
exports are more important; sustained growth therefore
requires a shift in export composition towards manufacturing, and human and physical capital must increase
relative to unskilled labor. Small countries can therefore be characterized as having a primary or an industry
orientation. Such information on the nature of economic
growth during the course of development might well be
included in models of fertility, since considerably
different labor force structures are involved in the two
paths of development described, and such differences could
logically be expected to be reflected in fertility.
Although the authors do not trace the demographic consequences of these contrasting patterns of development,
they do find that, in the cross section among developing
countries, higher levels of education and lower levels of
infant mortality are associated with a lower crude birth
rate.

Noneconomists have also examined the determinants of
fertility decline. One example is Mauldin and Berelson's
(1978) study of the relative role of development and
family planning programs. They define "demand" and
"supply" in a somewhat different manner from that used by
economists: "'demand' represents the basic determinants
of fertility--the fundamental socioeconomic, cultural,
social-structural factors that give rise to interest or
motivation to limit family size; 'supply' represents one
of the proximate determinants or intermediate factors"
(p. 90). Four variables are used to measure demand:
education (adult literacy and school enrollment), health
(mortality), economy (employment outside agriculture,
GNP), and urbanization. One variable--family planning

effort--is used to measure supply. Although it includes
a number of objective criteria, this variable appears to
be defined according to a somewhat qualitative evaluation
on the part of the authors. Furthermore, although it is
a summed scale, the variable appears to be ordinal, yet
enters the model linearly. As a consequence, it is difficult to know what meaning to attach to its estimated
coefficient. The dependent variable is the change in the
crude birth rate, which is decomposed into changes due to
age structure, to marriage patterns, and to marital fertility. The specification of temporal relations is somewhat unusual in that levels of the independent variables
for 1970 are used to predict change between 1965 and 1970
in the dependent variable; levels for 1960 are used with
similar empirical results. In the first case, this means
that, if the equation were rewritten with lagged values
of the dependent variable on the right hand side instead
of differences being used as the dependent variable, current (1970) values of the independent variables and lagged
(1965) values of the dependent variable would be expected
to predict current fertility; in the second case, lagged
values of the independent and dependent variables would
be expected to explain current fertility. The choice of
end points for computing fertility change and the selection of lags appears to be arbitrary. Mauldin and
Berelson find that the impact of family planning effort
outweighs that of the various economic indicators in
terms of contribution to the explained variance. In an
addendum using exploratory data analysis techniques,
Sykes finds that the program effort variable best describes the bimodal distribution of fertility change.

Tsui and Bogue (1978) carried out a study that in many
ways resembles the Mauldin and Berelson piece. Data for
113 developing countries for the period 1968-75 are
examined. The independent variables include per capita
GNP, percent urban, the infant mortality rate, life
expectancy, percent of the employed female population
working in agriculture, percent literate, and school
enrollment. These are "eight socioeconomic indicators
which represent factors in development that can be
presumed to be among the most important in affecting
fertility motivations" (p. 5). Tsui and Bogue also
include the Mauldin-Berelson family planning effort scale
among the independent variables. The dependent variables
are the total fertility rates for 1968 and 1975. Many of
the rates are estimated. One useful exercise they perform is to compare estimates of fertility from several

sources to show that the overall conclusions are generally similar.  They provide considerable descriptive
detail for the levels and trends of fertility, measures
of social and economic development, and information on
family planning programs, all broken down by region; they
also estimate a regression equation where fertility in
1975 depends on fertility and socioeconomic indicators in
1968 and the family planning score in 1972.  There is
little justification for their choice of years or lag
structure.  The analysis is performed for Africa, Asia,
and Latin America separately.  These cross-sectional
results show, not surprisingly, that the principal determinant of current fertility is past fertility.  No standard errors or tests of significance are presented, and
all results are discussed according to the fraction of
the variance explained.  As a consequence, it is difficult to evaluate their results.  They find that income is
sometimes positively, sometimes negatively related to the
total fertility rate; percent urban is negatively related
to fertility in Africa and Latin America but not in Asia;
infant mortality is positively associated with fertility;
the percent of the female labor force employed in agriculture is not related to fertility in a consistent manner;
and female school enrollment is negatively related to fertility, as is family planning effort.  They provide little
discussion of the sources of interregional differences or
the apparent instability of certain coefficients.

Finally, Entwisle and Winegarden's (1981) study of the
relationships between state-sponsored pension programs
and fertility change is of interest since it treats fertility and government expenditures on pension programs as
endogenous variables in a simultaneous system, then
examines direct and indirect effects with some care.  The
two dependent variables are the total fertility rate and
government expenditures for old age security as a fraction
of the gross domestic product.  Data come from about 50
countries for the period 1965-70.  Fertility is a function of past government expenditures on pension benefits,
life expectancy, per capita income, adult literacy, percent of the labor force employed in agriculture, family
planning effort (from Mauldin and Berelson, 1978), and a
dummy variable indicating those countries having a family
planning program that is at least ten years old.  Government expenditures on pension programs depend on past
fertility, a quadratic in life expectancy, per capita
income, the old age dependency burden, and the proportion
of gross domestic product originating in agriculture.  In

both equations, all right hand side variables are lagged five years. The specification is somewhat unusual in the choice of the time frame: although data appear to be available for at least three time points, suggesting a pooled time series of cross sections, only two cross-sectional equations are estimated. The fertility equation is estimated using rates for 1975, with 1970 values of the independent variables; the pension equation is estimated for expenditures in 1970, using values of the independent variables for 1965. It is difficult to see why a more general time index was not used and the cross sections pooled. It has already been noted that discrete lags in cross-sectional estimates may be biased because they include considerable long-run variability.[22]

Entwisle and Winegarden's results include estimates for both structural parameters and reduced form equations; only the former results are summarized here. They find that mortality is positively related to fertility in countries where life expectancy is less than 53 years and negatively where life expectancy exceeds 53 years; they conjecture that the positive association at lower levels of life expectancy may be due to initial health benefits associated with the early stages of mortality decline. They find further that pension expenditures, literacy, and family planning effort are negatively associated with fertility, as is the percent employed in agriculture. Although they are unable to account for the negative association between percent employed in agriculture and fertility, it may be the result of the cross-sectional nature of their estimates. When they estimate an equation where pension expenditures is the dependent variable, they find that expenditures are reciprocally related to fertility. However, it is not clear why fertility five years earlier ought to affect pension expenditures since children born at that time would just be entering the school system and should not strongly influence government decision making with regard to pension expenditures. Furthermore, it is difficult to draw conclusions about reciprocal causation from cross-sectional results. More extensive use of time series data might have provided better insight into the dynamics of these relationships, which would seem, at least potentially, to involve long delays.

SUMMARY AND SUGGESTIONS FOR FUTURE RESEARCH

This review of the literature has focused on determining what questions can be answered by a particular data set with a given set of analytical techniques. The discussion has therefore been more methodological than is common in such reviews. It was felt to be particularly important to determine when findings refer to cross-sectional differences, when they refer to temporal change, and when the former can be used to make inferences about the latter. It was found that, all too often, results are dominated by cross-sectional variability, and that, when results clearly based on cross-sectional variability can be compared with those clearly based on temporal variation, the two sets of results are often quite different. Considerable disagreement was noted among researchers over what portion of the variance ought to be examined, whether the long term or the short term demands explanation. In addition, many of the cross-national studies are, of course, plagued with data problems; the relatively small number of within-country studies demonstrates a similar difficulty in obtaining replicated cross sections.

The most conservative strategy requires display of the full analysis of covariance for within and between sums of squares for each classification (years and areal units) separately and for both classifications combined. Care must be taken that, when the response of the dependent variable is expected to follow a change in the independent variable five years earlier, the coefficient reflects the expected response over the five-year period rather than some long-run association of the two variables, where the latter need not imply a causal connection. At a minimum, this means that within-areal-unit estimates must be compared to those based on simple pooling of the data, and preferably to those based on cross-sectional variation as well. In addition, past research has shown that there are likely to be considerable nonlinearities in the relationships which must be more fully and systematically investigated.

Finally, it would seem desirable to develop a theory for aggregate fertility that reflects some of the nonlinearities and turning points revealed in empirical studies. Better account should be taken of the structure of development and possible implications for fertility. A logical starting point may be the new home economics theory of household choice, since this approach has been fruitful in linking microeconomic and demographic change to the costs and returns of childbearing. A version of this approach emphasizing social and economic structure might be worthwhile. Although it has not been discussed here, there is a considerable literature on the socio-structural and economic determinants of mortality change (see, e.g., Preston, 1980). Since mortality frequently enters the fertility equations, a simultaneous equations approach might be indicated. From a statistical point of view, recent years have seen an explosion of methodology for the analysis of time series of cross sections. Such new estimation procedures allow the specification of sophisticated dynamic models (see Mundlak, 1978, for example); however, their application awaits the development of more specific theoretical models.

## PROPOSITIONS

The above discussion was primarily methodological, focusing on what questions it is possible and proper to answer with a given data set and statistical procedure. This section will be more substantive, assessing the evidence related to questions raised by particular authors; to some extent, this will also serve as a summary of empirical findings. The section has been organized according to the variables included in the studies, divided into three groups: those referring to social and economic structure, demographic variables, and variables concerning family planning.

Because there is no driving theoretical perspective shared by the studies, the derived propositions are empirically based. As each variable is discussed, associated concepts and arguments will be noted. In nearly all cases, the variables included are proxies for other variables that should be measured at the individual level or for some broader concept of structural change. Results are separated according to whether estimates refer to time series or to cross-sectional variation, so that the two can be contrasted; cross-sectional results are taken only from studies including a temporal dimension (the purely cross-sectional literature has been reviewed elsewhere; see, e.g., Birdsall, 1977). Although there is no theory for aggregate fertility time series that is distinguishable from propositions concerning cross-sectional differentials, it is hoped that the results presented here may display some patterns to guide future theoretical efforts.

## Sociostructural and Economic Variables

**Proposition 1**  Fertility decline is influenced by industrialization, more precisely by compositional changes in the labor force involving a shift from agriculture to industry.

From an economic point of view, shifts in the labor force from agriculture to industry require investments in human and physical capital.  Thus the situation shifts from one in which many unskilled laborers are required and children are easily employed to one in which fewer, more skilled laborers are needed, children are less easily employed, and the economic returns from children are therefore be diminished.  From a sociological point of view, the salient characteristic is the separation of place of work from place of residence, leading to exposure to new ideas and the end of the family as simultaneously unit of production and unit of consumption.  At the same time, traditional values that may have fostered high fertility are replaced by more individualistic decision making.  (Note that industrialization is not to be confused with urbanization.)

**Measures**  Proportion of males employed in agriculture (and fishing); proportion of the labor force in agriculture.

**Concepts**  Schultz (1973) uses the percent of males in agriculture to measure relative price effects:  lower costs of rearing children and lower expected returns to the education of children in rural areas.  Hermalin (1975) uses the proportion of males employed in agriculture as one of several measure of modernization; Entwisle and Winegarden (1981) use it as a control variable.

**Cross-sectional Results**  Schultz (1973) finds a consistent positive association between proportion of males in agriculture and age-specific fertility rates in Taiwan. The largest estimated coefficient is for the age group 25–29, which may reflect different marriage patterns between agricultural and nonagricultural regions.  In contrast, Hermalin (1978) finds a negative relationship between the proportion of males employed in agriculture and the total fertility rate, a conflict in findings that does not seem resoluble.  Tsui and Bogue (1978) find that the relationship is negative once family planning effort

is added to the equation. Entwisle and Winegarden (1981)
find an inverse relationship using cross-national data;
however, since their measure refers to the entire labor
force, it may be contaminated by differential reporting
of female labor force participation in agriculture among
the countries sampled.

Time-series Results   Schultz (1973) finds no consistent, statistically significant relationship.  Using
differenced data for two time periods (1965-70 and
1965-72), Hermalin (1978) finds that the coefficient is
negative and significant in the first instance and
positive and insignificant in the second.  This points
out the dangers of choosing two arbitrary cross sections
for an analysis of first differences, as well as the need
to sample several time points if at all possible.

Other Results   Mauldin and Berelson (1978) find a
positive association between proportion of males employed
outside agriculture (levels) and fertility decline
(change).  Hermalin (1978) finds that the proportion
employed in agriculture is positively related to the
estimated rate of fertility decline in Taiwan.

Conclusions   There is no strong time-series evidence
to suggest that industrialization will lead to fertility
decline.  However, the hypothesis has really been tested
in only one instance.


Proposition 2   Rising incomes are expected to lead to
increases in fertility.
   Most arguments concerning this variable arise from
economic theory.  However, higher incomes may be associated with increases in the value of time, particularly
the mother's time, if income is a proxy for women's
wages, and this may lead to lower fertility.  In addition, tastes may shift so that, at higher incomes, fewer,
higher-quality children are preferred, or consumption may
shift away from children to other goods.  Thus, the
household decision-making model yields indeterminate
results (see Mueller and Short, in these volumes).
Empirically, this means there may be important nonlinearities or discontinuities in the relationship.

Measures   Gross national product (GNP) per capita;
gross domestic product (GDP) per capita; personal income.

Concepts  Chenery and Syrkin (1977) use per capita GDP
as an overall index of development.  Tsui and Bogue
(1978) use GNP to the same end.  Gregory and Campbell
(1976) expect fertility decisions to change with income,
ceteris paribus, with the sign depending on the relative
magnitude of income and substitution effects.  Nerlove
and Schultz  (1970) make a similar argument:  if children
are a normal good, increases in income will result in
increases in desired family size; if the costs of childrearing rise sufficiently rapidly with income, increases
in income will result in decreases in desired family size.

Cross-sectional Results  Analyzing cross-national data
for 1965, Chenery and Syrkin (1977) find that the fall in
the crude birth rate is greater than that in the crude
death rate at incomes above $200.  Gregory and Campbell
(1976) find a positive relationship between per capita
income and fertility when the percent urban is below 69
percent; this coefficient is large only at low levels of
urbanization.  When results are broken down by region,
Tsui and Bogue (1978) find that the estimated coefficient
is sometimes positive, sometimes negative, with the sign
depending on what other variables are included in the
equation.

Time-series Results  Nerlove and Schultz (1970) find
no relationship when instrumental variables (IV) estimates
are examined for the Puerto Rican data.

Other Results  Mauldin and Berelson (1978) find a positive relationship between the level of GNP and fertility
decline.

Conclusions  There is no strong time series evidence
that rising incomes lead to either increases or decreases
in fertility, although there may be important nonlinearities that have not been investigated.


Proposition 3  Urbanization leads to fertility decline.
    The economic arguments concern higher costs of
children in urban areas; the sociological arguments
concern implicit changes in life style, the breakdown of
traditional family structures, and the fact that urban
areas are a source of new ideas.  (As noted above,
urbanization is often confused with industrialization.)

<u>Measures</u>  Percent of the population living in urban areas; distance from the nearest city; density.

<u>Concepts</u>  Gregory and Campbell (1976) use urbanization as a measure of changes in attitudes associated with development.  Tsui and Bogue (1978) emphasize the increased opportunities for work and education, particularly for women, leading to delayed marriage and increased costs of childrearing.

<u>Cross-sectional Results</u>  Gregory and Campbell (1976) find that percent urban is an important interaction variable.  They also find that it has a consistent negative impact on the crude birth rate, net of the interaction effects.  Chenery and Syrkin (1977) find no effect of urbanization net of education, income level, and infant mortality.  Both sets of results are based on cross-national data.  Tsui and Bogue (1978) find the percent urban negatively related to fertility in Africa and Latin America, but positively related to fertility in Asia.  Hermalin (1978) finds that, in Taiwan, population density is negatively related to the total fertility rate, but distance to the nearest city is unrelated to the area's level of fertility.

<u>Time-series Results</u>  No studies of fertility change in developing countries include this variable.

<u>Other Results</u>  Hermalin (1978) finds that population density is positively related to the estimated slope of fertility change and that the strength of the relationship increases between the two subperiods (1961-65 and 1965-72) examined.  He also finds that distance to the nearest city is positively related to the estimated slope of fertility decline in the first subperiod, but that the relationship is insignificant in the second subperiod.  This suggests that the two variables may be alternative measures of the same thing.

<u>Proposition 4</u>  Increased education of the adult population leads to fertility decline.

Economic arguments concern the increased value of parents' time and rising opportunity costs.  Sociological arguments concern the emancipating effect of education and the decreasing impact of traditional values.  Increased education may also lead to later marriage.  Some economists separate the impact of mother's education from that of father's education (see Cochrane, in these volumes).

**Measures**   Male and female educational attainment; median education of adult population; percent literate.

**Concepts**   Schultz (1973) argues that educational attainment measures potential lifetime earnings.  He expects male educational attainment to have an income effect on fertility, whereas female educational attainment increases the opportunity costs of childbearing. Nerlove and Schultz (1970) emphasize the increased value of parents' time.  Gregory and Campbell (1976) also use educational attainment as a measure of potential wages, although their data do not allow separation of results by sex.  Entwisle and Winegarden (1981) use education as a control variable.

**Cross-sectional Results**   Schultz (1973) finds that male educational attainment depresses fertility for all age groups except 25-29; female education is negatively associated with fertility at 25-29, but is positively associated with fertility in the older age groups. Schultz suggests this may be due to a collinearity problem.  Hermalin (1978) finds that female educational attainment is negatively related to the total fertility rate.  Gregory and Campbell (1976) find that the elasticity of fertility with respect to the percent illiterate is positive until the population reaches about 60 percent urban, and suggest that literacy may be picking up changes in fertility control.  Entwisle and Winegarden (1981) find an inverse relationship between the percent literate and fertility.

**Time-series Results**   Schultz (1973) finds that the pattern of coefficients for the effects of male education on fertility is similar to the cross-sectional estimates when time-series variation alone is examined; however, the time-series estimates are considerably smaller.  Over time, female education has a consistent negative impact on the fertility of all age groups.  Nerlove and Schultz (1970) find an inverse relation between the education of adults and fertility.  Analyzing differences between 1965-70 and 1965-72, Hermalin (1978) finds no statistically significant relationships; this result may be due to the choice of cross sections, or to instability of the

model as the coefficients change signs with only slight
changes in the specification.

Other Results   Mauldin and Berelson (1978) find a
positive relation between levels of literacy and the
extent of fertility decline.  Hermalin (1978) finds a
positive relationship between female educational
attainment and the estimated slope of fertility decline
in Taiwan for 1961-65, but only a very weak relationship
for 1965-72.

Conclusions   Both in the cross section and over time,
fertility and the educational attainment of adults are
inversely related, although there may be important nonlinearities and considerable differences by sex.  Over
time, increased education of females depresses fertility
for all age groups.

Proposition 5   Increased female labor force participation
in the modern sector leads to fertility decline.
     Economic arguments concern increased value of women's
time and higher opportunity costs of childbearing and
rearing; sociological arguments add changes in the role
of women and increased equality between men and women in
the fertility decision-making process (see Standing, in
these volumes).

Measures   Proportion of women in the labor force;
proportion of employed women working in agriculture.

Concepts   Nerlove and Schultz (1970) emphasize
decreased time for home activities and consequently
smaller family-size desires.  Gregory and Campbell (1976)
point to increased costs of childbearing.  Tsui and Bogue
(1978) point out that the decline of female employment in
agriculture reflects both women's release from childbearing as more children survive and increases in opportunities to work in nonfarm situations.

Cross-sectional Results   Gregory and Campbell (1976)
find that the elasticity of fertility with respect to
female labor force participation changes from positive to
negative when the population is 28 percent urban.  They
suggest that, at low levels of modernization, female labor
force participation may be concentrated in agriculture
rather than in the modern sector, where work may be less

compatible with childbearing. Nerlove and Schultz (1970) find a positive association between female labor force participation and fertility when they examine estimates based on pooled data. Tsui and Bogue (1978) find a weak positive relationship between the proportion of employed females working in agriculture and fertility, but the coefficient is close to zero and negative once family planning effort is added to the equation.

Time-series Results  Nerlove and Schultz (1970) find an inverse relation between female labor force participation and fertility.

Conclusions  Cross-sectional evidence suggests there may be important nonlinearities in the relationship between female labor force participation and fertility, induced by the failure to separate employment in the traditional sector from that in industry. Time-series results suggest that increasing female labor force participation may be important for reducing fertility. However, better measures are needed for more definitive conclusions, and work in the modern sector must be separated from that in agriculture.


Proposition 6  Increasing education of children leads to fertility decline.
Economic arguments concern the conflict between schooling and labor force participation of children; these arguments often combine assumptions about the changing structure of production and opportunities for child labor. Sociologists and economists both emphasize the changing role of children in the family, evidenced by increasing investments in child quality (Caldwell, in these volumes; Lindert, in these volumes).

Measures  School enrollment.

Cross-sectional Results  Chenery and Syrkin (1977) and Hermalin (1978) find an inverse relationship between school enrollment and fertility.

Time-series Results  Nerlove and Schultz (1970) find a weak inverse relationship between increasing school enrollment and fertility; Hermalin (1978) finds a positive relationship using a differenced model.

Conclusions  School enrollment is at best a weak proxy
for parental investment in child quality.  Both cross-
sectionally and over time, this variable is contaminated
with differences and changes in the supply of schools, as
well as in parental demand for education.  Better measurements of investment in child quality are particularly
important for the analysis of fertility change in developing countries.  Bulatao (1980) is the only study that
includes data on child employment, school enrollment, and
perceived returns to and costs of children; unfortunately,
his analysis is not designed so that the various effects
can be disentangled.

## Demographic Variables

Proposition 7  Falling mortality leads to fertility
decline.

Parents value surviving children, not births, whether
as additional workers or as a possible source of support
in old age.  However, it can be shown that mortality
decline will not lead to compensating fertility decline
unless desired family size also declines (see O'Hara,
1975; also Heer, in these volumes).  Increasing probabilities of survival also increase the expected returns from
investment in child quality; this may in turn encourage
investment in child quality as opposed to child quantity,
thereby lowering fertility.

Measures  Life expectancy at birth ($e_0$); the infant
mortality rate; the crude death rate; child survival
rates.

Concepts  Schultz (1973) argues that the relationship
between child mortality and fertility embodies both a
decrease in the costs of rearing a surviving child and a
decline in the marginal return of additional children.
Gregory and Campbell (1976) claim that the expected sign
on the elasticity depends on whether the demand for surviving children is highly price elastic or not.  Mauldin
and Berelson (1978) use mortality as an index of the
health of the population.  Entwisle and Winegarden (1981)
allow mortality to have a nonlinear relationship to
fertility to allow for the proxy effects of morbidity:
initial rises in life expectancy may reflect improvements
in health conditions and have a fertility-enhancing
effect; as mortality decline progresses, the inverse
relationship between child survival and fertility emerges.

Cross-sectional Results Schultz (1973) finds a
moderately strong positive association between child
mortality and fertility for young women and for older
women, with considerable change between the two cross
sections for which estimates are given. Hermalin (1978)
finds a moderate positive association between child
mortality four years previous and the total fertility
rate. Gregory and Campbell (1976) find that the elasticity of fertility with respect to mortality is positive
for populations that are less than 80 percent urban,
after which it becomes negative; they interpret this to
mean that replacement effects dominate substitution
effects over most of the course of modernization.
Chenery and Syrkin (1977) find that infant mortality and
fertility are positively associated in less developed
countries, but that the relationship is not significant
in more developed countries. Entwisle and Winegarden
(1981) find that fertility is positively associated with
mortality up to a life expectancy of about 53 years.
Tsui and Bogue (1978) find a positive relationship between
the level of infant mortality seven years earlier and
fertility in Africa, Asia, and Latin America.

Time-series Results Schultz (1973) finds a consistent
positive relationship between fertility and child mortality (lagged three years) that is particularly marked
for older women. Nerlove and Schultz (1970) find a
positive association between the crude death rate (lagged
three and four years) and fertility. Using five- and
seven-year differences, Hermalin (1978) also finds a
positive relationship between the change in child
mortality five years earlier and the change in fertility.

Other Results Mauldin and Berelson (1978) find that
both high levels of infant mortality and low levels of
life expectancy are inversely associated with the amount
of fertility decline. Hermalin finds no relationship
between the level of child mortality and the estimated
slope of fertility change for the period 1961-65, but
finds a moderate negative relationship for the later
period; however, it is difficult to interpret this result
since the lag structures for the two subperiods are not
the same.

Conclusions The association between mortality and
fertility may reflect a wide variety of influences other
than the replacement effects that some researchers are

attempting to measure. There appears to be considerable confusion as to whether replacement or the general health status (morbidity) of the population ought to be examined. Contemporaneous correlations pick up a considerable portion of the proxy effect of morbidity; when mortality is lagged two to four years, both physiological and behavioral portions of the replacement effect are likely to be captured. Time-series results suggest that fertility decline and mortality decline (appropriately lagged) are positively associated.

## Family Planning

Proposition 8    Family planning programs are expected to reduce fertility by disseminating information on contraception and distributing contraceptives (see Hermalin, in these volumes).

Concepts   Economists are interested in the demand for children. They regard family planning efforts as an information variable that alters the costs of fertility regulation. Mauldin and Berelson (1978) call family planning effort a "supply" factor to indicate that such programs also supply contraceptives.

Measures   Number of family planning field workers (person months per 1,000 women aged 15-49); "family planning effort"; cumulative acceptance rate.

Cross-sectional Results   Although Schultz (1973) finds no consistent effects, results for different cross sections suggest that the impact of the program is more evident soon after the program has been initiated than several years later. Hermalin (1978) also finds that, although worker input was generally less in areas with low preprogram fertility than in other areas, acceptance rates in the first five years of the program tended to be higher. In addition, the acceptance rate is negatively related to fertility, and the relationship is strongest in areas where the preprogram fertility level was highest. This holds in a model where the cumulative acceptance rate is treated as endogenous. Entwisle and Winegarden (1981) find that Mauldin and Berelson's measure of family planning effort is associated with lower fertility; they also find that countries where the family planning program is at least ten years old have

lower fertility than those where the program is more
recent.

Time-series Results   Schultz (1973) finds a consistent
negative impact of family planning field workers on
fertility that is particularly marked for women aged
25-29 and 30-34.   In a model that analyzes differences
between 1965-70 and 1965-72, Hermalin finds that changes
in worker input are more important than changes in the
acceptance rate in predicting fertility decline.   This
may be due to collinearity between the two variables.

Other Results   Mauldin and Berelson (1978) find their
index of family planning effort to be more highly correlated with fertility decline than are socioeconomic
variables.   They also find that programs in place ten or
more years are associated with larger fertility declines
than are newer programs.

Conclusions   Although family planning programs appear
to be associated with fertility decline, cross-sectional
and within-country studies appear to yield conflicting
results.   Schultz's results for Taiwan suggest that the
impact is larger initially than several years later;
however, these results refer only to cross-sectional
differences.   Time-series results show a consistent
negative impact when the independent variable is lagged
one year.   Mauldin and Berelson's and Entwisle and
Winegarden's results suggest a ten-year delay before
national-level programs have an effect, although part of
this discrepancy may be due to the indirect way in which
Mauldin and Berelson's index is constructed.


                          NOTES

1.   There are of course variants to this general approach.
     Kirk (1971) and Oechsli and Kirk (1975) have empha-
     sized the holistic nature of the development process
     and have preferred to use composite indices of
     development rather than individual variables.
2.   A possible exception is McNicoll's (1980) work on
     community and institutional factors.
3.   Easterlin's work (1978) is one of the few exceptions
     which considers both the demand and the supply side.
4.   A good example of an application of the new home
     economics to the study of fertility change is Schultz

(1969, 1973). Williams (1976) summarizes much of the literature and does a particularly careful job of tracing the consequences of development for the costs of children. Cassen (1976) provides a good critique of the literature which examines the value of children as an investment. He makes the important point that, in many societies, children are the only possible investment, however low and uncertain their rate of return. O'Hara (1975) and Heer and Smith (1968) develop formal models of the effects of mortality decline, given the desire to have surviving children in one's old age.

5.  To test the worst case, Cavanaugh's (1979:289, Table 3) estimate of the minimum change in the crude birth rate for 24 countries between 1965 and 1975 from any two sources was correlated with the maximum change. This entailed considerable scrambling of data sources. The result was a respectable rank order correlation of 0.70 with approximate standard error 0.19. The various estimates of change in the crude birth rate were also examined as they relate to international expenditures on family planning programs (Cavanaugh, 1979:290, Figure 1). Again, regardless of the data source considered, the conclusion is largely the same: there is no or at most a very weak negative relationship. Of course, this is merely a test of internal consistency and not of the validity of the data. This is troublesome since many of the sources borrow information from one another.

6.  A counter example is Entwisle and Winegarden (1981).

7.  In the regression framework, this is the same as putting in dummies for region and for time.

8.  Random effects or error components models offer a compromise by weighting the two estimates (based on within and between sums of squares) inversely by their error variances. Unfortunately, the clarity of the decomposition is sometimes obscured as a result.

9.  A counter example to this is Preston's work (1980) on the socioeconomic determinants of mortality decline.

10. For example, if current values of the independent variable and lagged values up to ten years previous are appropriate and only the value five years earlier is included, the coefficient on the independent variable (lagged five years) will "pick up" both the effects that would have occurred in the five years between the value of the independent and the value of the dependent variable and some longer-term effects. However, the shorter- and longer-term effects may be

quite different, and results obtained from the inclusion of a single lag quite misleading.

11. This procedure is somewhat discomfiting given the smooth exponential trends that are necessarily fit to most of the independent variables. It would seem that this procedure would lead to quite a high degree of collinearity among the variables where values must be interpolated. Furthermore, this procedure leaves the within-region variance rather precariously defined.

12. This variable is designed to capture the effects of persisting high fertility on the age structure, but does not perform as expected. Nerlove and Schultz eliminate it in some estimations.

13. The IV estimates use all exogenous variables as instruments. However, there is little discussion of the choice of instruments or of the causal structure of the model.

14. Because of the high autocorrelation typically present in such data sets, deviations models and error components models tend to yield similar estimates. This is particularly true for the Nerlove and Schultz work, where there is heavy reliance on interpolated series.

15. Again, this instability of estimated coefficients may be due to collinearity induced by the interpolation procedure.

16. It is common in the economics literature to use education as a proxy for potential income.

17. In the analysis of the total fertility rate, Schultz (1973:237) finds that estimates based on intertemporal variability are much smaller than those based on cross-sectional differentials. He suggests that estimates of short-run response are biased upward in the cross-sectional estimates.

18. It is not clear that this procedure explicitly models the pattern of urban and rural decline, although such explicit modeling is possible.

19. In the preceding review of within-country studies, it was found that relationships that hold in the cross section need not hold when temporal variability is examined. Further, it was noted that estimates based on a simple pooled sample tend to be dominated by cross-sectional differences, some of which can be attributed to long-term variability. Thus Gregory and Campbell's results must be treated with some caution.

20. The use of percent of the population living in urbanized areas is a rather arbitrary choice as a measure of the attitudinal changes accompanying development. Gregory and Campbell also examine interactions of the other independent variables with literacy, but find that a model incorporating both sets of interactions does not perform as well as one which includes only interactions with the percent urban. It is not clear how much this may be due to collinearity problems and loss of degrees of freedom. Cassen (1976:75) proposes that urbanization represents "a concentrated form of those general societal developments which affect fertility." This supports Gregory and Campbell's contention that urban residence implies a change in life style. However, it seems odd that they also include industrialization as part of this same concept.

21. For an alternative look at turning points, see Kirk (1971).

22. This criticism also applies to their procedure for searching for the appropriate lag.

BIBLIOGRAPHY

Birdsall, N. (1977) Analytical approaches to the relationship of population growth and development. Population and Development Review 3:63-102.

Bulatao, R. A. (1980) The Transition in the Value of Children and the Fertility Transition. Paper presented at Seminar on the Determinants of Fertility, Bad Homburg.

Cassen, R. H. (1976) Population and development: A survey. World Development 4:785-830.

Cavanaugh, J. A. (1979) Is fertility declining in less developed countries? An evaluation analysis of data sources and population program assistance. Population Studies 332:283-293.

Chenery, H., and M. Syrkin (1977) Patterns of Development 1950-1970. Oxford, England: Oxford University Press.

Coale, A. (1973) The demographic transition. Pp. 53-72 in International Population Conference, Liege 1973, Vol. 1. Liege: International Union for the Scientific Study of Population.

Easterlin, R. A. (1978) The economics and sociology of fertility: A synthesis. Pp. 57-134 in C. Tilly, ed., Historical Studies of Changing Fertility. Princeton, N.J.: Princeton University Press.

Entwisle, B., and C. R. Winegarden (1981)  Fertility and
    Pension Interrelationships in Developing Countries:
    Econometric Evidence.  Research Report 81-9,
    University of Michigan, Ann Arbor.
Freedman, R. (1979)  Theories of fertility decline:  A
    reappraisal.  Social Forces 58:1-17.
Gregory, P. R., and J. M. Campbell, Jr. (1976)  Fertility
    and economic development.  Pp. 160-188 in M. C.
    Keeley, ed., Population, Public Policy and Economic
    Development.  New York:  Praeger.
Heer, D., and O. D. Smith (1968)  Mortality level,
    desired family-size and population increase.
    Demography 5:104-121.
Hermalin, A. I. (1975)  Regression analysis of areal
    data.  In C. Chandrasekaran and A. I. Hermalin, eds.,
    Measuring the Effect of Family Planning Programs on
    Fertility.  Liege:  International Union for the
    Scientific Study of Population.
Hermalin, A. I. (1978)  Spatial Analysis of Family
    Planning Program Effects in Taiwan, 1966-72.  Papers
    of the East-West Population Institute No. 48.
    Honolulu:  East-West Population Institute.
Janowitz, B. S. (1973)  An econometric analysis of trends
    in fertility rates.  Journal of Development Studies
    9:413-425.
Kirk, D. (1971)  A new demographic transition?  Pp.
    138-145 in Rapid Population Growth.  Baltimore, Md.:
    The Johns Hopkins University Press.
Mauldin, W. P., and B. Berelson (1978)  Conditions of
    fertility decline in developing countries, 1965-75.
    Studies in Family Planning 9:89-147.
McNicoll, G. (1980)  Institutional Determinants of
    Fertility Change.  Paper presented at Seminar on
    Determinants of Fertility Trends,  Bad Homburg.
Mundlak, Y. (1978)  Models with variable coefficients:
    Intergration and extension.  Annales de l'INSEE (no.
    30-31):483-509.
Nerlove, M., and T. P. Schultz (1970)  Love and Life
    Between the Censuses:  A Model of Family Decision-
    Making in Puerto Rico.  Rand Monograph RM-6322-AID.
    RAND Corporation, Santa Monica, Calif.
Oechsli, F. W., and D. Kirk (1975)  Modernization and the
    demographic transition in Latin America and the
    Caribbean.  Economic Development and Cultural Change
    23:391-420.
O'Hara, D. (1975)  Microeconomic aspects of the
    demographic transition.  Journal of Political Economy
    83:1203-1216.

Preston, S. (1980) Causes and consequences of mortality declines in LDC's during the Twentieth Century. Pp. 289-360 in R. A. Easterlin, ed., Population and Economic Change in Developing Countries. Chicago: University of Chicago Press.

Schultz, T. P. (1969) An economic model of family planning and fertility. Journal of Political Economy 77:153-180.

Schultz, T. P. (1973) Explanation of birth rate changes over time: A study of Taiwan. Journal of Political Economy, Supplement 81:238-274.

Teitlebaum, M. (1975) Relevance of the demographic transition for developing countries. Science (May 2).

Tsui, A. O., and D. J. Bogue (1978) Declining world fertility: Trends, causes, implications. Population Bulletin 33(4).

van de Walle, E., and J. Knodel (1980) Europe's fertility transition: New evidence and lessons for today's developing world. Population Bulletin 34(6).

Williams, A. D. (1976) Determinants of fertility in developing countries. Pp. 117-159 in M. C. Keeley, ed., Population, Public Policy and Economic Development, New York: Praeger.

Winegarden, C. R. (1978) A simultaneous equations model of population growth and income distribution. Applied Economics 10:319-330.

# Chapter 20

# Cohort and Period Measures of Changing Fertility

NORMAN B. RYDER

Fertility change over time is a central issue in demography. If data are available to calculate birth rates for successive (birth) cohorts in successive periods, those rates can be summarized either by adding the rates for each particular cohort over the span of periods in which it is engaged in reproduction, or by adding the rates in each period over the span of cohorts engaged in reproduction in that period. The time series of indices resulting from these two operations ordinarily differ; the focus of the present paper is that discrepancy.

The discrepancy is illustrated by the long time series of fertility data available for the United States (Heuser, 1976). The series of period and cohort total fertility rates differ in two distinct ways. First, period fertility is much more variable than cohort fertility from year to year. This is shown by the relative deviations of fertility for each year from a fitted value based on a five-term moving quadratic. For the years 1927-66, the average deviation per thousand is nine; for cohorts 1900-39, the average deviation per thousand is one. (The difference of 27 years in the time spans is based on an approximate mean age of fertility of 27 for cohorts during the era.) There is substantial dispersion in the deviations for periods: the values were 15 per thousand in 1929-34 and 20 per thousand in 1945-50. For cohorts, the only nontrivial deviations were 3 per thousand for the cohorts of 1917-21, and there is reason to suspect that those deviations reflect difficulties in estimating cohort size. Second, short-term changes in fertility are characteristically associated with changes in the environment within which reproduction takes place, an environment more or less shared by cohorts of childbearing age. From a period standpoint, the changing climate leads to fertil-

ity variations in one direction, followed shortly by
countermovements; from a cohort standpoint, the change is
manifested in a displacement of births from one period to
another, with little net influence on the eventual cohort
total fertility rate.

As ide from these short-term variations, there is also
a systematic tendency for period and cohort fertility to
diverge over the longer term. This divergence falls into
three phases in the available American experience:  relative to cohort fertility, period fertility was 9 percent
higher in 1917-30, 7 percent lower in 1931-44, and 15
percent higher in 1945-64. A simple explanation has been
proposed for these discrepancies (Ryder, 1979b):  change
in the age distribution of cohort fertility signifies a
change in the way cohorts are allocating their fertility
among the successive periods of their reproductive
experience; thus period fertility tends to swing around
cohort fertility as a manifestation of that change.[1]
The annual change in the mean age of cohort fertility
within the three time spans was -0.08, +0.06, and -0.15,
respectively. The discrepancy between period and cohort
fertility is approximately the complement of the annual
change in the mean age of cohort fertility. If the only
changing aspect of the distribution of cohort fertility
by age were its mean, this would be an exact relationship.
This point is developed more fully below.

The discrepancy between period and cohort time series
of fertility is of both practical and theoretical
interest.

From a practical standpoint, the prime consideration
is the kind of data available. There are essentially
three sources of fertility data. The first is birth
rates calculated from vital registration data. Unless
the registration system has been functioning effectively
for a long time, the only feasible measures of fertility
over the life cycle are period total fertility rates (and
associated indices). The second source is census data on
children ever born per ever-married woman. For women
beyond the maximum age of reproduction, the mean number
of children ever born multiplied by the proportion ever
married yields the equivalent of a cohort total fertility
rate. To determine the extent of fertility decline by
comparing these data sets, one must consider potential
discrepancies because the measures are based on different
modes of temporal aggregation. There are other sources
of difference as well:  the quality of reporting tends to
vary inversely with the length of recall required, and

the information available through enumeration is necessarily restricted to those women who are members of the cohort in question at the time (since the mortality and migration of which they are survivors may not be unselective with respect to reproductive characteristics). Because of incomplete registration and infrequent as well as incomplete enumeration, the third data source--the fertility survey, or a cross-sectional sample of women below the maximum age of reproduction at the time of interview (Ryder, 1975b)--has become important. For the oldest of these women, members of the earliest birth cohort represented, this provides the same kind of data as enumeration, that is, a cohort total fertility rate. If each respondent reports a birth history, it is also feasible to tabulate births by time of occurrence and age of mother at that time; this will yield the equivalent of a period total fertility rate for the most recent period prior to the survey date. Again, to determine fertility changes by comparing these two calculations, one must consider potential discrepancies due to mode of temporal aggregation.

From a theoretical standpoint, the issue is whether the available data are in a form appropriate to testing the hypotheses being investigated. The fertility of a cohort in a particular period can be seen as resulting from the interaction of two factors: the circumstances peculiar to the period in question, or the environment for the behavior, and characteristics descriptive of the cohort and its constituent actors, or the history and experience they bring with them into the period. Although there may be considerable controversy over the sources of temporal variations in fertility, some of them are unquestionably period-specific, whereas other are more aptly considered as properties associated with each particular cohort. Ideally, the form of the measure should be adapted to the nature of the hypothesis.

With respect to long-term change, the case for a cohort orientation, ceteris paribus, seems strong (Ryder, 1964a, 1965). The character of a cohort can be specified in two ways: according to the life of each individual member, and according to the distribution of the aggregate membership with respect to influential variables.

As for individual qualities, most fertility research considers these to be described by both demographic characteristics (such as age at marriage or parity) and sociocultural characteristics (such as religion or ethnic origin). In addition, an individual enters each period with mental constructs such as knowledge and attitudes, with an endowment of physical property, with long-term commitments, and with an established structure of relationships with others. To the extent that such considerations are important, the cohort orientation to fertility data is appropriate.

The integrity of the cohort as a unit of analysis also holds on the aggregate level. The distribution of individuals within a cohort with respect to various characteristics affecting fertility variables tends to be relatively fixed, and to differ between cohorts. An example would be the proportion of the cohort that has completed an elementary school education. Although the composition of the cohort can change over time, even for characteristics that for the individual are fixed for life--because of the selective effects of mortality and migration--the cohort tends empirically to maintain a distributional integrity through time. This also speaks for a cohort orientation to analysis.

Thus, although period measures are disproportionately represented in the literature, this does not reflect a theoretical judgment that the sources of temporal variation in fertility are period-specific (apart from short-term change). Rather, it reflects the relative ease with which the most recent evidence (ordinarily the most interesting, at least from a policy standpoint) can be aggregated to produce period measures. Because most of the cohorts responsible for this reproduction are far from having completed their fertile age span, the calculation of total fertility rates for them must necessarily be deferred. In a later section, an alternative approach that addresses this problem is explored.

### SOME FORMAL RELATIONS BETWEEN COHORT AND PERIOD FERTILITY MEASURES

The nature of the relationship between period and cohort total fertility rates can be indicated in the following way. Assume a group of cohorts born in the period from t-z to t, where z is any age greater than the maximum age of fertility. Assume further that they follow a pattern of fertility by age, say $g'(a)$, for which the total is $G'$ and the mean age of fertility $M'$. Then the amount of fertility in the period from t to t+z that is attributable to these cohorts is

$$\int_0^z ag'(a)da = G'M'.$$

Next, assume that all cohorts born in the period from t to t+z follow another pattern of fertility by age, say g"(a), for which the total is G" and the mean age M". Then the amount of fertility in the period from t to t+z that is attributable to these cohorts is

$$\int_0^z (z - a)g''(a)da = G''z - G''M''.$$

Then the average annual fertility in the period from t to t+z is

$$F = (G'M' + G''z - G''M'')/z.$$

This expression can be simplified to bring out its significance.
Let $(G' + G'')/2 = G$; $(M' + M'')/2 = M$; and $(M'' - M')/z = m$. Furthermore, since the value of z is arbitrary (provided only that it is large enough), it is convenient to let $z = (M' + M'')$. Substituting these values, we have

$$F = G(1 - m).$$

This suggests the basis for the empirical relationship observed in the first section.

Provided there is no change in the mean age of fertility from the earlier to the later cohort (if m = 0), the level of period fertility in the interim is the average of the levels of cohort fertility before and after. However, if the mean age is lower in the later cohorts (so that m is negative and [1 - m] is greater than unity), the average level of period fertility is inflated above the average level of cohort fertility. Period fertility just before the change (when the first member of the later cohort set appears in the youngest fertile age) is equal to G'; just after the change is completed (when the last member of the later cohort set appears in the oldest fertile age), period fertility is equal to G". It therefore follows that the time path of period fertility in such circumstances is concave relative to a straight line from G' to G". On the other hand, if the mean age of cohort fertility is higher for the later cohort set, the converse holds; in this case, the path of period fertility is convex relative to a straight line from G' to G". The nature of the time series of period fertility between t and t+z cannot be stated more precisely since it would depend on the particular shape of the cohort fertility functions (about which nothing was assumed above).

The import of this finding is that, given two populations with a common decline in the cohort total fertility rate, the mean age of fertility could be rising in one population and declining in the other. The period-by-period pattern in the former case would be more rapid decline at first and less rapid decline later (relative to the cohort series); in the latter case, it would be less rapid decline at first and more rapid decline later. This is clearly a matter for concern in conducting comparative analysis, and is explored in more detail in a later section.

Although the above demonstration has the advantage of simplicity, it is clearly unrealistic to posit that fertility change occurs in one discontinuous step. Moreover, the approach does not resolve the related question being addressed here of the respective time series of period and cohort mean ages of fertility.

The following model sheds light on this question (Ryder, 1964b). First, distinguish between the quantum of fertility, $G(T)$, and its tempo, or distribution by age, $D(a,T)$, where $D(a,T) = g(a,T)/G(T)$. Assume a linear change in $G(T)$ amounting to g per annum, and a linear change in $D(a,T)$ amounting to d(a) per annum. (A constraint on the latter assumption is that the proportions must remain between zero and one.)

The mean age of fertility is defined as follows:[2]

$$M(T) = \sum aD(a,T).$$

With linear changes in $D(a,T)$, there is also linear change in $M(T)$. The annual change in $M(T)$ is symbolized by m. Likewise, the variance in the age distribution of fertility is

$$V(T) = \sum a^2 D(a, T) - M^2(T).$$

With linear change in $D(a,T)$, there is quadratic change in $V(T)$. The annual change in $V(T)$ is symbolized by $v(T)$. Similarly, there is cubic change in the third moment about the mean, say $W(T)$, and the annual change in $W(T)$ is symbolized by $w(T)$.

Next, consider age to be coded in integral values, with the youngest age of fertility set at 1. Then let $F(X)$ be the total fertility rate for the period in which the cohort having total fertility rate G and distribution $D(a)$ is in age X:

$$F(X) = \sum (G - (a - X)g) * (D(a) - (a - X)d(a))$$
$$= (G + Xg) * (\sum D(a) + X\sum d(a) - \sum ad(a))$$
$$- g * (\sum aD(a) + X\sum ad(a) - \sum a^2 d(a)).$$

Now $\sum D(a) = 1$ ; $\sum d(a) = 0;$
$\sum aD(a) = M$ ; $\sum ad(a) = m;$
$\sum a^2 D(a) = V + M^2$ ; $\sum a^2 d(a) = v + 2Mm.$

Substituting, we have

$$F(X) = G(1 - m) + g((X - M) * (1 - 2m) + v).$$

Letting $X = M$, we have

$$F(M) = G(1 - m + rv),$$

where $r = g/G$, the rate of change in the cohort total fertility rate. This result is almost the same as the earlier expression, $G(1 - m)$, since the product $rv$ involves two derivatives and is thus of the second order of smalls.

Furthermore, we have the interesting result that the annual change in period total fertility rate, say f, equals $g(1 - 2m)$. Thus change in the cohort mean age of fertility causes twice as large a discrepancy in the change in the period total fertility rates as in the total fertility rate itself.

The same approach can be used to establish the relationship in this model between the period and cohort mean ages of fertility. The numerator of the period mean age of fertility is

$$\sum a * (G - (a - X)g) * (D(a) - (a - X)d(a)).$$

Noting that

$$\sum a^3 D(a) = W + 3MV + M^3 \quad \text{and}$$
$$\sum a^3 d(a) = w + 3mV + 3Mv + 3M^2 m,$$

we make the substitutions as before and arrive at the following expression for the period mean age of fertility:

$$M_p = M - \frac{Gv + g(V(1 - 3m) - w)}{G(1 - m) + gv}.$$

Although this is a clumsy expression that does not immediately evoke the sense of the situation, there is a close approximation: $M - Vr$, where $r = g/G$ as before. Likewise, the approximate derivative is $m - r(v - Vr)$.

The relationship between the period and cohort mean age of fertility signifies that, when the total fertility rate is declining from cohort to cohort ($r$ negative), the period mean age of fertility is higher than the mean age for the corresponding cohort.[3] This is an intuitively plausible result since fertility decline from cohort to cohort implies from a period standpoint that those in the younger ages will represent lower fertility overall, while those in the older ages will represent higher fertility overall.

These approximate expressions--$F = G(1 - m)$ and $M_p = M - Vr$--indicate the way in which cohort change is manifested period by period. They also suggest ways in which models predicated on cohort change will lead to period results that can differ markedly. The symmetry of the findings may also be noted: the tempo of period fertility is a distorted version of the tempo of cohort fertility when the quantum of cohort fertility is changing; likewise, the quantum of period fertility is a distorted version of the quantum of cohort fertility when the tempo of cohort fertility is changing.


SOURCES OF CHANGE IN THE MEAN AGE OF COHORT FERTILITY

It is evident from the above discussion that time series of period fertility measures depend on change in the mean age of cohort fertility, a subject seldom addressed in the literature. It is almost self-evident that the average age at which childbearing occurs depends on when the reproductive process begins, how many babies are born, and how long it takes to bear each child. More specifically, the total fertility rate can be divided into the equivalent calculation restricted to births of a particular order and the associated mean age at occurrence of births of that order. Let the nth-order total fertility rate and mean age of fertility be $G(n)$ and $M(n)$, respectively. For simplicity's sake, assume that $M(n + 1) - M(n) = J$; that is, the difference between the

time of occurrence of births of successive orders is
independent of the order. It is important to note that J
is not the length of the birth interval as that is ordinarily understood, but rather something shorter, since
those who progress to a birth of the next higher order
ordinarily have the preceding birth at a younger age than
those who do not.

Then, if we symbolize the mean age at marriage by
$M(0)$, we have $M(n) = M(0) + nJ$.

$$
\begin{aligned}
M &= \Sigma\, G(n) * M(n)/G \\
&= \Sigma\, G(n) * (M(0) + nJ)/G \\
&= M(0) + J * (\Sigma\, nG(n)/G),
\end{aligned}
$$

where the summations are over all birth orders. The
coefficient of J in this expression, and thus the number
of reproductive events going into the calculation of the
mean age of fertility, M, is the mean order of birth, say
$\phi$. That is closely related to the total fertility rate;
however, another facet of reproductive behavior (in the
aggregate) is involved. Let $p(i)$ be the proportion of
women in the cohort who have (completed) parity i. Then
$G(n) = \sum\limits_{i=n}^{z} p(i)$, where z is the highest parity.

$$
G = \sum_{n=1}^{z} G(n) = \sum_{n=1}^{z} \left( \sum_{i=n}^{z} p(i) \right) = \sum_{i=1}^{z} ip(i)
$$

$$
\sum_{n=1}^{z} nG(n) = \sum_{n=1}^{z} \left( n \sum_{i=n}^{z} p(i) \right) = \sum_{i=1}^{z} \frac{i(i+1)}{2} p(i)
$$

$$
= \left( \sum_{i=1}^{z} i^2 p(i) + \sum_{i=1}^{z} ip(i) \right)/2.
$$

Now mean parity is

$$
\sum_{i=1}^{z} ip(i) = G,
$$

and the variance in parity is

$$
\sum_{i=1}^{z} i^2 p(i) - G^2.
$$

It follows that

$$\phi = ( \sum_{n=1}^{z} nG(n))/G = (G(1 + c^2) + 1)/2,$$

where c is the coefficient of variation of the parity distribution (the ratio of the standard deviation to the mean).

Thus we see that the mean age of fertility depends on two parameters of the parity distribution: first, the quantum parameters--not only the mean of the parity distribution, G (the total fertility rate), but also its heterogeneity, as measured by the coefficient of variation (c); second, two temporal parameters--M(0), the mean age at marriage, and J, the time difference between birth orders. The influence of each of these parameters on change in the mean age of fertility, and thus on the relation between period and cohort total fertility rates, is discussed below.

## Change in the Quantum Parameters

If all components of the mean age of fertility except the total fertility rate are invariant over time, then the change in the mean age of fertility is equivalent to g * $(J(1 + c^2)/2)$, where g, as before, is the annual change in the total fertility rate. Consider a path of fertility change in which the total fertility rate follows a downward ogive, with decline reaching its maximum in the middle of the transition. Then the change in the mean age of fertility also reaches its maximum at that point, as does the relative discrepancy between the period and cohort total fertility rates.

A convenient functional form for a decline of the postulated type is a symmetrical cubic

$$G(T) = GA - (GA - GZ) * ((3T^2/N^2) - (2T^3/N^3)),$$

giving a decline from GA to GZ over the course of N years. The second column of Table 1 shows the pattern for an example in which GA = 6, GZ = 2, and N = 60. The value of g at the midpoint is -0.10. To derive the value of m, we need assumptions about J and c. Plausible values over a wide range of populations would be J = 2 and c = 0.6. Then m = -0.136, and F' = G(1 - m ) = 4 * 1.136 = 4.544

TABLE 1    Changes in the Cohort Total Fertility Rate (G)
and the Period Total Fertility Rate without Change in
Heterogeneity (F') and with Change in Heterogeneity (F")

| T | G | Change | F' | Change | F" | Change |
|---|---|--------|-----|--------|-----|--------|
| 0 | 6.000 | | 6.000 | | 6.000 | |
| | | -0.625 | | -0.077 | | -0.397 |
| 15 | 5.375 | | 5.923 | | 5.603 | |
| | | -1.375 | | -1.389 | | -1.195 |
| 30 | 4.000 | | 4.544 | | 4.408 | |
| | | -1.375 | | -1.651 | | -1.317 |
| 45 | 2.625 | | 2.893 | | 3.091 | |
| | | -0.625 | | -0.893 | | -1.091 |
| 60 | 2.000 | | 2.000 | | 2.000 | |

at the midpoint of the transition. The values of F'
associated with these assumptions are shown in the fourth
column of Table 1. Change in the period total fertility
rate is very small at first, but becomes large during the
last half of the transition. This is an artifact of the
changing time distribution of cohort fertility.

Note that period fertility is higher than cohort
fertility throughout the entire transition. This seems
problematic since the source of both calculations is the
same surface of fertility rates by age and time. However, if the two fertility series, period and cohort,
were integrated over the time span of the transition, the
ratio of the former to the latter would be (N + MA -
MZ)/N, where MA and MZ are the mean ages of fertility at
the beginning and end of the transition. In effect,
cohort fertility is being compressed into a smaller number of (period) years by the decline in its mean age.
The ratio just given is another form of the expression
(1 - m) for distributional distortion.

Of course, it is unrealistic to assume that the coefficient of variation of the parity distribution will
remain invariant during a decline in fertility. A more
plausible model would predicate a gradual decrease in the
proportion of the population following the initial
reproductive pattern, and a gradual concomitant increase
in the proportion adopting the final reproductive
pattern. This idea can be captured by rewriting the
previous expression for G(T) as follows:

$$G(T) = GA * P(T) + GZ * (1 - P(T)),$$
$$\text{where } P(T) = 1 - (3T^2/N^2) + (2T^3/N^3).$$

Although this is the same time series as before, one implication of the new formulation is that the coefficient of variation of the parity distribution increases during the early part of the transition; this is because variance between groups is being added to variance within groups. If each part of the population (that following the traditional and that following the modern pattern) has the same coefficient of variation of the parity distribution, c, then it may be shown that the coefficient of variation for the population as a whole, say k(T), is determined by the expression

$$(1 + k^2(T)) = (1 + c^2) * ((GA^2 * P(T)) + (GZ^2 * (1 - P(T))))/G^2(T).$$

In the previous model, in which the coefficient of variation was invariant over time, the values of m at T = 15, 30, and 45 were −0.102, −0.136, and −0.102, respectively. With the revised model, the values become −0.042, −0.102, and −0.178. The results are shown in Table 1 in the column labeled F". The change in the final quarter of the transition is even more pronounced than was the case with F'.

Two conclusions can be drawn from this exercise. First, there is reason to expect that fertility decline, as portrayed by period measures, will proceed more slowly in the first half of a transition and more rapidly in the last half, relative to the pattern portrayed by cohort measures. Second, the pattern of discrepancy can be substantially affected by the way different parts of the population participate in the decline, which will affect the heterogeneity of the parity distribution through time.

## Change in the Tempo Parameters

Because rising age at marriage is a common aspect of reproductive change in developing societies, its consequences for the discrepancy between period and cohort fertility are of considerable interest. If all factors in the equation for the mean age of fertility other than age at marriage were invariant over time, then the period total fertility rate would equal the product of the cohort total fertility rate and the complement of the annual change in the mean age at marriage. If, for example, age at marriage followed a symmetrical rising cubic (of the form specified above) from an initial value of 20 to a

final value of 24 over the course of two decades, the
slope of the mean age at marriage, and thus of the mean
age of fertility, would be +0.3 at the midpoint in this
change. Thus the period total fertility rate would
decline by 30 percent during the first decade, and then
rise to its original level by the end of the second
decade. To make this surprising result more plausible,
consider what would happen if all of a cohort's childbearing were concentrated in one year. Then a rise in
the (mean) age of fertility by one year would be manifested from a period standpoint in a year in which no
fertility occurred; a rise in the mean age of fertility
(associated with the postulated change in age at marriage)
of four years over the course of twenty years would be
equivalent to the allocation of only sixteen years of
cohort fertility to those twenty periods. Although much
better evidence than is currently available would be
needed to document the point, the recent rapid decline in
the crude birth rate (a period measure) in China may have
resulted at least partly from the reproductive strategy
of raising the age at marriage. It may further be
posited that cessation of the rise in age at marriage
would be accompanied by a rise in period fertility. It
should be emphasized that what is being described here is
a source of discrepancy between period and cohort fertility. From the standpoint of eventual population growth,
any reduction in the birth rate, whether or not it signifies a change in the quantum of cohort fertility, and
whether or not it is transitory, leads to a lower ultimate
population size than would otherwise be the case (Ryder,
1975a).

The implications of a lengthening or shortening of the
time difference between successive births (J) are comparable to those of a change in age at marriage. Although
the magnitude of change in J is likely to be much less
than that in M(0), any change becomes weighted by the mean
order of birth (O) and can therefore lead to an appreciable distortion of period fertility when fertility is
high.

To summarize, the key element causing the values of
period and cohort total fertility rates to diverge is the
annual change in the mean age of cohort fertility. Four
variables have been identified as responsible for that
change: the level of fertility and the heterogeneity of
the parity distribution, on the one hand, and the mean
age at marriage and mean time difference between births
of successive orders, on the other. Populations having

identical time series of their cohort total fertility
rates may therefore have very different time series of
their period fertility measures, depending on their
particular experience with these variables.

ESTIMATION OF COHORT PARAMETERS FROM DATA FOR PERIODS

The foregoing discussion indicates generally the kinds of
discrepancy between period and cohort fertility measures
that may be expected in various configurations of demographic change.  However, it is unresponsive to the
practical problem noted above that data for cohorts with
completed fertility are irrelevant to analysis of the
most recent reproductive experience of a population, and
period measures will therefore be used, giving a distorted
picture of temporal variations in cohort fertility.

To exemplify this problem and indicate one direction
for resolving it, one can draw on some results from the
1976 Colombian National Fertility Survey (Ryder, 1979a).
Figure 1 shows the period-specific and cohort-specific
fertility information provided by the Survey.  For each
cohort, births per woman are shown along a positively
sloping diagonal for each successive period of the
cohort's history up to interview (the upper right negative diagonal); successive cohorts proceed from left to
right by time of birth.  The fertility in each period is
represented along a negatively sloping diagonal, termi-
nated by the upper left positive diagonal (representing
the time of birth of the oldest respondent in the survey).
Four-year units are used for both cohorts and periods.
The birth date limits for the first cohort are 1926.5/
1930.5, for the second cohort 1930.5/1934.5, and so
forth; the time limits for the last period are 1973.0/
1977.0, for the second to last period 1969.0/1973.0, and
so forth.  For convenience, the cohorts are numbered from
1 to 9 and the periods from 2 to 10.  Age is defined
implicitly by the period/cohort intersection, so that the
first "age" for each cohort is coded "1" (the difference
between the period number and the cohort number).

Reasonably complete life-cycle information is
available only for the earliest cohort and the latest
period:  the earliest cohort has a total fertility rate
of 6.78 and the latest period a total fertility rate of
4.42.  The question is to what extent a comparison of
these numbers gives a flawed picture of the temporal
change in fertility that has been occurring in Colombia.

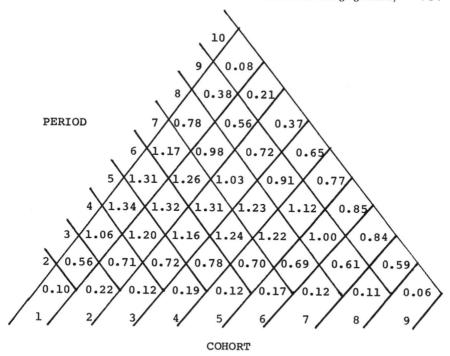

COHORT

FIGURE 1  Births per Woman by Cohort and Period, in
Four-Year Time Units, 1976:  Colombia

Note:  Cohort #1 was born 1926.5/1930.5.  Period #10 is
1973.0/1977.0.

Source:  Colombian National Fertility Survey (Ryder,
1979a).

(Other questions that are relevant to such a comparison,
like the quality of information for the earliest cohort,
which has the most difficult recall problems, are set
aside for the present discussion.)

One tempting procedure is to devise a projection for
each cohort of fertility in the periods subsequent to the
interview date, in effect turning the triangle into a
rhombus.  However, there are as many ways of performing
this procedure as there are demographers, and the result
would go well beyond what is ordinarily understood as
data analysis.  Another popular idea, also a projection
procedure, is to obtain from each respondent an estimate

of the number of her expected future births. However, experience with this approach over the last several decades in the United States has been disappointing: the future is no less unpredictable for the individual respondent than for the demographer (Westoff and Ryder, 1977). On the other hand, an interesting model has been developed to exploit such data for the analysis of period-specific change (Lee, 1977, 1980).

In an earlier section, a derivation of period parameters from assumptions about change in cohort fertility functions was presented. There is no formal difficulty in employing the same approach in reverse, that is, making assumptions about change in period fertility functions and deriving the consequent cohort parameters. Assume that the total fertility rate for period t is $F(t)$, and that it is changing linearly by $f$; assume that the proportion of the (period) total fertility rate occurring in age a is $D(a,t)$, and that it is changing linearly by $d(a)$. Then the fertility in age a, for cohort $T = t - M_p(t)$ (where $M_p(t)$ is the mean age of period fertility), is

$$(F(t) + (a - M_p(t))f) * (D(a,t) + (a - M_p(t))d(a)).$$

The development proceeds in the same fashion as before. The total fertility rate for cohort T is

$$G(T) = (F(t)) * (1 + m_p + r_p v_p),$$
with derivative $g = f(1 + 2m_p)$.

Similarly, we have as the mean age of cohort fertility

$$M(T) = M_p(t) + \frac{Fv_p + f(V_p (1 + 3m_p) + w_p)}{F(1 + m_p) + fv_p}.$$

In applying these formulae to the data in Figure 1, the values for the total fertility rate (F), the mean ($M_p$), and the variance ($V_p$) refer to period 10: $F = 4.42$; $M_p = 4.5023$; and $V_p = 3.3224$. The values for changes in the various functions are based on a comparison of the data for periods 9 and 10 (deleting from period 10 the experience of cohort 1, in order to ensure life-cycle comparability). The required values are $f = -1.08$; $m_p = 0.1273$; $v_p = 0.2836$; and $w_p = 0.0104$. Insertion of these values in the formulae gives the following values for cohort 5.50 ($T = t - M_p = 10 - 4.50$), which is the cohort born 1944.5/1948.5: $G(T) =$

4.1637; and M(T) = 3.6658. Thus the cohort total fertility is 6 percent less than its period counterpart, and the cohort mean age of fertility is 3.34 years less than its period counterpart (remembering that the unit is 4 years).

These results are what one would expect, drawing on the previous discussion, from substantial decline in both the cohort total fertility rate (which elevates the period mean age of fertility) and the cohort mean age of fertility (which elevates the period total fertility rate). The total fertility rate for cohort 1, referring to Figure 1, is 6.78; thus the decline per annum in cohort fertility is estimated to be about 2.7 percent. The mean age of fertility for cohort 1 is 4.8009 (in coded form); thus the decline per annum in the cohort mean age of fertility is estimated to be about 0.25 years. It should be noted that a direct comparison of the mean for cohort 1 (4.8) with the mean for period 10 (4.5) would have indicated no such rapid decline in the mean age of fertility.

In a previous section, it was noted that the translation formula for the total fertility rate, moving from cohort to period, can be simplified by ignoring the term rv. The equivalent approximation, moving from period to cohort, would be $G = F(1 + m_p)$. In the Colombian data, that would be a bad approximation, because the period functions being summarized showed large values for both $r_p$ and $v_p$. Accordingly, the approximation is not recommended as a general rule. On the other hand, the approximate formula for the mean age of fertility is quite convenient because of its relative simplicity; it may also be preferable because of the well-known sensitivity of the calculation of higher moments to vagaries in the data base. In the period-to-cohort direction, the approximation is $M = M_p + r_p v_p$. In the Colombian data, that gives 3.69 instead of the 3.67 yielded by the complete formula. Experimentation would be needed to determine whether this approximation is indeed as robust as this example suggests. It may be noted further that the formula for the change in the mean age of fertility, based on this approximation, is $m = m_p + r_p(v_p - r_p v_p) = 0.26$, essentially the same value as that reported above.

## PROPOSITIONS AND CONCLUSIONS

The following propositions can be derived from the foregoing discussion.

1.  The period total fertility rate ordinarily differs from the comparable measure for the cohort that is at its mean age of fertility in the period in question.  The relative difference is approximately the complement of the annual change in the mean age of cohort fertility.

2.  The period mean age of fertility ordinarily differs from the comparable measure for the cohort that is at its mean age of fertility in the period in question.  The difference is approximately the product of the rate of change in the cohort total fertility rate and the variance in the age of cohort fertility.

3.  Since the mean age of cohort fertility is ordinarily changing along with the cohort total fertility rate (because of its dependence on both the mean and the coefficient of variation of the parity distribution), the time series of period total fertility rates may be expected to diverge from the comparable series for cohorts during an era of fertility transition.

4.  Given the close dependence of the cohort mean age of fertility on the mean age at marriage, change in the latter may cause substantial divergence between the period and cohort total fertility rates.

5.  Fertility functions for recent periods may be used to estimate the contemporary cohort total fertility rate and mean age of fertility.

Although these propositions are presented according to fertility rates specific for age and time, they have a wider applicability since they are essentially mathematical in character.  Period measures of fertility may be defined as those in which the temporal identification is established by the time of occurrence of the births in their numerators.  This holds for the crude birth rate and the general fertility rate, for measures keyed to marital duration or interval since last birth, and so forth.  All such measures are responsive, mutatis mutandis, to the strictures specified for the period total fertility rate and mean age of fertility when they are used to draw inferences about changes in cohort reproductive behavior.

Moreover, the applicability of the propositions presented here extends beyond fertility to other demographic processes, such as nuptiality, mortality, and migration, and indeed to all changes of state during the life cycle.  In its most general form, an event of interest is identified as occurring at some interval of time after a preceding event, ordinarily selected because it signals in some way the beginning of exposure to risk of occurrence of the event of interest. Period measures are created by considering the distribution of the preceding event (the cohort-defining event) in relation to the succeeding event, with the temporal identification of the result the time of the succeeding event. Cohort measures are created by considering the distribution of the succeeding event in relation to the preceding event, with the temporal identification of the result the time of the preceding event. Thus two time series exist; ordinarily, the period series is available, but the cohort series is preferable. The above propositions apply in all such situations.

Two kinds of research suggestion flow from the above argument. First, because of the way changes in the tempo of cohort fertility and changes in its quantum interpenetrate the pattern of fertility from a period standpoint, much more knowledge is needed about the time distribution of reproductive behavior, and the processes which determine its shape. Second, the algebra of translation between cohort and period fertility functions requires further study. For example, it would be worthwhile to explore, perhaps through computer simulation, alternative translation formulae based on different models from those employed here, in part to discriminate between the essential and superficial aspects of the process. For another example, the formulae presented above apply solely to additive functions (like the total fertility rate), whereas most demographic processes are best described by risk functions, which are multiplicative (like the survival process represented in the conventional life table).

In conclusion, it is often the case that evidence about fertility comes in period form, whereas ideas about fertility come in cohort form. Although no formulae can be expected to resolve this problem fully, its recognition is essential to the integrity of our research procedures.

### NOTES

1. Ward and Butz (1978) have developed an analysis of American fertility based on the distribution of cohort fertility over time. A similar approach was used in Ryder (1980; first published in 1951).
2. Unless otherwise specified, all sums in this account are over the span of reproductive ages.

3. In all of these formulae, the period in question is the period when the cohort for whom the parameters are calculated is at its mean age of fertility.

BIBLIOGRAPHY

Heuser, R. L. (1976) Fertility Tables for Birth Cohorts by Color: United States 1917-73. DHEW Publication No. (HRA)76-1152. Rockville, Md.: National Center for Health Statistics.

Lee, R. D. (1977) Target fertility, contraception and aggregate rates: Toward a formal synthesis. Demography 14:455-479.

Lee, R. D. (1980) Aiming at a moving target: Period fertility and changing reproductive goals. Population Studies 34:205-226.

Ryder, N. B. (1964a) Notes on the concept of a population. American Journal of Sociology 69:447-463.

Ryder, N. B. (1964b) The process of demographic translation. Demography 1:74-82.

Ryder, N. B. (1965) The cohort as a concept in the study of social change. American Sociological Review 30:843-861.

Ryder, N. B. (1975a) Notes on stationary populations. Population Index 41:3-28.

Ryder, N. B. (1975b) Fertility measurement through cross-sectional surveys. Social Forces 54:7-35.

Ryder, N. B. (1979a) Notes on Fertility in Colombia. Reproduced and distributed (in Spanish) by CCRP (Corporacion Centro Regional de Poblacion), Bogota, Colombia.

Ryder, N. B. (1979b) Components of temporal variations in American fertility. Pp. 15-54 in R. W. Hiorns, ed., Demographic Patterns in Developed Societies. London: Taylor and Francis.

Ryder, N. B. (1980) The Cohort Approach. New York: Arno Press.

Ward, M. P., and W. P. Butz (1978) Completed Fertility and its Timing: An Economic Analysis of U.S. Experience Since World War II. Report R-2285-NICHD. Santa Monica, Calif.: Rand Corporation.

Westoff, C. F., and N. B. Ryder (1977) The predictive validity of reproductive intentions. Demography 14:431-453.

Part V
# CONCLUSION

Chapter 21

# An Overview of Fertility Determinants in Developing Countries

RODOLFO A. BULATAO and RONALD D. LEE

This chapter briefly summarizes the research evidence about fertility determinants in developing countries presented in the preceding papers. The goal here, as in the preceding papers, is not to break new ground, but rather to provide an analytically organized and balanced overview of what is already known, emphasizing empirical findings rather than theory.

The organization of this chapter follows that of these volumes as a whole. First, it reviews the analytical framework presented in Chapter 1. Expanding on the categories provided by the framework, the chapter then considers, in order, the supply of children, the demand for children, the fertility decision process, fertility regulation and its costs, nuptiality patterns and their effect on fertility, and the influence of social institutions.

Though this chapter does involve some selective sampling and interpretation, most of the information and evidence is drawn directly from the preceding papers. Passages that follow individual papers particularly closely (in some cases verbatim) are referenced. It is, of course, impossible to provide full references in a chapter of this sort; for comprehensive bibliographies the reader is referred to the papers themselves.

## THE FRAMEWORK

To organize knowledge about the complex interacting influences on fertility in the less developed countries (LDCs), a conceptual framework was developed. The framework groups influences on fertility according to three channels through which they operate: demand, supply, and regulation costs. "Demand" here refers to the family size and composition a couple would choose, abstracted from all concern with the childbearing process required to attain that outcome. Demand has many dimensions, such as number, gender, and spacing of surviving children. "Supply" refers to the surviving children couples would have if they did not regulate their fertility, or their children's survival, in parity-specific ways. Supply depends on natural fertility, which in turn reflects biology, culture, socioeconomic circumstances, and to some degree individual choice; supply also depends on child survival and on nuptiality patterns. The interaction of demand and supply considerations presumably determines whether and how strongly a couple wishes to have or to avoid a birth. Whether they actually take any steps to avoid it depends in addition on how undesirable or inaccessable contraception and induced abortion are. This latter kind of influence, referred to as "regulation costs," includes such considerations as the difficulty of obtaining contraceptive information, distance to a family planning clinic or other source, religious or moral attitudes, and perceived health consequences.

This three-part framework is developed at the level of the couple or household, on the assumption that actions by couples are ultimately crucial. At the community or societal level, fertility is the sum of the outcomes for numerous couples; influences on community and societal fertility, therefore, can also and will be treated within the categories of the framework.

The framework can accomodate all hypothetical influences on fertility; indeed, past fertility research appears to fall rather naturally into these three categories. Other means of categorizing past research are of course possible, but the present approach appear to be the most comprehensive and coherent of those so far suggested and allows treatment of research across disciplines. Although this framework may seem at first to assume an economic model in which couples make optimizing decisions, in fact no such assumption is necessary; indeed, "demand" and "supply" as used in the framework are only loosely related to the corresponding economic concepts. In principle, any particular influence--such as social norms, cultural practices, or nutrition levels--might dominate the fertility outcome.

For some purposes, it is useful to take the bold step of elevating the three categories to the status of variables which summarize in a single number the totality of subsumed concerns and influences. Such a "strong" version of the framework--as illustrated in Figure 1, for instance (following Easterlin, 1978)--amounts to a refutable theory and offers a distinctive view of how various influences interact to produce fertility outcomes. This version greatly simplifies the framework by implicitly ruling out certain kinds of interactions, thereby simplifying empirical work as well. However, it is not yet known whether the necessary assumptions are empirically appropriate; the framework is used here, therefore, primarily as a rough classification scheme, avoiding these substantive assumptions.

Any framework necessarily involves simplification, with some gain in clarity but also the risk of arbitrary or misleading structuring. Various key issues about the framework, such the question of whether couples make fertility decisions and whether these are one-time or sequential decisions, are discussed in Chapter 1, and some points about these issues are reviewed below. The framework may tend to direct attention away from some fruitful lines of inquiry, such as the study of deliberate spacing of children (Page and Lesthaeghe, 1981; United Nations, 1981), the substitution of modern contraceptives for traditional means of spacing, and the use of marriage delay as a family limitation strategy. To compensate for such possible biases, some explicit attention is paid to such areas either in the sections below or in the following chapter.

## THE SUPPLY OF CHILDREN[1]

The supply or potential output of children is defined as the surviving children a couple would have if family size were not deliberately limited. Supply thus depends directly on levels of natural fertility and child survival, and indirectly on the background variables which influence these levels. In contemporary more developed countries (MDCs), demand is well below supply, and is the principal determinant of observed fertility given the relatively low cost of fertility regulation. In contrast, in many poor developing countries, as well as in historical societies, the situation is unclear: demand may approach or exceed supply, or couples may not formulate any effective fertility goals, or fertility regulation may be thought too difficult or not considered at all. Fertility in these societies is determined

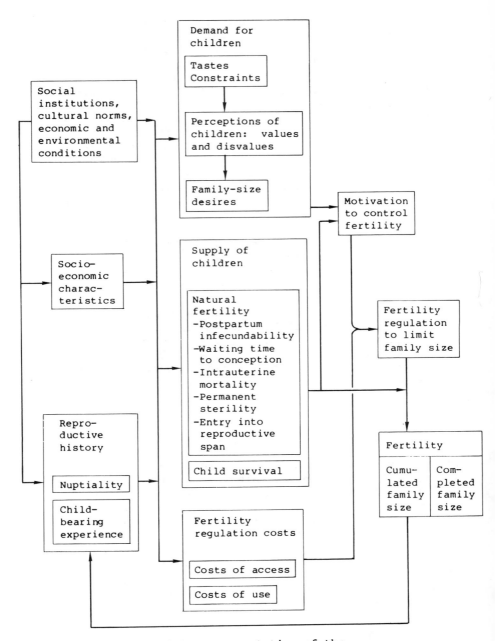

FIGURE 1  One Possible Representation of the
Interrelationships Among the Basic Components of the
Framework

primarily by supply factors, and natural fertility
obtains.

The sections that follow review the evidence regarding
the two direct determinants of the supply of
children--natural fertility and child survival--and their
effects on supply trends.

## Determinants of Natural Fertility

Natural fertility prevails in the absence of deliberate
attempts to limit family size; since this is difficult to
observe directly, the absence of any parity-dependent
limitation behavior, or the absence of any use of contraception or abortion, may be taken as approximations.
Natural fertility is a function of both behavioral and
biological proximate determinants through which background variables, including socioeconomic factors, health,
and nutrition, operate. The proximate determinants were
first identified independently by Henry (1953) and by
Davis and Blake (1956). Slightly modified, Henry's
approach yields the following set of five proximate
determinants of natural fertility: (1) postpartum
infecundability; (2) the waiting time to conception; (3)
spontaneous intrauterine mortality; (4) the onset of
permanent sterility; and (5) age at marriage (or at onset
of exposure to intercourse) and marital disruption.
Natural fertility differences among populations and
trends in natural fertility can always be traced to
variations in one or more of these five proximate
determinants.

Although each of the five does affect natural
fertility, their quantitative impacts are quite unequal,
as shown in the sensitivity analysis displayed in Figure
2. A standard value of 7 may be assumed for total
fertility in a natural-fertility setting. If each
proximate determinant is varied individually, holding the
other determinants fixed, this value for total fertility
will be affected. Each bar in the figure shows the range
of variations in total fertility that can be expected
from varying each determinant across its observed range
in populations of the world (though these variations are
not equally likely). It is clear that variations in age
at marriage and in postpartum infecundability dominate
the other sources of natural-fertility variations in this
exercise (Bongaarts and Menken, in these volumes).

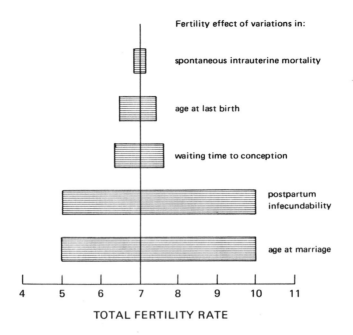

FIGURE 2   Variations in the Total Fertility Rate Induced
by Variations in Five Proximate Determinants of Natural
Fertility

Marriage age and its determinants will be discussed in
a later section.  As for postpartum infecundability, this
primarily reflects variations in breastfeeding practices:
in the intermediate range of breastfeeding durations, each
additional month of breastfeeding adds over half a month
to postpartum amenorrhea (Bongaarts, in these volumes).
This rough estimate does not take into account variations
in intensity of breastfeeding, which have considerable
effect.  In certain cultures, culturally induced restrictions on postpartum sexual intercourse are also important
in extending the infecundable period.

The influence of background variables on natural
fertility, starting with nutrition and health, may now be
considered.  Although the subject has been controversial,
the bulk of the evidence now indicates that the moderate
chronic malnutrition that is found in many parts of the
developing world has only a small physiological impact on
fertility.  Although famines unquestionably lead to

significant fecundity impairments, this is apparently not
the case for moderate chronic malnutrition. Several
studies have indicated that poorly nourished women may
have later menarche (perhaps by two or three years) and
that they have slightly shorter postpartum amenorrhea
intervals (typically by one or two months). However,
since the fertility effect of each of these factors is
small, chronic malnutrition is not a major fertility
determinant.

With regard to the physiological links between health
and fertility, Gray (in these volumes) points out that
malnourishment and ill health frequently occur together
and interact. He nevertheless concludes that only severe
morbidity is likely to inhibit reproduction, at worst
affecting a minority of disadvantaged women. There is
one important exception: the pelvic inflammatory diseases
that are almost certainly responsible for high levels of
primary and secondary sterility and consequent low
fertility in some areas, especially in parts of Africa
where venereal disease is widespread. However, it must
also be noted that low natural fertility in some settings
may result from deliberate spacing of births in response
to poor health and nutrition conditions (Knodel, in these
volumes).

Turning to socioeconomic and cultural influences on
natural fertility, the critical behaviors to address are
breastfeeding and postpartum abstinence (Nag, in these
volumes). Research into the way these influences affect
variations in breastfeeding and therefore in amenorrhea
is a rather recent response to recognition of the over-
riding importance of lactation as a determinant of
fertility in the developing world. It is now generally
accepted that, in many areas, breastfeeding becomes
shorter and less frequent as education increases; is
higher in rural than in urban areas; and exhibits marked
differences across regions and ethnic groups (Nag, in
these volumes). Although the role of changing economic
pressures and labor force participation in determining
breastfeeding practices is not well understood, there is
considerable concern that the net effect is increased
pressure to reduce lactation (Lesthaeghe, 1981). Controversy remains over whether the availability and
advertising of infant formula encourages earlier supplementation and weaning, resulting in deleterious
effects on the infant and contributing to an increase in
natural fertility. In general, mounting evidence from
widely separated parts of the developing world shows that

declines in breastfeeding are taking place, and these will cause fertility to rise unless countered by major increases in the use of contraception or other methods of fertility control.

Cultural influences are also important determinants of variations in postpartum abstinence. It has long been known that sexual intercourse may be restricted for cultural reasons during lactation, as in many societies in sub-Saharan Africa. Recent research has shown that, in some settings, postpartum abstinence is used by couples deliberately to space births for the health of both the children and the mother (Knodel, in these volumes). Available survey data indicate that postpartum abstinence is negatively associated with education, urbanization, and contraceptive use (Nag, in these volumes).

## Determinants of Child Survival

Considered next are influences on child survival, which has improved considerably in recent decades. It is recognized that infant and child mortality varies with the mother's age and parity; both parents' socioeconomic status, including education and income; the adequacy of drinking water; the availability of health care and the control of disease; nutrition; and a host of other factors. Yet there is some disagreement about the relative importance of these mortality determinants in the world today. Two views in particular are opposed: one asserts the primacy of "social action and techno-logical change," the second the primacy of "socioeconomic modernization" (Chen, in these volumes). Since infant and child mortality remain high in many developing countries, it is especially important to understand the factors involved, and to assess how these can be changed to promote improved survival.

## The Trend in Supply

Natural fertility and child survival together determine the supply of children; both factors vary widely among populations and over time. Their influence on the supply of children can be seen by considering supply trends over the course of a hypothetical demographic transition. The natural total fertility rate may rise from 5 or 6 to about 10 during the transition, primarily because breastfeeding is largely abandoned.  (However, actual fertility at the end of the transition is much lower because most couples deliberately control their fertility.)  Accompanying this trend in natural fertility is a sharp improvement in survival; an increase in life expectancy from 25 to 75 implies that the proportion of births surviving to age 20 rises from under 50 percent to about 98 percent.  The combined effect of these trends in natural fertility and mortality is roughly a fourfold increase in the supply of children, as measured by the number surviving to age 20. Clearly, increased natural fertility and improved child survival, whose effects are roughly equal in this example, can result in very large changes in supply.

## THE DEMAND FOR CHILDREN

Advances in the understanding of natural fertility like those just reviewed, together with better understanding of the effects of access to modern contraception, have improved the ability to explain the timing and pace of fertility decline, as well as apparently deviant cases of rising fertility.  Nonetheless, the demand for children still remains at the heart of most explanations of fertility decline in response to modernization.  Inevitably at some stage in the transition, and probably fairly early, change in demand becomes a key factor, if it has not been one all along.  It may be asked, of course, whether the concept of demand has any meaning in pre-transition populations.  In fact, the available evidence, though far from conclusive, suggests that it does:  most survey respondents are able to answer questions about family-size desires and justify their responses, although this may not be true in all societies.  Related issues, such as whether demand can be measured (McClelland, in these volumes), how it depends on the identity of the decision maker within the family (Hollerbach, in these volumes), and how it relates to behavior (Pullum, in these volumes) have not been entirely resolved.

Like supply, demand refers to surviving children.  It is assumed that couples generally set goals in regard to the family size they want to achieve, rather than the number of births necessary to achieve it.  However, improvements in child survival do not lead to perfectly offsetting decreases in births, because mortality also has some influence on demand for surviving children. Several studies show that losing a child increases a

couple's desired number of additional births.  This
effect varies by sex of the deceased child and by
achieved parity; however, it is less than unity, so that
couples on the average do not completely make up for the
lost children.  Strictly interpreted, the evidence
suggests that the experience of child mortality, while
increasing the number of desired births, reduces the
demand for surviving children (Heer, in these volumes).
There is also quite limited evidence that perceived, as
opposed to experienced, child mortality also has a
positive effect on the desired number of births.
     The four main classes of factors affecting demand may
now be discussed:  the direct economic costs and benefits
of children, their opportunity costs, the effects of
income and wealth, and norms and tastes for children.

### Direct Costs and Benefits of Children

The direct economic costs and benefits of children are
important considerations for parents in high-fertility
developing countries, as many attitudinal studies have
shown (Fawcett, in these volumes; Bulatao, 1979).
General financial and practical assistance and expected
help in old age are among the most frequently cited
advantages of children, rivaled only, in some cases, by
concern with preserving the family name or line.  The
same surveys also show that direct financial costs are
the predominant disadvantage attached to having children
in LDCs.  Instrumental benefits are of much less concern
in MDCs; within both LDCs and MDCs, they are less important in urban than rural areas.  Whether positive or
negative, the net value of a child varies, among other
things, by sex, number of siblings, size of landholding,
the extent to which other institutions provide substitute
services, the nature of labor markets, the desired level
of expenditures on the child, and the extent to which
costs of children can be passed on to a larger social
group.
     Painstaking time-use studies, particularly in Asia,
have in the last decade begun to give us a picture of
what children actually contribute economically.  Although
children in some settings begin quite young to contribute
many hours in agricultural labor and housework, the
cumulative value of these services (averaged across sex)
typically does not compensate for their cumulative
consumption before leaving home (Lee and Bulatao, in

these volumes; Cain, 1982). Children also provide other services, such as old age support and insurance against risk. Unfortunately, in the absence of acceptable market substitutes, it is not possible to assign a money value to these services. If they were valued according to the cost of providing them through efficient institutions (which, for example, would yield a positive return on investments for old age security), it is clear that they would be worth relatively little, and children's net economic contribution would still be negative. However, in the absence of such institutional alternatives, these services may be extremely valuable (Caldwell, in these volumes).

## Time Costs of Children

There is little direct evidence on the time costs of children in LDCs; nonetheless, it appears that these time costs are of much less consequence in LDCs than in MDCs, where they have often been stressed as the central influence on fertility. Attitudinal studies have shown that MDC women frequently report "feeling tied down" as an important cost of children; this is rarely so in LDCs (Fawcett, in these volumes). Compatibility between childbearing and work on the farm reduces time costs in agricultural settings, as does the availability and acceptibility of parental surrogates (Oppong, in these volumes). Indeed, children in LDCs are often net suppliers of time, rather than net consumers, and a general rise in wages may therefore initially raise the net value of children (Lindert, in these volumes).

During the course of modernization, time costs presumably become increasingly important in determining demand. It is not surprising, therefore, that the empirical association of fertility and female labor supply in LDCs is sometimes positive and sometimes negative (Standing, in these volumes); likewise, higher female wage rates in LDCs are sometimes associated with higher, rather than lower, fertility.

## Income and Wealth

In principle, whether children are net producers or net consumers, higher income or greater wealth should make them more affordable and therefore increase demand for

surviving children, with a subsequent increase in the
number of desired births. However, income increases may
lead to a demand for higher quality in children rather
than a larger number. Furthermore, higher incomes
provide parents with access to substitutes for child
services which would tend to mitigate the rise in the
demand for surviving children. Finally, higher incomes
may lead in various ways to a change in tastes away from
children toward competing material goods. Perhaps as a
consequence, the evidence on the effect of income on
demand is inconclusive (Mueller and Short, in these
volumes). It is striking that studies have consistently
found fertility to be positively associated with size of
landholding, and perhaps with rural incomes generally;
whether this reflects an influence of income on demand,
supply, or regulation costs is unknown (Mueller and
Short, in these volumes).

## Tastes and Norms

In addition to economic costs, benefits, and resources,
it is necessary to consider norms, tastes, or personal
preferences for children in contrast to preferences for
other goods or services. Although norms have frequently
been identified as central to understanding fertility
behavior, there is an absence of any direct supporting
evidence (Mason, in these volumes). Similarly, the
evidence for the influence of tastes is inferential,
since no direct attempts have been made to measure them
in LDCs. Although parents' reports of the psychosocial
values and disvalues attached to children imply
considerable variability in tastes, the sources of this
variability remain obscure. Tastes seem to vary across
religious, linguistic, and other ethnic boundaries;
whether they vary similarly across social classes is
difficult to determine. Tastes are also affected by
exposure to new consumer goods.

## The Trend in Demand

Modernization radically alters the demand for children.
First, children's economic contributions fall off
considerably, as education gains in importance, as the
tasks children do become obsolete or unnecessary, as the
labor force shifts out of agriculture, as children are

replaced by other institutions providing security against risk or old age, and as greater social mobility and weaker family ties reduce dependence on children. Second, direct costs of children rise in monetary terms, although incomes are also rising. There does in fact seem to be less concern about direct costs in later stages of development, possibly because of the improved financial situation of the typical household. Time costs, on the other hand, become heavier with modernization: substitutes for parental care become more costly, jobs become less compatible with childbearing, and the value of parental time rises. Time costs may therefore begin to have a significant effect in the later stages of modernization. The effect of rising incomes is not clear, since they are offset by rising costs and by various indirect effects, mainly negative, on demand. Finally, tastes may change against children and in favor of new material goods, including those necessary for better child quality, although other factors in tastes, such as those based on ethnic differences, may remain largely unaffected (Lee and Bulatao, in these volumes).

There are few good estimates of the magnitude of the resulting changes in demand. Taking survey measures of family-size desires to reflect demand, two illustrations of apparently falling demand may be noted: data for Taiwan show a drop from 4.0 to 2.8 in preferred number of children between 1965 and 1980 (Chang, Freedman, and Sun, 1981); data for South Korea show ideal family size falling from about 5 to about 2.5 in the last two decades (Cho, Arnold, and Kwon, 1982). In both cases the fall is exceeded by the fall in total fertility; however, surveys in other countries currently show larger preferred numbers (between 6 and 9 in several sub-Saharan countries [Lightbourne et al., 1982]) than the initial levels in these two cases.

## FERTILITY DECISIONS

Given an expected supply of children and some concept of demand, how does a couple go about making a fertility decision, or possibly avoid a decision? Some researchers see a couple's response to their supply-demand situation as entirely shaped by cultural norms; others prefer to see it as involving a multitude of deliberate decisions; still others divide couples according to these two levels of response. This section identifies different strategies a couple may use in fertility decision making in an attempt to synthesize the limited evidence, and then discusses the couple interaction involved.

## Six Strategies

A couple may use six different strategies, either singly or in combination. First, in what may be considered the null case, if there is no significant imbalance between supply and demand, no action is necessary. Of course, other fertility-related decisions are made--on marriage, on breastfeeding, on separation, and so on--though these generally do not result from the supply-demand balance and are typically not directed to controlling family size.

The other five strategies are activated only if there is some significant imbalance between supply and demand. The second strategy is to misperceive or deny such imbalance, as illustrated by a couple's rationalizing an unexpected birth or misperceiving the probability of an unwanted pregnancy or the likelihood of having a son or a daughter. The third strategy is to do nothing, recognizing the imbalance but "tolerating" it, perhaps out of passivity or fatalism. There may be various reasons for passivity, such as limited information about or high costs attached to fertility regulation, ambivalence about decision consequences, or a general feeling of powerlessness over one's life. Fatalism of this sort may be the dominant mode in environments of capricious productivity, high mortality, authoritarian politics, rigid stratification, and widespread poverty (Hull, in these volumes).

By contrast, the fourth strategy involves active coping:  making a conscious, considered attempt to deal with imbalance, deliberately seeking to make the best of the situation or maximizing the utility derived from it. This involves applying some decision rule (Hollerbach, in these volumes); some suggested rules have been shown to predict behavior in developed-country samples, though for developing-country couples the evidence is too scanty to allow conclusions.

The fifth strategy may be labeled "advanced coping." Instead of trying to extract the maximum out of a situation, one may use various means to economize on one's effort while still obtaining a satisfactory result. This includes such methods of simplifying decisions as satisficing (choosing an acceptable but not necessarily the best alternative); bounded rationality (evaluating only a subset of the possible consequences); and the development of routines and habits. Though attractive in concept, these advanced coping methods have not been illustrated with behavioral data.

The sixth strategy, which may be considered a form of advanced coping, is labeled "sequential coping," and involves adjusting one's behavior as the situation changes; one-time decisions are avoided in favor of continually modified decisions throughout the reproductive span. Sequential coping may be desirable because perceptions of demand, supply, and regulation costs change, and because fertility plans sometimes fail and require revision (Namboodiri, in these volumes).

These strategies form a rough hierarchy, from the simpler and more passive to the more complex and active. Since fertility regulation requires some effort, the strategies of denial and passivity cannot lead to regulation, whereas the other, more active strategies may.

When does a couple use one or the other strategy for a fertility decision? One important factor may be the degree to which supply exceeds demand: greater excess may require a more active strategy. The social situation is also important; it has already been suggested that traditional peasant settings may predispose toward a passive strategy. Personal characteristics also affect choice of strategy: a stronger sense of personal efficacy, a greater tendency to plan, and a future rather than a present time orientation may lead to adoption of a more active strategy. The factors determining choice among these active strategies are not known; however, it is suggested that maximizing will take place where there is more experience with the behavior and greater personal control over it and where fewer alternatives have to be considered, whereas advanced and sequential coping are more appropriate to situations with more options, more complex alternatives, less available information, and the possibility of sequential rather than simultaneous choices (Hollerbach, in these volumes).

## Couple Interaction

The six strategies generally involve different degrees of cooperation between partners. A passive strategy, for instance, does not require any discussion, whereas active coping may. Although interaction between partners has been studied more intensively in developed countries, some evidence is also available for developing countries. Considered here, first, are the effects on fertility of the partners' attitudes and their agreement with each other; second, the effects of communication between them; third, the effects of egalitarianism in the dyad; and, fourth, the effects of influence from others on the couple.

Agreement between partners need not result from discussion: in some samples, in fact, those who do not discuss the issue are more likely to think there is agreement, because they project their own attitudes onto their partners. Coincidental agreement, or concordance, is linked to passive decision making; agreement based on discussion, or consensus, is linked to more active decision making, and to a greater likelihood of fertility control (Beckman, in these volumes). The approval of both partners is often essential in decisions to control; if there is disagreement, the pronatal view is often taken by the man and the antinatal view by the woman.

Communication between spouses is essential to consensus, and suggests a more active than passive decision style. Although more frequent communication between spouses does not necessarily mean a greater likelihood of use of fertility regulation, more frequent discussion of regulation itself is consistently linked with more frequent use. Communication is often initiated by the woman. The amount of communication varies, however, by regulation method: in the case of abortion in particular the woman is somewhat more likely to make a unilateral, surreptitious decision (Beckman, in these volumes).

Communication is more likely, it might be argued, if the partners share decisions and consider each other social equals. A few studies suggest that decision sharing does lead to more frequent fertility control; other studies do not agree, however, possibly because patterns of decision sharing are difficult to determine accurately. Domestic egalitarianism in task distribution and sharing does relate to more frequent fertility control in some studies.

It has been assumed that the couple themselves make the fertility decision. It is difficult to tell how often this is not the case. Although it is sometimes alleged that mothers or mothers-in-law, grandparents or patriarchs are in fact making the fertility decisions (Caldwell, in these volumes), reliable supporting evidence has not been provided. Certainly others can

influence the couple--not only relatives, but also
members of peer groups and medical and paramedical
personnel.  Such influence may change a couple's demand
or alter their regulation costs, though the ultimate
decision remains their own.

## FERTILITY REGULATION

Particular decision strategies, it has been argued,
predispose toward the practice of fertility regulation.
One of the important factors considered in a decision is
the cost of regulation, especially of contraception and
induced abortion (on which the focus is placed in this
discussion), but also of other means like deliberately
prolonged breastfeeding, infanticide (Scrimshaw, in these
volumes), and abstinence.  These costs, it is important
to note, should be balanced against the costs of unwanted
pregnancy and childbirth incurred in the absence of
regulation.

### Costs of Regulation

A rough distinction is useful between the costs of access
to regulation and the costs of use, with the latter
including both health costs and psychosocial costs.
Obtaining access to contraceptive methods involves
purchase costs as well as information and travel costs.
Purchase costs from private sources are similar across
developing countries, and also roughly comparable for
different methods, ranging from U.S.$23 to U.S.$34
annually for four major methods (Schearer, in these
volumes).  For contraceptives from public family planning
programs, on the other hand, the purchase costs are
usually nil.  The costs of locating and traveling to a
family planning facility are more difficult to determine.
One study suggests that travel costs in rural areas are
over a dollar a trip; moreover, for those who have no
knowledge about contraception or about sources of
supplies and services, information costs might be assumed
to be prohibitive.  Monetary costs generally do not seem
to be a major barrier to contraceptive use:  few survey
respondents cite them as a barrier, many purchase
contraceptives from private sources even when public
low-cost sources are available, and price has not been a
major deterrent in experimental programs (Schearer, in

these volumes). Availability of information about contraception, on the other hand, and the psychosocial costs connected with obtaining access, are clearly important determinants of use.

Access to abortion depends partly on its legal status. Abortion is legal in less than 20 percent of countries worldwide (both developing and developed), and permitted with some restrictions, often fairly stringent, in another 60 percent. Legalization does not, however, require health authorities to ensure service availability, which can be complicated by many regulatory requirements, as well as by the reluctance of health personnel to provide abortions. Availability therefore varies, and the monetary costs of abortion are accordingly quite different.

Of the costs of use of fertility regulation, the most serious are probably the health risks of abortion. Mortality from illegal abortion is about 50 to 100 deaths per 100,000 operations, making it a major cause of maternal mortality in developing countries. However, where abortions are legal and easily available, the risks are dramatically lower: for instance, only around 1 death per 100,000 legal abortions was reported for Cuba during the 1970s (David, in these volumes). Similar if somewhat less dramatic differences between the morbidity effects of legal and illegal abortions are reported.

The psychic and social costs associated with abortion are often taken to be serious. Again, however, studies in countries where abortion is legal suggest that, for the vast majority of women, feelings of guilt and depression, when noticeable, are mild and transitory, and usually followed by a sense of relief associated with successful crisis resolution. Despite such costs, and even the serious health risks of illegal abortion, substantial numbers of women resort to this method. Crude estimates of the worldwide ratio range from 200 to 450 abortions per 1,000 livebirths (David, in these volumes).

The health risks associated with particular methods of contraception similarly exert only weak influence on method selection and contraceptive prevalence. Little effort is made to publicize these risks in developing countries, given the lack of adequate medical resources and the recognition of the risks of childbirth and the benefits of controlling fertility. However, fears about health effects, often based on misinformation and rumor, do have significant impact: they are often the major reason given for discontinuing contraception.

Besides actual and feared health costs, a few other psychosocial costs might be noted. It was stated earlier that communication between partners about contraception is related to the likelihood of its use. The difficulty spouses in traditional societies have in discussing this subject may be considered a cost of many methods. Misinformation about the reliability of methods may also impose costs: often there is overestimation of the effects of traditional methods and contrary underestimation of the efficacy of more modern methods. Then there are costs of social disapproval: the couple may be concerned about violating religious or moral standards, or about gossip and ostracism within their social group, or about the attitudes of their extended families. Other probably less significant psychic costs include possible interference with sexual enjoyment and the affront to some women's modesty represented by a gynecological examination (Bogue, in these volumes).

Many of the psychic and social costs connected with contraception might be seen as generated by an innovation before it has been fully integrated into the culture. These costs are mutable, as views about the innovation change, for instance under the impact of organized public information programs. When the innovation has been fully integrated into the culture and antinatal perspectives have become entrenched in a community, it is in fact possible for these costs to reverse, and for social disapproval and other kinds of costs to become attached to uncontrolled childbearing instead of to contraception.

## Diffusion and Family Planning Programs

The process of change in the acceptance of contraception might be studied as a process of diffusion. Besides affecting psychic and social costs, diffusion should also reduce the costs of access, as more information becomes available and as demand for contraceptives generates greater supply. The costs of access may be especially affected by organized family planning programs, designed to provide contraceptives at minimal monetary cost to large populations. Health costs, on the other hand, are affected in a more complex manner by diffusion and by family planning programs: health risks are not necessarily increased or decreased; rather, imagined risks are gradually replaced by more objective assessments.

Diffusion involves the flow of information and attitudes within interpersonal networks, and, on a wider scale, within social groups and societies. It is typically a complex multistage process, involving the mass media at some point but depending critically on local opinion leaders to validate, support, and sell the innovation. At the societal level, the degree of social integration strongly influences the rate of diffusion: cultural homogeneity, geographic compactness, a strong centralized political authority, and the absence of dissenting minorities all allow contraception to diffuse more readily and its perceived psychosocial costs to drop more quickly (Retherford and Palmore, in these volumes).

Family planning programs might be considered agents of diffusion. They have a massive effect in increasing access to contraception: by the late 1970s, the number of service points in national family planning programs was about 110,000 in thirty countries. Limited growth or antigrowth policies have been adopted in three dozen countries with 80 percent of the population of the developing world; another thirty countries (with an additional 15 percent of that population) do not have such policies but nevertheless promote family planning on other grounds (Mauldin, in these volumes; Ross, in these volumes). The effects of such large-scale programs on contraceptive costs are difficult to quantify: they have certainly reduced the travel time required to obtain services for many rural populations, though many other areas remain unserved. Family planning programs have contributed to contraceptive prevalence, as several analyses suggest; although it is difficult to distinguish this contribution from the level that would exist in the absence of a program, some program effect seems fairly certain even with the imperfect models that have been tried. However, it also appears that programs have much greater effect where the social setting is initially favorable, as one would in fact expect given the analytical framework used here (Mauldin, in these volumes).

The patterns of regulation use that have resulted from the diffusion process and from family planning programs, combined with the effects of the supply-demand balance, can be reviewed only sketchily here. Contraceptive prevalence among married women of reproductive age varies considerably in the developing world, from above 20 percent in three of the largest countries--China (where rates three or four times this have been reported),

Indonesia, and India--to below 10 percent in three other
large ones--Nigeria, Bangladesh, and Pakistan.  These
latter countries, as well as several others, have had
national family planning programs for years with no
notable effect.  In other countries, by contrast, the
rapidity of change has been notable:  much of the
dramatic rise in prevalence has  occurred within the last
two decades, and often only in the last decade.  This
increased prevalence has undoubtedly had significant
effects on fertility, though procedures for estimating
these effects do not always agree.

## FERTILITY EFFECTS OF NUPTIALITY PATTERNS

Among the sociocultural factors affecting supply, demand,
and regulation costs, marriage--and patterns of sexual
unions more generally--has a pervasive effect.  Three
characteristics of sexual unions are of greatest importance for fertility:  their stability; their composition,
including whether they are polygynous or monogamous and
whether families are extended or nuclear; and their
formation and dissolution.  For some of these characteristics, a strong and consistent link to fertility has
been found; for others, the evidence is equivocal.  Each
characteristic could affect fertility through a number of
channels, usually involving the supply of children but
also sometimes involving demand.  Moreover, each characteristic could have spurious relationships with fertility because of self-selection or because of reverse
causality.  Whereas something is typically known about
the impact of each characteristic on fertility, little if
anything is known about which of the possible channels
are operative in each case.

### Stability of Unions

From the standpoint of stability, three types of sexual
unions may be distinguished:  legal marriages; consensual
unions that are socially recognized and stable but have
no legal standing; and casual unions characterized by
discontinuous cohabitation.  Consensual and casual unions
are especially important in Latin America and the
Caribbean and in parts of Africa, though they are not
unknown elsewhere.  Type of union depends to a great
extent on the couple's age:  less stable forms are often

transitional to more stable ones. Though women in metropolitan Latin American areas may be an exception, it is fairly consistently reported that women in more stable unions have higher fertility (Burch, in these volumes). This association may be due partly to self-selection: apart from being older, women may be selected into stable unions because of their higher fertility. It may also be due to an effect on supply: casual unions are more likely to involve extensive periods with no exposure to intercourse. Finally, it may be due to demand differences: a woman may be more likely to avoid having children until her union is stable. It has not been determined which explanation, or what combination of them, is correct.

## Composition of Unions

For polygyny, the relation to fertility is more problematic (Burch, in these volumes). Polygyny involves substantial numbers in some societies: it is reported, for instance, that one in five West African men has more than one wife. Polygynous men clearly have more children, which may in fact be a major reason for the practice. For polygynous women, however, the evidence is mixed; the predominant view in the literature is that they have lower fertility, but many empirical studies find no consistent difference. A number of possible links between polygyny and lower female fertility can be identified: for instance, the polygynous wife may have intercourse less frequently and may observe postpartum taboos more strictly, or may on the average marry later than monogamous women. It may also be argued, however, that polygyny should raise fertility by leading to early and universal marriage for women. These and other opposing arguments (Burch, in these volumes) may help to explain the indeterminate empirical findings.

The other aspect of composition is the extended versus the nuclear family. Much research on this issue fails to find a relationship between household composition and fertility. It may be argued that most of this work is flawed because it generally focuses only on current household composition, not allowing for a couple's movement through several types of households in their married life; because it considers only joint residence rather than other links between members of an extended family; and because it fails to control for other variables that may affect fertility. Recent, carefully detailed data for Taiwan do support the thesis that extended families are related to higher fertility (Freedman, 1981). The arguments for such a link primarily involve the demand for children. Compared to the nuclear family, the economics of childbearing may be more favorable in the extended family: costs may be spread more widely, and more resources may be available to make children productive. In addition, the decision process may itself be affected if the locus of fertility decisions in the extended family lies not with the couple but with their elders or if the elders exercise very powerful influence. One linkage through supply has also been suggested: the extended family may promote or facilitate early marriage. The argument may also be made, however, that the relationship is spurious, in two senses: higher fertility in a particular society may itself lead to greater family extension (though not necessarily coresidence) because couples should have more kin with whom to maintain ties and may need family extension as a means of providing childcare; or the values and outlooks in a community with many extended families may induce high fertility, whether or not the particular couple lives in an extended family situation. Although there has been recent theoretical work on these linkages, most of the issues are still unresolved (Burch, in these volumes).

## Dissolution and Formation of Unions

There is less controversy on the effects of the dissolution of unions. Because attitudes toward and the incidence of divorce vary considerably across developing societies, the process of modernization induces no consistent trend in the divorce rate. The effect of dissolution depends on the frequency and speed of remarriage: if significant time is lost between unions, fertility is affected negatively because of lower exposure to intercourse. Where venereal disease is endemic, sequential unions may also contribute to secondary sterility.

The formation of unions has been left for last here because this is a complex issue on which the research is voluminous. The timing of marriage has an undisputedly strong association with fertility. Marriage prevalence (or the proportion ever marrying) also has some effect; it is generally believed that later marriage and lower prevalence are linked, so that their effects are parallel (Smith, in these volumes).

The major effect of a delay in marriage is lower exposure to intercourse in the early, more fecund years of the reproductive span. This is only partly counteracted by a tendency toward higher age-specific fertility rates among those more recently married (Knodel, in these volumes), for several possible reasons, such as higher intercourse frequencies early in a marriage, lower previous exposure to the risk of sterility, the absence of any postpartum amenorrheic interval, and, conceivably, deliberate attempts to catch up with those who started childbearing earlier. Marriage delay may also contribute to smaller families by reducing demand for children: delay may allow each partner the time to develop roles and commitments antithetical to large families. Some suggest that marriage delay should also be seen as a regulation factor, though there is little evidence to support this in LDCs. Finally, self-selection could also be at work, if greater fecundity or less effectiveness at contraception lead to earlier marriage. As with the other nuptiality factors, the validity of these alternative explanations is uncertain (Smith, in these volumes); it is clear, nevertheless, that, throughout the world, women who marry past their early 20s generally end up with fewer children.

## Trends and Determinants in Marriage Timing

Given the importance of marriage timing, a brief discussion of its trends and major determinants is in order. In the attempts that have been made to distinguish regional marriage patterns, northwestern Europe usually stands out as a region long characterized by late marriage, at least partly because of its stem-family tradition. During the demographic transition, age at marriage in this region fell with urbanization; the constraints imposed by the stem family were weaker in urban areas. By contrast, contemporary developing countries start the transition with early and usually near universal marriage; they all nevertheless show remarkably similar shifts to later marriage (e.g., Henry and Piotrow, 1979; Smith, in these volumes). These shifts, usually unaccompanied by any change in marriage prevalence, tend to occur before marital fertility begins to decline.

The factors behind these shifts are imperfectly understood, though a very diverse literature has been

devoted to the determinants of marriage timing. To
summarize briefly, three very general considerations in
marriage timing might be considered: the relative
attractiveness of staying single; the availability of a
mate; and the resources required and resource transfers
involved in getting married.

The attractiveness of staying single depends on
education and on employment opportunities. Given the
limitations in many cultures on married women working,
more education for women, particularly at higher levels,
raises the opportunity costs of marrying and leaving the
labor force. Education for men does not have this effect.
The attractiveness of singlehood may also be affected by
controls over sexual access. It has been hypothesized,
for instance, that male marriage is late where social
arrangements permit common-law liaisons or prostitution.
The attractions of the married state, such as the social
status that may be gained and the advantages of having
children, must also be considered (though, as previously
noted, there is little evidence about the use of marriage
timing to control family size). Legislation may affect
the relative attractiveness of marriage, and is more
likely to be effective if it attempts this than if it
simply sets some arbitrary minimum marriage age (Smith,
in these volumes).

The availability of a mate is determined partly by the
marriage market. The effect of sex ratios on age at
marriage has often been studied, generally with weak or
inconsistent results. Although such ratios can be considerably perturbed by sex-selective migration, marriage
markets show a flexibility that tends to override such
effects.

Where marriage involves the creation of a new household, the resource requirements and transfers mandated by
a marriage, including dowries and bridewealth, will be
major factors in timing. Marriage may require division
of land or other resources in accordance with inheritance
patterns, which therefore partly control marriage timing.
The implications of these and other necessary transfers
are complex: households with more resources may be able
to afford earlier marriages for their offspring; on the
other hand, they may also generate higher aspirations
among offspring that would tend to delay marriage, or
they may hang on to offspring longer because their labor
is more productive.

One other factor shown to affect marriage timing is
urban or rural residence. Urban residence led to earlier

marriage in the European transition, but is generally
associated with later marriage in the developing countries
today. Although some of the factors previously mentioned,
like education, the efficiency of marriage markets, and
the availability of resources, may be related to the
effect of residence, it is not clear if they entirely
account for it.


## FERTILITY EFFECTS OF SOCIAL INSTITUTIONS

The nuptiality factors just discussed have a dual
character: they may be considered either as personal
characteristics of couples or as social institutions.  In
principle, other personal characteristics and social
institutions could be similarly analyzed:  one might
identify the relevant features of an institution, discuss
the evidence relating each feature to fertility, consider
the possible channels for these effects, and discuss the
determinants of each feature. Although an extensive
discussion of all the relevant personal characteristics
and social institutions is not possible here, brief
consideration can be given to the fertility effects of
two of the most important personal characteristics--
education and urban or rural residence--as well as to the
broad effects of social institutions.


### Socioeconomic Characteristics

The effect of education on fertility is often observed to
be negative; this is more often true for female education,
which may have an effect about three times that of male
education. However, a positive effect on fertility is
also sometimes observed, more often for male than for
female education, more often in countries with low levels
of urbanization and development, and more often, finally,
at higher than at lower fertility levels (Cochrane, in
these volumes).  There are numerous channels through
which education could affect fertility.  It could
influence supply by its effects on age at marriage,
breastfeeding, noncontraceptive abstinence, and child
survival.  It could affect demand because of its linkages
to the benefits and costs of children, to income and
wealth, to female wage rates and labor participation, and
to a number of other variables.  Finally, it could affect
fertility regulation by modifying access to contraception

and abortion and by changing the perceived costs of using
them. This variety of possible linkages creates a problem
for empirical analysis: isolating the effect of education
from the effects of other socioeconomic characteristics
requires introducing statistical controls, but this often
results in holding constant some of the channels through
which education operates. Moreover, although the variety
of channels allows for many possible alternative explanations for education's effects, research to document these
explanations is limited.

The effects of urban vs. rural residence on fertility
are somewhat smaller than the effects of education.
Urban women generally have lower fertility than rural
women; this difference is greater the more urbanized a
country is. If marriage and marriage duration are controlled, the difference is often smaller and may even be
reversed, suggesting that nuptiality is a major reason
for the fertility effects of residence. As with education, there are many other possible channels related to
differences in features of urban and rural communities as
well as to differences between urban and rural households
that affect supply, demand, and regulation costs
(Cochrane, in these volumes).

Of other important socioeconomic characteristics,
some, like female employment and income, have been
discussed under demand because it is assumed that their
major impact is through this channel. Others, like
ethnicity and religion, have such different meanings
across societies that it is difficult to discuss them
without considering the effects of variations in social
settings.

## Social Institutions

Characterizing social settings and distinguishing those
that generate high fertility from those that generate low
fertility is a task that researchers have barely begun to
address. From descriptions of different settings and
from the limited analyses available, one might identify
three major institutions or complexes of institutions
that appear to have the greatest significance for
fertility variation (Potter, in these volumes).

First are the institutions that determine the economic
contributions children can make. It is argued by some
that the mode of production is critical: familial
production, in contrast to industrial production, means a

greater role for child labor and allows parents to reap
the benefits. Other institutions are also implicated in
this relationship, such as institutions that provide old
age security, welfare, or insurance against risk, which
by their absence may increase dependence on children;
landownership, which determines the availability of a
complementary factor of production; and the level of
technology, which must be low to make it profitable to
employ untrained children.

The second important class of institutions includes
those that create tastes for or against children.
Religion is primary here because it often validates
pronatalist ideals, though it also has important
additional effects on the normative and psychic costs of
regulation. On the other side might be the consumer
economy and complementary institutions like the mass
media and advertising because they generate material
expectations that compete with traditional family ideals;
other institutions that promote secularism and the decline
of traditional family values, particularly education,
might also be included here.

The third major class of institutions are political
institutions, which must be considered at two levels. At
the community level, they may be sufficiently strong if
the community is cohesive, and sufficiently motivated if
the community bears the costs of providing child welfare
and employment, to manipulate the incentives for childbearing, interfering fairly directly in couples' lives.
At the national level, strong political institutions are
essential in defining population goals and mobilizing the
resources to meet them, chiefly through making fertility
regulation available and reducing its costs.

Besides these three complexes of institutions, other
institutions were previously mentioned for 'their fertility
effects: public health and medical care for their effects
on natural fertility and child survival; the institutions
related to nuptiality and the family; and institutions
and cultural patterns that create barriers to or promote
the diffusion of fertility regulation.


## Fertility Change

The process of modernization involves major transformations in these institutions and, complementary to these,
in the socioeconomic characteristics of individuals and
households.

Very few time-series studies have attempted to substantiate the effects of changing institutions on fertility.  Although such studies provide limited confirmation for the impact of education, female employment, mortality change, and family planning programs on fertility, the effects of other factors have not so far been confirmed (Richards, in these volumes). There are no comparable studies that investigate the intermediate links, that is, the impact of institutional change on supply, demand, and regulation costs.

There is useful speculation, nevertheless, about the way fertility responds to the process of modernization (Easterlin, in these volumes).  Setting aside many complex problems, such as the relationship between period and cohort rates as fertility changes (Ryder, in these volumes) and the nature of the modernization process itself, the process might be described in this way.  In the premodern situation, marriage is early and, in most LDC settings, close to universal.  Many couples desire large families, often larger than they are able to have. The early stages of modernization bring a gradual rise in marriage age, but also an increase in the supply of children, with the rise in natural fertility as breast-feeding becomes less common and with declines in infant and child mortality.  At some point, supply begins to exceed fertility desires, which also begin to fall as children contribute less economically and as tastes change away from large families.  Then it becomes relevant to consider fertility regulation.  The costs of regulation have been declining simultaneously, not only because of family planning programs but also because of increased secularization; eventually, a threshold is reached at which these costs are sufficiently low, and the desire to limit families sufficiently strong, for substantial numbers to adopt fertility regulation.  This complements the effects of marriage delay, and also accelerates the fall in regulation costs; in addition, demand continues to decline, as opportunity costs of childbearing rise late in the transition, until an eventual equilibrium is reached, with fertility at a new low level.

This speculative picture is consistent with the arguments and evidence reviewed here, though it is far from being an established view.  It suggests that the current fertility situation of the developing countries is a complex of interrelated factors.  From this per-spective, the debate about whether development or family

planning is primarily responsible for lowering fertility
is largely beside the point; both are integral parts of
an intricate process that no two countries pass through
in exactly the same manner.


NOTE

1  The initial draft for this section was prepared by
   John Bongaarts and Jane Menken.


BIBLIOGRAPHY

Bulatao, R. A. (1979)  On the Nature of the Transition in
    the Value of Children.  Paper No. 60-A.  Honolulu:
    East-West Population Institute.
Cain, M. T. (1982)  Perspectives on family and fertility
    in developing countries. Population Studies
    36:159-176.
Chang, M.-C., R. Freedman, and T.-H. Sun (1981)  Trends
    in fertility, family size preferences, and family
    planning practice:  Taiwan, 1961-80.  Studies in
    Family Planning 12:211-228.
Cho, L.-J., F. Arnold, and T. H. Kwon (1982)  The
    Determinants of Fertility in the Republic of Korea.
    Washington, D.C.:  National Academy Press.
Davis, K., and J. Blake (1956)  Social structure and
    fertility:  An analytical framework.  Economic
    Development and Cultural Change 4:211-235.
Easterlin, R. A. (1978)  The economics and sociology of

    fertility:  A syntheses.  Pp. 57-113 in C. Tilly, ed.,
    Historical Studies of Changing Fertility.  Princeton,
    N.J.:  Princeton University Press.
Freedman, R. (1981)  Trends in Household Composition and
    Extended Kinship in Taiwan and Relation to
    Reproduction:  1973-1980.  Paper prepared for the
    IUSSP Seminar on Family Types and Fertility in
    Less-Developed Countries, Sao Paulo, Brazil.
Henry, A., and P. T. Piotrow (1979)  Age at marriage and
    fertility. Population Reports 7:105-159.
Henry, L. (1953)  Fondements theoriques des mesures de la
    fecondite naturelle.  Revue de l'Institut
    International de Statistique 21:135-151.
Leibenstein, H. (1981)  Economic decision theory and
    human fertility behavior.  Population and Development
    Review 7:381-400.

Lesthaeghe, R. (1981) Lactation and Lactation-Related Variables, Contraception and Fertility: An Overview of Data Problems and World Trends. Paper prepared for the Seminar on Breastfeeding and Fertility Regulation sponsored by the World Health Organization and the U.S. National Academy of Sciences, Geneva.

Lightbourne, R. Jr., S. Singh, and C. P. Green (1982) The World Fertility Survey: Charting global childbearing. Population Bulletin 37(1).

Page, H., and R. Lesthaeghe (1981) Childspacing in Tropical Africa: Traditions and Change. New York: Academic Press.

United Nations (1981) Variations in the Incidence of Knowledge and Use of Contraception: A Comparative Analysis of World Fertility Survey Results for 20 Developing Countries. New York: United Nations.

# Chapter 22

# An Agenda for Research on the Determinants of Fertility in the Developing Countries

The preceding chapters have reviewed the research on
determinants of individual fertility and fertility change
in the developing countries within a unified analytical
framework. Although progress in the scientific understanding of human fertility in the last two decades has
been substantial, significant areas of scientific
ignorance remain. This paper attempts to sift through
these areas of ignorance and identify some priority areas
for further research.

Following a brief review of several recent attempts to
provide such a research agenda for the field, the scope
and approach of the present paper are described. Next,
research priorities are discussed under the same general
headings used for these volumes: the supply of children,
the demand for children, fertility regulation and its
costs, decision-making processes, nuptiality, and the
effects of social institutions and modernization.


## PREVIOUS WORK

The five agendas for research on fertility determinants
in the developing countries reviewed here were prepared
in the last decade, and each appears to be still relevant.
Most of them focus on policy-relevant research; two do
not limit themselves to fertility but deal with broader
population issues. They shall be considered in chronological order.

The first agenda is a short paper entitled "Social
research and programs for reducing birth rates" (Freedman,
1974). The author lays out "what we need to know" and
"what we know" about six topics: fertility itself, the
"intermediate" variables affecting it, social norms

affecting both fertility and the intermediate variables, the specific social institutions affecting fertility, mortality change and its effects on fertility, and family planning programs. He concludes that the research has major shortcomings, yet provides sufficient knowledge for family planning programs to proceed without waiting for more scientific detail. He then gives six general principles to suggest where research can best assist family planning programs. First, as a general consideration, each country requires its own data and research; not enough is known about relationships among variables for general formulas to be reliably applied. Next, he identifies two types of data for which there is particular need: basic data on birth rates and their major components, at the national level and for major strata and local areas; and regular sample survey data on actual and potential family planning acceptors. Then he notes that family planning programs provide a special opportunity for research along the lines of natural or contrived social experiments. Finally, at the level of more basic research, he points to two areas deserving special attention: the influence of economic factors on fertility and the biosocial process of reproduction.

Also policy-oriented, though with less of a concentration on family planning, is a monograph by McGreevey and Birdsall (1974) on The Policy Relevance of Recent Social Research on Fertility. Where Freedman takes the perspective of the family planning administrator, McGreevey and Birdsall adopt the point of view of a government planner. First they review the evidence for the effects on fertility of a number of standard variables, including education, income, income distribution, employment, and infant mortality; in the process they provide a largely atheoretical catalog of verified and unverified relationships. They observe that knowledge of relationships varies in specificity: in some cases, one may have only a general idea that some relationship probably exists; in other cases, one may know exactly how much change to expect in fertility from some change in the determinant, how much it costs to produce the change in the determinant, and how cost-effective such a change is as a means of affecting fertility. Table 1 provides their useful hierarchy of the specificity of relationships. They believe that the more useful research for planners is at the more specific end, dealing with questions of elasticities, expenditures, and economizing.

TABLE 1   A Hierarchy of Research Findings Addressed to
Public Policy

| Type | Characteristic |
| --- | --- |
| Observation | Awareness of relationship between fertility and some other variable without specific examination of the nature, direction, or strength of the relationship. |
| Simple Correlation | Findings of relationship between a single ecological variable or a single personal or social characteristic and fertility; suggests a targeting procedure for population policy. |
| Multiple Correlation | Findings of relationship between multiple ecological, personal and social characteristics and fertility which may suggest targeting procedure for population policy. |
| Causation | Demonstration of correlation plus reasoned argument for the direction and scope of causation in such form as to indicate that a given policy act would produce fertility change in a predictable direction. |
| Elasticity | Given correlation and causation, an elasticity offers a specific prediction that a stated percentage change in an independent variable would produce a given percentage change in fertility. |
| Expenditure | At this level of analysis one could predict that a stated percentage change in public sector expenditure would produce a predicted fertility reduction. |
| Economizing | Research demonstrating that a given balance of resources between sectors could not be replaced by any alternative, more cost-effective mix of expenditures. |

Source:   McGreevey and Birdsall (1974:63).

    In keeping with this emphasis, the research they
recommend stresses the efficient use of public resources.
They favor research to justify and facilitate the
mobilization of external as well as local resources for
population activities; research on the population impact
of such government projects as rural development, expansion of educational facilities, and health, sanitation,
and related public works programs;   research on the
allocation of resources between family planning and
non-family planning programs; and research on the
efficiency of family planning programs.  On program
efficiency, three issues are considered critical:   "(1)
What fertility-reduction results could one anticipate

from a 'quality' family planning program?  (2) How
cost-effective are existing and quality family planning
programs?  (3) Are there means of reducing fertility that
are more cost-effective than family planning programs?"
In addition to these concerns with efficient resource
allocation, they offer one recommendation on more basic
research on fertility determinants:  they argue that the
household decision system should be studied more intensively, with attention to fertility choice behavior, the
resource constraints on it, the options that confront the
family, and the special character of decision making in
societies where fertility decline is taking place.

An emphasis on high-level policy also appears in
Mertens' (1978) paper entitled "Research Priorities for
Population and Socio-Economic Development:  Recommendations for UNFPA Inter-Country Programmes," which in fact
ranges beyond national to regional and global issues.
Mertens attempts to lay the foundations for an agenda by
criticizing certain perspectives in population work and
describing what he considers proper orientations.  Thus
he advocates a "needs of the people" approach, proposes
that the historical dimension not be forgotten in
population studies, attacks the belief that desirable
population changes will occur without some "blood and
sweat," objects to "floating skyscrapers" (meaning theory
without data), inveighs against the "circus" of proxy
variables, and cautions researchers against the sin of
Faustian omnipotence and the danger of the "single
research project neurosis."

Mertens' research recommendations are somewhat more
down-to-earth.  First, he favors national population
impact studies, by which he means studies more wide-
ranging than those recommended by McGreevey and Birdsall;
these would include description of the demographic
situation, discussion of factors influencing levels of
the demographic variables, analysis of consequences of
the demographic situation, and analysis of government
policies in relation to population.  Second, he sees the
need for research on alternative government policies to
influence each of the demographic variables.  Under these
general headings are a number of more concrete research
topics, including women's roles, decision making, and
intrafamily flows.  Third, he recommends work on integrating population concerns into development planning.
Fourth, he sees and applauds renewed interest in family
planning research, and lists seven related specific
priority areas:  the need for programs to promote family

planning; measures of family planning program effort;
comparisons of family planning programs with other development and welfare programs; the provision of family
planning services through indigenous institutions; the
identification of new client groups; consideration of
problems of unwanted pregnancy; and the contribution of
family planning programs to social change. Finally, he
points to a number of unexplored research areas, including ethical aspects of population issues and differential
growth rates in multiethnic countries.

At least equally ambitious is Miro and Potter's (1980)
report, Population Policy: Research Priorities in the
Developing World, the result of a three-year review of
population studies involving a substantial number of
population researchers from both developing and developed
countries. This report reviews both research and research
capacities in the major regions of the developing world,
and then attempts to describe the state of knowledge
about the demographic variables, specifically mortality,
fertility, internal migration, and international migration. Several appendices, published separately, provide
much more detail about population studies in each
region.[1] Research recommendations are made at several
levels: for specific regions, on specific topics, and
across all regions and topics.

Miro and Potter's general recommendations include a
balanced menu of research including description, theory
building, and policy-related work. Descriptive research,
they argue, is needed to provide information on levels,
trends, and differentials of the demographic variables; a
related enterprise is decomposing demographic indices, in
order to better understand what is involved in demographic
change. In addition, because of the complexity of demographic phenomena, theoretical research is needed to
provide suitable frameworks for analysis. They recommend
that evaluation of the demographic effects of public
policies and programs also receive high priority. Nor do
they neglect the political dimension in population
affairs: analysis of the political factors in policy
making, in research generation, and in research utilization is another part of their agenda. Finally, they
argue for an integrative perspective on population and
development, suggesting that "styles" of development have
a dominant impact on population policy, and therefore
merit special attention.

Several of these themes recur in their specific recommendations for fertility research, which include descriptive research, work on the components of fertility, and
the evaluation of the impact of particular development
programs.  Their other priority areas are even more
specific:  they recommend microlevel work on the family
economy, analyses of social institutions and how they
affect fertility decisions, work on the availability of
contraceptive services, and analyses of the effects of
fertility on income distribution.

Recommendations similar to these are provided in the
most recent research agenda, a statement adopted by a
research awards program at the Population Council (1981)
entitled "Research on the determinants of fertility:  A
note on priorities."  After a short and highly selective
review of determinants research, the paper identifies
five areas that merit special attention:  mathematical
models for the proximate determinants of fertility;
determinants of marriage patterns; the process of fertility decision making; cultural perceptions of fertility
settings; the economics of having children; effects of
institutional settings on fertility incentives and
disincentives; access to contraceptive services and
supplies, and evaluation of demonstration projects for
affecting access; and the fertility implications of
development programs and strategies.

In summary, the majority of these research agendas
call for monitoring levels and trends in fertility and
its components, though components are understood in
different ways; for studying the economics of fertility
and of household decision-making systems, sometimes
considered together; and for conducting family planning
research, the specifics being different in each case.
Other topics appearing on at least two lists include
access to contraception (which might be considered an
aspect of family planning research), biosocial or
proximate fertility determinants, and the effects of
social institutions and government programs on fertility.

## SCOPE AND APPROACH

The present paper differs in scope, approach, and emphasis
from each of these previous efforts.  The subsections
below discuss, first, what is and is not covered here;
second, the level at which priorities are defined; third,
the criteria used; and fourth, how this agenda might be
used.

## Coverage and Exclusions

This paper focuses entirely on fertility determinants, leaving out of consideration the consequences of fertility levels and trends, mortality and migration (which one also needs to study to understand population growth), and the wider field of population and development interrelations. Many of the issues raised by McGreevey and Birdsall, Mertens, and Miro and Potter are not addressed, not because they are unimportant but because they are beyond the scope of this paper.

The focus here is on social science research rather than biomedical research. A few of the preceding chapters do in fact refer to relevant research in reproductive biology; however, the present paper cannot adequately evaluate all the relevant biomedical work, and therefore does not consider it. This does not imply that behavioral research on fertility can safely ignore biomedical findings: in fact, closer collaboration on both sides would probably be fruitful.

Finally, this paper does not consider research concerned with the measurement of aggregate fertility. Such research is the subject of a separate series of recent reports (Coale, Cho, and Goldman, 1980, is the first in the series); an accompanying manual (United Nations, 1982) details the best available methods for making fertility estimates with data of uncertain quality. Although there is a need to collect better fertility data in many developing countries, as well as to extract as much fertility information as possible from each data set, the focus here is on determinants rather than on such measurement issues.

## Levels of Analysis

A research agenda might be developed at several different levels. The most general level might be labeled research areas, where an area covers a broad field of inquiry, such as breastfeeding and fertility. On a more specific level, priorities might be set among research questions (such as the research question: How do family planning programs affect breastfeeding?). Alternatively, priorities might be set among research approaches, used here to refer to distinct methodologies for investigating hypotheses (such as household studies or community surveys). At the most detailed level, priorities might be set among research prototypes, which can be defined by linking a specific research question to a specific research approach. For example, a research prototype might be developed along the lines of a household survey of breastfeeding practices across communities having different types of family planning inputs, with controls for other development inputs.

Ideally, priorities would be set at each of these four levels. That can be difficult, however: global comparisons among research areas can involve considerable subjectivity; at the other end, comparisons among prototypes require much more detail than can be furnished here. Therefore this paper remains at an intermediate level, attempting to identify priorities among research questions; where possible, comments about appropriate research approaches are added. The result is a more extensive agenda than any of those reviewed above. Forty important research questions are identified; these are then reviewed and placed in some order of priority.

These questions range widely, covering the need for both data and theory, the need for new measures of key variables and new methods of analysis, the need for descriptive studies and studies that test particular hypotheses. For many of the behaviors of concern, the determinants are numerous; in these cases, models or explanatory systems, mathematical or otherwise, are recommended to address various determinants simultaneously together with their interrelationships.

## Criteria for Setting Priorities

The basic criterion for selecting important research questions is the potential contribution of investigation of the topic to an increased understanding of fertility determinants. Unlike most of the agendas reviewed, which take potential impact on population policy or programs as their major criterion, the present paper adopts a scientific criterion because its objectives are different, in a sense more modest. (Nevertheless there are many points of convergence in the resulting priorities.)

How can potential gains in understanding be estimated? If there were a dominant theory or paradigm in the field, greater importance might be assigned to research that more directly confirmed or extended that theory. As the preceding chapters show, however, no current theory comes near being adequate for this purpose. On the other hand, it would be wrong to go to the other extreme and adopt purely statistical criteria, such as equating gains in understanding with explaining more of the variance in fertility. For example, one might explain a respectable portion of fertility variance with a variable like education, but if one does not know what education really means in this context and how it works on fertility, the gain in understanding may not be so great.

The present paper therefore estimates potential gains in understanding in relation to the analytical framework presented in Chapter 1. Though this framework is not a theory but a loose structure for holding together various ideas, it does encompass the field, and all the critical issues about fertility determination can be raised within it. It thus permits comprehensive and consistent discussion of the different factors affecting fertility, identification of obvious gaps, and an understanding of the extent to which different studies contribute evidence on related points. Research can be assigned importance if it (1) involves the testing of basic assumptions underlying the framework; (2) clarifies or provides measures for key concepts; (3) explicates fundamental relationships; or (4) provides data linking the framework to particular fertility situations. In addition, for a research question to have priority, methods to investigate it must be at least prospectively available.

## The Use of This Agenda

This agenda is intended to provide guidance to researchers, agencies that support research, and policy and program personnel concerned with fertility in the developing countries. However, the research priorities it provides have been chosen from a specific perspective; those using it should be aware of its limitations.

First, as noted above, several important issues are excluded from coverage, including the measurement of fertility and the consequences of particular fertility levels. Moreover, the focus is on scientific as opposed to policy criteria, though brief mention of policy implications is contained in the final section.

Second, some of the most productive research is the most difficult to anticipate. As Thomas (1979) writes about another field, "the safest and most prudent of bets to lay money on is surprise. There is a very high probability that whatever astonishes us . . . today will turn out to be usable, and useful, tomorrow." A research agenda is at best a complex projection from past research into the future, relying on guesses about developments in knowledge, and therefore may easily overlook the possibility of substantial breakthroughs that go beyond current theory.

Third, the quality of the research project is generally more important than its topic. Though this may appear obvious, especially to researchers, it has an important corollary: high-quality research on a topic that does not receive priority here may in fact be worth more, and in the long run may add more to knowledge, than research of lesser quality on a priority topic.[2]

Fourth, this agenda presents general priorities, without specifying which might be more important in a particular developing country or developing region of the world. These priorities involve increasing the general understanding of fertility, rather than promoting understanding of specific national or local situations.

Fifth, this paper does not discuss the institutional and human resources available for fertility research in the developing countries (see Miro and Potter, 1980). Improving and expanding these resources is essential; otherwise, work on and from the perspectives of the developing countries might not result from this agenda. Many issues raised here are also relevant to developed countries, and work on developed-country samples or with developed-country perspectives may be more likely and may be overall of higher quality, given the availability of greater expertise, better infrastructure, and more funding support. Efforts are clearly needed to remedy this asymmetry in the distribution of scientific resources between the developed and the developing worlds.

With these limitations in mind, this agenda is presented as one contribution in what is expected to be a continuing dialogue within the research community and among research users. Unexpected theoretical developments, should they occur, may suggest reordering the emphases here, and consensual judgments about the quality of research should temper the focus on specific topics. At the least, however, this agenda should be useful as a foil against which individual researchers might develop their own priorities.

The major elements of the analytical framework described in Chapter 1 are the supply of children, the demand for children, and fertility regulation and its costs. The following sections discuss important research

questions under each of these topics, and then focus on
the decision process in which couples consider these
three components together. The factors affecting each
component and modifying the decision process itself are
then discussed within two main categories: nuptiality
and social institutions.

## THE SUPPLY OF CHILDREN

The supply of children refers to the number of surviving
children that a couple would have in the absence of any
deliberate attempt to increase or decrease fertility.
Supply depends, first, on levels of natural fertility,
and, second, on levels of child survival. Surviving
children are specified on the assumption that number of
survivors is more salient to a couple than number of
births. However, the age to which children should survive
to be counted in a couple's reckoning is not specified;
different ages might be selected for different purposes.
Survivorship is determined by levels of age-specific
mortality.

It is convenient to list five components of natural
fertility (Bongaarts and Menken, in these volumes), the
first three affecting the length of the birth interval
and the last two the length of the entire reproductive
span:

   a.  postpartum infecundability, which is affected
       mostly by breastfeeding, possibly supplemented by
       postpartum abstinence;
   b.  the waiting time to conception, determined to some
       extent by frequency of intercourse and also by the
       fecundity of each spouse;
   c.  intrauterine mortality, including spontaneous
       abortions and stillbirths;
   d.  permanent sterility, whose incidence increases
       with age, and which may be preceded by terminal
       abstinence; and
   e.  entry into the reproductive span, which is
       influenced partly by age at menarche and age at
       puberty, but more strongly by age at marriage.

These factors are not of equal importance. Age at
marriage, through its impact on entry into the reproductive span, probably has as great an effect on
fertility differentials as any other factor; it is

accordingly treated in a special section on nuptiality below.  Breastfeeding may have a comparable effect; most attention is paid to it here, and some attention is also paid to intercourse, to pathological infertility, and to terminal abstinence.  The first four research questions apply to the supply factors in general; these are followed by questions about particular natural fertility components, and finally by a question on child survival.

1. How do levels and trends in the components of the supply of children vary across the developing countries? Precise data on the natural fertility components is missing for many population aggregates.  Consequently, these factors are often assumed to be constant in much current research, with values assigned to them from limited sample surveys.  It is desirable to obtain data from larger, nationally representative samples over time.  Having measures for all the natural fertility components together, though it would probably require supplementing social surveys with more intensive measurement efforts, would facilitate the investigation of many research issues.  One issue of particular importance is the trend in supply with modernization. Some have argued that the early stages of modernization produce a sharply upward trend in supply that is crucial in producing motivation to control fertility; reliable assessments of supply levels are essential for determining the validity of this argument.

2. What measures of natural fertility and of the natural fertility components are appropriate at the level of the individual or couple?  Much work on natural fertility has been concerned with comparing populations rather than understanding individual differences.  Work on natural fertility therefore contrasts with work on demand or on fertility regulation, which has at least some emphasis on understanding the individual or couple. Measures appropriate to individuals or couples are essential if supply factors are to be successfully incorporated into theories of household fertility.  It may be argued that natural fertility cannot be measured at the level of the individual or couple; however, a couple does form perceptions of their potential fertility, and what these perceptions are as well as what they are based on--whether the couple's own waiting times or their beliefs about group averages or about the factors affecting potential fertility--require investigation.

3. What models are appropriate--at both the aggregate and the individual levels--for the contributions of the

<u>natural fertility components to fertility levels</u>?  The
reproductive models currently attracting most attention
are mainly aggregate and deterministic, and have not been
tested thoroughly (Bongaarts, in these volumes).  Such
tests are needed; in addition, new models with stochastic
elements should be developed.  Models at the individual
level, interrelating the natural fertility components
within each birth interval and across successive
intervals, would make an important contribution.

4.  <u>How appropriate are the assumptions underlying the</u>
<u>concept of natural fertility</u>?  Although natural fertility
is a key concept in the framework, it is often misunder-
stood outside demography.  Even within demography, it has
two not entirely congruent definitions:  it may be defined
as fertility in the absence of any deliberate attempt to
limit births or as fertility in the absence of any variation in fertility-relevant behavior across parities
(Knodel, in these volumes).  The first definition, hinging
on the intent behind any practice of fertility regulation,
implies the need for research to distinguish regulation
meant for spacing from that meant for family limitation,
and possibly from that meant to serve both purposes
simultaneously, as well as on the relative prevalence of
each type of behavior.  The second definition assumes
that any behavior varying across parities involves
deliberate limitation, and that limitation always involves
different practices across parities.  It therefore needs
to be asked how constant behavior connected with the
natural fertility components is across parities.  Answers
to these questions should indicate how natural fertility
ought to be measured, and what part of regulation
behavior should be considered a supply factor.

5.  <u>What are the levels of and trends in duration of</u>
<u>postpartum infecundability and breastfeeding in various</u>
<u>national and subnational populations</u>?  Of the several
natural fertility components, the duration of postpartum
infecundability probably deserves most attention since it
is apparently responsible for the greatest variation in
fertility (Bongaarts and Menken, in these volumes).  In
addition, there is evidence that the duration of breastfeeding changes with modernization, a relationship that
is important to explore.  Since there is little good
demographic data on postpartum infecundability and
breastfeeding, the need for such data, implied in Q.1
above, is restated here.  In addition, appropriate and
easily applicable methods of measurement need to be
developed.

6. <u>How do variations in breastfeeding patterns and duration affect the duration of postpartum infecundability</u>? The effect of breastfeeding duration on postpartum infecundability has been estimated, and it is known that full breastfeeding is more effective than partial breastfeeding; however, further study is needed of the effects of variations in breastfeeding practices, including the effects of different schedules and patterns of feeding (Bongaarts, in these volumes). This includes the relation between suckling and prolactin release, as well as the relation between amenorrhea and anovulation and how it is affected by breastfeeding. Such information might clarify the reasons for variations in postpartum infecundability, and thus have the practical impact of allowing women to use breastfeeding more reliably for contraceptive purposes. Quasi-experimental work with small samples, or research based on time diaries or hormonal measurement of ovulation, might provide the most useful data.

7. <u>What behavioral models help account for variations in the practice of breastfeeding</u>? Behavioral models are stressed here because these should provide more adequate understanding than single-variable hypotheses. Such models should explain differences in breastfeeding among social groups, as well as the effects of market forces and government programs. This question might be broken down into a series of more specific questions about the determinants of breastfeeding, on some of which there is ongoing work: (a) How consistent are variations in breastfeeding by education, income, and rural-urban residence? What explains these variations? (b) What effect do labor market opportunities for women have on breastfeeding? What other factors modify this effect? (c) What cultural beliefs, values, and practices affect the duration and pattern of breastfeeding? How can the degree of individual participation in or committment to the relevant cultural patterns be measured? (d) Are women aware of the contraceptive effect of breastfeeding, and does this affect their use of it? How does the availability of contraceptives affect breastfeeding? (e) How do the local availability and prices of commercial infant foods and other substitutes affect breastfeeding? (f) How do beliefs about and attitudes toward breastfeeding diffuse in a population? What role do medical and hospital personnel play? Do family planning clinic personnel play any role? What is the role of education and the media in decreasing or increasing breastfeeding, and what role do advertisments for infant foods play?

On most of these questions, the evidence to date is quite meager. A variety of research approaches might therefore be taken; these include purely theoretical model building and simulations, intensive field observation, analysis of existing survey data sets and official records, quasi-experimental work with small samples, and the design of new surveys.

8. Under what circumstances does the length of postpartum abstinence exceed the anovulatory interval? Postpartum abstinence typically has much less effect than breastfeeding. In a few populations, however, it is practiced for prolonged periods, and might have measurable demographic consequences. Studies need to concentrate on these populations, paying careful attention to changes in practices over time.

9. How does frequency of sexual intercourse affect waiting time to conception? Waiting time to conception is a second natural fertility component of some importance, and its behavioral determinants include frequency of intercourse.[3] Although frequency of intercourse is typically found to decline across age groups, little if any reliable data are available from which to determine differences across populations. It is often assumed that these differences are so small that they have no important fertility effect; however, exceptions have been identified. Reports on frequency of intercourse can be difficult to obtain and may be quite undependable. This limitation, which is possibly due to the limited scientific effort in this area to date, hampers research at present. Plausible models for the relationship of frequency of intercourse to waiting time to conception are available; so far, however, they lack empirical confirmation.

A related question is: What behavioral models can account for variations in frequency of intercourse? If there are important differences in frequency of intercourse across social groups, populations, and time periods, the reasons for this require investigation. A number of more specific questions might also be posed: How does frequency of intercourse vary by type of sexual union? How does it vary by age, by age of spouse, by marriage duration? How often is it affected by physical separation (for such reasons as work outside the community) in different social settings? How does it vary in relation to cycles of work and the food supply? How is it affected by education, income, and other socioeconomic variables? How is it affected by cultural beliefs, values, and practices?

10.  What factors produce high levels of secondary sterility in some settings?  Both primary and secondary sterility may reach demographically significant levels in particular populations, especially in sub-Saharan Africa. Sterility is often associated with pelvic inflammatory disease resulting from sexually transmitted infections such as gonorrhea.  A number of related questions need to be investigated:  (a) How prevalent is secondary sterility in different settings?  (b) What are its causes?  How important is pelvic inflammatory disease resulting from sexually transmitted diseases, postabortal or postpartum sepsis, or female circumcision?  (c) What is the natural history of pelvic inflammatory disease and consequent infertility?  (d) What strategies are appropriate for the prevention and treatment of infertility in developing countries, and what would be the demographic consequences of control programs?

The remaining natural fertility components, though they produce less variation in natural fertility, may nevertheless be important in particular settings.  Fetal loss is estimated to occur in almost two out of three conceptions, increasing sharply in frequency for women in the mid-thirties, apparently because of higher rates of chromosomal abnormalities.  There is direct evidence linking venereal syphilis and indirect evidence linking malaria to spontaneous abortion rates, and this might deserve further assessment.  Despite the frequency of fetal loss, it has not been shown to have any other significant demographic determinants.

The possible fertility impact of age at entry into the reproductive span is much reduced by social factors:  age at marriage is usually well above age at menarche or age at puberty.  At the other end of the reproductive span, the possible impact of terminal abstinence is also much reduced by biological factors, including declining fecundity and the onset of terminal sterility.  For these factors, the significant research question seems to be whether and in what circumstances this practice might still have a significant fertility impact.

On the topic of child survival, the needed research is substantial and cannot be fully covered here (see Chen, in these volumes; Bell, 1980; Miro and Potter, 1980).  As an example, a better understanding of the proximate determinants of infant and child mortality, including their interactions and biosocial relationships, would be useful.  So would field epidemiological studies of the major infections and parasitic diseases of childhood, to delineate attack rates, prevalence, clinical spectra, and case-fatality rates. Evaluating all such possibilities for research would require a separate report. Focusing only on the interrelations between infant and child mortality and natural fertility components, one important research question might be identified:

11. How are birth interval length and infant mortality interrelated? Problems of definition and concept have somewhat clouded some previous research on this question. Very brief preceding intervals may be associated with higher mortality risk, which would in turn predispose toward shorter intervals. The mechanics of this relationship, however, are not entirely clear: shorter intervals may lead to low birth weights, limit time and resources devoted to infants, or reduce the frequency and duration of lactation. As a better and safer form of infant nourishment, breastfeeding could have a direct effect in reducing mortality; it might also have an indirect effect through increasing interval length. Maternal age and parity may also be implicated in these relationships, since shorter intervals imply that higher parities will be reached at a younger age. Even in well-nourished populations, there may still be a relationship between birth spacing and infant mortality. Disentangling these relationships and determining the magnitude of their effects does not seem difficult in principle.

## THE DEMAND FOR CHILDREN

The demand for children, as the term is used here, refers to the number of surviving children a couple wants to have. As was argued in previous chapters, couples in many settings seem to formulate such a number, and it often seems to be behaviorally meaningful. The problem of understanding exactly what demand means and measuring it properly leads to the first research question below. A couple's demand for children results from a number of considerations: their personal preferences between children and other competing goods (referred to as tastes); the benefits children provide, their cost, including the out-of-pocket costs and the time they take up, and the relative benefits and costs of competing goods (which might be said to define the "relative price" of children); and the income and wealth available to the couple to meet these costs. All of these components are included in the research questions that follow.

12. <u>How should demand for children be measured, and
what are the implications of using different measures?</u> A
number of measures of family-size desires have become
fairly standard in the literature, and some of these
appear to reflect demand for children (McClelland, in
these volumes). It is often unclear, however, what
constraints respondents have in mind in answering questions on family-size desires, and how much their responses
reflect personal desires or social norms. Measures like
desired family size should continue to be collected,
although research on the characteristics of these measures is also needed. The stability of such measures
needs to be established, as does the role played by
rationalization, the effect of family growth on stated
desires, and the way these relate to fertility behavior.
In addition, psychometric and survey work is desirable
into more sophisticated measures of demand, which should
follow more closely a delineation of the theoretical
criteria for such measures (see McClelland, in these
volumes).

13. <u>How does the desire for births respond to the
expected level of child survival?</u> The analytical
framework assumes that demand is connected with surviving
children, and that the desire for births should therefore
be entirely determined by demand coupled with the perceived level of infant and child mortality. This assumption invites testing. Much less research has been
devoted to this question than to the related question of
the effects on fertility of prior child loss (Heer, in
these volumes). Researchers have seldom attempted to
measure perceived survival levels directly. A related,
crucial issue is how preferred levels of childcare or
preferred investments in child quality respond to
perceived survival chances, and in turn affect child
mortality.

14. <u>How should tastes or relative preferences for
children be assessed?</u> There is very little useful
research directly on this question (Lee and Bulatao, in
these volumes). Some researchers assume tastes to be
constant and ignore them; others deal with concepts
linked with but not identical to tastes, like fertility
norms (Mason, in these volumes) or values and disvalues
of children to parents (Fawcett, in these volumes).
Although such work could provide important insights into
tastes for children and should therefore continue, it
should be supplemented with attempts to measure tastes
directly. A key problem in producing such measures is

selecting the competing goods or activities against which
relative preferences for children can be assessed.
Another problem is the difficulty (and perhaps the
advisability) of attempting to separate tastes from
perceptions of the economic costs and benefits of
children.

15. What explains tastes or relative preferences for
children: How do they vary across social groups, across
societies, and over time? How do they develop, and how
are they diffused? What models account for variations in
tastes? Given the uncertainties regarding assessment of
tastes, this series of questions is advanced tentatively,
and will require reformulation as these uncertainties are
clarified. The literature suggests that tastes for children vary in systematic ways; however, without standard
measures of tastes, firm generalizations are not possible.
Factors possibly related to variations in tastes that
need attention include: parent's sex, education, income,
rural-urban residence, family type, religion, ethnicity,
and level of community or societal development. On the
development of tastes, some work in population socialization is suggestive, but much remains to be done. The
diffusion of tastes, particularly of weaker rather than
stronger relative preferences for children (or of competing consumption aspirations), is an important related
issue; more information is needed about factors that
promote or retard diffusion and the manner in which it
occurs.

A related topic that overlaps somewhat with other
questions is the relative desire for sons and daughters.
Despite recent conceptual clarification (McClelland, in
these volumes), the contribution of son or daughter
preferences to actual fertility variation is difficult to
specify; however, this is thought to be significant in
some cultures, and some work on the fertility effects
might be useful.

16. What institutional factors and household characteristics affect the economic contributions of
children? Child labor, the old age support children
provide, and their value as risk insurance to parents all
depend on institutional arrangements that may make these
things important or costly or provide alternatives to
them. Such economic contributions from children also
vary with a family's wealth and position in the social
structure. There are some careful accounts of children's
economic contributions in particular settings (Lindert,
in these volumes; Caldwell, in these volumes; Lee and

Bulatao, in these volumes), as well as impressionistic
accounts of institutional arrangements promoting such
contributions (Potter, in these volumes).  However, much
remains to be done to specify the circumstances under
which particular contributions from children are more or
less important to parents:  what effect landownership has
on the productivity of child labor, whether social
security reduces reliance on children, how labor market
structures affect the relative contributions of sons and
daughters, whether local governments can manipulate
incentive structures to reduce children's net value, and
so forth.  Measuring specific contributions and how they
are perceived by couples is one research issue; a more
critical one seems to be how to represent the types of
institutional structures and interrelationships that
enable children to contribute economically and make
parents depend on such contributions.

     17.  How do the direct economic costs of children
vary--under what circumstances do parents spend more or
spend less on children?  Although this question is often
studied together with the previous one, the factors
determining the direct costs of children may be sufficiently distinct from those determining their economic
contributions to warrant separate listing.  Some
inventive research has attempted to quantify parents'
expenditures on children (Lindert, in these volumes);
however, understanding of the factors linked to variations
in expenditures is fragmentary.  This clearly involves
household decisions on matters like selecting levels of
investment in children, as well as factors external to
the household, such as the costs of childrearing inputs
like education and housing.  Allocative issues within the
household also arise:  what determines the division of
goods between parents and children and their distribution
among children (between sons and daughters, between first-
born and later-born, etc.), and how is joint consumption
to be taken into account?

     18.  How do couples in different social settings
assess, adjust for, and react to the time costs of
children?  Of the alternative activities with which
children interfere, women's work has received the most
attention.  The literature on women's work and fertility
in developing countries contains many inconsistent
findings (Standing, in these volumes); nevertheless, it
suggests that the time costs of children are light in the
developing countries or that parents find many ways of
coping with these costs, such as relying on relatives or

hired help, engaging in work that allows continual childcare, reducing the time they give to children, or cutting into their own leisure time. These strategies for coping are not costless, but they complicate the study of time costs and of the effects of women's work on fertility. Research is necessary on the actual magnitude of these costs, whether in lost work, leisure, or housework, and on the various strategies used to avoid or minimize them. Research should also address the effects of social settings on time costs: for instance, labor market organization, and particularly discrimination against women, may substantially affect time costs.

19. How should the economic contributions, the direct economic costs, and the time costs of children be combined into some net cost-of-children measure, and what determines the time path of this net cost in different social settings? It is useful for some purposes to reduce the economic contributions, direct costs, and time costs of children to some common metric so they can be combined and their total effect on the demand for children and on fertility assessed. One such net cost measure has been presented in the literature (Lindert, in these volumes), and deserves further attention. Research under the preceding three questions may suggest possible changes in this measure or other approaches to measurement; research on perceptions of costs is also critical. How the net cost changes is a critical question that requires investigating changes in each of its components. In general, it is widely accepted that net costs rise in the course of socioeconomic development; whether this rise is unbroken (or whether there might in fact be a temporary fall at an early stage of development), how rapid it is, and what factors, including government interventions, accelerate or retard it all deserve investigation.

20. What are the relative effects of tastes for children, their economic contributions and direct and time costs, and household income levels on the demand for children and on fertility? This is a complex question, and some of the preceding questions dealing with measurement of demand components will have to be answered before it can be tackled. Few if any studies have dealt with the impact on demand of all of these components simultaneously. Some theorists assign primacy to particular components (e.g., to net costs; see Caldwell, in these volumes), but empirical evidence establishing this has not been provided. How the relative effects of these

components vary across individuals, households, communities, and societies, as well as over time, and what causes one or another component to become more important also require investigation.

21. <u>Can the demand for children be modified by the availability or use of fertility regulation methods--and, if so, how does this occur?</u> The strict version of the analytical framework suggests that the demand for children is independent of fertility regulation costs. However, it is sometimes argued--and some psychosocial theories support the idea--that demand may adjust to rather than simply being a determinant of fertility control behavior. The perception that fertility can be controlled, the spreading belief 'that family limitation is legitimate, or the successful use of a fertility regulation method for birth spacing might lead to a downward adjustment in demand. Whether this does occur would seem difficult to establish, which may account for the lack of research on this point. If it does, however, the concept and measures of demand will require rethinking, and there are also fairly obvious practical implications. This question might equally well be listed under the next section, and provides a logical bridge to it.


## FERTILITY REGULATION AND ITS COSTS

The analytical framework assumes that a couple considers the costs connected with practicing fertility regulation; if these costs are reasonable (and their motivation to control fertility, defined by the excess of supply over demand, sufficiently strong), they engage in some form of regulation behavior. Fertility regulation therefore fits into the analytical framework in two distinct ways: its costs constitute one of the three sets of factors that couples weigh in deciding whether or not to use it. This distinction is implicit in past research on family planning: it is paralleled, for instance, by the distinction between knowledge of and attitudes toward family planning, on the one hand, and its practice, on the other. Nevertheless, the perspective on regulation provided by the framework differs somewhat from that in most previous family planning research, and leads to some research questions not commonly identified. Other questions in this section deal with standard concerns in the literature, although one common concern, the development of new contraceptive methods, is left out because biomedical research is not covered here.

   22.  **What are the levels of and trends in the practice**
**of fertility regulation in different countries, in differ-**
**ent areas within countries, and in different social**
**groups?** More information probably already exists on this
question than on any other question in this research
agenda. Nevertheless, it remains a critical question,
since fertility regulation has to be continually moni-
tored if variations in fertility are to be understood.
In addition, the data are not equally good for all
countries, or for all areas within most developing
countries, or for all methods of fertility regulation.
Data on abortion, in particular, are usually less
reliable than other data, and new approaches to measurement need to be developed. Data on prevalence of methods
are better than data on method continuation, and the
latter need additional work.

   23.  **How should the costs a couple bears in obtaining**
**access to and using fertility regulation be assessed?**
Researchers in this area have often been concerned with
the question of who adopts fertility regulation and why.
Given the analytical framework, these questions have to
be asked in a new way:  one should ask, both of those who
practice and those who do not, what costs they bear or
would expect to bear from practicing regulation, including
psychic, social, health, and economic costs. Although
some inferences about these costs can be drawn from
previous research (Schearer, in these volumes; Bogue, in
these volumes), the specific issue of how to measure and
aggregate such costs has seldom been raised. The costs
to be considered include those of obtaining access to and
actually using each method. Examples would be the time
and effort required to obtain a particular method, any
associated embarassment or social stigma, and the risk of
side effects and the fears they engender, whether valid
or not. Such costs may be expected to vary across
regulation methods, and may be related to effectiveness
of use. It is worth noting also that a couple may be
subject to other costs if they do not use regulation,
such as possible complications of pregnancy; these
negative costs should also be assessed. Whether an
appropriate measure can be developed to cover all these
costs or whether some other approach to assessment should
be taken requires study.

   24.  **How do different ways of delivering fertility**
**regulation services affect the costs to the couple?**
Fertility regulation services include not only formally
established family planning programs but also private

clinics, doctors, nurses, native healers, community
workers, and anyone else who provides advice, supplies,
or services connected with contraception or abortion.  A
critical measure of the effectiveness of these services
is their ability to minimize the costs among couples,
both those practicing and not practicing regulation.
Services have sometimes been assessed from the perspective of "user satisfaction" or their effect on fertility;
both of these are less appropriate than cost minimization
as output measures.  Types of delivery systems may affect
costs; some attention should be paid to such alternatives
as community-based distribution systems, integrated
community health and development programs, commercial
retail sales, mothers' clubs or other acceptor groups,
the simultaneous use of multiple distribution channels,
saturation projects, and generally any innovative systems
that appear to have greater success than parallel services
in the same area.  Specific features of a delivery system
may also be important:  which methods they provide, which
they promote, and how effective these are; whether they
provide a mix of methods or only a few; whether specific
incentives are provided for regulation;[4] how comfortable clients are with clinic personnel; and so on.  If
their impact on costs is to be determined, delivery
systems have to be properly classified and their relevant
features identified as well as measured, where possible.

Delivery systems for abortion also exist--the evidence
is that every significant decline in birth rates has
involved some recourse to abortion (David, in these
volumes)--though these systems may not be officially
sanctioned and may in fact be illegal.  The effects of
system design on abortion costs, particularly the legal
status of the delivery system, may be more dramatic than
in the case of contraception and also deserve study.

25.  What models can account for variations in the
costs to a couple of obtaining access to and using
fertility regulation?  Costs are affected not only by the
design of fertility regulation services but also by
characteristics of the individual or household (such as
their location within social networks that provide
information about or support for using regulation); by
aspects of the social and cultural setting (such as
religious prescriptions, medical folk beliefs, and public
opinion); and by characteristics of particular methods
(whether they require constant attention, are tied to
intercourse, involve more or fewer health risks, etc.).
In the absence of adequate measures of regulation costs

(Q.23), research on the determinants of these costs is so far quite limited. Much detailed investigation of such factors is needed before adequate integrative models can be formulated.

26. <u>What considerations affect a couple's use or nonuse and the effectiveness of their use of fertility regulation?</u> The analytical framework assumes that attempts to limit family size follow from consideration of the supply of children, the demand for children, and fertility regulation costs. However, a couple may practice regulation not only to limit family size but also to space births or to avoid a birth at a particular time or in particular circumstances. Decisions to limit and to postpone births have to be distinguished, if possible, and the major considerations in each case investigated.[5] Use and nonuse of regulation need not be considered simply as a dichotomy; there are degrees of effectiveness in the use of many methods, often related to the underlying motivation. A common approach in this area is to attempt to identify the characteristics of users and nonusers; this allows inferences about but fails to get directly at the considerations underlying use and nonuse. Another way to investigate these questions would be to describe and analyze individual thought processes and couple decision processes.

Other aspects of the use of regulation, such as timing and choice of method, are considered under separate questions because of their importance.

27. <u>What models can represent and account for spells of use and nonuse of fertility regulation methods?</u> A few generalizations can be made about patterns of use of fertility regulation: for instance, the longer a contraceptive user continues with a given method, the less likely is discontinuance. More precise representations of this and similar relationships would be useful, but require better data on duration of use and spells of use and nonuse, or, essentially, detailed contraceptive histories. Even more important then representing the relationships, perhaps, is understanding the factors related to timing of initial use, to continuation and discontinuation, to method switching and readoption, and how these factors change as the couple nears, reaches, or exceeds their family-size goals. This question is linked with the previous one, since spells of use and nonuse depend partly on the intent behind use and the effectiveness of use; it is also linked with the following question, since they also depend on the particular method chosen.

28. <u>What models can account for choice of particular</u>
<u>fertility regulation methods</u>?  Choice of method depends
on relative costs, both of access and of use.  Characteristics of a method may make it more acceptable in
particular cultures, more suitable for some people or at
particular stages of the family cycle, more convenient or
cheaper to use, and so on.  Choice may be dictated by
availability; it may also be affected by the information
provided and the influence exercised by medical and
paramedical personnel and the members of one's reference
group, as well as by personal tastes.  Method shifting is
a related matter of some interest.  The costs perceived
by different people for different methods need to be
specified, and models developed for the factors influencing costs and the effects of costs on method choice.

29. <u>What models properly represent and explain the</u>
<u>process of diffusion of fertility regulation</u>?  The spread
of fertility regulation among households shows patterns
similar to those for the diffusion of other innovations.
Fertility regulation diffuses within interpersonal networks, flowing from opinion leaders to followers, being
interrupted by barriers like geographic and social
distance and differences in language and religion, and
being aided or retarded by specific characteristics of
regulation methods (Retherford and Palmore, in these
volumes).  Within and across societies, similar diffusion
patterns have sometimes been suggested:  diffusion may be
facilitated by social and cultural homogeneity, might be
more rapid in island societies, or may be impeded by
ethnic and linguistic barriers.  Diffusion seems to be a
major factor in changing the perceived costs and increasing the adoption of regulation.  The study of diffusion
patterns, whether at the micro or the macro levels, is of
both theoretical and practical interest; diffusion is
accomplished partly through fertility regulation services
(Q.24), but also involves various psychological and
interpersonal mechanisms that can modify their effect.

30. <u>What policies and programs for fertility</u>
<u>regulation have the most fertility impact in different</u>
<u>social settings</u>?  Studies of family planning programs
demonstrate a diversity of effects, indicating that
program impact varies not only with the character of the
program but also with the social setting.  The effect of
a fertility regulation program depends not only on its
impact on regulation costs but also on other factors that
interact with costs in affecting fertility.  Specific
fertility regulation policies and programs are unlikely

to be equally effective across social settings, and it
remains to be seen whether some match can be made between
particular settings and the policies and programs optimal
in each.

FERTILITY DECISION MAKING

A key assumption underlying the analytical framework is
that a couple makes some decision about their preferred
family size and tries to implement this decision. Some
research on fertility decision making accepts this assumption and tries to characterize the process; other research
investigates the validity of this assumption and the
utility of some alternative. This work contains a variety
of suggestions for "nondecisional" perspectives or alternate decision rules, but provides few solidly supported
propositions (Hollerbach, in these volumes). The research
questions worth further investigation must therefore be
posed in rather general terms; the payoff from investigating these questions is probably less certain than for
other questions in this agenda.

    31. What explicit models might better account for
differences in individual fertility than utility
maximization models? The dominant models in the economics
of fertility assume utility maximization; alternatives
have sometimes been suggested, but whether they would
work any better is not known. An alternative model might
assume that couples do make fertility decisions but use
other decision rules, that decisions are made in some
settings but not others (e.g., after the demographic
transition but not before it), or that individual
decisions are not made at all (Hull, in these volumes).
No such models have been sufficiently developed to provide testable hypotheses. For example, discussions of
the influence of social norms on fertility sometimes imply
a model in which individual decisions are not made;
however, no one has provided a satisfactory way to
identify norms or an adequate account of how they relate
to sanctions and to socialization, how they affect reproductive behavior, and how these effects can be distinguished from the effects of other factors (Mason, in
these volumes). The primary need, therefore, is to spell
out in more detail models that are often merely implicit
in sociological and anthropological writing (and some
economic work) about fertility and that might compete
with individual utility maximization models. It will

then be possible to determine what the new models add to understanding and how well they fare empirically.

32. <u>What regularities are there in the process in which fertility decisions are made</u>? The analytical framework addresses the issue of what decisions are made, not the behavioral and psychological steps and social interactions involved. Empirical investigation of this process has so far mainly used developed-country samples (Beckman, in these volumes). Several aspects of this process deserve investigation: the timing of decisions, how decisions about fertility regulation and regulation methods relate to decisions on family size, who participates in the decision process and with what influence, what search process is involved in investigating alternative choices, how information inputs affect decision making, and how marital satisfaction and other aspects of a marriage color the process. Regularities in the process are important in themselves, and may also relate to what decisions are finally made. One aspect of the process—how decisions are modified in response to changing circumstances—appears important enough to include under a separate research question.

33. <u>How do fertility plans and decisions change in response to changing family circumstances, and what effect do such changes have on fertility</u>? It has been demonstrated that fertility plans and decisions, and the factors underlying them, undergo transformation throughout the years of a marriage (Namboodiri, in these volumes): family-size goals may change, sterility and the probability of intrauterine mortality rise, parental resources available for childrearing may increase or decrease, the role successive children play in the family varies, knowledge of and the ability to practice regulation effectively improves. The community setting, including all the external forces acting on the decision process, may also change. Given the time required to follow a family through its developmental cycle, little research has systematically addressed the issue of the effect of such changes on fertility. Besides empirical work, theoretical modeling of the sequential decision process and its effects would be useful. It may be critical, depending on the results of such work, to reformulate the analytical framework in accordance with this rather than a single-decision perspective.

## NUPTIALITY

This heading encompasses research on the timing and forms of sexual unions. Both formal and informal unions are included: though legal marriages often predominate, informal unions are demographically significant in some cultures. Both the initiation and the dissolution of unions deserve scrutiny, as do the various stages a union may pass through. Although marriage, divorce, and family forms serve many important social functions and are worth scientific study for a variety of reasons, the perspective here is limited to their fertility-relevant aspects.

34. What models can account for variations in age at marriage across societies and social groups and over time? Variations in age at marriage have been identified as a prominent reason for differences and changes in fertility levels (Smith, in these volumes). However, explaining these variations has proved difficult. There are few integrative models that take into account all the relevant factors--such as the search costs of finding a culturally acceptable mate, the sex ratio in the marrying ages, the likelihood and costs of establishing a new household, and the status rewards and economic benefits from marriage. Such models need to be developed and tested cross-culturally using multidisciplinary perspectives. Although this research question refers specifically to age at marriage, a readily identifiable point that usually represents the critical transition, it might be interpreted more broadly to refer to age at first entry into a sexual union. Another factor that needs explaining is variations and changes over time in the proportion who never marry.

35. How do the demand for children and premarital pregnancy affect timing of marriage? The assumption is often made that fertility decisions are separate from and follow marriage decisions. This simplifying assumption, which allows marriage to be omitted from discussions of fertility regulation, needs systematic investigation. Several specific points need examining: whether and how frequently timing of marriage represents an attempt to control fertility; how often, in different settings, a marriage is contracted because of a previous pregnancy; and how often changes in form of sexual union result from decisions to have children or from pregnancy. Fertility decisions may also be interdependent with decisions on subsequent marriages, as when the norm dictates having children in each of one's marriages; this too requires investigation.

36.  How do form of sexual union and frequency of
leaving and entering successive unions affect frequency
of intercourse, and what factors modify the effects?  The
major forms of sexual union of concern, in contrast to
monogamous legal marriage, are polygyny and consensual
and visiting unions, the former of possible demographic
significance in Africa and the latter two in the
Caribbean and Latin America, and possibly in Tropical
Africa.  Whatever other effects these forms of sexual
union may have, they should affect frequency of intercourse and therefore have some impact on fertility
(Burch, in these volumes).  However, there is little
reliable data on frequency of intercourse (Q.9), and
essentially none on the effect of forms of sexual union
on frequency.  Divorce and other forms of dissolution of
sexual unions should also affect frequency of intercourse, but again the magnitude of the effect and how it
varies are unknown.  Obtaining reliable data about
intercourse is quite difficult, and it may be worth
trying simulation studies first to quantify the possible
fertility effects of forms of union.  A second possible
effect of forms of sexual union and frequency of divorce
on the supply of children is through the incidence of
secondary sterility (Gray, in these volumes).  There is
very little evidence about this effect, but it is probably
smaller than the effect of frequency of intercourse.

37.  How do family structure and household composition
affect the demand for children and the process of
fertility decision making?  Much previous research has
failed to establish any reliable link between household
composition and fertility.  Various attempts have been
made to rescue the hypothesis that extended families
produce higher fertility by broadening the focus beyond
household composition to include the network of kin
relationships (Burch, in these volumes).  The essential
research required here appears to be on the specific ways
an extended family might increase the demand for children:  because of the sharing of childrearing costs,
because of better opportunities for utilizing child
labor, because of differences in tastes for children that
are somehow generated by the family structure, because
decisions about children are made in a different manner
or by different individuals, or for some other such
reason.  This question is obviously complex:  it requires
attention to changes in household composition through the
life cycle as they affect and are affected by fertility;
it may also require examination not only of family

structures by themselves but also of the other social
institutions and the communities in which families are
embedded. It is this wider societal context that is
discussed in the next section.

## EFFECTS OF SOCIAL INSTITUTIONS

The farther back one moves from the most immediate or
proximate determinants of fertility, the more difficult
it is to determine the relative importance of different
lines of research. The issue of how social institutions
affect fertility is obviously critical, since major fertility change is often linked with substantial alterations
in these institutions. However, the more that is learned
about the immediate determinants of fertility, the more
difficult it is to identify the effects of particular
social institutions, since the number of channels through
which they might affect fertility seems to proliferate
and the possibilities for complex offsetting or pyramid-
ing effects to increase. It also becomes increasingly
difficult, as broader social patterns are addressed, to
segregate a concern with fertility determinants from a
concern with other demographic linkages of social
institutions. Therefore, the research questions
identified in this section are posed at a fairly general
level, rather than dealing with specific effects of
particular institutions.

    38. <u>Through what channels do a couple's socioeconomic
characteristics affect their fertility</u>? The socioeconomic characteristics of concern include, but are not
limited to income, education, urban-rural residence,
women's employment, ethnicity, religion, and migration
and social mobility experience. For each of these
factors, there is a considerable literature showing, at
some times a stronger, and at other times a weaker link
to fertility. Further studies of this sort seem almost
inevitable. It would be of much greater scientific
interest, however, to concentrate on unraveling the
various possible links between each of these factors and
fertility. How much of the fertility impact of a given
factor is due to its effect on breastfeeding, on tastes
for children, on the balance of economic benefits and
costs of children, and on perceptions of the costs of
fertility regulation? Although questions like this have
been asked about some of these factors, particularly
education, income, and female employment (Cochrane, in

these volumes; Mueller and Short, in these volumes;
Standing, in these volumes), much more work remains to be
done. A better understanding and more accurate representation of the intervening processes, covered in
earlier sections of this paper, should generate improved
research on these questions. A good portion of the work
may be theoretical and integrative, involving piecing
together results from a variety of existing studies and
making inferences about the mechanisms involved. Some
empirical testing of specific models for all the effects
of particular factors will eventually be desirable, but a
more immediate need is to develop alternative models.

   39. What variations in institutional and community
settings are consistently and reliably related to higher
or lower fertility? If adequate answers were available
to all of the previous research questions, it would be
possible in principle to build up, piece by piece,
descriptions of institutional and community settings
most conducive to high and to low fertility. One could
take models for the determinants of breastfeeding, of
tastes for children, of fertility regulation costs, and
of the decision process, extract those determinants at
the institutional or community level, and combine them
appropriately. It is also advisable, however, to have
some research that begins at the other end, not with
individual or household models, but with types of institutional and community settings, distinguishing and
cataloging them and determining which are linked to
differences in fertility. Little beyond impressionistic
descriptions of such settings has been completed so far.
It has been suggested, for instance, that fertility might
be lowered by families becoming integrated into the
capitalist mode of production, economic institutions that
make child labor uneconomical, institutions that provide
alternate forms of risk insurance, and communities that
have the political will and capacity to control their
populations; however, the evidence in each case is fairly
limited (Potter, in these volumes). Systematically
relating settings to fertility should lead to identifying
the most important variations in setting, and could be
followed eventually by analysis of the various channels
by which each setting affects fertility.

   One important aspect of institutional and community
settings is the set of government policies and projects
that affect fertility, including those that affect infant
feeding, infant and child mortality, incentives for
childbearing, female employment, the availability of

contraception, and age at marriage. Study of such
programs may be advantageous if they serve to manipulate
variables of key interest. However, for the majority of
relevant programs the obstacles to satisfactory research
are considerable: the key interventions (from the
perspective of fertility) are difficult to separate from
others; program implementation is often at variance with
program design; and program success may depend on latent
receptivity produced by extraneous factors whose effect
is difficult to determine. For these reasons, evaluation
of the fertility effects of development projects and
policies requires considerable scientific effort and much
close collaboration between researchers and project
personnel.

40. What role do particular institutional changes
play in the dynamics of aggregate fertility in the course
of modernization? Research on the previous question
should provide some understanding of variations in
fertility across institutional settings. However,
understanding the dynamics of fertility in the course of
modernization also requires time-series studies, to which
this question refers. A better understanding is needed
of the interrelationships among fertility measures in the
course of modernization (see Ryder, in these volumes), as
well as of the impact that particular institutional
changes have on different measures (Richards, in these
volumes). Adequate data for time-series studies are very
limited, severely constraining the kind of work that can
be done.


CONCLUSION

The agenda provided by these forty questions covers a
wide range of research interests, theoretical problems,
and social science disciplines. Nevertheless, the list
is meant to be selective rather than comprehensive; a
number of possible questions have been left out or
deemphasized, such as the effect of terminal abstinence
on fertility (generally slight and likely to decrease),
the effect of sex preferences (listed only as a subques-
tion, because its magnitude is problematic), the role of
infanticide (no solid evidence exists that it is frequently used for regulation), and the effects of factors
like women's employment and urban residence (deemphasized
in favor of studies of the channels through which these
operate).

It is desirable to establish priorities among the questions listed. For this purpose, the questions are classified into several groups, priorities within groups are discussed, and the relative importance of each group considered. The questions have already been classified by topic; they are now reclassified by the general type of research indicated.

## Priorities for Each Type of Research Question

On the main components of the supply of children, the demand for children, and fertility regulation costs, three types of questions can be distinguished: (a) levels and trends in some components; (b) the development of measures of other components; and (c) integrative models to represent the combined effects of components on fertility. On the determinants of these components, four additional types of questions can be distinguished: (d) models for these determinants; (e) specific relationships or linkages between variables; (f) fertility decision-making processes; and (g) global influences on fertility. The questions are classified according to these seven types in Table 2; priorities for each type of question may now be discussed.

### Levels and Trends

Three questions deal explicitly with levels and trends: in components of the supply of children (Q.1), postpartum infecundability and breastfeeding (Q.5), and the practice of fertility regulation (Q.22). It is assumed, of course, that levels and trends in fertility itself will also continue to be assessed. Questions corresponding to these on levels and trends in the demand for children and in nuptiality were not included among the forty questions. In the case of demand, research must proceed first on the development of satisfactory measures; in the case of nuptiality, some data seem to be available, and the relatively neglected study of determinants should take precedence.

Research on these three questions is desirable in each developing country for which data are not available; priority among these questions depends partly, therefore, on the specific country or region. In general, however, it may be argued that Q.5, which deals with the most important of the supply components in Q.1, takes priority over the latter. Q.22 may seem more relevant to policy decisions than Q.5, but there is less work on Q.5, and it may deserve slightly higher priority. On the other hand, there is no reason why all three of these questions could not be addressed within the same study or set of studies, as is the case to some extent in the World Fertility Survey.

Development of Measures

The five questions that address the development of new measures are listed in Table 2. Q.4 is not strictly about measurement, but it does involve the assumptions behind the key concept of natural fertility and may imply possible changes in measures.

An important criterion in comparing these five questions is the potential gain from better measures. Since measures of demand (Q.12) are currently the closest to being adequate, the gain from improving these is probably less than the gain from improved measures of tastes (Q.14) or regulation costs (Q.23), to which higher priority is therefore assigned. Measuring the natural fertility components at the individual level (Q.2) is considerably more problematic, and for this reason does not receive high priority.

Integrative Models of Components

The next set of questions addresses the proper way to combine sets of components, of natural fertility (Q.3), of the demand for children (Q.20), and of their net cost (Q.19). No parallel question was listed for the supply components as a whole because these include the natural fertility components, which are already listed, and child survival, whose addition does not pose major problems. Nor is there a parallel question for fertility regulation costs: a distinction has been made between costs of access and costs of use as well as among psychic, social, health, and economic costs, but not enough work has been done on these classifications for the manner of combining costs to be a specific concern.

Of the three questions listed, the net cost of children is probably less urgent to study, given the presence in the literature of one well-considered measure; the other two questions seem about equally important.

TABLE 2   Research Questions Classified by Type and Priority

| Type | High Priority | Medium Priority |
|---|---|---|
| Levels and trends | Postpartum infecundability and breastfeeding (Q.5)<br>Practice of fertility regulation (Q.22) | Components of the supply of children (Q.1) |
| Development of measures | Tastes for children (Q.14)<br>Costs of regulation (Q.23) | Natural fertility components (Q.2)<br>Assumptions of natural fertility (Q.4)<br>Demand for children (Q.12) |
| Integrative models | Natural fertility components (Q.3)<br>Demand for children (Q.20) | Net cost of children (Q.19) |
| Models for determinants | Breastfeeding (Q.7)<br>Tastes for children (Q.15)<br>Economic contributions of children (Q.16)<br>Costs of regulation (Q.25)<br>Use and effectiveness of regulation (Q.26)<br>Diffusion of regulation (Q.29)<br>Age at marriage (Q.34) | Secondary sterility (Q.10)<br>Direct costs of children (Q.17)<br>Time costs of children (Q.18)<br>Spells of use (Q.27)<br>Choice of regulation methods (Q.28) |
| Specific relationships | Availability or use of regulation and demand (Q.21)<br>Delivery systems and regulation costs (Q.24) | Breastfeeding and postpartum infecundability (Q.6)<br>Postpartum abstinence and anovulatory interval (Q.8)<br>Frequency of intercourse and waiting time (Q.9)<br>Interval length and infant mortality (Q.11)<br>Desire for births and expected survival (Q.13)<br>Demand or pregnancy and timing of marriage (Q.35)<br>Form of union or dissolution and frequency of intercourse (Q.36)<br>Family structure and demand or decision process (Q.37) |
| Decision processes | Changes in plans and decisions (Q.33) | Nonmaximizing models (Q.31)<br>Regularities in process (Q.32) |
| Global influences | Regulation policies and fertility (Q.30)<br>Channels for effects of socio-economic characteristics (Q.38)<br>Institutional variation and fertility (Q.39)<br>Institutional change and fertility (Q.40) | |

Models for Determinants of Components

Where the previous questions deal with combining components, these twelve questions deal with the influences
upon particular components and how influences should be
combined.  (The questions on diffusion and on age at
marriage do not strictly involve basic components, but
are sufficiently similar to be included here.)  Numerous
possible questions are left out of this list, such as
determinants of the frequency of intercourse, of the
costs of alternatives to children, and of types of sexual
unions.

Most of the questions listed explicitly mention the
need for models, in recognition of the multiplicity of
influences on each immediate determinant and the importance of interactions among these influences.  However,
this does not imply that only model-building research is
appropriate; in most cases, much work is also needed to
identify and describe influences, to confirm them, and to
estimate effects before these influences can be combined
in a satisfactory model.

Priorities among these questions are most easily
discussed within subsets.  Of the two questions on
supply, the question on breastfeeding (Q.7) is clearly
more important than that on secondary sterility (Q.10),
since breastfeeding has a greater effect in the aggregate.  Of the four questions on demand, those on tastes
(Q.15) and on economic contributions of children (Q.16)
have priority over those on direct economic costs (Q.17)
and on time costs (Q.18), since variation in the former
factors is more significant in developing countries.  Of
the four questions on regulation, those on regulation
costs (Q.25) and on use and effectiveness (Q.26) are more
basic than those on spells of use (Q.27) and on method
choice (Q.28).  The last two questions on diffusion
(Q.29) and on age at marriage (Q.34) both seem of very
high priority, diffusion because of the wide impact of
the process and the potential that a scientific understanding holds for exercising control over it, and age at
marriage because of the considerable fertility variation
that can be traced to this single factor.  Thus seven
questions out of these twelve have priority; further
narrowing the list is difficult and will not be attempted.

Specific Relationships or Linkages

The next set of ten questions addresses particular relationships or linkages between variables rather than sets
of determinants. These questions are diverse. Three
(Q.11, 13, and 35) deal with linkages that are critical
in the analytical framework, though substantively the
effects involved may not be large. Three others (Q.8, 9,
and 36) involve secondary components that might have
significant effect, though the evidence is poor. The
remaining four questions probably deserve higher
priority; of these, the questions on the effect of the
availability and use of regulation on demand (Q.21) and
on the effects of delivery systems on regulation costs
(Q.24) appear slightly more important than those on the
effects of breastfeeding on postpartum infecundability
(Q.6) and on the effects of family structure on demand
and decision making (Q.37).


Decision Processes

The three research questions on fertility decision
processes are distinctive and do not fit in any of the
other groups. The question on nonmaximizing models
(Q.31) is the most speculative and not likely to produce
immediate concrete results; the question on regularities
in the decision process (Q.32) could lead to useful
descriptive research, but not, in the short run, to much
evidence relating to fertility variation; the third
question, on sequential decision making (Q.33), appears
to be the main priority here.


Global Influences on Fertility

Under global influences are included questions about
determinants that affect fertility through a variety of
different channels. All three of the questions on social
institutions are included here, as is one question on
fertility regulation. These questions are all composite,
referring to multiple variables affecting fertility
through multiple channels of influence. All four seem to
deserve high priority.

Table 2, summarizing this discussion, shows more items
with high priority than in the agendas reviewed earlier;
however, these research questions are considerably more
specific than the items in the other agendas.

Priorities Across Types of Research Questions

What type of research is given highest priority depends
critically on the point of view adopted toward the analytical framework. Three points of view are possible:
(a) to take the framework, or some more intricate version
of it, seriously as a strong statement of the factors
involved in fertility; (b) to accept the framework as
useful, but only as a loose conceptual structure within
which different theoretical perspectives and problems can
be held together; and (c) to reject the framework and
replace it with some other perspective.

From the first point of view, that of taking the
framework literally, the most important type of research
is developing and testing integrative models for components of supply, demand, and regulation costs. More than
research of any other type, this could lead directly to
confirmation, rejection, or modification of the framework.

From the second point of view, testing the framework
is less important than using it heuristically, particularly to identify and classify variables of interest.
The key task is to elaborate on fertility determinants
using the framework, and the priority questions are
therefore those on determinants of the components, and
possibly those on global influences and how they work
their way through the framework.

The third point of view involves abandoning the framework; what is put in its place determines the priorities.
If the perspective of a particular discipline or a
particular research tradition were adopted, the priority
questions would cut across types and refer instead to
subject areas. From the perspective of family planning
research, the questions might address regulation; from
the perspective of psychology, demand and decision
making; from the perspective of public health, supply and
regulation; and from the perspective of macrosociology,
global influences. Alternatively, a policy perspective
might be adopted; highest priority might then be given to
the questions on global influences, because they deal
with possible policy instruments, and to some questions
on fertility regulation.

The implications of these different perspectives for
each type of research question can be briefly summarized.
(a) The questions on levels and trends generally receive
high but not top priority; such data are less crucial for
theoretical development, though continual data collection
is indispensable for research on many of the other ques-

tions.    (b) The questions on development of measures lead
to necessarily innovative forms of research, whose
potential payoff is less certain.    Since research on
these questions is a high-risk enterprise, top priority
is difficult to justify.    (c) The questions on integrative
models of the components get to the core of the framework, and deserve top priority if verifying the framework
is considered crucial.    (d) The questions on models for
the determinants of the components deserve top priority
if extending the framework and giving it substance are
primary concerns.    (e) The questions on specific relationships or linkages are a motley set; some of them get at
core issues in the framework, whereas others are slightly
more peripheral.    More than for other groups, it is
difficult to assign a priority for this group as a
whole.    (f) The questions on decision processes, like
those on measures, involve innovative approaches; the
payoff, again, is uncertain, and may well be delayed.
(g) The questions on global influences on fertility,
finally, deserve top priority if extending the framework
is considered critical, and may also be assigned top
priority from a policy perspective.

## Research Approaches

It remains to ask what the priorities discussed here
imply about research approaches.    Many different
approaches are required to investigate all of the
priority questions; those useful for some questions are
often inappropriate for others.    This volume has not
reviewed developments in data collection, data analysis,
and theory construction; it therefore cannot provide
recommendations about the most recent or most sophisticated approaches (see, e.g., National Research Council,
1981; Brillinger, 1982).

Three possible approaches nevertheless seem worthy of
mention.    First, large, general-purpose surveys, possibly
with changing special modules, are an efficient mechanism
for providing data on many topics simultaneously.    For
tracking levels and trends, for exploiting new measures
as they are developed, and for testing models that involve
large numbers of variables, such surveys present many
advantages, and are desirable to conduct periodically in
at least a few countries.

Second, and perhaps more important, are cross-national
studies that focus on particular fertility determinants.

Much mention has been made in the preceding chapters of two such studies, the Princeton European Fertility Project (Watkins, forthcoming) and the Value of Children Project (Fawcett, in these volumes). Some chapters have also made use of the World Fertility Survey, though many of its results are coming out too late for inclusion here. The insights provided by cross-national comparisons, when they involve not simply comparing fertility rates but unravelling determinants, have been especially important in the recent increase in understanding of fertility, generating many of the important hypotheses reviewed in the these volumes. Carefully designed cross-national studies, despite the considerable time and resources they require, need to be encouraged.

A third approach, that of randomized experiments, is often advocated as the proper means of investigating causal hypotheses about fertility. The experimental approach has much to recommend it, and greater ingenuity and inventiveness is desirable among fertility researchers in designing appropriate experimental or quasi-experimental tests. Government interventions often provide settings that can be utilized for natural experiments. Nevertheless, important areas for research seem so far impervious to this approach, and it remains more of a scientific ideal, in many cases, than a practical possibility.

## NOTES

1. One of these appendices, by Berelson (1978), provides a perspective on policy and research issues slightly different from that of the main report but equally provocative.
2. It seems reasonable to ask how one identifies quality research. Unfortunately, there is no easy answer. Sophisticated methodology does not guarantee quality, nor does the ability to attract research funds. Judgments on quality have to be made consensually within the research community in the context of the most recent research developments.
3. Timing of intercourse within the menstrual cycle should be, if anything, more important than frequency, but may be subject to too many random influences to merit study.
4. Some incentive schemes are meant to affect demand rather than regulation costs, and fall under Q.19 instead.

5. Spacing decisions may be considered to fall under
   supply. The interaction between spacing and limiting
   decisions is also critical to investigate.


## BIBLIOGRAPHY

Bell, D. E. (1980) Introduction: Special issue on
   health and population in developing countries. Social
   Science & Medicine 14C:63–65.

Berelson, B. (1978) Social Science Research for
   Population Policy. (Appendix 1 to Population Policy:
   Research Priorities in the Developing World). Mexico
   City: IRG, El Colegio de Mexico.

Brillinger, D. (1982) Statistics in fertility research:
   Its contributions, its limitations. Department of
   Statistics, University of California at Berkeley.
   Unpublished paper.

Coale, A. J., L.–J. Cho, and N. Goldman (1980)
   Estimation of Recent Trends in Fertility and Mortality
   in the Republic of Korea. Washington, D.C.: National
   Academy of Sciences.

Conference on Social Science Research on Population and
   Development (1974) Social Science Research on
   Population and Development. New York: Ford
   Foundation.

Freedman, R. (1974) Social research and programs for
   reducing birth rates. In Social Science Research on
   Population and Development. New York: Ford
   Foundation.

International Conference on Family Planning in the 1980's
   (1981) Family planning in the 1980's: Challenges and
   opportunities. Studies in Family Planning 12:251–256.

McGreevey, W. P., and N. Birdsall (1974) The Policy
   Relevance of Recent Social Research on Fertility.
   Occasional Monograph Series, No. 2. Washington,
   D.C.: Smithsonian Institution.

Mertens, W. (1978) Research Priorities for Population
   and Socio-Economic Development. Recommendations for
   UNFPA Inter-Country Programmes. Unpublished paper,
   United Nations Fund for Population Activities, New
   York.

Miro, C. A., and J. E. Potter (1980) Population Policy:
   Research Priorities in the Developing World. London:
   Francis Pinter.

National Research Council (1981) Collecting Data for the
   Estimation of Fertility and Mortality. Panel on Data

Collection, Committee on Population and Demography. Washington, D.C.:  National Academy Press.

Population Council (1981)  Research on the determinants of fertility:  A note on priorities.  Population and Development Review 7:311-324.

Thomas, L. (1979)  The Medusa and the Snail.  New York: Viking Press.

United Nations (1982)  Indirect Techniques for Demographic Estimation.  Manual X.  New York:  United Nations.

Watkins, S., ed. (forthcoming)  Proceedings of a Conference on the European Fertility Project. Princeton, N.J.:  Princeton University Press.

# ABSTRACTS

Volume 1

SUPPLY AND DEMAND FOR CHILDREN

INTRODUCTION

1  A Framework for the Study of Fertility Determinants

A household decision framework is developed within which the research evidence regarding fertility determinants can be summarized.  The basic components of the framework are the supply of surviving children (determined by natural fertility and child survival), the demand for children (determined by tastes and constraints), and fertility regulation costs (including costs of access and costs of use), which combine in couples' decisions on fertility regulation.  These basic components are affected by nuptiality and childbearing experience, socioeconomic characteristics, and social institutions and culture.  Several key questions about the framework are discussed, including the separability of the basic components, whether couples actually make decisions, and if they do whether these are single or sequential.

THE SUPPLY OF CHILDREN

2  The Supply of Children:  A Critical Essay
   John Bongaarts and Jane Menken

Two main factors in the supply of children, natural fertility and child survival, are considered.  Of the

proximate determinants of natural fertility, it is shown
that postpartum infecundability and age at marriage
produce the greatest variation, with waiting time to
conception, age at last birth, and spontaneous intrauterine mortality having progressively less fertility
effect. The determinants of these proximate determinants,
specifically nutrition and health and socioeconomic and
cultural factors, are briefly discussed. It is demonstrated how many children families would have in natural
fertility conditions, under various assumptions about
child survival probabilities.

### 3    Natural Fertility:    Age Patterns, Levels, and Trends
John Knodel

The concept of natural fertility is discussed: the
age-pattern of natural fertility is described and factors
affecting this pattern considered, particularly breastfeeding, postnatal abstinence, terminal abstinence,
declines in pathological infertility, age differences
between spouses, age at marriage, and premarital
pregnancy. Hypothetical examples are used to illustrate
the potential impact of these factors on the age pattern.
Finally, trends in natural fertility and the way they
relate to modernization are discussed. Reference is made
throughout the paper to material from contemporary
developing countries and from historical demography.

### 4    The Proximate Determinants of Natural Marital Fertility
John Bongaarts

Natural marital fertility is below the biological maximum
because of several factors which operate in all societies
but vary widely in impact. These are the postpartum
infecundable period (largely, if not entirely, affected
by breastfeeding), the waiting time to conception (a
function of the length of the fertile part of the menstrual cycle and frequency of intercourse), intrauterine
mortality, and permanent sterility. Variations in the
duration of postpartum amenorrhea are the main cause of
variations in levels of natural marital fertility among
different populations. An examination of the biological
and demographic evidence indicates that the duration of
the fertile period in each menstrual cycle is approximately two days and leads to some estimates of the
probability of conception given varying coital frequency.

## 5  The Impact of Health and Nutrition on Natural Fertility
Ronald Gray

The effects of health and nutrition on the proximate determinants of natural fertility (including breastfeeding and postpartum amenorrhea, fecundability, sterility, age at menarche and menopause, and intrauterine mortality) are examined. With the exception of pelvic inflammatory disease (PID), health and nutrition have not been shown to have a significant direct demographic effect on fertility among large populations in the developing world. Among agricultural populations and hunter-gatherers subject to severe malnutrition, health and nutrition may have some significant demographic effect.

## 6  The Impact of Sociocultural Factors on Breastfeeding and Sexual Behavior
Moni Nag

The sociocultural determinants of three main components of natural fertility are considered. Breastfeeding is examined as a function of education, urbanization, income, and female labor force participation. The availability of powdered milk and modern health services may also affect it. Both terminal and postpartum abstinence are examined, with the emphasis on postpartum abstinence, which has a much greater effect on natural fertility and varies greatly across societies. Finally, variation in frequency of coitus among sociocultural groups, by marriage type, and across age groups is considered.

## 7  Child Survival:  Levels, Trends, and Determinants
Lincoln C. Chen

There is wide divergence in mortality levels and trends in various regions of the developing world. A framework is developed to analyze the factors responsible for these variations. Four determinants are hypothesized to affect child survivorship: parental factors, nutrition and diet, infection factors, and health care. These are in turn affected by socioeconomic and environmental factors at the family, community, and national levels. The implications of this framework for mortality control policies and health care programs are discussed.

8  The Demand for Children:  A Critical Essay
   Ronald D. Lee and Rodolfo A. Bulatao

The concept of the demand for children is discussed:  Is
it meaningful in LDCs?  Does it affect behavior?  Is it
properly measured by family-size desires?  Then the
factors involved in demand are considered:  the economic
costs and benefits of children, their time costs, tastes
for children, and the effects of income and wealth.
Evidence for the magnitude of the costs and benefits is
evaluated, as well as evidence that each factor affects
demand and, through it, fertility.  How costs, benefits,
and tastes change in the course of modernization is also
discussed.  The effects of childbearing experience on
demand are briefly covered.

9  Family-Size Desires as Measures of Demand
   Gary H. McClelland

What the "demand" for children means within a microeconomic model is explicated.  Fertility demand is
interpreted as a conditional decision process responding
not only to objective economic conditions but also to
subjective beliefs.  As potential measures of demand,
family-size desires are investigated for their face
validity, their stability, their ability to reflect
demand itself rather its determinants like preferences,
norms, or economic constraints, their exclusion of
natural-fertility and regulation-cost considerations, and
their relation to fertility behavior.  Two appendices
consider gender preferences and levels and trends in
family-size desires.

10 Correlates of Family-Size Desires
   Thomas W. Pullum

Among the correlates of family-size desires considered,
life-cycle factors are treated most prominently.  It is
argued that family-size desires exhibit some stability
over the life cycle, but rationalization tends to shape
desires to fit actual fertility experience.  Attention is
also paid to gender preferences and to the knowledge and
use of family planning.  Finally, socioeconomic charac-

teristics of couples are considered as correlates of family-size desires; the evidence for their effect, once life-cycle factors, gender preferences, and family planning are controlled, is not strong.

## 11 Infant and Child Mortality and the Demand for Children
David M. Heer

Two major questions are considered: whether fertility responds to the actual experience of a child death and whether fertility responds to the perceived probability of child death. Prior loss does lead to increased fertility, particularly where the costs of birth control are low; however, under no circumstances does this increased fertility fully compensate for the loss. The evidence about the effects of perceived survival probabilities is thin; higher survival probabilities may contribute to lower fertility, but this has not been established.

## 12 Norms Relating to the Desire for Children
Karen Oppenheim Mason

The general nature of norms and two approaches to them, the Parsonian approach and the social construction approach, are discussed. It is shown that what evidence about norms is considered acceptable depends greatly on one's theory of norms. The evidence about family-size norms is considered: responses to survey questions about perceived sanctions linked to alternative family sizes, about respondents' approval for alternative sizes, about how many children are too many or too few, about ideal and desired family size, as well as responses to projective questions and analyses of social network agreement are all considered. It is argued that the importance of norms depends on the role they are assigned in intervening between social conditions and fertility.

## 13 Perceptions of the Value of Children:  Satisfactions and Costs
James T. Fawcett

Findings from cross-national studies of the value of children are discussed. Socioeconomic characteristics of

couples affect positive values in consistent ways across
cultures:  lower-status urbanites and more rural couples
emphasize children's economic and practical contributions;
higher-status, more educated couples stress their psychosocial benefits.  Cultural factors, sex roles, and life
cycle factors also partly determine the values emphasized.
Perceived economic costs of children do not vary consistently across groups, but opportunity costs do, especially
the psychosocial dimensions involving loss of freedom and
flexibility.  Some evidence links particular values to
fertility, and also suggests that a pattern of transition
with modernization takes place in values and disvalues.

## 14 Direct Economic Costs and Benefits of Children
John C. Caldwell

It is argued that children make many contributions to
their families, including defense against threat and
investment for the future, that no other institution in
pretransition societies can provide.  These benefits flow
especially to the elders, who control family labor and
consumption, which is generally unequal.  Fertility
decline results from a reversal of this "wealth flow,"
caused by a change in emotional relationships within the
family with consequences for economic relations among its
members, and by such external changes as the provision of
education, all of which tend to make children more costly.

## 15 The Changing Economic Costs and Benefits of Having Children
Peter H. Lindert

At all phases of development, couples are roughly aware
of the economic consequences of childbearing.  Fertility
falls when, fairly late in development, the relative
costliness of extra children rises.  A relative cost
measure is developed taking into account the need to
assess child costs relative to other forms of consumption
and to discount expected future costs.  This measure
suggests that children are seldom ever a net asset.  They
may be time-supplying in less developed countries,
eventually becoming time-intensive and even more costly
as development proceeds.

16 <u>Women's Work Activity and Fertility</u>
   Guy Standing

The hypothesis that women's employment reduces fertility
has not been consistently supported in LDC studies.  It
is necessary to examine more closely the characteristics
of types of work that make them incompatible with childcare:  possibly only work away from home, or urban jobs,
or employment in the modern sector, are incompatible.
Characteristics of childcare also affect compatability,
including the availability of parental surrogates, the
desired level of care, and the ability to adjust the time
allocated to leisure.  Other aspects of the women's
work-fertility relationship discussed are the effects of
work experience, job interruption, labor discrimination,
and labor substitution.

17 <u>Women's Roles, Opportunity Costs, and Fertility</u>
   Christine Oppong

The impact of children on a woman is traced through their
impact on each of the major roles she plays in her life,
as a mother, a wife, a member of a household, a worker, a
kinswoman, a member of a community, and an individual.
Children provide various economic, political, social, and
psychic rewards, but women may have alternative sources
for these available, and children also impose various
opportunity costs and create role conflicts.

18 <u>Effects of Income and Wealth on the Demand for Children</u>
   Eva Mueller and Kathleen Short

Macro-level studies and micro-level studies of the effect
of income on fertility are separately reviewed.  No
consistent effect is found.  The "pure" effect of income
as a constraint on the household's ability to afford
goods or children cannot be observed because of such
indirect effects as the impact of income on tastes, its
relation to female employment, and the way it raises the
economic cost of children, each of which may operate to
counter or reinforce the pure effect.  Source of income
may also be important:  in rural areas, landownership is
related to higher fertility.  No good evidence for the
effect of income inequality on fertility has so far been
presented.

Volume 2

FERTILITY REGULATION AND INSTITUTIONAL INFLUENCES

## FERTILITY REGULATION AND ITS COSTS

### 1  Fertility Regulation and Its Costs:  A Critical Essay
Albert I. Hermalin

Hypotheses concerning the relation of motivation and costs to fertility regulation are reviewed.  The costs of fertility regulation to the couple are discussed, covering the costs of access (which include costs of purchasing services and information and travel costs) and the costs of use (health costs and psychosocial costs).  Methods of measuring and analyzing the concepts of motivation and costs are described and illustrated.  Attention is given to distinguishing the role of individual socioeconomic characteristics from the impact of development, diffusion, and family planning.  In this context, the research on evaluation of family planning programs is reviewed.

### 2  Birth Control Methods and Their Effects on Fertility
John A. Ross

Data on the prevalence of contraceptive methods and abortion are presented.  Countries vary by contraceptive prevalence levels, with some of the largest LDCs being above 30 percent but others being below 10 percent.  The pill and sterilization are the leading methods overall, though the ranking varies by country.  For method continuation, sterilization and the IUD outrank the pill. The use-effectiveness of the methods is considered, and links to fertility are discussed in a brief review of the relevant literature.

### 3  Monetary and Health Costs of Contraception
S. Bruce Schearer

The monetary costs of contraception are analyzed and new survey data used along with existing data to estimate their magnitude.  It is concluded that monetary costs have a substantial indirect impact on contraceptive use: they significantly restrict availability of supplies and

services in many developing countries.  However, people's
ability to pay for contraception may be much greater than
generally believed, permitting important public sector
cost reductions and more efficient design of both public
and private distribution systems in the future. Health
costs are also reviewed; it is concluded that these
costs, although substantial, exert little impact on
overall contraceptive use or fertility in developed
countries.  In developing countries, however, largely due
to limited familiarity with contraception and lack of
scientific and health knowledge in general, fears about
side effects are a significant deterrent to contraceptive
use.  In countries where knowledge and experience become
more widely diffused, however, this barrier rapidly
diminishes.


4   Normative and Psychic Costs of Contraception
    Donald J. Bogue

An inventory is presented of the normative and psychic
costs attached to contraception, and illustrated at
several points with Egyptian data.  The major normative
and psychic costs, it is argued, are fears of side
effects and of long-term health effects (often unrelated
to objective risks), anxiety over contraceptive failure,
the need for discussion with the spouse, and the need for
internal control over behavior.  These costs, and other
less important ones, can be reduced by well-planned
programs of public information.


5   Abortion: Its Prevalence, Correlates, and Costs
    Henry P. David

The legality of abortion and its incidence worldwide are
described.  No country has achieved fertility decline
without some recourse to abortion.  Mortality from
illegal abortion is very high, making it a major cause of
maternal mortality; for legal abortion under proper
clinical conditions, however, rates are lower than for
normal deliveries.  Psychological costs are difficult to
assess, but generally, where abortion is legal, do not
seem to be serious.

6 <u>Infanticide as Deliberate Fertility Regulation</u>
Susan C. M. Scrimshaw

Deliberate infanticide and passive infanticide
(infanticide through neglect) are discussed as means by
which couples may attempt to control family size and
composition. There is little good statistical evidence
on these practices, but some indirect evidence (such as
imbalanced sex ratios or mortality within a closely
spaced pair of births) as well as many ethnographic
accounts exist. The available evidence indicates that
infanticide as deliberate fertility control existed in
predindustrial times, but has increasingly been replaced
by differential care in industrializing societies.

7 <u>Population Programs and Fertility Regulation</u>
W. Parker Mauldin

During the past two decades, a substantial number of LDCs
have adopted population policies and programs designed to
reduce rates of population growth. Contraceptive
prevalence has risen considerably in many of these
countries, and fertility rates have declined appreciably,
although the changes have been quite uneven across
countries. Both improvements in social and economic
sectors and the implementation of family planning
programs have influenced fertility declines, but it is
difficult to disentangle the effects of these factors.
Availability of contraceptives does seem to promote their
use, however. The consensus seems to be that family
planning programs, when well-managed, do have a substantial effect independent of the influence of
socioeconomic factors.

8 <u>Diffusion Processes Affecting Fertility Regulation</u>
Robert D. Retherford and James A. Palmore

Diffusion of birth control is a process integral to
fertility transition. Diffusion proceeds more readily
where there is greater cultural homogeneity and social
integration, and it can advance the timing and accelerate
the pace of transition. Diffusion operates through a
hierarchy of networks at several levels: the local or
personal, the national or family planing, and the
international. Utility-cost concepts are useful in

explaining the timing and rate of diffusion and provide a means of integrating difusion concepts into fertility transition models.

## FERTILITY DECISION-MAKING PROCESSES

### 9 Fertility Decision-Making Processes:  A Critical Essay
Paula E. Hollerbach

The literature, mainly social-psychological, on fertility decision-making processes is reviewed. Different types of decisions, such as passive and active, are defined, and the decision processes characterizing pretransitional and posttransitional societies distinguished. Some decision models focus on the perceived supply of children, others on the demand for children, still others on the perceived costs of fertility regulation; a few combine all these elements. Rules such as subjective expected utility and expectancy x value specify how individuals combine and weigh decision factors. Sequential models focus on different stages of the family life cycle. The manner in which competing decisions among family, kin, and others are reconciled is also examined.

### 10 Cultural Influences on Fertility Decision Styles
Terence H. Hull

Decisions affecting fertility are ubiquitous: they involve not only ultimate family size but also marriage, breastfeeding, intercourse, and many other culturally patterned behaviors. A complex web of cultural knowledge and symbolism surrounds these decisions, which sometimes, or for some parts of a decision sequence, may take on a routine or habitual pattern. The argument that no decisions are made is considered and rejected. Different fertility-related decisions are classified according to a variety of criteria, including whether the individual is usually aware that choices are available, whether either habit or custom make the decision routine, whether joint decisions are necessary or likely, and whether decisions are morally sensitive.

11 Communication, Power, and the Influence of Social
   Networks in Couple Decisions on Fertility
   Linda J. Beckman

Couple agreement and couple interaction are examined as
they affect fertility decisions. Agreement more often
reflects projection in the absence of discussion, and is
therefore more often linked to high fertility. Couple
discussion promotes lower fertility, partly because
discussion is necessary for some forms of contraception.
Egalitarianism may also promote lower fertility, possibly
because it encourages communication, but the evidence is
unclear. The influence of others--members of the
extended family, peer groups, medical and paramedical
personnel--on couple decisions is also discussed.

12 Sequential Fertility Decision Making and the Life
   Course
   N. Krishnan Namboodiri

Fertility decisions are discussed as a sequential process
interacting with the couple's passage through the stages
of the life course. Motives for having children change;
fertility plans require reformulation after failures due
to fecundity impairment, marital breakdown, or unintended
pregnancies; and the social position, household arrangements, employment plans, and marital relationships of the
couple are altered by unforeseen events. The effect on
reproduction depends on the timing of each event.

NUPTIALITY AND FERTILITY

13 The Impact of Age at Marriage and Proportions Marrying
   on Fertility
   Peter C. Smith

Areal variation in marriage patterns across and within
nations is reviewed, and trends are compared for the
historical European transition and contemporary LDCs.
The effects of marriage pattern on fertility depend on
reduced exposure to intercourse, but also involve the
shifting of childbearing to older ages and such aggregate
effects as changes in the mean length of a generation.
Determinants of marriage timing are covered in a very
diverse literature, which includes work on the avail-

ability of spouses, changes in family institutions from agricultural to industrial settings, and the effects of urban residence, education, and different types of employment.

## 14 The Impact of Forms of Families and Sexual Unions and Dissolution of Unions on Fertility
Thomas K. Burch

Several characteristics of marriages (sexual unions) or kin groups are investigated for their effects on fertility. First, polygyny has a positive impact on male fertility but an indeterminate impact on female fertility; several possible reasons for this are discussed. Second, stability of unions tends to increase fertility; consensual and visiting unions may involve restrictions on exposure to intercourse and may also involve lower demand for children. Third, marital dissolution tends to reduce fertility if remarriage is infrequent or delayed. Fourth, the extended family may promote higher fertility; the evidence on this is mostly inconclusive, but more recent work has begun to deal with many of the methodological problems. The prevalence and determinants of these different patterns are also discussed.

## SOCIAL INSTITUTIONS AND FERTILITY CHANGE

## 15 Modernization and Fertility:  A Critical Essay
Richard A. Easterlin

The components of the analytical framework are considered as intervening links between modernization and the fertility transition. Various aspects of modernization, including improved public health and medical care, urbanization, new goods, and growth in formal education, affect supply, demand, and regulation costs. These, in turn, are linked to the adoption of fertility control. It is demonstrated that this approach could help explain differences in the timing of fertility decline and changes in fertility differentials by age and other social characteristics. Changes in demand and regulation costs are recognized as important in the transition, but changes in supply are also critical, as couples move from an era of social control over fertility to an era in which individual control is needed.

## 16 Effects of Education and Urbanization on Fertility
Susan H. Cochrane

The various channels through which education and residence affect fertility, through modifying supply, demand or regulation costs, are outlined. Determining the fertility effects of education and residence is difficult because introducing statistical controls often results in limiting the channels considered. Education often has a negative effect; circumstances under which a positive effect is more likely are identified. Urban residence usually leads to lower fertility, more often at higher levels of urbanization.

## 17 Effects of Societal and Community Institutions on Fertility
Joseph E. Potter

In the study of fertility determinants, much more attention has traditionally been paid to the characteristics of individuals, households, and families than to the characteristics of their environments. Some of the questions that arise when the emphasis is reversed are explored here; the concern is with the effect on reproductive behavior of the economic incentives, administrative sanctions, ideological influences, and social pressures that emerge from the institutional setting. The institutions considered range from concrete entities like schools, churches, and local governments to less tangible aspects of economic organization like land tenure arrangements and the social relations of production. Illustrations of their effects are drawn fro a variety of contemporary and historical contexts. For future research, heavily clustered samples are recommended to permit an adequate appreciation of contextual variables while still providing nationally representative results.

## 18 Effects of Culture on Fertility: Anthropological Contributions
Robert A. LeVine and Susan C. M. Scrimshaw

A guide is provided to the anthropological literature on human fertility, with specific attention to the concepts of culture and natural fertility and to the processes by which fertility patterns are linked to human adaptation

at the societal and family levels.  Anthropological
research methods are discussed as complementary to
demographic approaches in the understanding of factors
affecting fertility in developing countries.  The review
includes historical and contemporary perspectives and
also covers the cultural acceptability of intervention
programs.

## 19 Statistical Studies of Aggregate Fertility Change: Time Series of Cross-Sections
Toni Richards

A small set of statistical studies have investigated the
determinants of fertility change, either within countries
or across countries.  These studies are reviewed, with
careful attention to their methodological aspects.  Cross-
sectional results are distinguished from time-series
results; these are often quite different.  The effects of
standard sociostructural and economic variables--
industrialization, income growth, urbanization, infant
mortality, family planning programs--are summarized for
the few studies available.

## 20 Cohort and Period Measures of Changing Fertility
Norman B. Ryder

The mathematical relationship between cohort and period
fertility is explicated.  These two measures generally
diverge as fertility changes; economic conditions may
displace births from one period to another but not affect
cohort rates, or the mean age of childbearing may change
over the long term, again with greater impact on period
than cohort rates.  Understanding these relationships is
essential if apparent changes in fertility are to be
properly interpreted.

### CONCLUSION

## 21 An Overview of Fertility Determinants in Developing Countries
Rodolfo A. Bulatao and Ronald D. Lee

An overview is provided of the research evidence summarized in the other papers in these volumes regarding

fertility determinants in developing countries. The topics briefly touched on include: natural fertility and child survival, their determinants, and consequent trends in the supply of children; direct costs and benefits and time costs of children, the effects of income and wealth and of tastes and norms, and consequent trends in demand for children; strategies that are used to make fertility decisions; the regulation costs considered in such decisions and the diffusion of fertility regulation, including the role of family planning programs; the fertility effects of different nuptiality patterns; and the fertility effects of social institutions and consequent changes in fertility with modernization.

## 22 An Agenda for Research on the Determinants of Fertility in the Developing Countries

Following a review of other research agendas, 40 priority research questions on fertility determinants in developing countries are identified. The basic criterion for choosing the questions is the potential for research in these areas to add to scientific understanding. The questions cover all the major categories provided by the analytical framework, and involve research of many types: into levels and trends in the components of the framework; on the development of measures of key variables; on the development of models for combining components and models for the determinants of components; and on other issues like decisions processes and global influences on fertility.

# STUDIES IN POPULATION

*Under the Editorship of:* H. H. Winsborough

*Department of Sociology*
*University of Wisconsin*
*Madison, Wisconsin*

*Samuel H. Preston, Nathan Keyfitz, and Robert Schoen.* **Causes of Death:** *Life Tables for National Populations.*

*Otis Dudley Duncan, David L. Featherman, and Beverly Duncan.* **Socioeconomic Background and Achievement.**

*James A. Sweet.* **Women in the Labor Force.**

*Tertius Chandler and Gerald Fox.* **3000 Years of Urban Growth.**

*William H. Sewell and Robert M. Hauser.* **Education, Occupation, and Earnings:** *Achievement in the Early Career.*

*Otis Dudley Duncan.* **Introduction to Structural Equation Models.**

*William H. Sewell, Robert M. Hauser, and David L. Featherman (Eds.).* **Schooling and Achievement in American Society.**

*Henry Shryock, Jacob S. Siegel, and Associates.* **The Methods and Materials of Demography.** *Condensed Edition by Edward Stockwell.*

*Samuel H. Preston.* **Mortality Patterns in National Populations:** *With Special Reference to Recorded Causes of Death.*

*Robert M. Hauser and David L. Featherman.* **The Process of Stratification:** *Trends and Analyses.*

*Ronald R. Rindfuss and James A. Sweet.* **Postwar Fertility Trends and Differentials in the United States.**

*David L. Featherman and Robert M. Hauser.* **Opportunity and Change.**

*Karl E. Taeuber, Larry L. Bumpass, and James A. Sweet (Eds.).* **Social Demography.**

*Thomas J. Espenshade and William J. Serow (Eds.).* **The Economic Consequences of Slowing Population Growth.**

*Frank D. Bean and W. Parker Frisbie (Eds.).* **The Demography of Racial and Ethnic Groups.**

*Joseph A. McFalls, Jr.* **Psychopathology and Subfecundity.**

*Franklin D. Wilson.* **Residential Consumption, Economic Opportunity, and Race.**

*Maris A. Vinovskis (Ed.).* **Studies in American Historical Demography.**

*Clifford C. Clogg.* **Measuring Underemployment: Demographic Indicators for the United States.**

*Doreen S. Goyer.* International Population Census Bibliography: *Revision and Update, 1945-1977.*

*David L. Brown and John M. Wardwell (Eds.).* New Directions in Urban–Rural Migration: *The Population Turnaround in Rural America.*

*A. J. Jaffe, Ruth M. Cullen, and Thomas D. Boswell.* The Changing Demography of Spanish Americans.

*Robert Alan Johnson.* Religious Assortative Marriage in the United States.

*Hilary J. Page and Ron Lesthaeghe.* Child-Spacing in Tropical Africa.

*Dennis P. Hogan.* Transitions and Social Change: *The Early Lives of American Men.*

*F. Thomas Juster and Kenneth C. Land (Eds.).* Social Accounting Systems: *Essays on the State of the Art.*

*M. Sivamurthy.* Growth and Structure of Human Population in the Presence of Migration.

*Robert M. Hauser, David Mechanic, Archibald O. Haller, and Taissa O. Hauser (Eds.).* Social Structure and Behavior: *Essays in Honor of William Hamilton Sewell.*

*Valerie Kincade Oppenheimer.* Work and the Family: *A Study in Social Demography.*

*Kenneth C. Land and Andrei Rogers (Eds.).* Multidimensional Mathematical Demography.

*John Bongaarts and Robert G. Potter.* Fertility, Biology, and Behavior: *An Analysis of the Proximate Determinants.*

*Randy Hodson.* Workers' Earnings and Corporate Economic Structure.

*Ansley J. Coale and Paul Demeny.* Regional Model Life Tables and Stable Populations, Second Edition.

*Mary B. Breckenridge.* Age, Time, and Fertility: *Applications of Exploratory Data Analysis.*

*Neil G. Bennett (Ed.).* Sex Selection of Children.

*Rodolfo A. Bulatao and Ronald D. Lee (Eds.).* Determinants of Fertility in Developing Countries. Volume 1: *Supply and Demand for Children;* Volume 2: *Fertility Regulation and Institutional Influences.*

In preparation

*Kenneth G. Manton and Eric Stallard.* Recent Trends in Mortality Analysis.

*Joseph A. McFalls, Jr., and Marguerite Harvey McFalls.* Disease and Fertility.